Endodontic Treatment, Retreatment, and Surgery

ueen Elizabeth Hospita

withdrawn

Bobby Patel

Editor

Endodontic Treatment, Retreatment, and Surgery

Mastering Clinical Practice

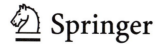

Springer

Editor
Bobby Patel
Forrest
Aust Capital Terr
Australia

ISBN 978-3-319-19475-2   ISBN 978-3-319-19476-9   (eBook)
DOI 10.1007/978-3-319-19476-9

Library of Congress Control Number: 2016947839

Printed on acid-free paper

This Springer imprint is published by Springer Nature
The registered company is Springer International Publishing AG Switzerland

This book is dedicated to my endodontic mentor:

Ms Serpil Djemal

Preface

The discipline of endodontics and its principles have undergone a vast array of changes over the last 100 years shaped by evolving advances in both our understanding of the biological aetiology of periapical disease and rationale for treatment as well as improved technology, instruments, materials and techniques to achieve this purpose.

From a clinical standpoint we are often faced with a decision to decide whether to adopt these newer and "proven" techniques requiring some period of disruption to our daily routines or remain sceptic with the knowledge that our traditional views will continue to impart the best level of care to our patients.

To master any given subject one must be able to reflect on current views and opinions that are based on the best evidence provided. In order to determine whether these views are accurate, reliable and relevant, one must therefore be able to critically evaluate and understand at a deeper level trying to get to the heart of the matter.

It is with this concept of critical thinking in mind that I offer this compact yet comprehensive text with emphasis placed on both traditional and newer materials and techniques that can offer the potential for endodontic success.

Similar to my first book *Endodontic Diagnosis, Pathology and Treatment Planning*, each chapter describes many of the techniques and methods available for practitioners who wish to undertake the planning and treatment of complex endodontic cases. Numerous illustrations with high-quality photographs and radiographs highlight clinical cases, which serve to demonstrate practical non-surgical and surgical techniques. The text is referenced to provide a comprehensive source of scientific evidence and principles that underline these techniques.

It is hoped that readers will be provided with a concise literature-based approach to clinical problem-solving rather than a quick fix "recipe book" for everyday problems. Certainly it is not a replacement for existing contemporary textbooks but further serves as an accompaniment with emphasis placed on clinical hints and tips that may not be covered in standard endodontic textbooks.

The reader is reminded that this text is also aimed at allowing deep learning for students, dental practitioners and specialists alike. The understanding of key concepts will allow the reader to appertain to and consolidate knowledge from other parts of their study, from which they can hopefully derive solutions to novel problems. Deep learning involves the critical analysis of new ideas, linking them to already known concepts and principles, and leads to understanding and long-term retention of concepts so that they can be used for problem-solving in unfamiliar contexts.

I hope this text stretches you towards excellence recognizing the importance of attention to multiple dimensions and enabling you to progress towards establishing clinical and academic understanding of the subject *par excellence*!

Canberra, ACT, Australia   Bobby Patel

Acknowledgements

Firstly I would like to thank my associate editor Antonia von Saint Paul and project co-ordinator Wilma McHugh at Springer DE for bringing this project to fruition and above all their patience whilst I completed this second endeavour. I would also like to express my deepest appreciation to the Production Editor, Abha Krishnan and Project Manager, Suganya Selvaraj, who were responsible for perfecting the language, design and layout of the book and final copy-editing of the completed text. I also acknowledge Gursharan Minhas, Robert Fell, John Cho, Roberto Sacco, Sarita Atreya, Anthony Greenstein and Mark Stenhouse for allocating time out of their busy schedules in order to contribute to their respective chapters and numerous proofreads along the way.

I would like to express my gratitude to the staff (Kathleen, Julie, Jess R, Jess Ellis and Deb) for their endless help throughout including photography skills using various Android and Apple phones and patients at *Canberra Endodontics* who agreed to be photographed for illustrative material; I would also like to thank both Dr Luke Maloney and Ms Serpil Djemal for providing me with their trauma presentations and access to images. Special mention also goes to Dr Kim Mai Dang, Dr Daniel Felman and Dr Aovana Timmerman for providing many of the excellent trauma images throughout the "Traumatic Injuries" *chapter*; I must also mention special thanks to Kim for providing me with full access to all journals and articles throughout the preparation of this manuscript and providing numerous passwords at short notice! I must also give recognition to Phil Gaff who provided me with many images courtesy of Dentsply. I would like to thank Steven W Dahlstrom my first mentor in specialist clinical practice who gave me full clinical freedom as well as support in those early years.

I thank my parents for their faith in me and allowing me to fulfil my dreams. It was only through their hard work, sacrifice and determination that I was able to achieve what I have from the very beginning. I must also thank Sarita's parents who have provided us with unending encouragement, support and love. To my wife Sarita whose unwavering love has been the bedrock upon which the last 23 years of our lives have been built. She has been my true inspiration and motivation and brings out the very best in me even in the worst of times. Without her none of this would have ever been conceivable. Finally to my three all-inspiring children Raya, Sofia and Iyla, for always making me laugh, the realization of the true purpose of life and the reason to escape from my daily workload. I hope that these books are a testimony to you that one day you too can follow your dreams with some hard work and conviction to make them a reality.

The great pleasure in life is doing what people say you cannot do. *Walter Bagehot*

Contents

About the Editor

Bobby Patel, BDS, MFDS RCS (ED) MClinDent (ENDO) (Dist) MRD RCS (ENG) MRACDS (ENDO), graduated from Bart's and the London Medical and Dental School in 1999. He subsequently gained experience as a dentist in general practice and the community dental services. He gained further experience within the hospital settings working as a restorative senior house officer at Bart's and the London Medical and Dental School. He then completed a 12-month surgical posting at Basildon hospital working as a clinical fellow in oral maxillofacial surgery. He was accepted onto the UK monospeciality endodontic training pathway at the Eastman Dental Institute where he completed his MClinDent in 2006. He was awarded a distinction for his academic achievement during this time. In 2006, the British Endodontic Society awarded him a poster prize for his innovative research entitled "Development of an in vitro model for the study of microbial infection in human teeth". In 2007, he was awarded membership in restorative dentistry, the highest formal qualification in the UK and registered on the specialist list for endodontics thereafter. He then moved to Australia to work in specialist referral practice from 2007 to present. In 2012, he was awarded membership of the Royal Australian college of Dental Surgeons (Endodontics). He is very active in continuing education programs, with a particular interest in hands-on courses dealing with diagnosis, treatment planning, root canal therapy, and surgical endodontics. He is a Dentsply Maillefer key opinion leader and certified trainer, regularly giving lectures to general dentists regarding the latest endodontic Ni-Ti rotary file techniques. His particular interests are with surgical endodontics, intentional re-implantation procedures, and endodontic re-treatment.

Contributors

Sarita Atreya, BDS MFDS RCS (ED) Private Practice, Canberra, ACT, Australia

John Cho, BDS (Hons) MDSc (Prosthodontics) University of Sydney, Canberra, ACT, Australia

Robert Fell, BDS DClinDent FRACDS FRACDS Specialist Periodontist, Canberra, ACT, Australia

Anthony Greenstein, BM BS MRCS BDS MFDS RCS (ED) Oral and Maxillofacial Surgery, Pan Scotland Rotation, Honorary Lecturer at University of Aberdeen School of Medicine and Dentistry, Aberdeen, UK

Gursharan Minhas, BDS BSc MSc MFDS MOrth FDSOrth Specialist Orthodontist, The Royal Surrey County Hospital, Hampshire, UK

Hampshire Hospitals NHS Foundation Trust, Basingstoke, UK

Bobby Patel, BDS MFDS MClinDent MRD MRACDS Specialist Endodontist, Brindabella Specialist Centre, Canberra, ACT, Australia

Roberto Sacco, CDT DDS MSc PG Cert Sed Oral Surgery Specialist, Senior Clinical Teaching Fellow, UCL-Eastman Dental Institute, London, UK

Oral Surgery Specialist Dentist, King's College Hospital NHS Trust, London, UK

Mark Stenhouse, BDS DClinDent (Endo), FRACDS Specialist Endodontist, Charlestown, NSW, Australia

Access Preparation

1

Bobby Patel

Summary

The main objective of access preparation is to identify all canal anatomy prior to preparation and obturation of the root canal system. Correct access preparation is a key to successful treatment outcome and avoidance of mishaps. Inappropriate access preparation can lead to inadequate cleaning and shaping and subsequent obturation mishaps. Iatrogenic errors such as instrument separation, canal transportations, zipping and possible perforation may also result as a consequence of inadequate access design.

Clinical Relevance

An appropriately designed pulp chamber opening represents the most important step in order to locate and negotiate root canals optimally. A correct opening should provide complete removal of the pulp chamber roof and all internal interferences such as calcifications and restorations. Straight-line access is key to avoiding instrumentation mishaps particularly in curved root canals where the propensity for canal transportation or instrumentation failure is high. An important prerequisite for achieving success is the fundamental understanding of root canal anatomy gained through knowledge of normal anatomy and the deviation from the norm that exists within specific teeth

types. Visualisation of the three-dimensional anatomy using more than one film when using plain radiography or cone beam CT scanning will provide valuable information before access preparation is initiated.

1.1 Overview of Endodontic Access Design Preparation

Cavity design preparation can trace its roots back to the principles heralded by GV Black including outline form, convenience, retention and resistance forms [1]. Traditional endodontic ideal access preparations, often described in textbooks, have been focused primarily on the operator needs rather than the restorative needs showing easily identifiable canal entrances at the base of a large pulp floor. Recently proponents for minimally invasive endodontics (MIE) aimed at directed

B. Patel, BDS MFDS MClinDent MRD MRACDS
Specialist Endodontist, Brindabella Specialist Centre,
Canberra, ACT, Australia
e-mail: bobbypatel@me.com

© Springer International Publishing Switzerland 2016
B. Patel (ed.), *Endodontic Treatment, Retreatment, and Surgery,*
DOI 10.1007/978-3-319-19476-9_1

dentine conservation have tried to shift the focus towards the tooth, whereby maximal tooth conservation has been heralded as the primary aim in an effort to maintain optimal strength and fracture resistance of the tooth [2–4]. Care must be taken when adopting the concepts of MIE in that there are proponents that would have you believe that MIE exists solely with the framework of preserving a few millimetres or less of cervical tooth structure whilst their empirical claims lack documented and meaningful longer term studies [5].

The endodontic access preparation influences all ensuing steps and provides the opening for ideal shaping of canals, cleaning root canal systems, and three-dimensional obturation [6].

Good knowledge of canal morphology in mandibular and maxillary teeth will guide clinicians in creating correct pulp chamber openings necessary for location of all canals [7, 8]. Radiographic assessment should always be integrated with this knowledge to recreate a mental image of the proposed access cavity before any drilling is begun. A minimum of two diagnostic periapical radiographs should be taken, giving a two-dimensional image of a three-dimensional root canal system. The radiographs should be taken parallel and with either a mesial or distal horizontal tube shift to visualise superimposed roots. A parallel radiograph will allow minimal distortion and enable the clinician to correctly identify the coronal pulp chamber location with respect to the furcal floor and the cement-enamel junction. Both of these landmarks are helpful when trying to locate the level of the pulpal floor and location of canal entrances. The author routinely uses a beam-aiming device to ensure that minimal image distortion occurs and reproducible radiographs can be taken throughout the procedure. Cone beam CT (CBCT) scans may be available that can demonstrate anatomical features three-dimensionally. CBCT projection data can be reconstructed to provide images in three orthogonal planes (axial, sagittal and coronal) demonstrating true spatial relationships. Tooth morphology assessment can easily be visualised in 3D including the number of root canals and their interrelationship (see Figs. 1.1 and 1.2). In young patients, large pulp chambers will be noted with obvious canal spaces. Older patients whose teeth have undergone repeated insults will often have secondary or tertiary dentine deposited reducing pulp chamber volume and root canal lumens and increased calcifications encountered making access preparation even more challenging. Any sudden changes in the radiographic density of the pulp space will usually indicate an additional canal. Furthermore a sudden narrowing or disappearance of the root canal space may indicate a bi- or trifurcation [9–11].

The anatomical laws formulated by Krasner and Rankow should be taken into consideration when opening pulp chambers because they give clinicians general anatomical landmarks that are very useful when localising all canal anatomy [12].

Several studies have concluded that the dental operating microscope provides and enhances lighting and magnification, which are essential for the clinicians' ability to correctly localise and negotiate canals [13–15].

The use of an ultrasonic unit (magnetostrictive or piezoelectric) with an appropriate tip confers unique advantages for refinement of access cavities, location of canal orifices and removal of obstructions such as calcifications. Magnetostriction ultrasonic unit devices operate between 18 and 4 kHz, converting electromagnetic energy into mechanical oscillation when an alternating magnetic field is applied to metal strips in a stack. Piezoelectric units operate between 28 and 36 kHz, converting electrical energy into mechanical energy through a crystalline piezoelectric

Fig. 1.1 Note (**a**) and (**b**) clinical periapical radiographs demonstrating nonsurgical root canal treatment of tooth 25. Note they reveal limited two-dimensional view of the true three-dimensional image. Insert shows (**c**) access preparation, (**d**) limited volume cone-beam computed tomography reconstruction of the projection data providing axial and sagittal views of tooth 25 demonstrating extent of periradicular pathology and internal root canal anatomy, and (**e**) sagittal view and various slices (apical (*A*), middle (*M*), and coronal (*C*) dotted lines) highlight anatomy of the root canal space further seen in Fig. 1.2 axial views

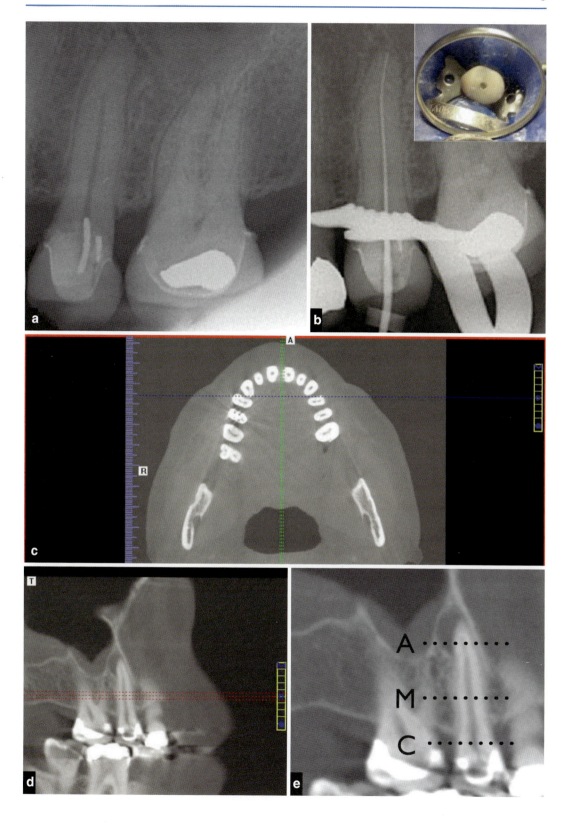

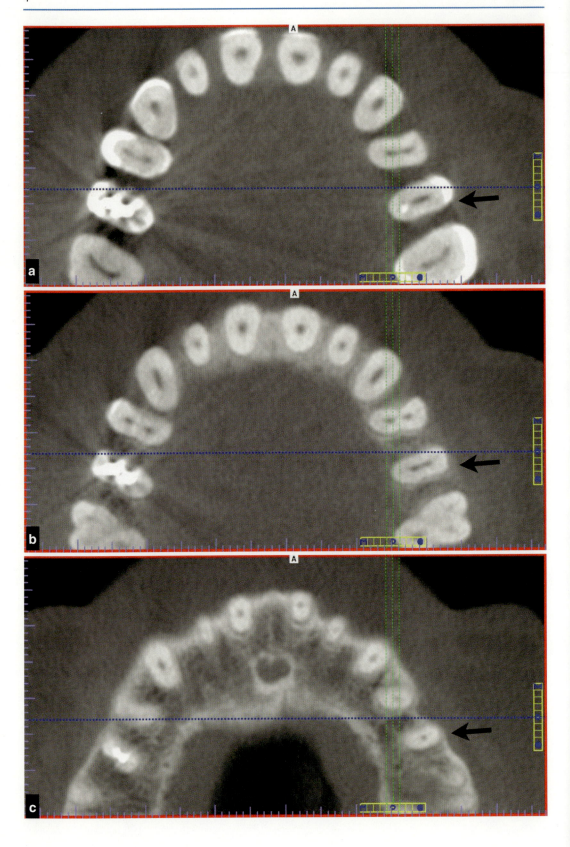

material. This mechanical energy is transferred to the cutting tips resulting in micro-vibratory movements in the ultrasonic frequency range. The tips should be used with a light brush and touch action, selecting a medium power setting under direct control using the operating microscope [16–18].

Ultrasonic tips are available in different lengths, diameters, angles and designs used with or without water. Length of tip is critical when determining whether the tip is to be used solely in the coronal aspect of the pulp chamber or within the root canal itself. Longer thinner tips are ideal in the case of the latter. Tip design is further classified according to whether it is constructed from stainless steel or titanium alloy. Stainless steel tips may be coated with zirconium nitride (ProUltra ultrasonic instruments; Dentsply, Tulsa, Oklahoma) or diamond grit (Spartan CPR instruments, Fenton, Missouri), which increases efficiency and durability. Most current available systems are designed to function either wet or dry. The former come with water ports to increase washing and cooling effects [19, 20].

Patients with cardiovascular implantable electronic devices, such as pacemakers, and the use of ultrasonics has been a concern. Dental equipment, which can pass a current to a patient, can potentially interfere with the pacemaker. Current guidelines recommend the avoidance of magnetostrictive devices, whereas the use of piezoelectric devices does not seem to have an affect on pacemakers [21, 22]. In the best interests of the patient, it would be prudent to discuss the case with the patients' cardiologist to ensure that there are no undue concerns with this regard.

1.2 Opening the Pulp Chamber

A front surface mirror, a Hu-Friedy DG16 endodontic probe, illumination and magnification are essential for preparation of the tooth for endodontic treatment. Caries and failing restorations must be completely removed prior to endodontic access cavity preparation. Where there is any doubt in relation to the restorability of the tooth in question, then dismantling of the existing restoration and preliminary assessment of the remaining tooth structure is an essential first step.

Removal of existing restorations also allows the examination of axial walls and the presence of any hairline cracks which could also influence the endodontic outcome. A restorability assessment is made in order to ensure that the planned future permanent coronal cast restoration is feasible.

Unsupported cusps are removed, and where any axial wall crack-lines are evident or a diagnosis of cracked tooth syndrome is suspected, then the tooth should be protected by placement of an orthodontic band during and following completion of treatment.

The roof of the pulp chamber should be penetrated through the central portion of the crown at a point where the roof and floor are at the widest (e.g. the palatal canal of a maxillary molar). An EndoZ bur, which has a non-end cutting tip, is ideal once the roof is penetrated, preventing potential damage to the floor of the pulp. All dentine ledges and lips should be removed.

Once the roof, in its entirety, has been removed, then the floor of the pulp chamber can be inspected. In cases, which are not calcified, dark developmental lines may be identifiable linking canal entrances. Following this 'road map' may reveal additional undetected canal entrances, and further probing with the DG16 may confirm a 'sticky' feeling.

Typical textbook description of pulp chamber anatomy is based on teeth with complete crowns and pulp chambers that are ideal in terms of position and width. Most clinical situations are far from ideal where teeth have been previously treated resulting in large restorations, cast restorations or dystrophic calcifications, which significantly alter the normal anatomy. Ideal access

Fig. 1.2 Cone-beam CT axial projection demonstrating (**a**) coronal, (**b**) middle, and (**c**) apical root anatomy. Access preparation could be carried out with confidence confirming a Vertucci 1-2-1 root canal anatomy. Note *black arrow* showing tooth 25

preparation may lead to iatrogenic errors due to inadequate or over-aggressive preparations. Access cavities should be prepared according to the internal anatomy of the tooth and refined according to the individual tooth and its unique anatomy accordingly (Fig. 1.3).

Krasner and Rankow evaluated the pulp chamber anatomy of 500 extracted teeth, and based on their findings, the following laws pertaining to general anatomical guidelines were made:

1. The floor of the pulp chamber is always a darker colour compared to the surrounding dentinal walls. This colour difference creates a distinct junction where the axial walls and floor of the pulp chamber meet (law of colour change).
2. The orifices of the root canals are always located at the junction of the axial walls and floor (law of orifice location 1).
3. The orifices of the root canals are located at the angle in the floor-wall junction (law of orifice location 2).
4. The orifices of the root canals lie at the terminus of developmental fusion lines, if present (law of orifice location 2).
5. The developmental root fusion lines are darker than the colour of the floor.
6. Except for maxillary molars, the orifices of canals are equidistant from a line drawn in a mesial-distal direction through the pulp chamber floor (law of symmetry 1).
7. Except for the maxillary molars, the orifices of canals lie on a line perpendicular to a line drawn in a mesial-distal direction across the centre of the floor of the pulp chamber (law of symmetry 2).

These generalised laws should be taken into consideration when preparing access cavities since they give clues to generalised landmarks independent of the crown anatomy (Fig. 1.4).

1.3 Access Through a Crown

It is not uncommon to carry out endodontic treatments in teeth already restored with crowns. Access preparations through existing crowns

whose margins are deemed good require careful consideration and diligence. It is necessary to mentally visualise the pulp chamber position from preoperative parallel radiographs. The distance of the pulp chamber floor from the most coronal aspect of the crown can be premeasured and noted. The angulation and any rotation of the tooth should be assessed and initial access preparation without the use of rubber dam may be advisable to ensure that penetration is carried out correctly without risk due to mis-angulation resulting in perforation. The position of the cement-enamel junction and furcation should also be noted as these landmarks help the clinician locate the level of the pulpal floor and likely position of canal entrances.

Tungsten carbide burs are ideal for cutting through metal such as full gold crowns. When mapping out the access through initial porcelain, a diamond bur should be used to reduce the likelihood of porcelain fracture. If the canals cannot be identified, then removal of the crown may be indicated to prevent iatrogenic perforation and unnecessary removal of sound dentine (see Figs. 1.5, 1.6 and 1.7).

1.4 Straight-Line Access

Once the canal entrances have been identified, it may be necessary to refine the outline shape of the access cavity to allow endodontic instruments unimpeded straight-line access in the coronal 1/3rd of the canal. Straight-line access will prevent or reduce the likelihood of unfavourable iatrogenic mishaps such as canal transportation including ledging, zipping and perforation. Straight-line access will also reduce file distortion, particularly important when using rotary nickel-titanium instruments, which may undergo unnecessary torsional loading and cyclic fatigue leading to instrument fracture (see Chap. 11). Access openings must be designed to preserve sound tooth structure and is fundamentally important to prevent unintentional gouging laterally, cervically or into/beyond the floor of the pulp chamber (see Fig. 1.11). Conversely, access that is too restricted may impact on correct identification of all internal

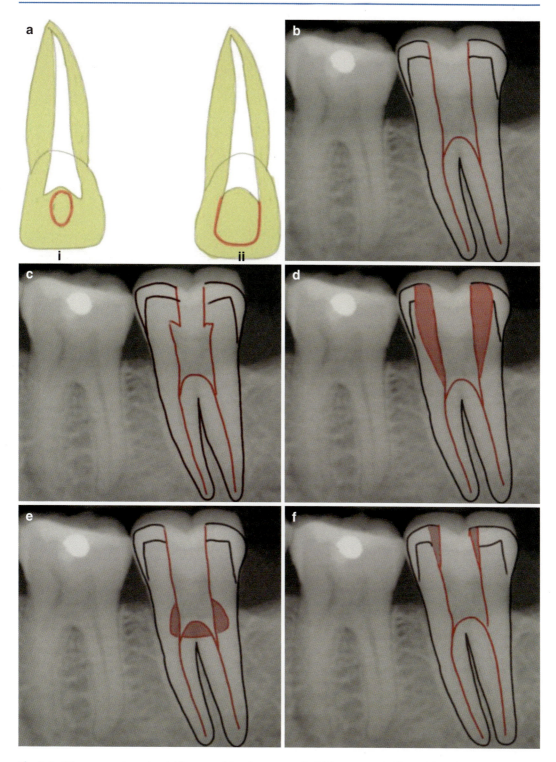

Fig. 1.3 Diagrams representing (**a**) incorrect (*i*) and correct (*ii*) removal of the pulp chamber in an incisor tooth. (**b**) Correct and (**c**) incorrect straight-line access in a posterior molar tooth. (**d**) Excessive removal of tooth structure leading to weakening and potential fracture of the tooth. (**e**) Damage to the floor of the pulp chamber will not only risk possible perforation but also hinder location of canal entrances. (**f**) The walls of the coronal access should not deflect an instrument placed in the canal

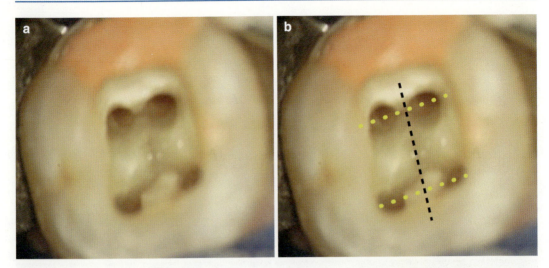

Fig. 1.4 Clinical photographs showing (**a**) internal anatomy of a tooth. Note dark developmental grooves on the floor of the pulp and darker color associated with root canal orifices. (**b**) As described by Krasnoe and Rankow Law of symmetry 1 and 2

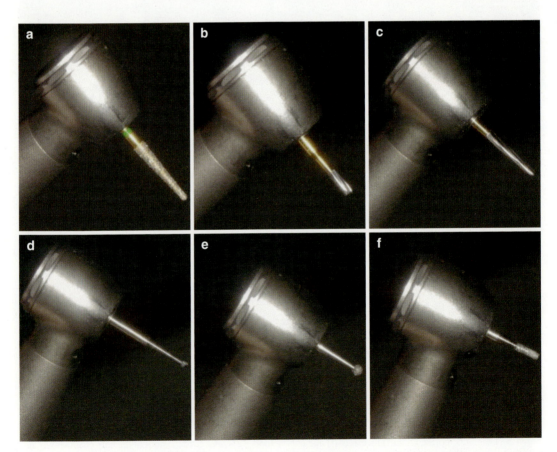

Fig. 1.5 Clinical photographs showing typical armamentarium of burs used for access preparations: (**a**) diamond grit tapered bur, (**b**) tungsten carbide bur, (**c**) non-end cutting Endo-Z bur, (**d**) long shank diamond, (**e**) diamond grit round diamond, and (**f**) parallel tapered short diamond bur

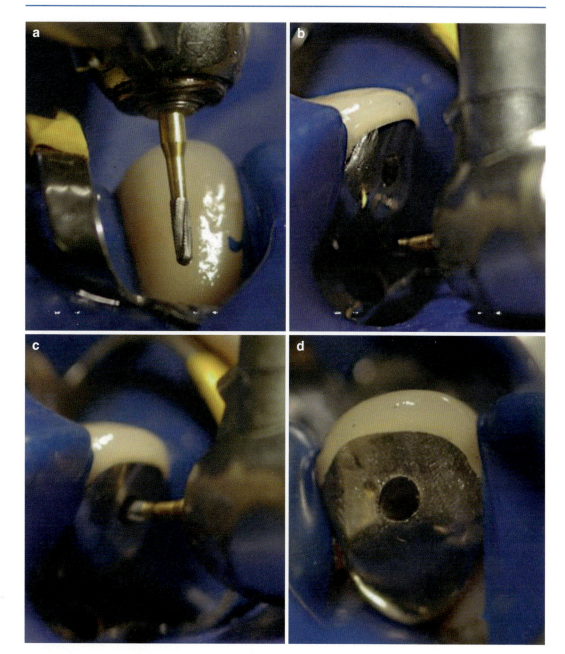

Fig. 1.6 Clinical photographs showing access preparation through a porcelain-metal crown. (**a**) Tungsten carbide bur is selected and (**b**) carefully aligned to long access of the tooth to (**c**, **d**) gain initial access through the metal infrastructure. Preoperative radiographs and clinical assessment of the tooth-root relationship is important to prevent misalignment. Occasionally, access can be carried out prior to placement of rubber dam if the long axis tooth is difficult to ascertain or the crown-root relationship is of concern

anatomy leading to iatrogenic errors during subsequent preparation as discussed earlier (Fig. 1.8).

Whilst unmistakable orifice location and careful canal penetration are warranted, efforts should be made to minimise excessive removal of cervical tooth structure in the canal orifice. Commonly used instruments such as Gates Glidden drills should be avoided since these instruments tend to

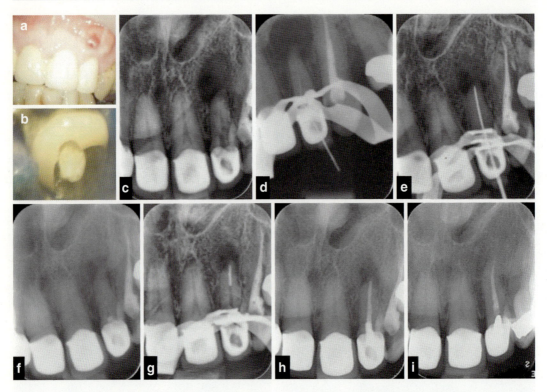

Fig. 1.7 Clinical photographs and radiographs demonstrating nonsurgical endodontic treatment through a ceramic-metal crown. Note (**a**) draining sinus in relation to tooth 22 and (**b**) prior endodontic access carried out by the general dental practitioner. (**c**) Preoperative radiograph confirming endodontic access. The dentist was unable to locate the canal orifice. Note access preparation extends below the cervical margin of the tooth and an obvious root canal can be seen. An extensive periradicular radiolucency is evident. (**d**) IAF demonstrating successful canal negotiation after careful access refinement. Initial access was misaligned due to orientation difficulties arising from the cast restoration in place.

Access had been directed towards the facial aspect but no perforation was noted. Access refinement was carried out using ultrasonic troughing under constant guidance using magnification. (**e**) MAF radiograph following working length determination. (**f**) 3-month follow-up radiograph showing intra-canal medicament dissolution and significant reduction in the pre-operative radiolucency. (**g, h**) Obturation was completed using a warm vertical compaction technique using AH plus cement. (**i**) The patient was reviewed a further 9 months later. The radiograph demonstrates an intact periodontal ligament space associated with the peri-apex of tooth 22 correlated with complete healing

straighten the canal and weaken the root canal walls, and overzealous use in some cases may lead to irreparable defects such as stripping or perforation.

Straight-line access is achieved by firstly correct access preparation with correct axial wall refinement. Once the floor of the pulp chamber has been identified, the use of a non-end cutting bur (Endo Z) is excellent for gross refinement and removal of dentinal overhangs that prevent unimpeded orifice location. Finer refinement can be carried out using ultrasonic tips under magnification allowing precision removal with minimal damage when carried out correctly. Creating straight-line access within the coronal 1/3rd of the canal can be achieved by introduction of initial rotary instruments that can be safely used in a brushing action, away from the danger areas, removing cervical dentine efficiently. Initial pre-flaring with the S1 ProTaper file can effectively remove this triangle if dentine is commonly encountered coronally. The angle of the inserted instrument within the canal is a good indicator as to whether straight-line access has been achieved

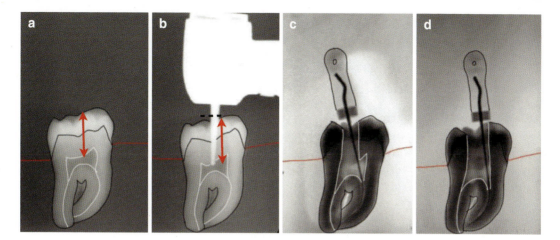

Fig. 1.8 Diagrammatic representation of straight-line access preparation in a mandibular molar tooth. A parallel preoperative radiograph is obtained, and (**a**) an initial measurement is calculated as to the depth of the pulp chamber in relation to the occlusal surface (*red arrow*). (**b**) This length is used as a guide for initial penetration into the pulp chamber. (**c**) Initial access preparation is incomplete with inadequate extension distally. Note file deflection as a result causing increased stress and potential for iatrogenic errors. (**d**) Correct access extension using appropriate non-end cutting to refine distally. Note file is now no longer deflected and therefore less likely to result in iatrogenic errors such as apical canal transportation or file separation

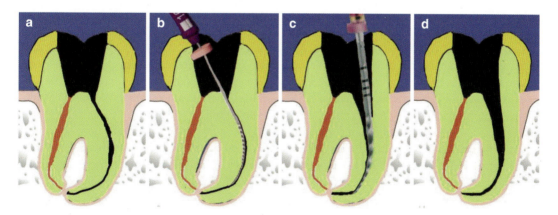

Fig. 1.9 (**a–d**) Clinical diagrams representing use of ProTaper shaping file S1 in a brushing action to aid removal of coronal interferences that prevent straight-line access. A lateral cutting action on withdrawal is recommended away from the danger area such as the furcation

(i.e. the instrument should stand upright). Radiographic imaging of initial apical file placement will also indicate whether any further coronal dentine removal is indicated. Once straight-line access is achieved, the clinician can be assured that iatrogenic errors such as transportations, which are common in any curved canal space, can be minimised with subsequent apical preparation and introduction of files of greater taper (Fig. 1.9).

1.5   Use of Ultrasonics

Ultrasonic tips are an excellent tool for refining access cavities, removing calcifications and finding canal orifices often hidden by deposition of secondary or tertiary dentine. The tips should be used with a light brush stroke and medium power setting and under constant vision using a dental operating microscope. Tips can be selected according to intended use, which can be broadly classified as bulk removal, access refinement or troughing (see Fig. 1.14).

Bulk removal

Bulk removal of dentine and core material such as amalgam or composite that can often obstruct the initial access preparation can be carried out using specifically designed tips. Axial wall refinement can be carried out using Start-X tip 1, CPR2D or BUC 1 tips. The Start-X tip number 1 has a non-end cutting tip diameter of 0.8 mm, a maximum diameter of the active portion of 1.6 mm and a blade length of 12 mm. The main indication for using this tip is for refinement of the axial walls. The tip can be used to remove restorations, filling material, caries and dentine interferences that may be present on the axial walls without altering the morphology of the pulpal floor due to its non-end cutting tip (Fig. 1.10).

Access refinement

Use of ultrasonic tips to enhance access can be carried out with precision with no hand-piece head to obscure indirect vision, allowing progressive cutting of dentine with minimal risk of danger. Dentine can be brushed away in smaller increments with greater control compared to traditional use of burs. Traditional techniques employed to unroof a pulp chamber advocated using large stainless steel round burs which would simply drop into the pulp chamber remove the roof by a back and forth action without damaging the floor. Unfortunately most endodontic cases are not carried out in young adults with pulp chambers that are so large that they can easily accommodate such burs. Typically teeth requiring endodontic treatment have often undergone multiple insults resulting in calcifications and a diminished pulp volume. Overzealous use of burs in these cases will typically result in gouging laterally, cervically and towards the furcation and beyond (see Figs. 1.11 and 1.12).

Ultrasonic tips can be used to uncover the floor of the pulp chamber with less risk of unfavourable damage to the tooth. A number of tips are available to refine the access cavity. The uncovering of the floor of the pulp chamber can be accomplished using the help of the Start-X tip 2 or 3, CPR2D or BUC 1 tips (see Fig. 1.10).

If the dark floor of the pulp chamber is not visible, it may often be obscured with pulp stones or tertiary dentine deposits. Removal of these interferences is not only important to enable location of canals but also prevent stones from blocking apical anatomy during preparation stages later.

The calcified deposits can be carefully vibrated or planned away until the dark coloured dentinal floor is visible (see Fig. 1.10). A sharp, tapered point at its end characterises the Start-X number 3 tip. The diameter of the tip at the base of the end is 0.64 mm; the maximum diameter of the active portion is 0.9 mm and has a blade length of 8 mm. It is very useful when removing calcifications from the floor of the pulp chamber or from the coronal 1/3rd of the root canal. Additionally this tip is useful for the removal of fibre posts encountered in retreatment cases. Note the tip is aggressive and should only be used in a very light touch to avoid iatrogenic damage.

Troughing

During fine refinement of the floor of the pulp chamber, dentinal overhangs may be removed in order to reveal additional or hidden anatomy. Maxillary molars commonly have second mesiobuccal canal orifices located in a bucco-palatal groove overlying the mesiobuccal root. Mandibular molars may have an additional middle-mesial canal located between the mesiobuccal and mesiolingual groove. Careful troughing of these areas is required to remove overlying dentine to safely expose the hidden orifice, which may often be present. The Start-X tip number 2 has an end-cutting tip diameter of

Fig. 1.10 Showing step-by-step access refinement using ultrasonics. Note (**a**) preoperative view showing calcifications present in the coronal pulp chamber typically overlying the canal orifices (*yellow*). (**b–e**) Ultrasonic files can be used in an axial and bucco-lingual direction to carefully remove calcific material and refine the access cavity preparation. Overzealous tooth removal is avoided ensuring (**f**) correct canal orifice identification without damaging the floor of the pulp and iatrogenic perforation

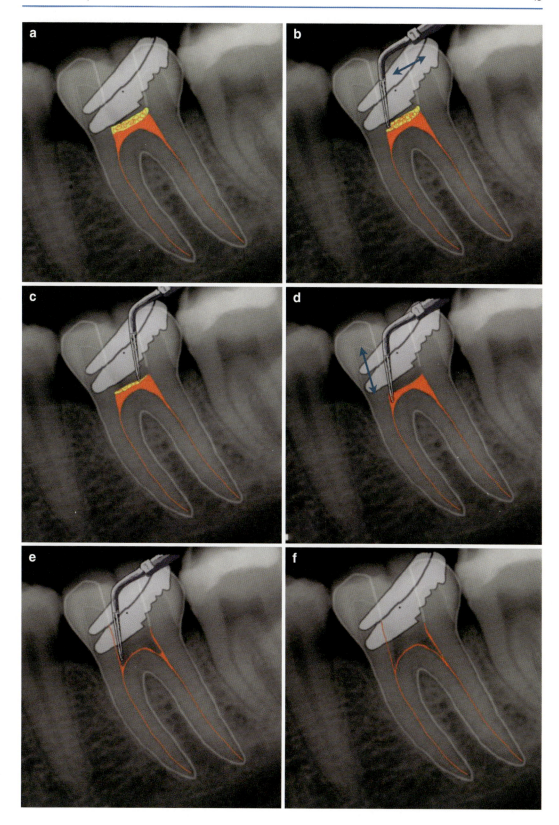

1.0 mm, a maximum diameter of the active portion of 1.54 mm and blade length of 8 mm. This tip is particularly useful for removal of dentine or calcifications overlying the floor of the pulp chamber and creating grooves allowing the removal of all dentinal interferences such as MB2 orifice location (see Fig. 1.13).

Troughing must be carried out diligently since removal of dentine in areas such as the floor of the pulp chamber can lead to irreversible damage. The clinician must be aware of the spatial relationship in terms of the danger area and where dentine is actively being removed. This is based on anatomical knowledge, radiographic pre- and

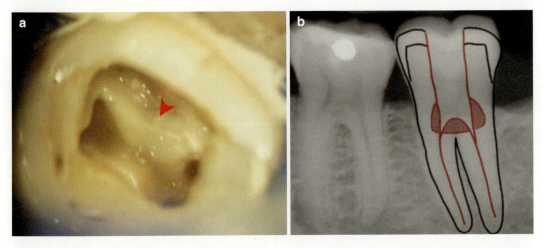

Fig. 1.11 Clinical photograph showing (**a**) excessive lateral dentine removal with gouging of the flow (*red arrow*) and (**b**) diagrammatic representation showing areas at risk which can be avoided (*red shaded*) by the use of ultrasonic instrumentation and microscopic visualization

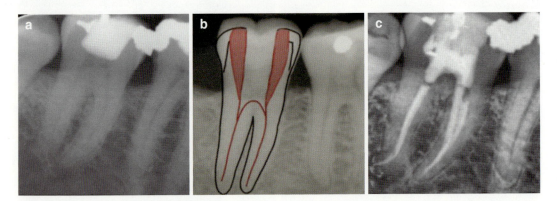

Fig. 1.12 Clinical radiographs and diagrammatic representations showing (**a–c**) pre- and postoperative view of a case with prior access where overzealous access preparation has resulted in excessive dentine removal. Axial wall refinement with selection of appropriate ultrasonic tips with non-end cutting properties would have been more suited to prevent this occurrence

Fig. 1.13 Clinical radiographs and photographs demonstrating (**a**) MB1, DB, and P canal working lengths, (**b**) additional MB2 located, (**c–f**) MB2 canal orifice (*arrow*) located using ultrasonic troughing in a buccopalatal direction (*dashed line*) followed by careful preparation. Care must be exercised when carrying out troughing in this area due to risk of perforation of the mesial root floor of the pulp chamber

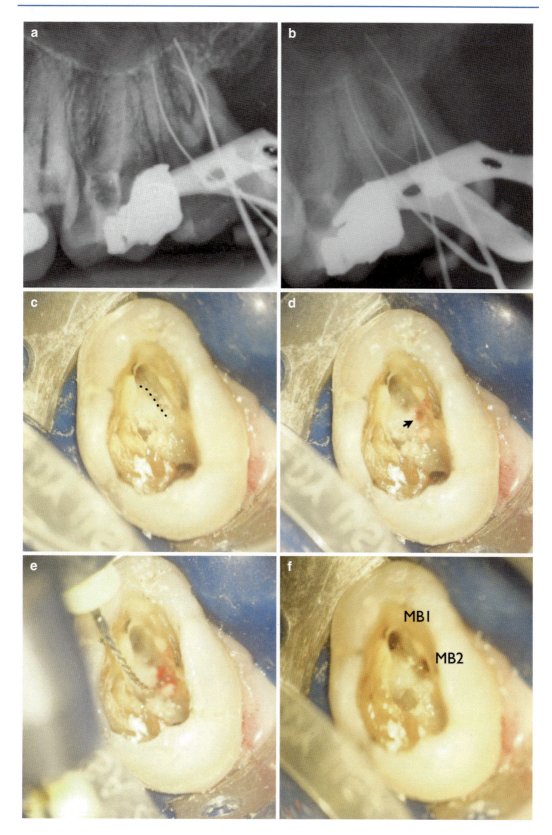

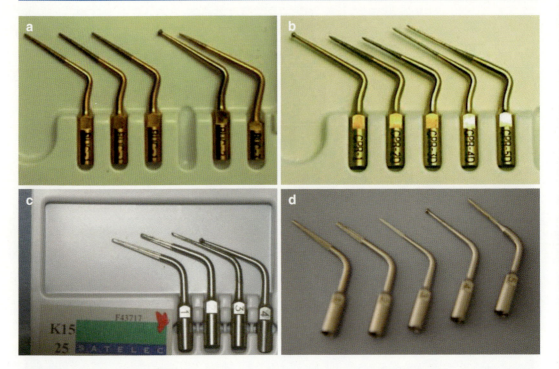

Fig. 1.14 Clinical photographs showing ultrasonic tips typically used in endodontics. (**a**) BUC tips, (**b**) CPR tips, and (**c**, **d**) Start-X tips

peri-assessment and clinical spatial assessment of the site of troughing, and its relationship to internal (dentine colouration and pre-existing roadmap) and external landmarks (axial walls and long axis of the tooth). When in doubt, it may be best to stop and take a further radiograph to help determine positioning within the tooth (Fig. 1.14).

1.6 Calcified Canals

Calcified canal systems are a consequence of ageing and the cumulative effects of restorative procedures and previous insults. The pulp chamber will often be reduced in volume due to the deposition of secondary dentine (yellow/grey colour) resulting in greater risk of pulpal floor iatrogenic errors during access preparation procedures. Tertiary dentine deposition (whiter and more opaque in appearance) in response to caries or micro-leakage may also be encountered, further reducing the overall pulp volume. The natural dome-shaped floor of the pulp chamber may appear flatter resulting in narrower canal

entrances, which are more difficult to locate. Pulp stones and calcifications are best removed using ultrasonic tips (see Figs. 1.15 and 1.16).

1.7 Clinical Cases

Case 1 Endodontic treatment of tooth 16 heavily calcified and restored with a ceramic metal crown

A fit and healthy 73-year-old patient was referred for endodontic treatment of tooth 16. The general dental practitioner had carried out an indirect pulp capping procedure on the mesiobuccal canal 2 years ago. A crown had been placed thereafter. Recently the tooth had become sore to touch and exacerbated with chewing/biting. Clinical examination confirmed tooth 16 was tender to percussion. Radiographic examination revealed a peri-radicular radiolucency associated with the palatal root. The root canals appeared calcified. A decision was made to carry out conventional non-surgical root canal therapy through the existing cast restoration, which had good marginal integrity. Access cavity preparation was carried out

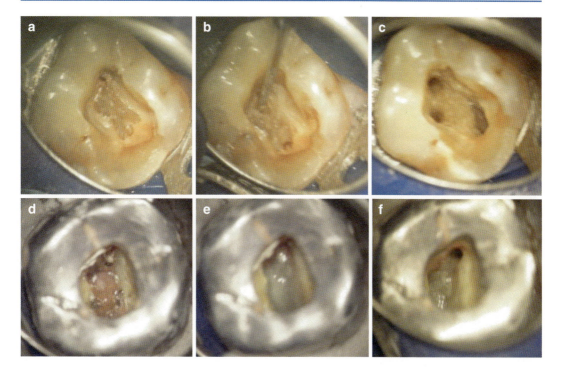

Fig. 1.15 Showing (**a–f**) clinical photographs of access refinements in cases with calcifications overlying the canal orifices. Careful removal using ultrasonic files eventually reveals canal orifices. Following canal preparation, canal orifices can be visualized line access

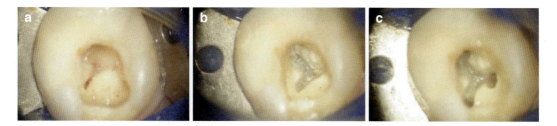

Fig. 1.16 Showing clinical photographs of access refinement using ultrasonics in tooth 36. Note (**a**) highly calcified root canal system with (**b**) multiple pulp stones which following removal reveals the (**c**) darker road map in the floor of the pulp chamber that leads to canal orifices

initially using a tungsten carbide bur confirming a completely calcified pulp chamber. Ultrasonic preparation was carried out and the palatal canal was located first (Fig. 1.17). Previous pulp capping material was identified and removed. Following extensive troughing mesially, the MB1 and DB canals were identified. Patency was achieved in all the canals and manual glide path preparation completed using stainless steel endodontic files. Chemomechanical preparation was completed using 1 % sodium hypochlorite solution. Rotary files were used to prepare the canals (ProTaper Universal) with recapitulation and patency filing throughout. All three canals had acute apical curvatures, which were maintained. An intra-canal dressing of calcium hydroxide was placed for a period of 4 weeks. Obturation was completed using a warm vertical compaction technique using AH Plus cement. The access cavity was temporarily sealed and the patient was discharged back to the referring dentist for permanent coronal restoration (Fig. 1.18).

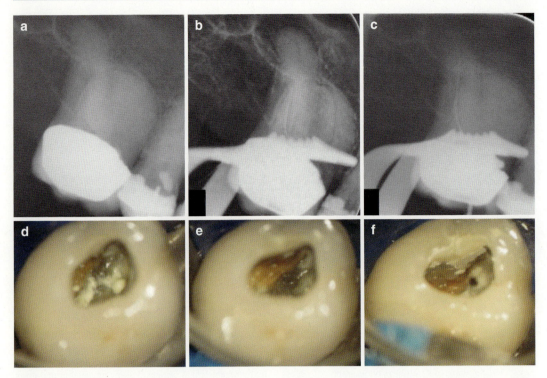

Fig. 1.17 Clinical radiographs and photographs demonstrating (**a**) preoperative x-ray showing crowned tooth 16 with completely calcified roof canal system. The patient had undergone a direct pulp capping of the MB root 12 months previously and then a crown preparation. (**b**) Initial access preparation revealed a palatal canal which could initially be partially negotiated. (**c**) Palatal canal negotiated to length (note DB and MB canals remain unlocated). Following further ultrasonic debridement and (**d**) removal of pulpal floor calcifications (*white areas*), the darker pulpal floor anatomy starts to become visible (**e**). (**f**) Successful MB1 canal orifice located and negotiated

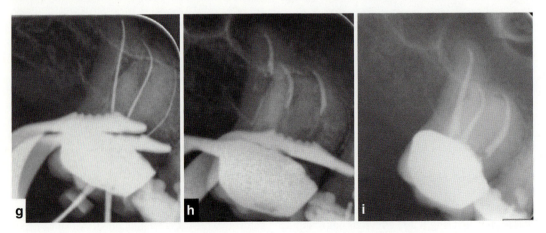

Fig. 1.18 Clinical radiographs demonstrating (**g**) MAF radiographs following successful negotiation of the MB1, DB, and P canals, (**h**) mid-fill x-ray demonstrating apical 1/3 obturation, and (**i**) final postoperative radiograph showing completed case. This case had all the ingredients of difficult access preparation through a metal-ceramic crown, calcified pulp canal system, and acute apical curvatures. Correct access design and preparation from the outset case to be completed without any iatrogenic errors along the way

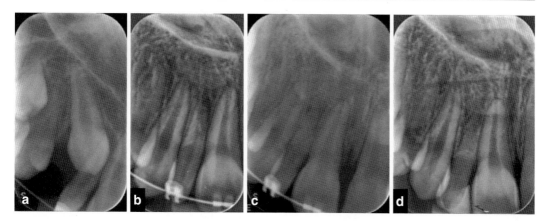

Fig. 1.19 Clinical radiographs demonstrating preoperative views of tooth 12. Note (**a**) radiograph taken in 2012 showing the impacted canine (tooth 13) and peg-shaped lateral incisor (tooth 12). Tooth 13 was brought into the line of the arch using surgical exposure and bracket and chain attachment. (**b**) Radiograph taken in 2013 showing tooth 13 in the line of the arch. Note orthodontic fixed appliance therapy was started. Note tooth 12 has a normal root canal space and volume at this time. (**c**) Further radiographic examination taken in 2014 showing pulp canal obliteration in tooth 12. The tooth was asymptomatic at this stage. (**d**) Radiographic examination taken in 2015. Orthodontic fixed appliance therapy was completed, brackets have been removed and tooth 12 has been masked with a composite restoration for aesthetic purposes. The root canal appears heavily calcified with a widened periodontal ligament space noted at the peri-apex. The patient was experiencing symptoms of irreversible pulpitis and an endodontic referral was made for further management

Case 2 Endodontic treatment of tooth 12 peg-shaped lateral masked with composite restoration and severely calcified

A fit and healthy 14-year-old patient presented with severe localised pain and discomfort associated with tooth 12. The patient had initially presented to her general dental practitioner in 2012 with an unerupted impacted canine tooth. The patient was seen for orthodontic treatment including canine exposure and alignment using a bracket and chain. Further fixed orthodontic appliance therapy was carried out over a period of 2 years. The tooth had been reshaped with a final composite restoration to improve the final aesthetics (Fig. 1.19).

Radiographic examination revealed a widened periodontal ligament space associated with the peg-shaped lateral incisor (tooth 12) and severe calcification of the pulp chamber. The tooth had undergone progressive pulp canal obliteration following orthodontic fixed appliance therapy (Fig. 1.19). A decision was made to attempt orthograde root canal treatment. The patient was forewarned of the inherent risks when attempting to locate canals and that the case was further complicated by the composite coronal restoration that masked the true orientation of the crown and root. Careful alignment was made parallel to the long axis of the tooth and initial coronal access preparation was completed using a small tapered diamond bur. The access cavity was deepened with an ultrasonic tip under the use of the dental operating microscope. To gain access through the calcified dentine, a #08K-file was modified with the final 1 mm removed using a sterile pair of surgical scissors. This modification allowed an improved cutting efficiency of the file with more resistance to both deformation and fracture. The file was carefully advanced 1–2 mm increments apically and an apex locator was used to confirm no perforation was evident. Irrigation was carried and performed using copious amounts of 1 % sodium hypochlorite solution throughout. Once the file was engaged within the canal, its presence was further verified by the observation of 'bubble' formations indicating contact with organic pulp tissue remnants under the dental operating microscope. Patency was eventually achieved and chemomechanical preparation completed using rotary files. An intra-canal medicament of calcium hydroxide was placed for 4 weeks and

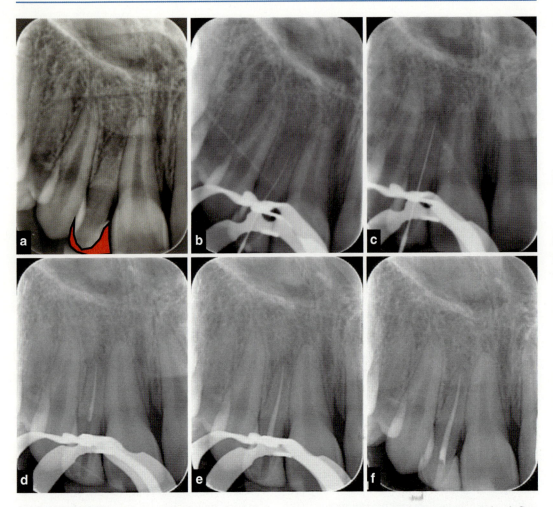

Fig. 1.20 Clinical radiographs demonstrating root canal treatment of tooth 12. Note (**a**) preoperative view with obvious pulp canal obliteration. A composite resin restoration (*red*) has been placed to mask the peg-shaped lateral to mimic a normal lateral incisor tooth. Access in this tooth is fraught with danger. (**b**) Initial apical file size radiograph following correct access preparation and use of ultrasonic troughing. Patency is eventually achieved using small K files (08 and 010). (**c**) Master apical file radiograph. Chemo-mechanical preparation has been completed. Care was taken to ensure that canal enlargement was carried out bearing in mind the overall size of the tooth in question. (**d–f**) Obturation is completed using a warm vertical compaction technique using AH Plus cement. The access cavity is restored with IRM and glass ionomer cement. The patient is discharged back to her general dental practitioner for placement of a permanent coronal restoration and further follow-up is arranged in 6 months

the patient was seen again for review. At the review appointment, the patient was asymptomatic and a decision was made to proceed to obturation. Root canal obturation was completed using AH Plus cement and a warm vertical compaction technique. A temporary double-seal restoration of IRM and glass ionomer cement was placed and the patient advised to see her general dental practitioner for placement of a permanent coronal restoration (see Fig. 1.20).

Case 3 Non-surgical root canal treatment of tooth 36 with minimal occlusal access

A fit and healthy 60-year-old patient was referred for non-surgical endodontic therapy of tooth 36. At the consultation appointment, the patient was complaining of pain and tenderness in relation to tooth 36. Radiographic examination revealed a supracrestal coronal restoration with degenerative pulpal changes.

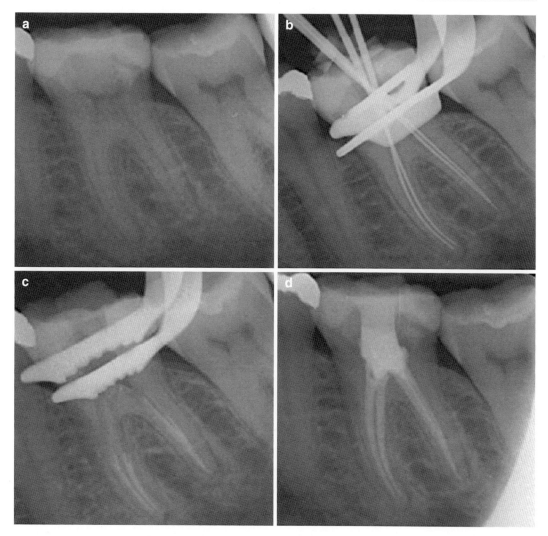

Fig. 1.21 Clinical radiographs demonstrating nonsurgical root treatment of tooth 36 with minimal occlusal access cavity preparation. Note (**a**) preoperative view showing calcified coronal pulp chamber and sclerosed canals with periradicular radiolucent lesions. (**b**) MAF preparation (DB and DL canal confluent in the apical 1/3. (**c**) Mid-fill radiograph following warm vertical compacting using AH Plus cement and gutta-percha. (**d**) Postoperative view showing completed obturation and coronal temporary restoration. Minimal access preparations aimed at dentine conservation serve to maximize tooth longevity. The clinician must balance this aim with the additional risks of iatrogenic problems such as file deformation and fracture and obturation difficulties that can arise as a result

The coronal pulp chamber appeared diminished in volume with sclerosed root canals. Peri-radicular radiolucencies were noted with both mesial and distal apices. Access preparation was completed through the coronal restoration directed at preserving as much dentine as possible. Use of the dental operating microscope was essential in being able to visualise internal anatomy and location of four canals. Ultrasonic preparation was used to refine both the axial walls and removal of pulp calcifications obscuring canal orifices. Chemomechanical preparation was completed using 1 % NaOCl solution. A manual glide path was created to size .20 before introducing rotary instrumentation. Following completion of preparation, an interim dressing of calcium hydroxide was placed for 4 weeks (Fig. 1.21).

Obturation was completed using a warm vertical compaction technique using AH Plus cement and gutta percha. A temporary coronal double seal was placed using IRM and glass ionomer cement. The patient was referred to his general dental practitioner for placement of a cast cuspal coverage restoration.

Case 4 Non-surgical endodontic treatment of tooth 42 requiring improvised access cavity preparation

A well-controlled hypertensive 46-year-old female patient was referred for endodontic management of tooth 42. The patient had previously seen his general dental practitioner for extensive caries treatment in the lingual aspect of the tooth. The patient had been warned of the deep restoration and possible pulpal sequelae. Following this treatment procedure, the patient recalled progressive pain and discomfort with the tooth exacerbated initially with chewing/biting and thermal stimulus. She recalled recent spontaneous dull pain from the tooth, which was relieved by analgesics. The patient had seen her dentist who prescribed some oral steroids (dexamethasone 4 mg) and a referral was sought. The dentist mentioned difficult access due to labial incisor imbrication in the area. Clinical examination revealed tooth 42 was restored with a lingual restoration. Tooth 43 was impacted against the lingual surface making conventional access impossible (see Fig. 1.23). Tooth 42 was tender to percussion. Radiographic examination revealed an extensive coronal restoration overlying the pulp chamber. Two canals were noted with no obvious signs of apical pathology (Fig. 1.22).

The patient was keen to try and retain the tooth and understand the difficulties with conventional access preparation. The patient was advised that a labial approach would be the alternative, requiring some aesthetic masking following endodontic completion. The patient was advised to stop taking the oral steroids and a further emergency treatment appointment was scheduled. After adequate anaesthesia, the tooth was isolated under rubber dam and a labial access preparation created. Access cavity was refined with an EndoZ bur to ensure that both labial and lingual canals were accessible. Working length radiograph was taken confirming the presence of two canals with separate apical foramina (Fig. 1.22). Chemomechanical preparation was completed using 1 % NaOCl solution. An intracanal dressing of calcium hydroxide was placed and the patient reviewed a week later. At the review appointment, all the patients' symptoms had resolved and tooth remained asymptomatic.

The patient was seen for a second treatment appointment 3 weeks later for completion of endodontic treatment. Obturation was completed using AH Plus cement and a warm vertical compaction technique. A coronal double-seal Biodentine/GIC temporary restoration was placed prior to discharging the patient back to her general dental practitioner (Fig. 1.23).

This final case highlights that every case should keep in mind the basic principles of cavity design procedures discussed but occasionally an alternative unconventional access design may be required to enable adequate treatment to be carried out.

Clinical Hints and Tips for Access Preparations

- **Use of magnification, illumination and ultrasonic equipment**
  Greatly improves the ability to successfully identify all the root canals in any tooth.
- **Preoperative parallel radiographs**
  Allows the clinician to mentally visualise the precise location of the canals. Assess the angulation and rotation of the tooth. Identify the position of the cement-enamel junction, which indicates the location level of the pulpal floor. Also identify where the

Fig. 1.22 Clinical radiographs and photographs demonstrating nonsurgical root canal treatment of tooth 42 with unconventional buccal access cavity. Note (**a**) preoperative view, (**b**) initial apical file (IAF) in buccal canal, (**c**) master apical file size # 25 in buccal canal and IAF # 010K file in lingual canal, (**d**) MAF buccal and lingual canals, (**e**) buccal access cavity, and (**f**) MAF files in place

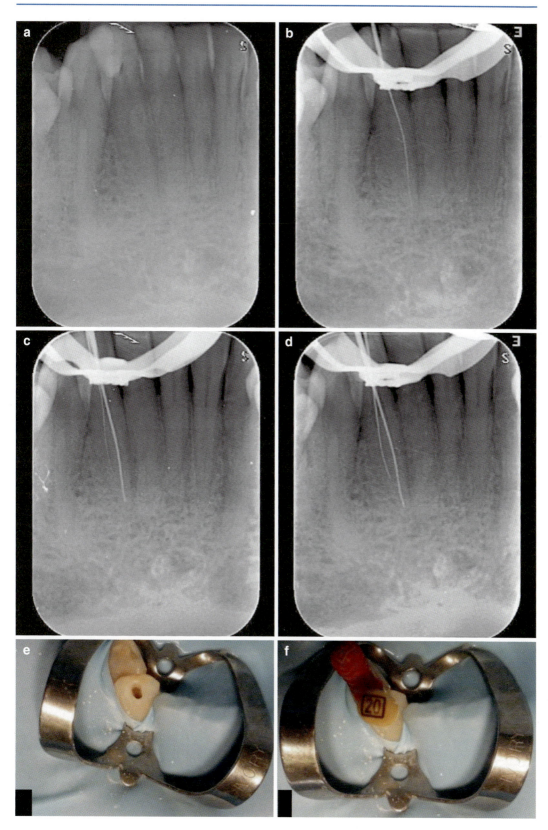

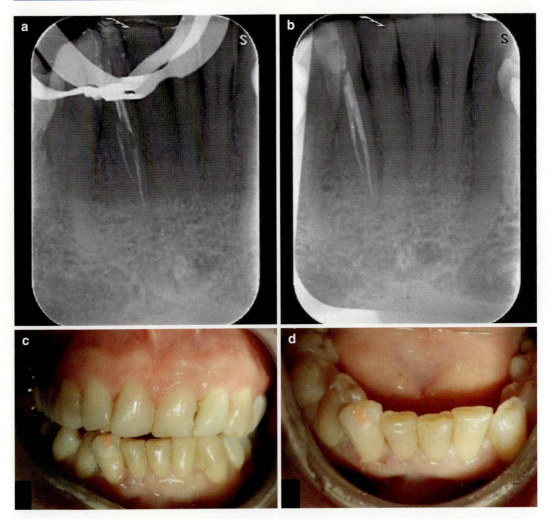

Fig. 1.23 Clinical radiographs and photographs demonstrating non-surgical root canal treatment of tooth 42 with unconventional buccal access cavity due to imbrication with tooth 43. Note (**a**) mid-fill radiograph following warm vertical compaction using AH plus cement and gutta-percha. (**b**) Completed endodontic treatment following backfill using Obtura. A final coronal restoration of Biodentine and glass ionomer cement (GIC) was placed. Pink GIC was selected so the general dental practitioner would not disturb the Biodentine seal overlying the root canal orifices. (**c**, **d**) Completed buccal access cavity. The patient was discharged back to her general dental practitioner for a permanent tooth coloured restoration

furcation is and to approximately what length preventing iatrogenic damage.

- **Anatomical knowledge**
  Pretreatment knowledge and experience of what to expect in individual teeth will give the clinician the ability to ensure that he can locate all anatomy.

- **Straight-line access**
  The importance of gaining straight-line access into the root canals prevents iatrogenic damage or problems occurring with subsequent cleaning, shaping and obturating procedures.

References

1. Black GV. Operative dentistry, vol. II. 7th ed. Chicago: Medico-Dental Publishing; 1936.
2. Clark D, Khademi J. Modern molar endodontic access and directed dentin conservation. Dent Clin North Am. 2010;54:249–73.

3. Clark D, Khademi J, Herbranson E. Fracture resistant endodontic and restorative preparations. (120–3). Dent Today. 2013;32:118.
4. Clark D, Khademi J, Herbranson E. The new science of strong endo teeth. (116–7). Dent Today. 2013;32:112–4.
5. Gutmann JL. Minimally invasive dentistry (Endodontics). J Conserv Dentist. 2013;16(4):282.
6. Ruddle CJ. Endodontic access preparation: an opening for success. Dent Today. 2007;26(2):114.
7. Vertucci FJ. Root canal anatomy of the human permanent teeth. Oral Surg Oral Med Oral Pathol Oral Radiol Endod. 1984;58:589–99.
8. Vertucci FJ. Root canal morphology and its relationship to endodontic procedures. Endod Topics. 2005;10:3–29.
9. Slowey RR. Root canal anatomy. Road map to successful endodontics. Dent Clin North Am. 1979;23:555–73.
10. Castellucci A. Endodontic radiography. In: Castellucci A, editor. Endodontics. vol 1, 2nd ed. Italy: Tridente Florence; 2006, pp. 66–119.
11. Patel S, Rhodes J. A Practical guide to endodontic access cavity preparation in molar teeth. BDJ. 2007;203:133–40.
12. Krasner P, Rankow HJ. Anatomy of the pulp chamber floor. J Endod. 2004;30:5–16.
13. Kulild JC, Peters DD. Incidence and configuration of canal systems in the mesio-buccal root of maxillary first and second molars. J Endod. 1990;16:311–7.
14. Coehlo de Carvalho MC, Zuolo ML. Orifice locating with a microscope. J Endod. 2000;26:532–4.
15. Baldassari-Cruz LA, Lilly JP, Rivera EM. The influence of dental operating microscopes in locating the mesio-lingual canal orifices. Oral Surg Oral Med Oral Pathol Oral Radiol Endod. 2002;93:190–4.
16. Clark D. The operating microscope and ultrasonics: a perfect marriage. Dent Today. 2004;23:74–81.
17. Tomson P, Lea SC, Lumley PJ, Walmsley AD. Performance of ultrasonic retrograde systems. J Endod. 2007;33:574–7.
18. Plotino GL, Pameijer CH, Grande NM, Somma F. Ultrasonics in endodontics: a review of the literature. J Endod. 2007;33:81–95.
19. Iqbal MK. Non surgical ultrasonic endodontic instruments. Dent Clin N Am. 2004;48(1):19–34.
20. Park E. Ultrasonics in endodontics. Endodont Topics. 2013;29:125–59.
21. Rezai FR. Dental treatment of patient with a cardiac pacemaker: review of the literature. Oral Surg Oral Med Oral Pathol. 1977;44:662–5.
22. Stoopler ET, Sia YW, Kuperstein AS. Does ultrasonic dental equipment affect cardiovascular implantable electronic devices? J Can Dent Assoc. 2011;77:b113.

Temporary and Interim Restorations in Endodontics

2

Sarita Atreya and Bobby Patel

Summary

One of the fundamental aims of root canal treatment is to reduce the microbiological load from within the root canal system to sufficiently low levels below a critical threshold that wil! allow an environment conducive to healing. This aim is achieved through the various stages of root canal treatment including interim temporary restorations that help prevent recontamination. Many different materials and techniques have been proposed based on numerous in vitro and in vivo studies. The clinician must ensure that a suitable material is selected and placed based on the type of endodontic procedure carried out and taking into considerations occlusal factors, length of intended time, material thickness and placement technique.

Clinical Relevance

Teeth that are undergoing root canal treatment or following completion are susceptible to microbial recontamination if adequate steps have not been taken. Temporary restorations are essential to preventing coronal leakage, both in the short and long term during and immediately following completion of treatment. During multi-visit treatments, appropriate intra-canal inter-appointment medicaments are recommended. The use of orthodontic bands and copper bands may be indicated for cracked teeth and badly broken-down teeth. Following completion of treatment, orifice barriers can be used as secondary seals overlying the three-dimensional gutta-percha root filling. Permanent restorations are recommended to ensure the long-term success of treatment.

2.1 Review of Materials Used for Temporization in Endodontics

Pulpal and peri-radicular disease develops when microorganisms and/or their by-products invade the root canal system, resulting in contamination

S. Atreya, BDS, MFDS RCS (ED)
Private Practice, Canberra, ACT, Australia

B. Patel, BDS MFDS MClinDent MRD MRACDS (✉)
Specialist Endodontist, Brindabella Specialist Centre,
Canberra, ACT, Australia
e-mail: bobbypatel@me.com

© Springer International Publishing Switzerland 2016
B. Patel (ed.), *Endodontic Treatment, Retreatment, and Surgery,*
DOI 10.1007/978-3-319-19476-9_2

27

Table 2.1 Percentage success determined by the absence of periapical pathology in relation to quality of endodontic treatment and coronal restoration [9]

Quality of the endodontic treatment	Quality of the coronal restoration	% success (absence of peri-radicular inflammation (API))
Good	Good	91.4
Good	Poor	44.1
Poor	Good	67.7
Poor	Poor	18.1

and ensuing infection [1–5]. The major aim of root canal treatment is to remove these irritants from within the root canal system and prevent future recontamination following adequate cleaning, shaping and obturating procedures which provides a three-dimensional seal against bacterial ingress [6–8].

Prevention of contamination of the root canal system by saliva, often referred to as "coronal leakage" or "coronal microleakage", is imperative to the long-term success and is highlighted by the need for providing an adequate coronal restoration following completion of endodontic therapy. Ray and Trope correlated the quality of both the root filling and the permanent coronal restoration in 1010 teeth with the periapical status assessed by radiographs. A stronger correlation was found between the presence of a periapical lesion and poor coronal restoration than poor quality of endodontic treatment. The combination of good endodontic quality (GE) and good coronal restoration (GR) had the highest absence of peri-radicular inflammation (API) at 91.4 %. These findings concluded that the technical quality of the coronal restoration was more important than the technical quality of the endodontic treatment (see Table 2.1). Poor restorations, determined radiographically by signs of overhangs, open margins or recurrent decay, had a negative impact on outcome. They suggested that leakage of bacteria and their by-products along the margins of restorations or root fillings was responsible for instigating or sustaining apical periodontitis. The interrelationship between coronal restoration and periapical health nevertheless is not clear-cut. Tronstad and colleagues evaluated the periapical status of 1001 teeth using full mouth radiographs randomly

selected from patient charts. Where the quality of the endodontic treatment was poor, then the quality of the coronal restoration had no significance. Hommez and colleagues, randomly investigating 745 root-filled teeth, found that both the quality of the coronal restoration (judged radiographically) and the length of homogeneity and the root canal fillings significantly influenced periapical status. It seems that suboptimal root canal fillings and deficient restorative treatment both have a negative impact on treatment outcome [9–14].

A retrospective study carried out over 3 years on 55 patients who had adequately root-filled teeth that had inadequate coronal restorations due to decay or that had been lost were investigated. At the end of the observation period 78 % of the teeth showed identical periapical conditions compared to the preoperative status showing no signs of apical periodontitis [15]. A further histological examination using Brown and Brenn staining of longitudinal sections of 39 root specimens in 32 extracted teeth was used to determine the role of coronal bacterial leakage and periapical health outcomes. All teeth had been lacking coronal restorations for a minimum of 3 months and in some specimens for several years. They concluded that despite prolonged exposure to the oral environment, bacterial penetration only seemed to occur in the coronal portion of roots in the majority of cases. It thus appears that well prepared and optimally sealed root canals resist bacterial penetration even after long exposures to the oral environment [16] (Fig. 2.1).

Numerous in vitro studies, using radioisotopes, dyes and microbes, have shown that exposure of coronal gutta-percha to bacterial contamination can lead to migration of bacteria and bacterial by-products to the apex in a matter of days. In 1990 Torabinjead and colleagues studied the penetration of *Staphylococcus epidermidis* and *Proteus vulgaris* on 45 single-rooted extracted teeth sealed by lateral condensation and Roth's sealer, but without coronal restorations. In 19 days, 50 % of teeth were contaminated to their full length after exposure to *S. epidermidis*. In 52 days, 50 % of teeth were contaminated to full length after exposure to *P. vulgaris*. Magura and colleagues evaluated the effect of salivary percolation in 150 single-rooted extracted teeth over a time period of

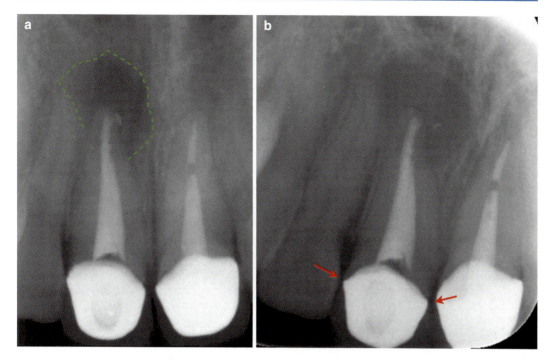

Fig. 2.1 Preoperative radiographs demonstrating root canal treatments of teeth 11 and 21. (**a**) Tooth 21 has a technically deficient root canal filling with a void in the apical 1/3rd. The coronal restoration is nevertheless deemed good with no marginal discrepancies noted. An intact periodontal ligament space is observed. Tooth 11 has a well obturated root canal with an obvious peri-radicular radiolucent lesion (*dotted green line*). (**b**) A horizontal tube shift radiograph confirms marginal discrepancies (*red arrows*) which may account for bacterial ingress and recontamination of the root canal space

3 months. The teeth were sealed by lateral condensation and Roth's sealer prior to salivary exposure. Teeth were evaluated by means of dye and histology. They concluded that retreatment should be considered in any case that has been exposed to the oral environment for over a 3-month period prior to placement of a definitive coronal restoration. In 1993 Khayat and colleagues showed that when the coronal 3 mm of root filling was removed and sealed with sticky wax, no leakage of bacteria occurred, whereas all root fillings sealed by lateral condensation and Roth's cement without a coronal orifice barrier were penetrated within 30 days. Although both in vitro and in vivo studies have questioned this correlation, taken together it seems essential to prevent coronal leakage secondary to restorative failures, both during endodontic treatment and following completion. Both temporary/interim and final definitive restorations must be placed, keeping in mind not only the capability of withstanding the physi-cal, chemical and thermal stresses within this harsh oral environment but also to provide a further barrier against the rich resident microflora that exists [17–21].

Prior to commencing endodontic therapy, it is essential to minimize potential bacterial ingress into the tooth via caries, cracks, exposed dentine and broken-down restoration margins. Complete removal of caries and defective restorations, establishment of sound supragingival tooth margins (required for optimal rubber dam placement) and restorability assessment are mandatory for all cases. Potential cracks and fracture lines should be identified using dyes or fibre optics to ensure that long-term success is both predictable and achievable. If the existing restoration, crown or onlay appears to be clinically and radiographically satisfactory and replacement is not planned, then the internal chamber and restorative material should be carefully inspected using magnification to ensure that neither caries or marginal gaps exist [22–27].

Many different temporary materials and techniques have been proposed for the restoration of teeth during endodontic therapy (see Table 2.2). Commonly used materials within endodontics include gutta-percha, glass ionomer cements (GIC), resin-modified GIC, composite resin, amalgam, reinforced interim restorative material in a zinc oxide eugenol base (IRM, Dentsply Caulk, Milford, USA) and calcium sulphate-based filling material (Cavit, 3 M ESPE, Seefeld, Germany). Cavit and IRM have withstood the rigours of testing and evaluation and can be used in combination to produce a "double seal". Alternatively GIC can be used in conjunction with Cavit as the external material of this desirable "double seal" [28–37].

Table 2.2 Various materials used for temporization in endodontics

Situation	Materials
Temporization of access cavity	Gutta-percha, zinc phosphate cement, polycarboxylate cement, zinc oxide/calcium sulphate, zinc oxide eugenol, GIC, composite resin
Broken-down teeth	Copper bands, orthodontic bands, temporary crown, pin-retained amalgam, GIC, composite resin
Nonvital walking bleach	IRM, polycarboxylate, zinc phosphate, GIC, Cavit
Long-term temporization	GIC, composite resin, amalgam cuspal coverage restorations

Prior to temporary filling placement during multi-visit endodontic treatment, an intra-canal inter-appointment medicament such as calcium hydroxide can be placed in the root canal to act as a barrier to the ingress of microorganisms. A dry cotton wool pledget can be placed to occlude the canal orifices preventing temporary filling material from displacing into the canals. The cotton wool can also act as a guide when reaccessing the tooth preventing iatrogenic errors such as inadvertent over-drilling and possible perforation, thus simplifying access for subsequent endodontic or restorative procedures. The cotton wool should also be thin enough to allow for sufficient space between the cotton wool and cavosurface margin of the access preparation permitting placement of an adequate thickness of temporary filling material. Some authors do not believe there is an indication for cotton wool pledget use with an increased inadvertent risk of fibres adhering to cavity walls and serving as a wick [28, 38, 39] (Fig. 2.2).

Stainless steel orthodontic bands have been recommended for the use of endodontically treated posterior premolar and molar teeth in conjunction with the placement of interim restorations. The main purpose of using bands is to protect the tooth from cuspal fracture (particularly in cracked teeth) and aid in strengthening and retaining the interim restoration during the endodontic phase of treatment [29, 40].

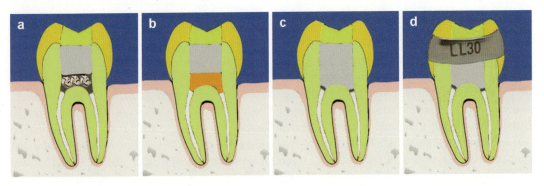

Fig. 2.2 Diagrammatic representation of various methods of interim restorations. Note (**a**) cotton wool pledgets placed over the canal orifices (dressed with medicament) to prevent dislodgment of overlying temporary restorations into the canals. The cotton wool must not have fibers adhering to the adjacent walls and externally that can result in a salivary wicking effect and recontamination. (**b**) Gutta-percha material placed over medicated canals to prevent material extrusion, (**c**) no temporary barrier used below the "double seal" restoration of IRM and glass ionomer cement, and (**d**) example of an orthodontic molar band with equal mesial and distal heights supragingi

The copper band provisional restoration is an ideal choice for ensuring adequate sealing and isolation of badly broken-down teeth. Its use can often transform a complex endodontic access preparation with minimal retentive walls into a class I cavity with adequate retention and strength for the interim temporary core [41, 42].

Following dismantling of a cuspal coverage cast restoration, the use of a well-fitting provisional restoration is desirable to prevent both tooth movement and coronal microleakage during endodontic procedures. A multitude of materials are available including direct chairside materials such as preformed crowns (made of plastic or metal), self-cured or light-cured resins or resin composites and cements. Laboratory-formed temporaries are generally made in self-cured or heat-cured acrylic or cast metal. Common self-cured or light-cured resins used either directly or indirectly include polymethyl methacrylate (e.g. Snap, Trim), bis-acryl composite (e.g. Protemp) and restorative composite. Bis-acryl composites produce less heat and shrinkage during polymerization than other resins, resulting in better marginal fit. Proprietary temporary cement materials are used to retain the provisional restoration in place and allow for easy removal if required (e.g. Tempbond) [43, 44].

When a custom-made post and core restoration is planned, a temporary post crown restoration may be required. Due to the inadvertent risk of further bacterial contamination of the root canal space, the temporary post and core restoration should be left in place for as short a time as possible. The use of prefabricated post and core systems immediately after completion of endodontic treatment has the advantage of minimizing microleakage and recontamination. An alternative method to reduce the possibility of coronal seal disturbance would be the use of a full coverage vacuum-formed retainer to replace the missing coronal tooth structure. These types of removable prosthodontics options have been used for temporization in the aesthetic zone after implant fixture placement [45–47].

Temporization for internal bleaching (walk-in bleach technique) requires the use of both a protective barrier overlying the orthograde gutta-percha material and suitable temporary restorative materials to be placed over the bleaching agent in between bleaching appointments. Polycarboxylate, zinc phosphate, glass ionomer, IRM or Cavit of at least 2 mm thickness are recommended for the purpose of barrier protection. Cavit and Coltosol with sufficient bulk can be used as interim restorations during the bleaching procedures (see Chap. 18).

After completion of endodontic treatment gutta-percha can be cut back to within the canal orifices, and an intra-orifice barrier can be placed to protect it. The uses of intra-orifice barriers, which are restorative materials placed over the canal orifices and covering the pulp chamber floor, have been advocated to provide a secondary seal. Criteria have been proposed for the ideal intra-orifice barrier. They should: (a) be easily placed and bond to tooth structure (retentiveness), (b) seal effectively against coronal microleakage, (c) be easily distinguished from the natural tooth colour and (d) not interfere with the final restoration of the access preparation. This material can be any material that will bond or seal the dentine and have a distinguishable colour from dentine. Common orifice barriers include Tetric Chroma (Vivadent), Permaflow Purple (Ultradent), Flow-it clear (Pentron) or resin-modified glass ionomer material [48, 49].

No current restorative material can claim to prevent microleakage completely. Interim temporary restorations serve to reduce contamination of the root canal system until permanent restorations have been placed. Due consideration when selecting a temporary material should be given based on the amount of remaining tooth structure, occlusal forces likely to be placed and length of intended time prior to three-dimensional obturation and permanent restoration procedures. Adequate thickness of material and accurate placement are crucial in minimizing recontamination. Clinicians should consider all factors and ensure that optimal temporary/interim restorations are placed to ensure optimal clinical outcomes.

2.2   Specific Materials for Temporization

Cavit

Cavit is a premixed temporary filling material that contains zinc oxide, calcium sulphate, zinc sulphate, glycol acetate, polyvinyl acetate resins, polyvinyl chloride acetate, triethanolamine and pigments. It is a hygroscopic material, and its ability to attract and hold water molecules results in a high coefficient of linear expansion with excellent marginal sealing ability. At least 3–4 mm of thickness is required to ensure optimal sealing ability. The material is ideal when used in conjunction with glass ionomer cement as a "double seal" restoration during root canal treatment and following completion prior to permanent restoration.

Coltosol

Coltosol is a zinc oxide, zinc sulphate and calcium sulphate hemihydrate-based material that hardens within 20–30 min when in contact with moisture. According to the manufacturer, the temporary filling can be subjected to masticatory forces within 2–3 h of placement. This material is recommended for short-term temporization not exceeding 2 weeks.

Zinc oxide eugenol

Zinc oxide eugenol is a widely used temporary restorative material consisting of powder (zinc oxide, pulverized glass or silica) and liquid (zinc chloride and borax). Reinforced zinc oxide eugenol preparations (Kalzinol) using a polystyrene polymer results in doubling of the compressive strength important in areas subjected to mechanical loading. Reinforced zinc oxide eugenol preparations (IRM) using polymethyl methacrylate provide improved compressive strength and hardness. During inter-appointment temporization, the use of a low powder to liquid ratio of zinc oxide eugenol preparations including IRM can provide adequate resistance to microbial penetration. A double seal technique using glass ionomer cement to overlay an adequate thickness of IRM will be effective in maintaining a good marginal seal.

Glass ionomer cement

Conventional glass ionomer cements contain a fluoroaluminosilicate ion leachable glass and a water-soluble polymer acid, which reacts to form cement. Current materials may contain a poly(alkenoic acid), which contains a copolymer of acrylic acid with itaconic or maleic acid. The polymer is often supplied as a dry powder blended with the glass. The powder is either hand mixed with water or supplied as capsules for mechanical mixing. Tartaric acid is often added to provide a clinically acceptable setting time. On mixing an acid-base reaction between the aqueous poly(alkenoic acid) and glass occurs. The outer layers of the glass particles decompose, releasing calcium and aluminium ions. These ions migrate into the aqueous phase forming cross-linked polyalkenoate chains, resulting in gelation and setting of the material. The set cement consists of a core of unreacted glass particles surrounded by a salt-like hydrogel bound by the matrix of reaction products. Glass ionomer cements can chemically bond to tooth structure, further reducing any marginal discrepancies between restorative and tooth interface. In endodontics they are ideal temporary restorations but need to be replaced over the long term due to low tensile strengths making them unsuitable in load-bearing areas of the mouth.

Composite resin restorations

Composite restorations consist of four main components, namely, the resin (organic polymer matrix), filler particles (inorganic), coupling agent (silane) and the initiator-accelerator of polymerization. The most common resin monomers used in composite restorations is BisGMA. To accommodate better filler load, triethylene glycol dimethacrylate (TEGDMA) or urethane dimethacrylate (UDMA) is added. Filler particles provide dimensional stability for the soft resin matrix and vary in size. Common filler particles include crystalline quartz, silica and glasses such as barium and strontium silicate. The size of the filler particles incorporated in the resin matrix has evolved over the years. Filler particles determine the mechanical properties of the composite material including wear, translucency, opalescence, radiopacity, surface roughness and polishability. Filler particle sizes can be classified into microhybrid, microfill or nanofiller. Microhybrid filler particles consist of glass or quartz particles ranging in sizes of 0.2–3 and 0.04 μm microfine particles. Microfill particles sizes range from 0.02 to 0.04 μm and nanohybrids are 0.01–0.04 μm. The coupling agent silane helps form a bond between the resin matrix and filler particles during the polymerization setting reaction. Initiators and accelerators are added for either chemical (aromatic tertiary amines) or photo-activated light curing (camphorquinones).

Enamel consists of 96 % inorganic hydroxyapatite prisms, 1 % organic material and 3 % water. In 1971 Buonocore showed that it was possible to bond resin to enamel after etching with 20–50 % phosphoric acid. Dentine consists of approximately 70 % inorganic hydroxyapatite, 20 % organic material (mainly collagen) and 10 % water. Dentine also consists of dentinal tubules that contain water making the hydrophobic resin difficult to penetrate. In addition the cut surface of dentine is covered by a smear layer composed of deranged dentine and bacteria, further reducing the potential adherency of resin to the underlying dentine. In 1982 Nakabayashi treated the dentine surface with an acidic primer, resulting in a demineralized dentine surface of approximately 10 μ prior to application of the bonding resin 4-META (4-methacryloyloxyethyl trimellitate). This resulted in micromechanical interlocking of the resin by collagen mesh, termed the hybrid layer.

Numerous bonding systems have evolved, broadly classified into either resin-based systems with an etch and rinse approach or self-etch adhesive systems. The fourth-generation bonding systems (Scotchbond 1, 3 M, ESPE, St Paul, MN, USA, or Optibond, Kerr, Orange, CA, USA) allowed for the removal of the smear layer using 30–40 % phosphoric acid involving several steps of etching, washing with water, drying, application of a primer or adhesion-promoting agent and finally applying a dentine-bonding agent. The fifth-generation dentine-bonding agents aimed at reducing/simplifying the number of steps by combining the primer and bonding agent in one bottle. The sixth-generation self-etch adhesive systems were introduced that differ from the previous etch and rinse systems by the use of an acidified resin which is not washed off like the previous phosphoric acid in the etch and rinse systems. Two types of dentine-bonding agent systems are available. A two-step application of self-etching primer followed by bonding agent application (Prime&Bond NT, Dentsply, Wybridge, UK) and one-step application where the etching and bonding components are mixed, prior to their application as one solution (One-up Bond F, Tokuyama, Tokyo, Japan). The sixth-generation one- and two-step adhesives dissolve the smear layer, and their components become incorporated into the hybrid layer in contrast to previous generations where the smear layer was removed by washing following application of phosphoric acid.

Resin-modified glass ionomer cements

These materials have two setting mechanisms: a glass ionomer acid–base reaction and a resin light-activated polymerization reaction. The resin-modified glass ionomer cement shows better aesthetic results and is less technique sensitive and soluble compared to conventional glass ionomer cements as a result of the resin content.

Amalgam

Dental amalgam has stood the test of time and has been successfully employed as a direct posterior restorative filling materials for over a century. Despite its popularity amongst general dental practitioners, including ease of manipulation, cost-effectiveness, strength, durability and long-term clinical performance, the issue of mercury toxicity remains a concern. The development of high-copper amalgams (whereby 30 % of the silver was replaced by copper) has resulted in improved corrosion and creep resistance and reduced ditching attributed to the tin-mercury (Y2 phase) formed in the set amalgam. Dental amalgam alloys contains silver (40–70 %), tin (12–30 %), copper (12–30 %) and trace elements including indium (up to 4 %), palladium (0.5 %) and zinc (up to 1 %). The inclusion of zinc has been reported to delay the expansion of amalgam on setting. The major disadvantage of dental amalgam has been its inability to adhere to tooth structure. Mechanical retention by means of slots, grooves and pins has been recommended and alternative bonded amalgam techniques to ensure preservation of tooth structure. The use of amalgam as an interim restoration in endodontics has been advocated, utilizing the coronal pulp chamber for added retention (Nayyar cores) and provisional cuspal coverage restorations where the long-term prognosis is questionable.

2.3　Orthodontic Bands

The cementation of orthodontic stainless steel bands around cracked teeth to prevent catastrophic fracture and aid in the endodontic diagnosis remains a widely accepted management technique. Bands can also be useful when used in conjunction with interim temporary restorations in large cavities that are missing cusps or where cusps are susceptible to fracture during the course of endodontic treatment (Fig. 2.3).

Before banding, space is created interproximally to allow for band fitting and cementation. This can be achieved by either placement of elastomeric separators mesially and distally or the use of a bur to remove tooth/restorative material interproximally. Care must be taken when using the latter approach to avoid damage to the adjacent tooth.

Separators are placed with the help of an instrument that spreads the elastomeric module to allow threading the separator between the contacts of neighbouring teeth (using a separator plier). Dental floss can also be used to pass the separator under the interproximal contact and then popping one side up through the contact. Separators usually need to be in place for 4–7 days to achieve adequate space.

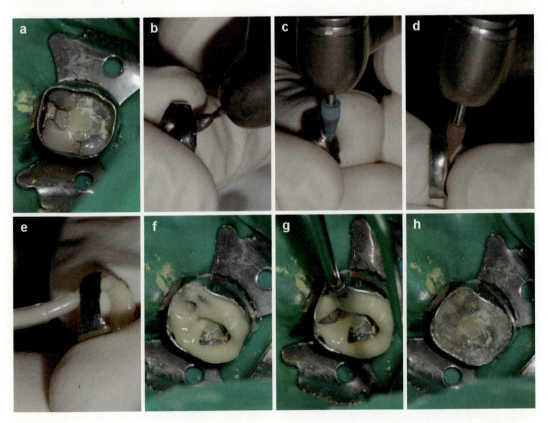

Fig. 2.3 Clinical photographs demonstrating stainless steel orthodontic band placement on a mandibular second molar tooth. Note (**a**) the band is seated with finger pressure to check correct size. The band is seated in the same amount (1–2 mm) below the marginal ridge heights of mesial and distal contact. (**b**–**d**) Band adjustment is carried out and trimmed to ensure there is no occlusal interference and then polished accordingly. (**e**) Placement of glass ionomer cement around the band prior to seating. (**f**) Band cementation, (**g**) seating, and (**h**) trimming of excess material

The clinical steps associated with orthodontic band placement are as follows:

1. Separation of interproximal contacts is achieved by use of either band separators or use of the thinnest diamond tapered bur or disc.
2. A preliminary molar/premolar band size is selected and checked in the mouth. The band is passively seated on the tooth ensuring the contacts are free and adequate separation has been achieved.
3. A correct band size selected should passively go over all cusps but should not seat down completely with just finger pressure. Once the correct size has been determined, the band is initially seated using a band pusher using a mesial and distal rocking motion. A bite stick can be used to facilitate the completion of the seating process with the patient biting on facial and lingual aspects of the band.
4. Often there may be a need to adjust the occlusal edge of the band to avoid occlusal interference, and this should be done during the trial seating stage. The adjusted band edges should be polished and trimmed to ensure comfort for the patient.
5. Once trial seating is completed and band adjustment completed, the band can be cemented in place using the same technique. Glass ionomer cement can be placed on the internal aspects of the band for cementation purposes. Excess cement is removed.
6. A final check should be made to ensure that the band is correctly seated without any gingival impingement and occlusal interference is absent.
7. The band can easily be removed prior to final definitive restoration by cutting the band on either facial or lingual aspects using a diamond bur. Residual cement can be easily removed using an ultrasonic scaler.

2.4 Copper Bands

Severely broken-down teeth may require the use of a copper band to aid retention of temporary restorative materials and ensure adequate sealing during endodontic procedures. With care and skill, a copper band can be adapted, secured and customized to fit the tooth tightly ensuring a good interim restoration is in place prior to completion of endodontic treatment and definitive restorative treatment. The step-by-step procedure for placement of a copper band is as follows:

1. The restoration is removed and the tooth is made caries-free. Restorability is assessed ensuring sufficient biological width and ferrule is available.
2. A polishing strip is used to ensure that interproximal contacts are relieved. A copper band is selected that is slightly smaller than the circumference of the middle one third of the clinical crown and is pushed down onto the tooth. A pencil can be used to mark the free gingival margin and occlusal surface (Fig. 2.4).
3. The band is removed, and crown scissors are used to trim the marked gingival margin on the band to ensure the band contacts when seated. Next the occlusal surface is trimmed to ensure that no occlusal interference is present on both lateral and protrusive excursions.
4. Occlusal and gingival margins of the band that have been adjusted are smoothed and polished using a brown and green stone.
5. Prior to final cementation, the band is reseated and checked for fit. Zinc phosphate cement or glass ionomer restorative material is manipulated according to manufacturers' instructions and placed around the band. The band is seated into position and excess material removed accordingly.

2.5 Clinical Cases

Case 1 Endodontic management of tooth 15 requiring a cast cuspal coverage restoration

A fit and healthy patient was referred for cracked tooth syndrome associated with tooth 15. The patient had recently sustained a fall, resulting in an avulsion injury of tooth 44. The patient had been experiencing sharp pain on biting and

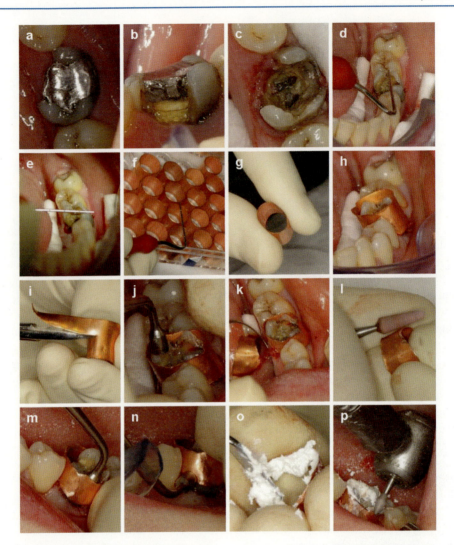

Fig. 2.4 Clinical photographs demonstrating placement of a copper band on a mandibular lower left molar tooth. Note (**a, b**) preoperative views of an extensive amalgam restoration that has fractured on the mesio-lingual aspect. (**c**) Restorability assessment is carried out following complete dismantling of the existing restoration. (**d, e**) Measurement of mesiodistal and bucco-lingual dimensions of the tooth enabling (**f, g**) appropriate band selection. (**h**) Initial try-in of the copper band. (**i**) Trimming of the band and (**j**) further try-in to check occlusal and (**k**) gingival marginal fit. (**l**) Band adjustment and final trimming prior to final (**m, n**) rechecking final fit. (**o**) Cementation of band using zinc phosphate cement and (**p**) final adjustments following band cementation

tenderness to percussion with tooth 15. Pulpal tests revealed negative responses to both electric pulp testing and thermal stimulus. Radiographic assessment revealed an unrestored tooth with no obvious periapical changes. A provisional diagnosis of acute apical periodontitis was made and endodontic treatment commenced. Following access preparation and inspection for any internal crack lines, a decision was made to place a stainless steel orthodontic band to prevent catastrophic cusp fracture.

Following pulp canal preparation and intracanal calcium hydroxide dressing placement, a temporary restoration of cotton wool, IRM and glass ionomer cement was placed. Obturation was carried out 4 weeks later. A warm vertical compaction technique was used using guttapercha and AH plus cement. The coronal guttapercha was cut back to allow for placement of a secondary orifice barrier (Permaflow). A double seal restoration of IRM and glass ionomer was placed as an interim restoration prior to definitive

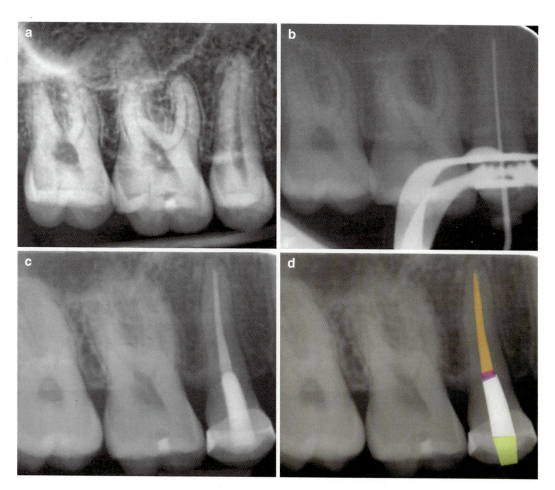

Fig. 2.5 Clinical radiographs of endodontic treatment of tooth 15 diagnosed as acute apical periodontitis with suspected crack tooth syndrome. An orthodontic band was placed to protect the cusps. Note (**a**) preoperative radiograph demonstrating unrestored tooth 15, (**b**) MAF prepa-ration, and (**c**) postoperative radiograph. (**d**) Completed endodontic seal from apex to coronal end consisting of gutta-percha root filling (*orange*), secondary orifice seal barrier (*purple*), IRM restoration (*white*), and glass iono-mer cement (*yellow*)

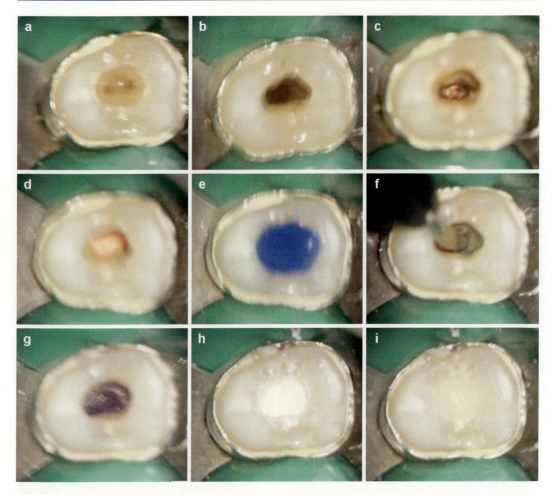

Fig. 2.6 Clinical photographs demonstrating temporization of tooth 15 following completion of obturation at second appointment. Note (**a**) final rinsing of canal space using 1 % NaOCl solution and 17 % EDTA. An intracanal medicament of calcium hydroxide was placed for four weeks, and the cusps were protected with an orthodontic band. (**b**) Final drying of canal prior to obturation; (**c**) apical plug of gutta-percha following down pack using System B; (**d**) backfill completed using Obtura; (**e**) phosphoric acid etch treatment; (**f**) placement of orifice barrier following wash, drying, and dentine bonding agent placement; (**g**) completed orifice barrier (PermaFLOW); (**h**) 4 mm IRM base; and (**i**) overlying glass ionomer cement restoration completed

cast restoration with the general dental practitioner (see Figs. 2.5 and 2.6).

Case 2 Endodontic management of tooth 15 requiring a cast post and core restoration

A fit and healthy patient was referred for endodontic treatment of tooth 15. The patient had presented to his general dental practitioner with a fractured tooth. Restorability assessment was carried out, and the dentist was planning to restore the tooth with a cast post and core restoration following completion of endodontic treatment. Access preparation revealed a necrotic canal system with an apical curvature. Chemomechanical preparation was completed using a combination of hand stainless files and rotary files using 1 % sodium hypochlorite solution. An interim dressing of calcium hydroxide was placed for a 4-week period. The tooth was temporized with IRM and glass ionomer cement. At the obturation appointment, the tooth was asymptomatic. A warm vertical compaction technique was used using gutta-percha and AH plus cement. The gutta-percha was cut back leaving 7 mm of gutta-percha. The remaining post space was dressed with calcium hydroxide. A temporary coronal restoration of IRM and glass iono-

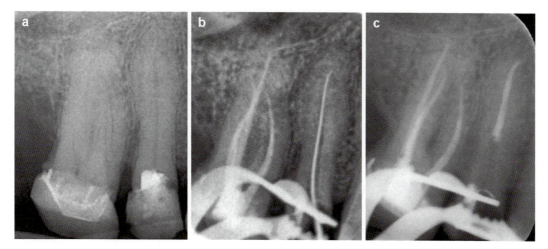

Fig. 2.7 (**a**) Preoperative radiograph demonstrating temporized tooth. Remaining tooth structure was assessed confirming the need for a post-retained restoration to support the overlying core and cast restoration. (**b**) Chemomechanical preparation completed using a combination of hand and rotary files. Apical patency was maintained and the acute apical curvature negotiated with a # 15 stainless steel hand file. (**c**) Obturation was completed following an interim period of 4 weeks. An intra-canal dressing of calcium hydroxide had been placed. A warm vertical compaction technique using AH Plus cement and gutta-percha was used. 7 mm of gutta-percha was left to maintain the apical seal. The remainder of the root canal was left for post space preparation

Fig. 2.8 (**a, b**) Post-operative radiographs demonstrating completed endodontic treatment. Note gutta-percha root filling (*orange*), post space dressed with calcium hydroxide (*blue*) and double temporary seal overlying root canal orifice using IRM (*red*) and glass ionomer cement (*yellow*)

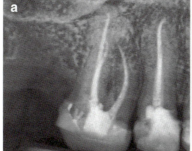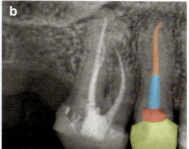

mer was placed and the patient discharged back to his general dental practitioner for permanent restoration of the tooth (Figs. 2.7 and 2.8).

> **Clinical Hints and Tips in Regard to Temporary Restorations During Endodontic Procedures**
> - **Pretreatment procedures to minimize bacterial ingress**
>   Complete removal of caries and defective restorations and placement of a temporary restorative material desirable

- **Orthodontic band placement**
  The use of bands in endodontically treated premolar and molar teeth may be desirable to protect the tooth from cuspal fracture (particularly in cracked teeth) and strengthening/retaining the interim restoration during the endodontic phase of treatment.
- **Copper band placement**
  In badly broken-down teeth, the use of a copper band is an ideal choice to ensure adequate sealing and isolation and providing additional

strength and retention of the interim temporary core.

- **Interim temporary endodontic restorations**
The use of a "double seal" restoration such as IRM and glass ionomer cement in the access cavity will prevent microleakage.
- **Temporary post and core restorations**
The use of prefabricated post and core systems can be fabricated chairside to minimize bacterial ingress into the root canal system. Alternative vacuum-formed retainers can be made but these will incur additional laboratory fees.
- **Temporization for internal bleaching procedures**
Following completion of endodontic treatment gutta-percha should be cut back below the cement-enamel junction. A protective barrier of at least 2 mm of IRM should be placed above the gutta-percha root filling to minimize diffusion of bleaching products and risk of external cervical root resorption. Following bleach placement IRM or Cavit can be used as an interim restoration to prevent washing out of bleaching product into the oral cavity

References

1. Kakehashi S, Stanley H, Fitzgerald R. The effects of surgical exposures of dental pulps in germ-free and conventional laboratory rats. Oral Surg Oral Med Oral Pathol. 1965;20:340–9.
2. Moller A. Microbiological examination of root canals and periapical tissues of human teeth. Methodological studies. Odont Tidskr. 1966;74(Suppl):1–380.
3. Sundqvist G. Bacteriological studies of necrotic dental pulps. Umea University Odontological Dissertations No. 7. Umea: Umea University, Sweden; 1976.
4. Möller A, Fabricius L, Dahlen G, Ohman A, Heyden G. Influence on periapical tissues of indigenous bacteria and necrotic pulp tissue in monkeys. Scand J Dent Res. 1981;89:475–84.
5. Fabricius L, Dahlen G, Holm S, Möller A. Influence of combinations of oral bacteria on periapical tissues of monkeys. Scand J Dent Res. 1982;90:200–6.
6. Sjrogren U, Hagglund B, Sundqvist G, Wing K. Factors affecting the long term results of endodontic treatment. J Endod. 1990;16:498–504.
7. Sjrogren U, Figdor D, Persson S, Sundqvist G. Influence of infection at the time of root filling on the outcome of endodontic treatment of teeth with apical periodontitis. Int Endod J. 1997;30:297–306.
8. Nair PNR. On the causes of persistent apical periodontitis: a review. Int Endod J. 2006;39:249–81.
9. Ray HA, Trope M. Periapical status of endodontically treated teeth in relation to the technical quality of the root filling and coronal restoration. Int Endod J. 1995;28:12–8.
10. Tronstad L, Asbjornsen K, Doving L, Pedersen I, Eriksen HM. Influence of coronal restorations on the periapical health of endodontically treated teeth. Endod Dent Traumatol. 2000;16:218–21.
11. Hommez GM, Coppens CR, De Moor RJ. Periapical health related to the quality of coronal restorations and root fillings. Int Endod J. 2002;35:680–9.
12. Chong BS. Coronal leakage and treatment failure. J Endod. 1995;21:159–60.
13. Bishop K, Briggs P. Endodontic failure – a problem from top to bottom. Br Dent J. 1995;179:35–6.
14. Saunders WP, Saunders EM. The root filling and restoration continuum. Prevention of long-term endodontic failures. Alpha Omegan. 1997;90:40–6.
15. Ricucci D, Grondahl K, Bergenholtz G. Periapical status of root-filled teeth exposed to the oral environment by loss of restoration or caries. Oral Surg Oral Med Oral Pathol Oral Radiol Endod. 2000;90:345–9.
16. Ricucci D, Bergenholtz G. Bacterial status in root-filled teeth exposed to the oral environment by loss of restoration and fracture and caries. A histobacteriological study of treated cases. Int Endod J. 2003;36:787–802.
17. Torabinejad M, Ung B, Kettering JD. In vitro bacterial penetration of coronally unsealed endodontically treated teeth. J Endod. 1990;16:566–9.
18. Magura ME, Kafrawy AH, Brown Jr CE, Newton CW. Human saliva coronal microleakage in obturated root canals: an in vitro study. J Endod. 1991;17:324–31.
19. Khayat A, Lee SJ, Torabinejad M. Human saliva penetration of coronally unsealed obturated root canals. J Endod. 1993;19(9):458–61.
20. Swanson K, Madison S. An evaluation of coronal microleakage in endodontically treated teeth. Part I. Time periods. J Endod. 1987;13(2):56–9.
21. Madison S, Wilcox LR. An evaluation of coronal microleakage in endodontically treated teeth. Part 3. In vivo study. J Endod. 1988;14:455–8.
22. Lovedahl PE, Gutmann JL. Periodontal and restorative considerations before endodontic therapy. J Acad Gen Dent. 1980;28:38–45.
23. Roulet J. Marginal integrity: clinical significance. J Dent. 1994;22(Suppl):S9–12.
24. Lynch CD, McConnell RJ. The cracked tooth syndrome. J Canad Dent Assoc. 2002;68(8):470–5.
25. Bishop K, Kelleher M, Briggs P, Joshi R. Wear now? An update on the etiology of tooth wear. Quintess Int. 1997;28(5):305–13.
26. Abbott P. Assessing restored teeth with pulp and periapical diseases for the presence of cracks, caries and marginal breakdown. Aust Dent J. 2004;49:33–9.
27. Smith C, Schuman N. Restoration of endodontically treated teeth: a guide for the restorative dentist. Quintess Int. 1997;28:457–62.

28. Naoum HJ, Chandler NP. Temporization for endodontics. Int Endod J. 2002;35:964–78.
29. Jensen AL, Abbott PV, Salgado CJ. Interim and temporary restorations of teeth during endodontic treatment. Aust Dent J Suppl. 2007;52:S83–99.
30. Galvan Jr RR, West LA, Liewehr FR, Pashley DH. Coronal microleakage of five materials used to create an intracoronal seal in endodontically treated teeth. J Endod. 2002;28(2):59–61.
31. Vail MM, Steffel CL. Preference of temporary restorations and spacers: a survey of diplomates of the American Board of Endodontists. J Endod. 2006; 32(6):513–5.
32. Buonocore MG. Caries prevention in pits and fissures sealed with an adhesive resin polymerized by ultraviolet light: a two-year study of a single adhesive application. J Am Dent Assoc. 1971;82(5):1090–3.
33. Nakabayashi N, Kojima K, Masuhara E. The promotion of adhesion by the infiltration of monomers into tooth substrates. J Biomed Mater Res. 1982;16:265–73.
34. Nakabayashi N, Nakamura M, Yasuda N. Hybrid layer as a dentine bonding mechanism. J Eesthet Dent. 1991;3(4):133–8.
35. Burke FT. What's new in dentine bonding? Self etch adhesives. Dent Update. 2004;31:580–9.
36. Mitchell RJ, Koike M, Okabe T. Posterior amalgam restorations – usage, regulation and longevity. Dent Clin North Am. 2007;51(3):573–89.
37. Ngo H. Glass ionomer cements as restorative and preventive materials. Dent Clin North Am. 2010;54(3): 551–63.
38. Messer HH, Wilson PR. Preparation for restoration and temporization. In: Principles and practice of endodontics. 2nd ed. Philadelphia: W.B Saunders & Co; 1996. p. 260–76.
39. Siqueira JF. Aetiology of root canal treatment failure: why well-treated teeth can fail. Int Endod J. 2001; 34(1):1–10.
40. Ehrmann EH. The use of stainless steel bands in posterior endodontics. Aust Dent J. 1968;13:418–21.
41. Linden R. Using a copper band to isolate severely broken down teeth before endodontic procedures. J Am Dent Assoc. 1999;130:1095.
42. Lai YY, Yu DC, Chen CP. Application of copper band in complex endodontic access preparations. J Dent Sci. 2006;1:44–6.
43. Burke FJT, Murray MC, Shortall ACC. Trends in indirect dentistry: 6. Provisional restorations, more than just a temporary. Dent Update. 2005;32:443–52.
44. Perry RD, Magnuson B. Provisional materials: key components of interim fixed restorations. Compend Contin Educ Dent. 2012;33(1):59–62.
45. Fox K, Gutteridge DL. An in-vitro study of coronal micro-leakage in root canal-treated teeth restored by the post and core technique. Int Endod J. 1997; 30:361–8.
46. Demarchi MG, Sato EF. Leakage of interim post and cores used during laboratory fabrication of custom posts. J Endod. 2002;28(4):328–9.
47. Ray-Chaudhuri A, Mirza Z, Searson L. Technique tips – options for temporization in the aesthetic zone after implant fixture placement. Dent Update. 2014;41:377.
48. Wolcott JF, Hicks M, Himel VT. Evaluation of pigmented intra-orifice barriers in endodontically treated teeth. J Endod. 1999;25:589–92.
49. Chailertvanitkul P, Saunder WP, Saunders EM, MacKenzie D. An evaluation of microbial coronal leakage in the restored pulp chamber of root canal treated multi-rooted teeth. Int Endod J. 1997;30:318–22.

Cleaning and Shaping Objectives

3

Bobby Patel

Summary

Canal preparation is an integral and important stage during root canal treatment. Access to the root canal system from a crown-down approach must be achieved ensuring the canal terminus is negotiated. Preparation of the root canal system is then further enlarged and shaped to enhance both disinfection and final obturation of the complex root canal space.

Clinical Relevance

Correct shaping procedures with maintenance of original anatomy (with reference to the apical constriction) without iatrogenic deviation (canal transportation) facilitate optimal and effective irrigant deposition and predictable placement of intra-canal medicament and facilitate permanent root fillings without risk of overfilling. Clinicians should be aware of the controversies surrounding the concept of cleaning and shaping canals including the terminal end point of preparation, master apical file size, patency filing and methods of preparation used (stainless steel or nickel-titanium rotary).

3.1 Overview of Cleaning and Shaping Objectives

Root canal preparation is recognized as one of the most important stages in root canal treatment [1]. In primary root canal treatment, it includes the removal of vital and necrotic tissues and infected dentine. In root canal retreatment (revision), it may also include the removal of additional metallic and non-metallic canal materials and/or obstructions including a variety of root canal filling materials.

The root canal system may be mechanically prepared to a debatable size and taper that facilitates both disinfection and obturation procedures using a plethora of instruments of various metallurgy, cutting designs, tips and tapers. A number of manual root canal preparation techniques have evolved over time including the standardized technique [2], step-back technique [3], circumferential filing [4], anticurvature filing [5], step-down technique [6], double flare technique [7], crown-down pressureless technique, balanced

B. Patel, BDS MFDS MClinDent MRD MRACDS
Specialist Endodontist, Brindabella Specialist Centre,
Canberra, ACT, Australia
e-mail: bobbypatel@me.com

force technique [8] and the modified double flare technique [9]. Step-back and step-down techniques are the two major approaches to cleaning and shaping procedures. The former commences apical preparation at the apex with small instruments that are progressively increased in size to enlarge the apical preparation diameter followed by sequential canal preparation coronally in a step-back manner of 0.5 or 1 mm increments depending on the desired taper. The step-down technique commences preparation using larger instruments from the coronal end towards the apex with progressively smaller instruments. The advantages of the latter include a reduction in necrotic extruded debris, minimal root canal straightening, less canal transportation and quick and efficient canal shaping and allow for better penetration of irrigant [6].

Most root canals are curved in multiple positions and planes, and the ability of endodontic instruments to shape the canal without deviation from the original canal position is dependent on the anatomical position, radius and degree of these curvatures. Any deviation from this original canal position is termed canal transportation. To minimize canal deviation in curved canals, Roane and Sabala described the balanced force technique associated with specially designed stainless steel or NiTi K-type instruments (Flex-R files) with modified tips used in a step-down manner [8].

Complications such as blockages, ledge formation, zip-and-elbow formation, strip perforations or excessive thinning of canal walls are possible results of canal transportation that can reduce overall success of treatment. The impact of canal transportation is the end result of the inability to adequately clean the canal with the possibility of persistent apical pathosis or excessive thinning of canal walls leading to eventual vertical root fracture [10].

Over the years, a number of different NiTi instrument systems have been designed and introduced on the market. The two main characteristics of this alloy are memory shape and superior elasticity making it possible to engineer file designs of greater taper than traditional 2 % stainless steel files. Manufacturing processes and design features such as cutting angle, number of blades, tip design (active or passive), cross section and taper will all influence the instruments individual flexibility, cutting efficiency and torsional resistance (see Chap. 4) [11]. Inherent in the material used, stainless steel files have a high rigidity that increases with increasing instrument size. In curved canals, this stiffness is responsible for straightening and resulting transportation and canal aberrations (ledging, zipping and perforations) [12–14]. Consequently, a size #15 nitinol hand file has been shown to have 2–3 times more elastic flexibility in bending and torsion, as well as superior resistance to torsional fracture when compared to a #15 stainless steel file manufactured by the same process [15, 16].

Several studies investigating the effects of root canal preparation when using NiTi systems have been carried out. Methods of investigation include the Cardiff experimental design using simulated root canals pre-curved with silver points of either curvature 20° or 40° with location of curvature at either 8 or 12 mm from the orifice [17–26]. The Zürich experimental design group used high-resolution micro-CT (μCT) to measure change in canal volume and surface area as well as pre- and post-preparation root canal anatomy differences using maxillary molars embedded into resin and mounted on SEM stubs to aid reproducible positioning into the μCT [27–30]. The Göttingen experimental design group investigated several endodontic handpieces and NiTi systems using a modified version of Bramante's muffle model [31–33]. The Münster experimental design group investigated several rotary NiTi systems using two types of plastic blocks with different degrees of curvature (28° and 35°) for the evaluation of straightening and working safety as well as extracted teeth with severely curved root canals (25°–35°) for the evaluation of working safety, working time and canal cleanliness following preparation [34, 35]. Taken together, these studies confirmed that although there were differences between the brands in that some do not proceed as others when comparing canal straightening, working time, blockages and file fractures, overall most

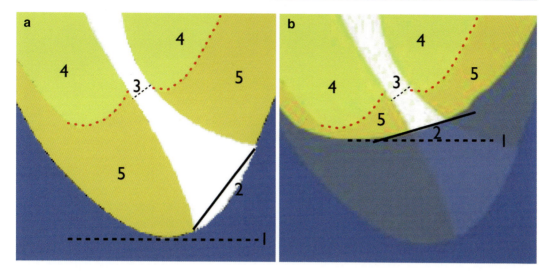

Fig. 3.1 Diagrammatic representation of the apical anatomy in a tooth (**a**) without apical root resorption and (**b**) a tooth with apical root resorption. Note (*1*) radiographic apex (*dash line*) as judged on a radiograph, (*2*) major diameter or apical foramen (AF) (*solid line*), (*3*) minor diameter or apical constriction (AC) (*green dash line*), (*4*) dentine, and (*5*) cementum. The *red dotted line* is the CDJ

systems differed only slightly and were highly constant. The use of NiTi instruments resulted in less straightening and better-centred preparations of curved root canals. With μCT, it has been shown that the amount of mechanically prepared root surface and perhaps equally distributed biofilm in the main root canal, depending on canal type, is frequently below 60 % of the canal surface [27, 28]. This means that the use of stainless steel or NiTi instruments alone does not result in complete cleanliness of the root canal walls. Cleanliness decreases from the coronal to apical portion of the root canal. The use of a special motor with constant speed, low torque and torque control is recommended.

The determination of an accurate working length (WL) is one of the most pivotal steps in achieving successful endodontic treatment. WL is defined as "the length between a coronal reference point and the apical limit of preparation" [36]. An erroneous WL, either long or short, can lead to long-term failure and outcome for any case. A short WL can lead to uncleaned and unfilled canal space that may contain microorganisms and their by-products that can sustain endodontic pathosis. Likewise over-instrumentation and overfilling as a consequence of too long a WL

can lead to postoperative discomfort and possible foreign body reaction and persistent inflammation following completion of a case. The apical extent of root canal instrumentation has been a long-standing debate with much disagreement in the endodontic field.

Anatomically, the apical region of a tooth has been classically described in terms of the apical constriction (AC), the cement-dentinal junction (CDJ) and the apical foramen (AF) (Fig. 3.1). Kuttler showed that the root canal tapers from the canal orifice to the AC, which is generally 0.5–1.5 mm inside the AF. The AF is defined as the region where the canal leaves the root surface next to the periodontal ligament [37]. The AC is the narrowest part of the root canal with the smallest diameter of blood supply and is the reference point most dentists' use when terminating cleaning, shaping and obturation procedures [38]. Termination of root canal preparation and obturation at the AC has been shown to give the best prognosis for success [39, 40]. Sjögren and colleagues demonstrated that obturation ending 0–2 mm short of the radiographic apex rendered significantly improved long-term results in teeth affected with apical periodontitis compared to overextended obturations (success

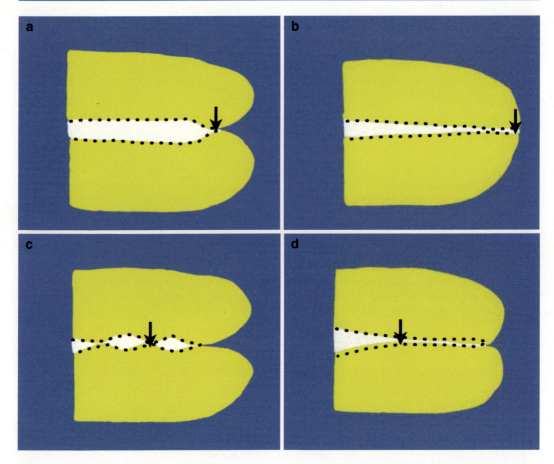

Fig. 3.2 Diagrammatic representation of classification of apical constriction. *Arrow* indicated narrowest portion of canal and point of measurement. Note (**a**) type A traditional single constriction, (**b**) type B tapering constriction, (**c**) type C multi-constriction, and (**d**) type D parallel constriction (Adapted from Dummer et al. [42])

rates of 94 % compared to 74 %, respectively) [41]. Dummer and colleagues further classified the AC into four distinct types (Fig. 3.2) [42]. Traditional teachings of determining WL to be 1–2 mm short of the anatomic apex as seen on the radiograph could lead to under-preparation (type B) or over-preparation (type D).

Traditional methods for determining WL have been the use of tactile sensation [43], the observation of bleeding points or moisture using a paper point technique [44, 45] and radiographic length determination [46].

The paper point technique used conventional absorbent paper points to determine WL. The technique is used as a method to determine final working length prior to obturation. It can only be used after initial shaping of the canal has been completed and where the patent canal is dry. WL is determined by the tip of the paper point and by the presence of either blood or tissue fluid indicating insertion beyond the foramen. Repeated points are used to determine the wet/dry points within the canal before final refinement of canal preparation [44, 45].

The radiographic apex is defined as the anatomical end of the root as seen on the radiograph [37]. Since this is visible radiographically, it has been widely used as a reference for determination of WL. Commonly 0.5–1 mm short of the radiographic apex has been used as a guide for determining termination of root canal preparation, and this is only an estimate. The radiographic apex and the anatomical canal terminus (where the canal exits the root) do not coincide. Frequently, canals exit short of the radiographic apex, and curvatures in the bucco-palatal/lingual plane will not be assessed using a two-dimensional image. Conversely when a file can be seen beyond the radiographic apex (such as the use of patency filing), we can be sure, without doubt, that we are beyond the confines of the canal. Radiographic determination of WL is subject to magnification, distortion, inter- and intra-observer variability and lack of three-dimensional representation. Despite inaccuracies, the use of radiographic length determination in combination with other techniques will give you the most accurate information as to the correct WL [53].

None of the aforementioned traditional techniques can truly satisfactorily determine the WL. The CDJ is a practical and anatomic termination point for the preparation and obturation of the root canal, and this cannot be determined radiographically. Modern electronic apex locators can determine this position with accuracies of greater than 90 % with some limitations. Knowledge of apical anatomy and the use of radiographs in combination with the correct use of an apex locator will assist practitioners to achieve predictable results [47]. The first electronic device for root canal length determination was constructed by Sunada using direct current based on the principle that the electrical resistance of the mucous membrane and periodontium registered 6.0kΩ in any part of the periodontium [48].

A number of electronic apex locator devices have been developed measuring resistance or impedance using frequencies (high, two or multiple) or low-frequency oscillation and/or a voltage gradient method to detect the canal terminus when an endodontic file penetrates inside the canal and approaches the apical constriction (minor apical foramen) [49]. Third-generation apex locators such as the Root ZX (J. Morita, Tokyo, Japan) were developed to calculate the ratio of two electrical impedances in the same canal using two different current frequencies to determine the canal length precisely even in the presence of electrolytes (root canal irrigants, serous intra-canal fluids, purulent exudate, haemorrhagic exudate) or vital pulp tissue in the root canal [50]. The Root ZX has been shown to be 90 % accurate to within 0.5 mm of the apical foramen and 100 % if accurate if 1.0 mm is accepted [51, 52]. Based on the majority of studies carried out in the endodontic literature, 0.5 mm should be subtracted from the length of the file at the point when the device suggests the file tip is in contact with the PDL (zero reading). This measurement does not indicate that the apical constriction has been located but rather that the instrument is within the canal and is close to the periodontal ligament [49]. Even though apex locators appear to be excellent tools for the determination of WL, they should be used as an adjunct and not as a substitute for radiographs. In fact, the combined use of electronic apex locators and radiographs of the initial or master apical file has been shown to be more accurate than the use of radiographs alone [53].

Apical patency is a technique in which the apical portion of the canal is maintained free of debris by recapitulation with a small file through the apical foramen [54]. Proponents of maintaining patency throughout the cleaning and shaping procedures are based on the belief that this helps to control debris accumulation in the apical portion of the canal preventing ledge formation, transportation and apical perforation [55]. In the teeth with necrotic and infected pulps, the use of patency filing ensures that mechanical and biological goals of cleaning and shaping are achieved by ensuring that cleaning and shaping procedures are carried out to the full extent of the canal (Fig. 3.3). In vital cases, apical patency is intended to prevent compaction of dentine chips into the apical region forming a plug that can interfere with WL [56]. The use of this technique is a matter of controversy, and antagonists claim this type of filing beyond the confines of the canal is biologically unacceptable with risks of over-enlargement of the apical foramen [57], damage to the periapical tissues [40] and inadvertent extrusion of contaminated dentine chips or bacteria leading to postoperative pain and sequelae [58].

Both stainless steel and nickel-titanium rotary instruments carry the risk of instrument fracture either as a result of flexural (fatigue fracture) or torsional (shear failure) stresses. Canal curvatures are thought to be the predominant risk factor for

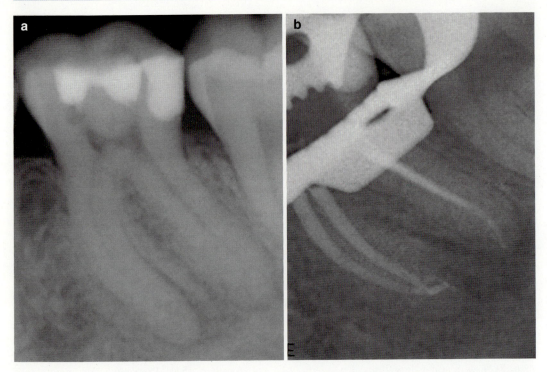

Fig. 3.3 Clinical radiographs demonstrating (**a**) preoperative view and (**b**) postoperative view of tooth 36. Note the use of apical patency filing ensures that complex apical anatomy has been satisfactorily treated

instrument failure through flexural stresses. To reduce the risk of file fracture when using rotary instrumentation techniques, coronal preflaring and the use of a manual or rotary glide path can help reduce stresses on the instrument [59]. The new PathFile NiTi rotary instruments (Dentsply Maillefer, Ballaigues, Switzerland) for mechanical preflaring have been recently introduced on the market and have demonstrated significantly less modification of canal curvature and fewer canal aberrations when compared to manual preflaring with stainless steel instruments [60].

The ideal final size of apical canal preparation remains controversial. The apical portion of the root canal system can harbour microorganisms that account for periapical pathosis and persistent inflammation; therefore, treatment interventions that allow for maximum reduction of pathogens should be indicated in the treatment of infected root canal systems [41]. Traditionally, final apical preparation techniques advocating enlarging the apical part of the root canal to three-four sizes larger than where the first file bound have

been recommended [61]. However, this concept has been questioned as a result of recent studies, which indicate up to 60 % of untouched canal walls that could contain biofilm [28]. Furthermore, Wu and colleagues demonstrated that in 75 % of root canals, the first instrument to bind at the apex had contact on the canal wall on one side only, and in 25 % the instrument tip had no contact with the canal wall at all [62]. A second school of thought from North America aimed to keep the apical diameter and preparation as small as practically possible. This concept of root canal preparation included establishing and maintaining patency using a small #10 K file 1 mm through the foramen and finishing the apical one-third to at least a size #20 [1]. Corresponding to this technique, modern rotary instruments such as ProTaper Universal finishing instruments have apical diameters ranging from 0.20 to 0.30 mm.

Classical bacteriological studies indicated that mechanical instrumentation alone resulted in significant reduction of bacteria but could not pre-

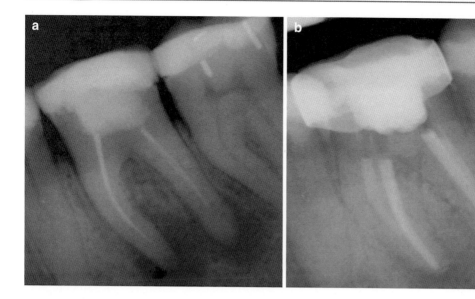

Fig. 3.4 Clinical radiographs demonstrating nonsurgical endodontic re-treatment of tooth 36. Note (**a**) preoperative film demonstrating incomplete suboptimal obturation that reflects inadequate cleaning and shaping procedures. Note extensive periradicular pathology associated with both apices. (**b**) 6 months posttreatment radiograph demonstrating complete healing of the case. Apical preparation sizes were #50 in mesial and distal canals

dictably achieve bacteria-free root canals [63]. Even combining mechanical preparation, antibacterial irrigants and intra-canal antimicrobial dressings did not achieve bacteria-free root canals, demonstrating the limited antibacterial effect of chemomechanical preparations [64, 65]. Ørstavik and colleagues studied the effects of chemomechanical root canal preparation in 23 teeth with apical periodontitis. Following a step-back technique and irrigation with sterile saline, 14 teeth yielded positive cultures at the end of the first appointment. Following a 7-day dressing of calcium hydroxide, this number was reduced to eight teeth [66]. Dalton and colleagues studied the effects of both stainless steel and nickel-titanium instruments in a clinical study of 48 teeth with apical periodontitis. In terms of bacterial reduction, no difference could be found with either technique although increasing instrument size reported increased bacterial reduction. Nevertheless, it was not possible to achieve bacteria-free root canals [67].

Rollinson and colleagues compared the removal of radioactively labelled bacteria using two different rotary NiTi preparation techniques. Preparations to size #50 (using Pow-R instru-ments) resulted in reduced bacterial counts compared to size #35 (using GT rotary and profile) (see Figs. 3.4 and 3.5) [68]. A recent systematic review suggested that contemporary chemomechanical debridement techniques with canal enlargement techniques do not eliminate bacteria during root canal preparation at any size [69]. The same authors carried out a similar systematic review assessing healing outcomes related to small and large master apical file sizes. They concluded that with the limited information available, the best current available clinical evidence suggests that for patients with necrotic pulps and periapical lesions, enlargement of the apical size would result in an increased healing outcome in terms of clinical and radiographic evaluation [69, 70].

Irrigation type, volume and depth of penetration are all crucial factors related to effectiveness and hence microbial reduction. Irrigants commonly delivered by syringe and needle devices indicate that successful irrigation delivery is related to canal diameter and curvature, and contemporary needle gauges used (27 and 30 gauges) require 0.42 and 0.31 mm diameter preparations, respectively. Therefore, the minimum canal size

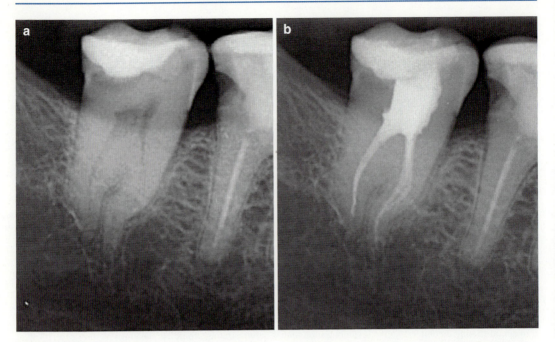

Fig. 3.5 Clinical radiographs of an S-shaped curvature in tooth 47. Note (**a**) preoperative radiograph and (**b**) postoperative radiograph following chemomechanical preparation procedures and final obturation. Apical preparation size mesially was to a size #20 to prevent iatrogenic canal transportation which could lead to failure

preparation when using a 30-gauge needle is 0.31 mm for the needle and therefore irrigant to reach within 1 mm of the WL (for more detailed discussion, see Chap. 5).

The uses of antimicrobial inter-appointment intra-canal dressings such as calcium hydroxide are also regarded as important adjuncts to optimize cleanliness and disinfection within the root canal system. Cleaning and shaping procedures facilitate placement of a suitable dressing that can further reduce microbial flora by virtue of its antimicrobial effects combined with its ability to suppress the nutritional supply that may allow further growth and multiplication of any remaining organisms (see Chap. 6 for more detailed discussion).

In summary, the goal of effective cleaning and shaping procedures is to remove all necrotic and vital organic tissue as well as some infected hard tissue from the root canal system. Correct shaping procedures with maintenance of original anatomy (with reference to the apical constriction) without iatrogenic deviation (canal transportation) facilitate optimal and effective irrigant deposition and

predictable placement of intra-canal medicament and facilitate permanent root fillings without risk of overfilling. Mechanical preparation techniques in terms of correct WL and master apical file size must be carried out with antimicrobial chemical treatments in mind (Fig. 3.6).

3.2   Radiographic Working Length Determination

The radiographic technique for determining WL is probably the most widely used technique to determine the end point of cleaning and shaping to facilitate final obturation. Clinicians should be aware of the limitations when carrying out such procedures and methods to ensure accuracy for interpretation. It is essential to have a preoperative diagnostic film (conventional or digital) using a paralleling cone beam-aiming device to ensure minimum distortion.

The use of digital radiography allows for easy and quick determination of the WL film with a file in position. The radiation dose is reduced

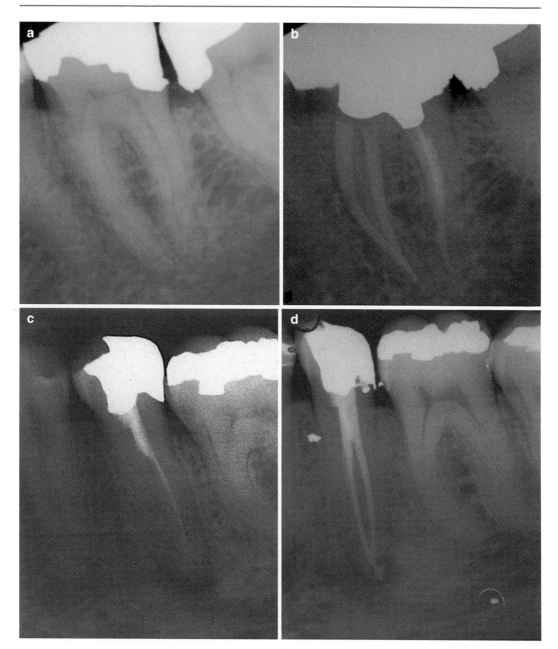

Fig. 3.6 Clinical radiographs demonstrating (**a**) pre- and (**b**) postoperative radiographs of primary root canal treatment carried out with nickel-titanium rotary files and (**c**) pre- and (**d**) postoperative radiographs of root canal re-treatment using stainless steel files. Cleaning and shaping procedures were carried out successfully irrespective of file design used. Key concepts utilized in both cases to ensure overall success include apical patency filing, recapitulation, working length determination (using radiographic and electronic methods), use of chemical disinfectants, and intracanal medicaments. Obturation procedures not only serve to prevent bacterial recontamination but also reflect the overall cleaning and shaping procedures carried out

when compared to conventional plain film radiography. Imaging software programs used with these devices allow for image modification including colour, contrast and magnification, which can be very helpful when assessing the apical limit of preparation. One must bear in

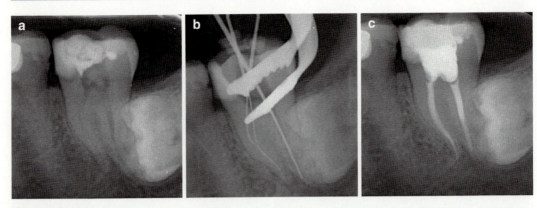

Fig. 3.7 Clinical radiographs demonstrating superimposition of a horizontally impacted wisdom tooth that makes radiograph determination of the working length difficult. Note (**a**) preoperative view demonstrating difficulty assessing distal root of tooth 37. (**b**) Working length files confirmed using an electronic apex device to determine master apical file and end point of preparation procedure. (**c**) Final obturation carried out with confidence without any risk of iatrogenic overfilling that could result in potential inferior dental nerve damage

mind with any conventional radiographic technique that the image is only a two-dimensional representation of a three-dimensional object, and so curvatures typically present in the buccal to palatal/lingual direction will remain undetected. Superimposition of anatomical structures such as the zygoma or zygomatic arch in the maxillary molar region or screws/plates/orthograde or retrograde fillings or overfills can also make WL interpretation difficult when using radiographs (Fig. **3.7**).

Radiographic determination of WL should therefore always be complimented with the use of an electronic apex locator to determine the correct WL based on the results of both techniques. Occasionally, the electronic apex locator method may not be possible requiring the sole use of a radiographic technique to estimate correct length. A typical example may be when you are working through a metallic restoration or metal crown, which results in short-circuiting and inaccurate readings.

To determine accurate WL's radiographically, the following guidelines are recommended:

1. All files should be placed in each canal that have been identified to correct estimated working length corresponding to reference points on the tooth (in multi-rooted teeth, this is preferable to taking multiple X-rays with separate files ensuring minimum radiation exposure).

2. Correct working length in each canal should be confirmed with the use of an electronic apex locator (see later) to verify 0.5 mm from 0 reading.

3. When using conventional film radiography, fresh developer and fixer must be available and developing carried out according to recommendations (time and temperature dependant).

4. The clinician must set the correct exposure for the film according to anatomical site and size of patient to ensure the resultant film is not under- or over-exposed resulting in poor image interpretation.

5. A parallel beam-aiming device should be used. This allows for minimal distortion of the WL film and comparable films that are useful during the later stages of treatment (an example is when further adjustments are required during the obturation phase).

6. Working length films should be reviewed, and if the distance between the file tip and root apex is greater than 1 mm, then another film is recommended with adjustments made accordingly.

7. When the file is seen beyond the radiographic apex, there is no doubt that the file is beyond the canal terminus.

8. When treating teeth with buccal and lingual canals, the use of the buccal object rule (SLOB same lingual opposite buccal) is essential when making distinctions between the canals, which may require length adjustment. Remember as the X-ray tube moves from

posterior (distal) to anterior (mesial) objects imaged on the film that are on the lingual aspect (disto-lingual, mesio-lingual and palatal roots) will be positioned mesially.

3.3 Electronic Working Length Determination

The cement-dentinal junction is the point at which the pulp tissue changes into the apical periodontal tissue and is the most ideal physiological apical limit of preparation. This point is also referred to as the apical constriction. The apical constriction does not coincide with the anatomic apex and is often deviated such that in a bucco-lingual plane, it will be impossible to confirm radiographically the exact position the file exits the tooth. The electronic apex locator, functioning on direct current, has proven to be a reliable method for determining the point at which the file exits the canal meeting the periodontal tissues. Furthermore, superimposition of certain anatomic structures (impacted teeth, tori, zygomatic arch, excessive bone density and overlapping roots) makes radiographic confirmation of working length difficult at times. Electronic apex loca-

tors are a reliable method of determining working lengths in addition to conventional radiography. Frequently, treatment time and radiation dose exposure to the patient can be routinely reduced when compared to working length determination using conventional radiography alone.

The Root ZX based on the "ratio method" for measuring the root canal length measures the impedances of 0.4 and 8 kHz at the same time, calculating the quotient of the impedances and expressing this quotient in terms of the position of the file within the canal. A built-in microprocessor automatically controls the calculated quotient to have a relationship between the position of the file within the canal and the digital readout when the file is placed in the coronal portion of the tooth. When the file is in the canal, the apex locator cannot tell you accurately what distance it is from the canal terminus even though most apex locators display a numeric value as the file progresses towards the apex (see Fig. **3.8**). However, when the file reaches the canal terminus, the screen will display "0", and the clinician can accurately determine that the tip of the instrument is at the apical constriction (Fig. **3.9**).

This feature is not only helpful for accurately determining the point at which pulpal and

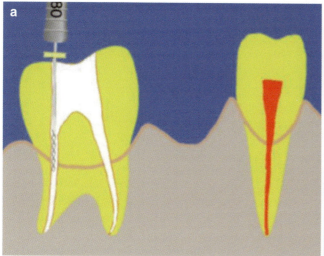
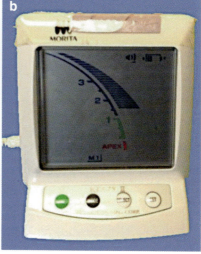

Fig. 3.8 (**a**) Diagrammatic representation and (**b**) clinical photograph of Root ZXII apex locator demonstrating digital reading when the file is placed in the canal. The graphic representation of the arbitrary units '3-2-1' displayed on the apex locator does not give you any reliable distance from the apex. The clinical technique of working length determination is to advance the file until the unit reads 'APEX'. At this point an audible alarm changes from a beep to a full tone

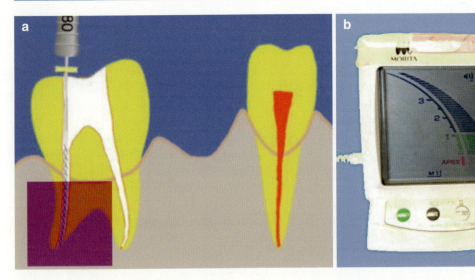

Fig. 3.9 (**a**) Diagrammatic representation and (**b**) clinical photograph of Root ZXII apex locator showing the digital reading when the file is at the apical constriction. If the file is advanced further then the unit reads 'APEX' with an audible alarm. The working length is then determined by subtracting 1 mm from the length measured when the meter flashes the first bar at the "Apex" and the sound first changes from a beep to a full tone. A radiographic image should be exposed with a small diameter files in the tooth at the electronically determined working length for verification

periodontal tissues (PDL) meet but also a reliable method when radiographic information at the apex is limited due to superimposition of other surrounding structures. The clinician should subtract 0.5 mm from the length of the file at the point when the device suggests the file tip is in contact with the PDL (zero reading). This measurement does not indicate that the apical constriction has been located but rather that the instrument is within the canal and is close to the periodontal ligament.

Although reliable, accurate and simple to use, some precautions and points of interest that are noteworthy when using the devices include the following:

1. A preoperative diagnostic parallel radiograph is essential for determining an estimate of working length prior to file insertion.
2. The lip hook should be placed under the rubber dam.
3. Metallic parts from the crown of the tooth including amalgam or crown should not come into contact with the file when using an apex locator. If contact occurs, the current is shunted resulting in an unstable electrical signal with rapid wandering signs.
4. The access cavity and pulp coronal pulp chamber should be relatively fluid-free although some fluid should be retained within the canals themselves.
5. The second electrode clip is attached to the file, and the file is placed within the canal and slowly advanced apically using a watch-winding movement (see later). The file is advanced until a stable "O" reading is achieved. The most stable reading is readily achieved when the file size approaches the natural apical constriction size. The file must fit snugly within the canal and have good electrical contact with the canal walls. Erratic readings suggest the file used is too small and the clinician is advised to change to a larger file size until the reading stabilizes.
6. The measurement should be checked and confirmed at the "O" reading. The file should be advanced slightly beyond the "O" reading and then slowly pulled back into the apical constriction to find the exact point at which pulp and periodontal tissue meet (Fig. 3.10). The rubber stopper should be placed at a reliable reference point on the tooth prior to file removal. The working length is calculated as 0.5 mm from the "O" reading length. Once all the canals have been measured, a working length radiograph is taken to confirm lengths.

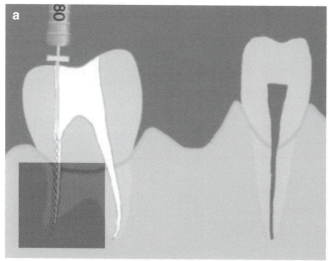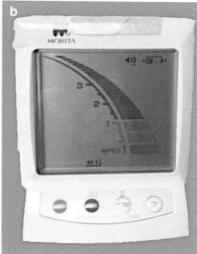

Fig. 3.10 (**a**) Diagrammatic representation and (**b**) clinical photograph of Root ZXII apex locator showing the digital reading when the file is passed beyond the apical constriction. At this point, we are certain that the file meets the periodontal apical tissues and we have confirmed canal patency. The file should be slowly pulled back confirming the exact point where an audible alarm for 'APEX' is reached. Care should be taken to advance small k files to ensure that apical foramen enlargement does not inadvertently occur when confirming working length. A reliable stable reading should be reproduced using the smallest file size possible

7. The measurement should be checked and confirmed at the "O" reading. The file should be advanced slightly beyond the "O" reading and then slowly pulled back into the apical constriction to find the exact point at which pulp and periodontal tissue meet. The rubber stopper should be placed at a reliable reference point on the tooth prior to file removal. The working length is calculated as 0.5 mm from the "O" reading length. Once all the canals have been measured, a working length radiograph is taken to confirm lengths.

8. In the case of preparing curved canals, it is recommended to recheck the working lengths following apical canal preparation since inherent straightening of the canal will result in working length changes of up to 1 mm.

9. Premature readings when the file has not advanced to the estimated working length calculated from preoperative diagnostic radiographs may indicate perforations within the root canal or can be associated with a wide-open apex. Occasionally, excessive fluid, exudate, pus or bleeding may interfere with the readings requiring removal using absorbent paper points. Conventional plain film or digital radiography may help confirm whether the file is indeed within the root canal or has exited prematurely suggesting perforation (see Fig. 3.11).

3.4 Hand Instrument Preparation Techniques (Fig. 3.12)

Step-back technique

1. Working length is determined prior to apical preparation of the canal to a minimum size #25.

2. Stainless steel files should be pre-curved in the apical 2–3 mm and inserted in the same direction as the canal curvature.

3. Recapitulation is recommended using a smaller file to working length with copious irrigation to prevent loss of working length.

4. Patency filing can be used to ensure that apical dentine debris does not block access at the apical constricture. A small #06 or 08K file can be passed 1 mm beyond the apical constricture to ensure patency is maintained.

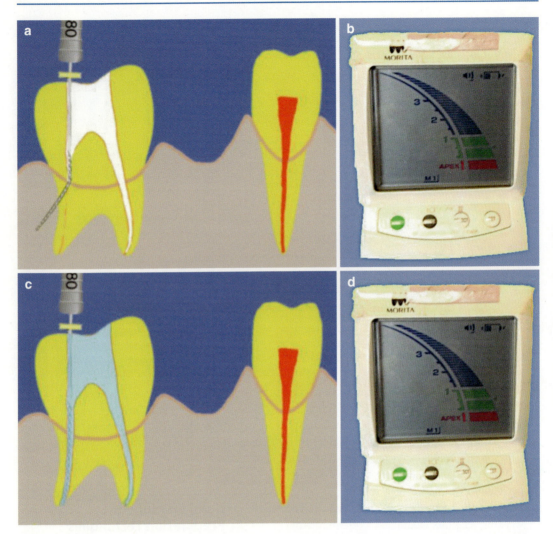

Fig. 3.11 Clinical diagram and photographs demonstrating (**a**) and (**b**) placement of a file into a perforation. Strip perforations can be detected and their position measured when 'APEX' is reached well short of the working length. Furcation perforations can also be detected if 'APEX' is registered when a file is inserted into a would-be-canal. Apical perforations may also be detected indicated by a sudden change in working length previously verified by the apex locator. Note (**c**) and (**d**) inaccurate readings on the apex locator as a result of excessive fluid (blood, irrigants, pus) within the canal or coronal pulp chamber. If the advancing file comes into contact with metallic restorations in the coronal pulp chamber instant and erroneous 'APEX' readings can also occur

5. Once apical enlargement has been achieved, serial step-back preparation can be carried out using successively larger files at either 1 or 0.5 mm increments. The latter allows for a greater apical taper if desired.
6. Recapitulation should be carried out with the master apical file (the last file used at the working length prior to step-back preparation).
7. The canal walls can be circumferentially filed using a 25H file to smooth the walls and steps created ensuring a constant taper is achieved.

8. Once preparation is completed, the master apical file radiograph can be taken to confirm working length.

Watch-winding technique

1. The use of K-type files is recommended.
2. A size 10# K file can be inserted into the canal until resistance is met. The file is turned 30–60° in a clockwise rotation which advances the file further into the canal engaging dentine.

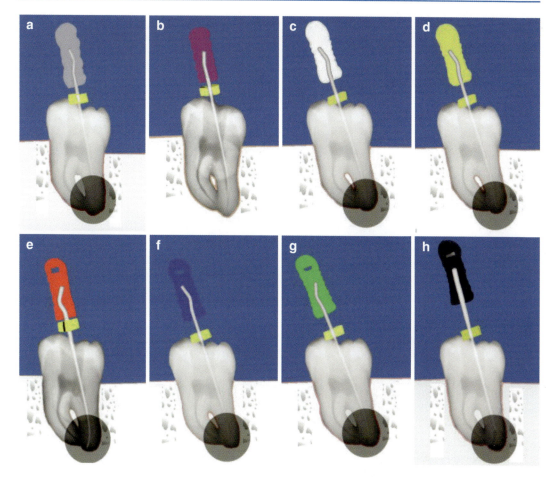

Fig. 3.12 Clinical diagrams representing step-back preparation technique. (**a–e**) After coronal flaring and determining the master apical file (initial file that binds slightly at the corrected working length), (**f–h**) the succeeding larger files are shortened by 0.5 or 1.0 m increments from the previous file length. This step-back process creates a flared, tapering preparation while reducing procedural errors. The step-back preparation is superior to standardized serial filing and reaming techniques in debridement and maintaining the canal shape

3. The file is turned 30–60° counter clockwise to partially cut away the engaged dentine.
4. Each clockwise and counter clockwise file motion results in further canal space opening and allowing the instrument to advance deeper into the canal (Fig. 3.13).

Balanced force technique

1. Flex-R files or Flexofiles with a modified noncutting tip should be used.
2. The coronal two-thirds of the canal should be prepared using a crown-down technique prior to apical preparation.
3. The file is placed in the canal (uncurved) and rotated clockwise from 90° to 180° with light apical pressure to engage dentine. If apical force is excessive, the file may prematurely "lock" predisposing to file separation on counter clockwise movement.
4. The file is rotated at least 120° counter clockwise with apical pressure to cut the engaged dentine. You may hear a "click".
5. A combination of clockwise turns and counter clockwise turns with apical pressure is carried out until working length is reached. The file can be withdrawn from time to time to ensure the cutting flutes loaded with dentine debris are cleaned.
6. Care must be taken when attempting to enlarge canal curvatures greater than 20°. Files larger than size #30 will have inherent inflexibility resulting in straightening of the canal and predisposition to canal stripping.

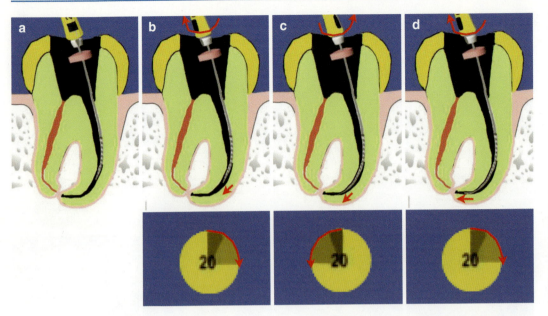

Fig. 3.13 (**a–d**) Diagrammatic representation of the 'watch winding technique'. Watch winding is reciprocating back and forth (clockwise/counter-clockwise) rotation of the instrument in an arch of 20°. It is useful for canal negotiation and file advancement to the apex. Light apical pressure is applied to move the file deeper into the canal

7. Any files that show signs of defects such as unwinding should be discarded on inspection (Fig. 3.14).

Crown-down technique

1. Hedstrom file sizes #15, 20 and 25 can be used with light apical pressure in the coronal two-thirds of the canal. Files should never be forced and placed short of the point of binding. If the canal is extremely calcified or exhibits a significant curvature, then smaller #08 and #010K files can be used to ensure patency. Circumferential filing motion with the H files ensures dentine interferences and pulpal tissue remnants are removed prior to pre-enlargement using Gates-Glidden burs (Fig. 3.15).
2. Copious irrigation should be used to ensure dentine debris and pulp tissue remnants are flushed out preventing apical blockage.
3. A No.2 and No.3 Gates-Glidden bur can be used in the coronal two-thirds just short of the apical one-third or curvature.
4. Working length is established, and the apex is enlarged (preferably minimal size #25 or #30 to ensure optimal irrigation).

5. A step-back preparation is carried out to blend the apical one-third and coronal two-thirds preparation.
6. Recapitulation and patency filing is recommended to ensure patency is maintained and no dentine debris/mud blocks the canal apically. Copious irrigation should be carried out using sodium hypochlorite solution.
7. Circumferential filing with a H file equivalent to the master apical file size to remove dentine interferences in the canal wall and ensure a smooth tapered preparation.
8. Working length radiograph is recommended to confirm desired length of preparation.

3.5 Creating a Glide Path

Over the last thirty years, the use of manual and rotary nickel-titanium instrumentation has revolutionized the field of endodontics and the way in which canals are cleaned and shaped. A concern regarding the use of any instrument that is rotated within the canal is the risk of either torsional or flexure fatigue that can lead to instrument separation. Torsional failure occurs when the instrument tip or any part of the rotating

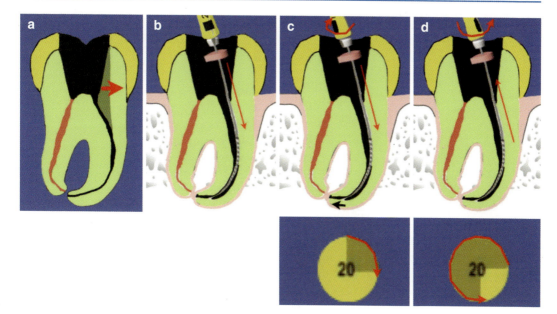

Fig. 3.14 Diagrammatic representation of the 'balanced force technique'. Note (**a**) before preparation is carried out all coronal interferences are removed to ensure straight-line access. This reduces iatrogenic preparation errors and excessive file deformation and propensity to fracture (especially in curved canals). The balanced force concept of instrumentation consists of (**b**) placing a file to length and (**c**) rotating the file clockwise to engage dentine followed by (**d**) rotation of the file counter-clockwise with apical pressure. The degree of apical pressure varies from light pressure with small instruments to heavy pressure with larger instruments. The clockwise rotation pushes the instrument into the canal in an apical direction. The counter-clockwise cutting rotation forces the file in a coronal direction whilst cutting circumferentially. Following the cutting rotation the file is repositioned and the process is repeated until adequate enlargement to working length is achieved. The balanced force technique has been shown to reduce canal transportation and ledging in curved canals

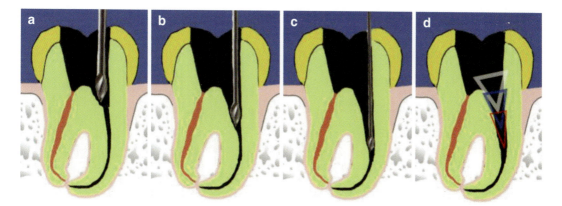

Fig. 3.15 (**a–d**) Diagrammatic representation of the crown-down technique whereby root canal preparation is completed from a coronal to apical direction. Traditional stainless instruments (K files or Gates Glidden burs) are used from larger to smaller files and advanced in an apical direction. Modern nickel-titanium rotary file preparation utilizes a crown down approach. Advantages include early debris removal coronally, deeper penetration of irrigants, reduced procedural errors such as ledging and zipping and less apical debris extrusion. During any corona-apical preparation frequent irrigation is essential and any forceful instrumentation may result in canal ledging, transportation, blockage or instrument separation

instrument binds to the canal wall, whilst the remainder of the instrument keeps rotating. The end result is fracture of the file due to excessive forces placed on the file beyond the elastic limit. Flexural fatigue relates to an instrument that is not bound within the canal but freely rotates resulting in weakening of the instrument due to excessive forces at the .point of maximum flexure. This usually occurs in canals with curvatures where undue stress is placed on the rotating instrument. Coronal pre-enlargement and creation of a "glide path" minimize the risk of instrument fracture. Glide path creation involves the use of either small flexible stainless steel hand files (sizes 10, 15 and 20) or rotary files to create sufficient space for the rotary instrument to follow. PathFile NiTi rotary instruments consist of three instruments with 21-25-31 mm lengths and 0.02 taper. The PathFile #1 (purple) has an ISO 13 tip size; the PathFile #2 (white) has an ISO 16 tip size; the PathFile #3 (yellow) has an ISO 19 tip size. The recommended technique for creating a rotary glide path is as follows:

1. Ensure straight-line access and removal of all coronal interferences within each root canal.
2. Negotiate the canal to WL (confirmed with apex locator and radiograph) and establish patency using pre-curved stainless steel K files (sizes 06, 08 or 10).
3. Establish an initial manual glide path using K files in a watch-winding movement.
4. Do not proceed with PathFiles until a size 10 K file has been established as an initial glide path. Verify this by inserting a size 10 K file at working length, withdraw 2 mm by hand and then reposition to WL. Repeat withdrawing a further 5–7 mm to ensure a smooth reproducible glide path is present.
5. PathFile #1 (ISO 0.13 mm at the tip) is introduced into the root canal at a rotation speed of 300 rpm in a slow in and out movement until full WL is achieved. It is important to never push the instrument or keep the instrument rotating in the same position, especially in

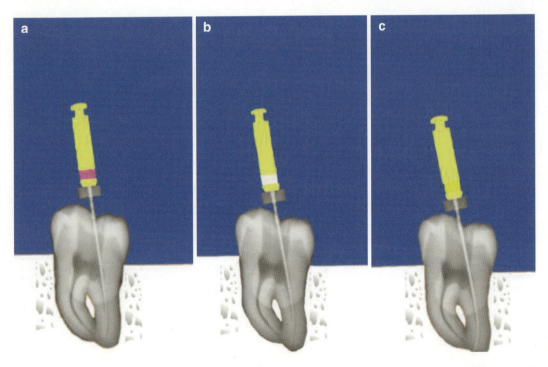

Fig. 3.16 Diagrammatic representation of a mandibular molar tooth undergoing reproducible glide path preparation using nickel-titanium rotary Pathfiles. Note (**a**) Pathfile #1 (*purple*) has an ISO 13 tip size. (**b**) Pathfile #2 (*white*) has an ISO 16 tip size. (**c**) Pathfile #3 (*yellow*) has an ISO 19 tip size

severely curved canals which can lead to ledging or fatigue and file separation.

6. Copious irrigation is recommended during glide path preparation and between each file use. Recapitulation with a 10 K file is important to maintain patency to full WL.

7. Proceed with PathFile #2 (ISO 0.16 mm at the tip) and PathFile #3 (ISO 0.19 mm at the tip) using the same protocol described before.

8. Proceed with NiTi rotary preparation according to manufacture guidelines (Fig. 3.16).

3.6 Loss of Working Length and Patency Filing

During root canal cleaning and shaping procedures, dentine chips produced by instrumentation and compaction of pulp tissue remnants into the apical foramen can occur leading to apical blockage and loss of working length. The combination of copious irrigation throughout and the repeated penetration of the apical foramen with a small file during instrumentation can prevent the accumulation of debris in this area leaving the foramen unblocked, e.g. patent. This concept has been described as apical patency. Maintaining apical patency throughout the root canal instrumentation procedure ensures that the working length is not altered and that optimal cleaning and shaping objectives are achieved (Fig. 3.17).

3.7 Recapitulation

Recapitulation is defined as "the reintroduction of small files during root canal preparation to keep the apical area clean and patent". The step-back technique and use of stainless steel hand files require the sequential placement of smaller-sized instruments to confirm WL is maintained prior to the introduction of a larger-sized instrument. This prevents packing of dentine debris or dentinal mud in the apical portion of the canal

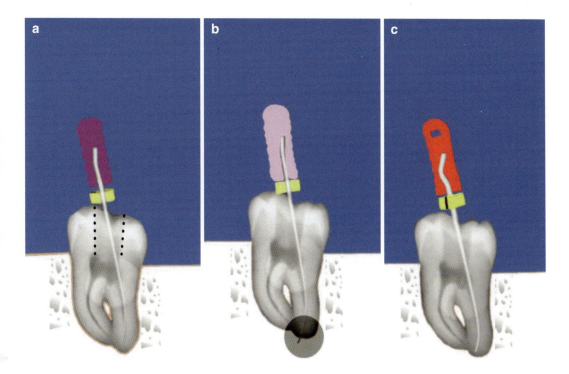

Fig. 3.17 Clinical radiographs of a mandibular molar tooth demonstrating (**a**) straight-line access (*dotted lines*), initial apical file size 10 K used to negotiate canal to working length, (**b**) 06 K patency file beyond apical foramen, and (**c**) master apical file 25 K working length

during preparation. Recapitulation ensures patency to the apical foramen, whereas patency filing ensures that the file is not only able to pass to the apical foramen but also beyond into the surrounding periapical tissues. Recapitulation should be used in any instrumentation technique prior to the introduction of a larger sequential file in the preparation steps. Suffice to say irrigation is an essential requirement during the process of instrument recapitulation.

3.8   Determination of Final Canal Preparation Size

The final apical size preparation has been a long-standing debate and is still focus of much disagreement in the endodontic field. From a biological standpoint, the aim of cleaning and shaping procedures is to ensure that all microorganisms and their by-products and necrotic pulp tissue remnants and infected dentine have been disinfected to allow for periapical healing to occur. From a mechanical perspective, a tapered canal with a minimum ISO size #30 will not only ensure that biological objectives are adhered to (through effective irrigation, disinfection and antimicrobial dressings) but also the end stage of final obturation can be carried out predictably with ease. Complex root canal anatomy such as canal curvatures greater than 20°, multiple canal curvatures (S shaped), confluent canals with abrupt merging or sharp exits at apical foramen will ultimately dictate final apical preparation size (Fig. 3.5). The astute clinician must be able to gauge early canal configuration and limits of preparation techniques that can be safely used without aberrant iatrogenic damage such as canal transportation and ultimate perforation.

3.9   Under-preparation and Under-instrumentation

Root canal under-preparation and under-instrumentation refer to the failure to adequately remove pulp tissue, dentinal debris and microor-

ganisms from the root canal system. Suffice to say inadequate preparation not only lends itself to failure of achieving the biological aims of cleaning and shaping but also inadequate shape necessary for three-dimensional obturation. Underprepared canals are best managed by adhering to the principles necessary when determining correct WL, adequate cleaning and shaping, use of patency filing and recapitulation and copious irrigation.

3.10   Over-preparation and Over-instrumentation

Over-preparation refers to excessive removal of tooth structure. During canal cleaning and shaping procedures, both coronal and apical preparation should correspond to the respective size, shape and curvature of the root. Overzealous preparation, particularly near danger zones such as the furcal region of molar teeth, canal curvatures greater than 20° or inappropriate instrument use such as a Gates-Glidden crown-down approach, can lead to not only apical transportation and zipping or ledging but also stripping and iatrogenic perforation. Modifications to the preparation technique to be used should be made according to pre-existing canal anatomy. Conservative use of any instrument within the canal is recommended without excessive preparations that can lead to further weakening of tooth structure and ultimate demise of the tooth by way of root fracture.

Over-instrumentation refers to instrumenting beyond the confines of the apical constriction leading to excessive apical enlargement. Careful use of patency files ensuring only small 06 or 08 files are passively passed 0.5–1 mm beyond the apical constriction will not lead to this undesirable outcome. On the other hand, disregard and poor attention to WL will lead to large file sizes preparing beyond the apical constriction leading to irreversible damage and an open apex with an increased likelihood of overfilling, inadequate apical seal and pain and discomfort for the patient. Clinically, the clinician may be alerted to this fact by bleeding in the apical portion of the canal. Often in canals with curvatures, the WL will be altered with inevitable straightening of the canal following canal preparation with a reduction in the WL. If the clinician fails to recognize this and continues to proceed with the initial WL, over-instrumentation will occur.

3.11 Blockage Versus Calcification

Blockage refers to an obstruction in a previously patent canal system. Access to the apical constriction is prevented and is commonly as a direct consequence of inappropriate cleaning and shaping principles. The cause of the blockage may be due to packing of dentine chips/debris or pulp tissue remnants from within the canal. Blockages can also occur as a result of restorative materials, cotton wool pledgets, paper points or separated instruments that can become introduced into the canal system and subsequently pushed in an apical direction if not recognized early. Renegotiation of the canal following packing of dentinal debris (mud) and pulp tissue remnants can be particularly troublesome. The best management is prevention by the use of copious irrigation, recapitulation and patency filing. To avoid restorative materials entering the root canal space correct access preparation, extension and dismantling of restorations is advisable prior to canal shaping and cleaning procedures. Removal of amalgam particles from within the root canal may be achieved by irrigation. Specific treatment protocols for instrument removal are discussed in Chap. 11.

If dentinal debris or pulp tissue remnants are suspected to be the cause of blockage, the following protocol may help removal:

1. A small stiff K file (size 10 or 15) can be used to try and negotiate through the blockage or seek to find space around the blockage.
2. The use of copious irrigation and sodium hypochlorite whenever any instrument is introduced into the canal should allow for removal of necrotic pulp tissue remnants and organic debris created by the smear layer effect.
3. The use of EDTA is recommended for smear layer removal and inorganic tissue remnants.
4. Care must be taken when introducing a file for removal of metallic amalgam filling materials, dentine debris or pulp stones/calcifications since too large a file may result in advertent pushing of debris further apically. It may be best to try and negotiate to WL using small files with copious irrigation followed by successively larger instruments.
5. Once the file has reached the original WL, it may be necessary to carry out circumferential filling in small amplitudes of 1–2 mm to the WL to ensure that patency is maintained. This may also help dislodge further blockage material.
6. Insertion of a small size H file to WL can help dislodge blockage material on the outstroke movement engaging the material as the file is withdrawn.
7. Occasionally, the blockage may not be bypassed or removed requiring alteration in WL and a possible surgical approach if healing does not occur.

Calcified canals are often encountered resulting in the inability to reach the apical limit of preparation due to a previously irritated pulp, which attempts to mount a reparative response prior to eventual pulp demise. Isolated pulp stones, diminished coronal pulp volume and diffuse root canal calcification may all be evident on preoperative radiographs. In most cases through careful treatment approaches, these obstructions can be overcome (see Chap. 4).

3.12 Canal Transportation

Canal transportation is defined as the "removal of canal wall structure on the outside of the curve in the apical half of the canal due to the tendency of files to restore themselves to their original linear shape during root canal preparation; may lead to ledge formation and possible perforation". This phenomenon is attributed to a number of variables including the properties of any metal alloy that lends itself to straightening when placed in a curved canal. Due to these restoring forces, the cutting edges of the instrument will be forced against the outer aspect of the curve (convexity) in the apical one-third and against the inner aspect of the curve (concavity) in the coronal and middle one-third of the canal. As a result, apical canal areas will tend to be over-prepared on the convexity of the canal, whereas more coronally greater amounts of dentine removal will occur on the concavity of the canal walls. This phenomenon will lead to various degrees of canal transportation or straightening including apical foramen damage, zip formation, elbow formation, ledging, perforation and stripping. The clinician must be aware of the dangers when carrying out cleaning and shaping procedures and necessary steps to minimize risk of occurrence.

Damage to the apical foramen

Original canal curvature deviation at the apical foramen can lead to excessive over-preparation and irreversible damage. As a consequence, the periapical tissues may be irritated by over-instrumentation, over-preparation and risk of extruded dentine debris, irrigants or obturating materials.

Zipping

Zip formation is defined "as an elliptical shape that may be formed in the apical foramen during preparation of a curved canal when a file extends through the apical foramen resulting in transportation of the outer wall". This will often produce an "hourglass", "a teardrop" or "foraminal rip" at the apical foramen, which can be difficult to seal and obturate.

Elbow

Elbow formation results in a narrow portion of root canal at the point of excessive over-preparation that occurs at the inner aspect of the curvature apically and outer aspect of the curvature more coronally. The resultant taper of the canal is insufficient with difficulties associated with cleaning, shaping and obturation.

Ledge

Ledge formation is defined as "an artificial irregularity created on the surface of a root canal wall that impedes the placement of an instrument to the apex of an otherwise patent canal". Ledging of curved canals is a common instrumentation

error that usually occurs on the outer aspect of the curvature due to careless manipulation and excessive cutting (Fig. 3.18).

Perforation

Perforation is defined as "the mechanical or pathological communication between the root canal system and the external root surface". This can occur in any part of the canal where a reproducible glide path has not been achieved and careless overzealous use of a sharp cutting instrument is forced to create an artificial pathway and eventual communication with the external root surface. Apical perforations can lead to irritation of the peri-radicular tissues and unfavourable healing.

Strip perforation

Strip perforation is defined as "a complete penetration of a root canal wall due to excessive lateral tooth structure removal during canal preparation; usually occurs in curved canals or roots with surface invagination's". These types of perforations commonly occur in the inner side of the curvature in the coronal and middle 1/3rd of the canals resulting in a communication between the root canal system and periodontal ligament in mandibular molars at the furcal aspect known as the "danger zone".

3.13 Clinical Cases

Case 1 Endodontic treatment of tooth 16 with calcified canals, long roots and abrupt apical curvatures

A 46-year-old patient was referred for non-surgical endodontic treatment of tooth 16 (Figs. 3.19 and 3.20). Clinical examination confirmed the tooth had an extensive tooth coloured restoration, which was tender to percussion. Radiographic examination revealed an extensive pin-retained coronal restoration. The pulp chamber appeared diminished in size with a calcified root canal system. Following straight-line access preparation and ultrasonic troughing, four canal orifices were located. The canals were calcified, long and tortuous in nature (working lengths of 27 mm in MB1 and MB2), and abrupt curvatures were confirmed in the mesiobuccal canals with

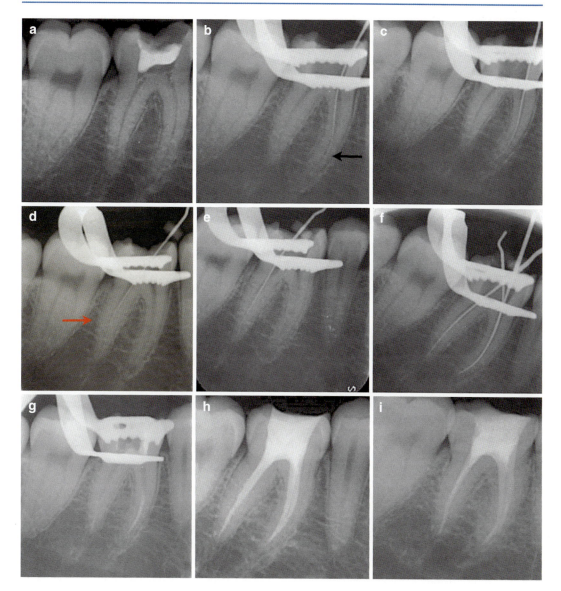

Fig. 3.18 Clinical radiographs demonstrating management of ledges in tooth 46. The general dental practitioner was unable to negotiate the mesial and distal canals to length. Note (**a**) preoperative view of tooth 46 showing previous endodontic access. (**b**) Initial apical file (IAF) in MB canal could not be negotiated to length. A ledge was confirmed at this point (*black arrow*). (**c**) Working length following ledge negotiation. (**d**) Ledge in distal canal (*red arrow*). (**e**) Ledge negotiation. (**f**) Master apical file working length radiograph. (**g**) Mid-fill radiograph and (**h**) and (**i**) completed obturation of canals

confluence. Apical patency was maintained throughout, and initial glide path was created using rotary nickel-titanium PathFiles. Chemomechanical preparation was completed using rotary files using a hybrid technique. Following an intra-canal dressing of calcium hydroxide for 4 weeks, the patient was seen for completion of treatment. Obturation was completed using a combination of warm vertical and warm lateral compaction.

Case 2 Endodontic retreatment and intentional reimplantation of tooth 27 with canal transportation

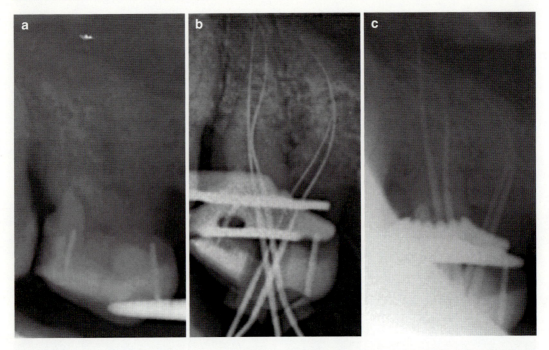

Fig. 3.19 Clinical radiographs demonstrating nonsurgical root canal treatment of tooth 16. Note (**a**) preoperative film demonstrating calcified canal system. (**b**) Initial apical radiograph demonstrating abrupt curvatures in all canals. A hybrid rotary technique was used maintaining apical patency filing throughout. (**c**) Master apical file radiograph demonstrating final apical sizes. A decision was made to limit apical preparation size due to the abrupt curvatures seen

A 78-year-old fit and healthy lady was referred for endodontic retreatment of tooth 27 (Fig. 3.21). The patient recalled endodontic treatment had been carried out many years previously. Recently, she had become aware of localized pain and discomfort in relation to this tooth. Clinical examination revealed significant palpation tenderness with the tooth. A 7 mm probing profile was noted with the mid-buccal aspect of the tooth. A cast cuspal coverage restoration was present with good marginal integrity. Radiographic examination confirmed previous endodontic therapy. The MB1 and P canals were transported. A periradicular radiolucency was associated with the mesial root. A decision was made to attempt nonsurgical root canal retreatment.

An access cavity was prepared through the existing crown, core material dismantled and MB1, DB and P canals identified. Previous gutta-percha was removed using a combination of heat and solvents. The MB1, DB and P canals were blocked and could not be negotiated to length. Ultrasonic troughing revealed an additional untreated MB2 canal. Chemomechanical preparation was completed and an intra-canal dressing of calcium hydroxide placed. The patient was reviewed a month later, and the sinus had not resolved. A decision was made to undertake an intentional reimplantation procedure.

The tooth was extracted using an atraumatic extraction technique. The roots were assessed for any evidence of root fractures. The MB root was fused to the DB root. All four roots were resected, and retrograde ultrasonic preparation was completed prior to retrograde filling using MTA. The tooth was bathed in saline throughout the entire procedure (total time 15 min). The tooth was atraumatically replanted. The patient was advised a soft diet for 1 week and analgesics as required.

At the review appointment 1 month later, the tooth had settled down, and all her symptoms had resolved. The tooth was reaccessed and orthograde obturation completed using a warm

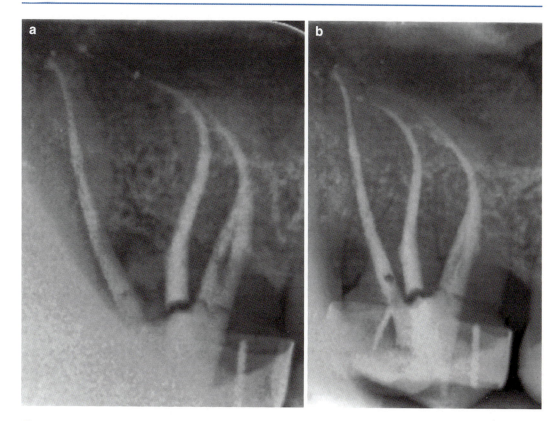

Fig. 3.20 (**a, b**) Clinical radiographs demonstrating final obturation of tooth 16. A warm vertical and warm lateral compaction technique was used with AH cement. Note sealer puffs confirming maintenance of apical patency throughout the treatment. The purpose of shaping is to facilitate cleaning and provide space for placement of the obturating material. The main objective of shaping is to maintain a continuously tapering funnel from the canal orifice to the apex. This decreases procedural errors when cleaning and enlarging apically. The degree of apical enlargement is often dictated by canal anatomy and the risk of canal transportation

vertical compaction technique. The patient was reviewed at 3 and 6 months at which time the buccal pocketing had resolved. The tooth remained asymptomatic with normal probing profiles. The patient has been placed on long-term review to ensure there are no signs of replacement resorption.

> **Clinical Hints and Tips to Minimize Iatrogenic Errors Such as Canal Transportation**
>
> - Correct straight-line access cavity preparation with removal of coronal interferences results in uninterrupted access to the apical one-third and curvature.
> - Creation of a reproducible glide path to ensure that larger tapered rotary files can follow a smooth path to the apex of the tooth.
> - Avoiding the use of inflexible large-size stainless steel instruments (ISO size 25 and above) in moderate curved canals (curvatures greater than 20°).
> - Preparation of moderate to severe canal curvatures. The degree of canal curvature and radius of curvature must be assessed. In general, the greater the degree of canal curvature and the smaller the radius of curvature, the greater the risk of canal transportation. Instrumentation techniques need to be modified according to canal anatomy.

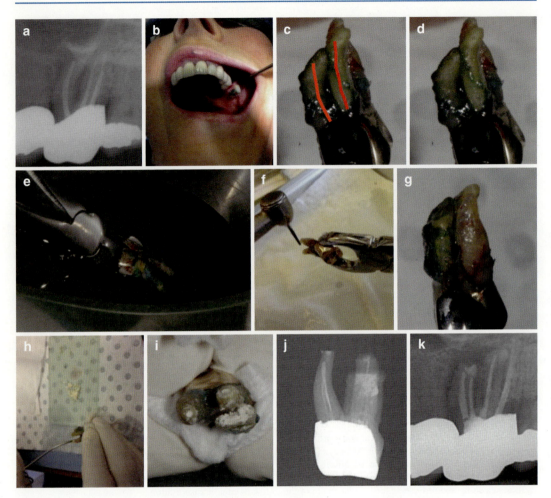

Fig. 3.21 Clinical photographs and radiographs demonstrating intentional reimplantation procedure for tooth 27. (**a**) Preoperative radiograph showing canal transportation of the MB1 canal. DB and P canals appeared to be obturated short of respective apices. A periradicular radiolucency was noted with the MB root. (**b**) Atraumatic extraction of tooth 27. (**c**) Canal transportation in MB and DB roots and (**d**) root morphology showing fusion of MB and DB roots. (**e**) Saline bath used throughout to ensure periodontal ligament cells remain viable. (**f**) and (**g**) Root resection. (**h**) and (**i**) MTA retrograde placement. (**j**) Radiographic confirmation of resection and retrograde obturation. (**k**) Postoperative radiograph at 1 month following procedure with completed orthograde warm vertical compaction

- Copious irrigation to prevent accumulation of dentinal debris within the canal.
- Instrumentation techniques used. Crown-down and balanced force techniques may be better when preparing curved canals compared to traditional step-back techniques.
- Avoid forcing any instrument in the canal.

References

1. Schilder H. Cleaning and shaping the root canal. Dent Clin North Am. 1974;18:269–96.
2. Ingle JI. A standardized endodontic technique using newly designed instruments and filling materials. Oral Surg Oral Med Oral Pathol. 1961;14:83–91.
3. Clem W. Endodontics in the adolescent patient. Dent Clin North Am. 1969;13:483–6.

4. Lim S, Stock CJ. The risk of perforation in the curved canal: anticurvature filing compared with the stepback technique. Int Endod J. 1987;20:33–9.
5. Abou-Rass M, Frank AL, Glick DH. The anticurvature filing method to prepare the curved root canal. J Am Dent Assoc. 1980;101:792–4.
6. Goerig AC, Michelich RJ, Schultz HH. Instrumentation of root canals in molars using the step-down technique. J Endod. 1982;8:550–4.
7. Fava L. The double flared technique: an alternative for biomechanical preparation. J Endod. 1983;9:76–80.
8. Roane JB, Sabala CL. Clockwise or anticlockwise? J Endod. 1984;10:349–53.
9. Saunders WP, Saunders EM. Effect of non-cutting tipped instruments on the quality of root canal preparation using a modified double flared technique. J Endod. 1992;18:32–6.
10. Jafarzedeh H, Abbott PV. Ledge formation: review of a great challenge in endodontics. J Endod. 2007;33(10):1155–62.
11. Baumann MA. Nickel-titanium: options and challenges. Dent Clin N Am. 2004;48:55–67.
12. Weine FS, Kelly RF, Lio PS. The effect of preparation procedures on original canal shape and apical foramen shape. J Endod. 1975;1:255–62.
13. Lim KC, Webber J. The effect of root canal preparation on the shape of the curved root canal. Int Endod J. 1985;18:233–9.
14. Eldeeb ME, Boraas JC. The effect of different files on the preparation shape of severely curved canals. Int Endod J. 1985;17:1–7.
15. Walia H, Brantely WA, Gernstein H. An initial investigation of the bending and torsional properties of nitinol root canal files. J Endod. 1988;14:346–51.
16. Schafer E. Root canal instruments for manual use: a review. Endod Dent Traumatol. 1997;13:51–64.
17. Thompson S, Dummer PMH. Shaping ability of profile.04 taper series 29 rotary nickel-titanium instruments in simulated root canals: part I. Int Endod J. 1997;30:1–7.
18. Thompson S, Dummer PMH. Shaping ability of profile.04 taper series 29 rotary nickel-titanium instruments in simulated root canals: part II. Int Endod J. 1997;30:8–15.
19. Thompson S, Dummer PMH. Shaping ability of Lightspeed rotary nickel-titanium instruments in simulated root canals: part I. Int Endod J. 1997;23:698–702.
20. Thompson S, Dummer PMH. Shaping ability of Lightspeed rotary nickel-titanium instruments in simulated root canals: part II. Int Endod J. 1997;23:742–7.
21. Thompson S, Dummer PMH. Shaping ability of Quantec series 2000 rotary nickel-titanium instruments in simulated root canals: part I. Int Endod J. 1998;31:259–67.
22. Thompson S, Dummer PMH. Shaping ability of Quantec series 2000 rotary nickel-titanium instruments in simulated root canals: part II. Int Endod J. 1998;31:168–274.
23. Bryant ST, Thompson SA, Al-Omari MAO, Dummer PMH. Shaping ability of profile rotary nickel-titanium instruments with ISO sized tips in simulated root canals: part I. Int Endod J. 1998;31:275–81.
24. Bryant ST, Thompson SA, Al-Omari MAO, Dummer PMH. Shaping ability of profile rotary nickel-titanium instruments with ISO sized tips in simulated root canals: part II. Int Endod J. 1999;31:275–81.
25. Thompson S, Dummer PMH. Shaping ability of HERO 642 rotary nickel-titanium instruments in simulated root canals: part I. Int Endod J. 2000;33:248–54.
26. Thompson S, Dummer PMH. Shaping ability of HERO 642 rotary nickel-titanium instruments in simulated root canals: part 2. Int Endod J. 2000;33:255–61.
27. Peters OA, Laib A, Gohring TN, Barbakow F. Changes in root canal geometry using high resolution computed tomography. J Endod. 2001;27:1–6.
28. Peters OA, Schönenberger K, Laib A. Effects of four Ni-Ti preparation techniques on root canal geometry assessed by micro computed tomography. Int Endod J. 2001;34:221–30.
29. Paqué F, Ganahl D, Peters OA. Effects of root canal preparation on apical geometry assessed by micro-computed tomography. J Endod. 2009;35:1056–9.
30. Paqué F, Ballmer M, Attin T, Peters OA. Preparation of oval shaped root canals in mandibular molars using nickel titanium instruments: a micro-computed tomography study. J Endod. 2010;36:703–7.
31. Bramante CM, Berbert A, Borges RP. A methodology for evaluation of root canal instrumentation. J Endod. 1987;13:243–5.
32. Briseno BM, Sobarzo V, Devens S. The influence of different engine driven instruments on root canal preparation: an in-vitro study. Int Endod J. 1991;24:15–23.
33. Paqué F, Musch U, Hülsmann M. Comparison of root canal preparation using RaCe and ProTaper rotary Ni-Ti instruments. Int Endod J. 2005;38:8–16.
34. Shäfer E, Vlassis M. Comparative investigation of two rotary nickel-titanium instruments: ProTaper versus RaCe. Part I. Shaping ability in simulated curved canals. Int Endod J. 2004;37:229–38.
35. Shäfer E, Vlassis M. Comparative investigation of two rotary nickel-titanium instruments: ProTaper versus RaCe. Part 2. Cleaning effectiveness and shaping ability in severely curved root canals of extracted teeth. Int Endod J. 2004;37:239–48.
36. Simon S, Machtou P, Adams N, Tomson P, Lumley P. Apical limit and working length in endodontics. Dent Update. 2009;36:146–53.
37. American Association of Endodontists. An annotated glossary of terms used in endodontics. Chicago: American Association of endodontists; 1984. p. 1–3.
38. Kuttler Y. Microscopic investigations of root apexes. J Am Dent Assoc. 1955;50:544–52.
39. Riccuci D. Apical limit of root canal instrumentation and obturation, part I. Literature review. Int Endod J. 1998;31:384–93.

40. Riccuci D, Langeland K. Apical limit of root canal instrumentation and obturation, part 2. A histological study. Int Endod J. 1998;31:394–409.
41. Sjögren U, Hagglund B, Sundqvist G, Wing K. Factors affecting long-term results of endodontic treatment. J Endod. 1990;16:498–504.
42. Dummer PMH, McGinn JH, Rees DG. The position and topography of the apical canal constriction and apical foramen. Int Endod J. 1984;17:192–8.
43. Chandler NP, Bloxham GP. Effects of gloves on tactile discrimination using an endodontic model. Int Endod J. 1990;23:97–9.
44. Rosenberg DB. The paper point technique. Part 1. Dent Today. 2003;22:80–6.
45. Rosenberg DB. The paper point technique. Part 2. Dent Today. 2003;22:62–7.
46. Williams CB, Joyce AP, Roberts S. A comparison between in vivo radiographic working length determination and measurement after extraction. J Endod. 2006;32:624–7.
47. Gordon MPJ, Chandler NP. Electronic apex locators. Int Endod J. 2004;37:425–37.
48. Sunada I. New method for measuring the length of the root canal. J Dent Res. 1962;41:375–87.
49. Nekoofar MH, Gandhi MM, Hayes SJ, Dummer PMH. The fundamental operating principles of electronic root canal length measurement devices. Int Endod J. 2006;39:595–609.
50. Kobayashi C, Suda H. New electronic canal measuring device based on the ratio method. J Endod. 1994;20:111–4.
51. Pagavino G, Pace R, Baccetti T. A SEM study of in vivo accuracy of the Root ZX electronic apex locator. J Endod. 1998;24:438–41.
52. Shabahang S, Goon WW, Gluskin AH. An in vivo evaluation of the Root ZX electronic apex locator. J Endod. 1996;22:616–8.
53. Fouad AF, Reid LC. Effect of using electronic apex locators on selected endodontic treatment parameters. J Endod. 2000;26:364–7.
54. Glossary of endodontic terms 2003. 7th ed. Chicago: American Association of Endodontists.
55. Buchanan LS. Management of the curved root canal. J Calif Dent Assoc. 1989;17:18–27.
56. Souza RA. The importance of apical patency and cleaning of the apical foramen on root canal preparation. Braz Dent J. 2006;17:6–9.
57. Goldberg F, Massone EJ. Patency file and apical transportation: an in vitro study. J Endod. 2002;28:510–1.
58. Siqueira Jr JF. Microbial causes of endodontic flare-ups. Int Endod J. 2003;36:453–63.
59. West JD. The endodontic glidepath: "Secret to rotary safety". Dent Today. 2010;29(9):86, 88, 90–3.
60. Berutti E, Cantatore G, Castelluci A, Chiandussi G, Pera F, Migliaretti G, Pasqualini D. Use of nickel-titanium rotary pathfile to create the glide path: comparison with manual preflaring in simulated root canals. J Endod. 2009;35(3):408–12.
61. Walton RE, Torabinejad M. Principles and practice of endodontics. 2nd ed. W.B. Saunders Company; 1996. Chapter 13 Cleaning and shaping, p. 210.
62. Wu MK, Barkis D, Roris A, Wesselink PR. Does the first file to bind corresponds to the diameter of the root canal in the apical region? Int Endod J. 2002;35:264–7.
63. Byström A, Sundqvist G. Bacterial evaluation of the efficacy of mechanical root canal instrumentation in endodontic therapy. Scand J Dent Res. 1981;89:321–8.
64. Byström A, Sundqvist G. Bacteriological evaluation of the effect of 0.5% sodium hypochlorite solution in endodontic therapy. Oral Surg Oral Med Oral Pathol. 1983;55:307–12.
65. Byström A, Claesson R, Sundqvist G. The antibacterial effect of camphorated paramonochlorophenol, camphorated phenol and calcium hydroxide in the treatment of infected root canals. Endod Dent Traumatol. 1985;1:170–5.
66. Ørstavik D, Kerekes K, Molven O. Effects of extensive apical reaming and calcium hydroxide dressing on bacterial infection during treatment of apical periodontitis: a pilot study. Int Endod J. 1991;24:1–7.
67. Dalton CB, Ørstavik D, Philips C, Petiette M, Trope M. Reduction of intracanal bacteria using nickel-titanium rotary instrumentation. J Endod. 1998;24:763–7.
68. Rollinson S, Barnett F, Stevens RH. Efficacy of bacterial removal from instrumented root canal in vitro related to instrumentation technique and size. Oral Surg Oral Med Oral Pathol Oral Radiol Endod. 2002;94:366–71.
69. Aminoshariae A, Kulild J. Master apical file size – smaller or larger: a systematic review of microbial reduction. Int Endod J. 2015;48(11):1007–22.
70. Aminoshariae A, Kulild J. Master apical file size – smaller or larger: a systematic review of healing outcomes. Int Endod J. 2015;48(7):639–47.

Non-surgical Root Canal Treatment

4

Bobby Patel

Summary

A plethora of new technology in endodontics has been available over the last 30 years, yet the outcome measures of success have changed very little. The clinician must be aware that the goal of non-surgical root canal treatment is fundamentally a biological one and the instrumentation of the canal serves to facilitate this approach. Adequate irrigation, disinfection, antimicrobial medication and subsequent obturation and final restoration all play key roles in preventing reinfection. Key factors that can have a negative impact on outcome are discussed.

Clinical Relevance

Non-surgical root canal treatment requires careful preoperative assessment to determine whether the tooth to be treated is of moderate or high risk requiring referral. Satisfactory canal preparation during non-surgical root canal treatment can be carried out with nickel-titanium instruments using a variety of systems. Canal curvatures (specifically radius of curvature and angle of curvature) and calcified canals warrant particular attention, and a good understanding allows appropriate management without the risk of iatrogenic errors of canal transportation or file separation.

B. Patel, BDS MFDS MClinDent MRD MRACDS
Specialist Endodontist, Brindabella Specialist Centre,
Canberra, ACT, Australia
e-mail: bobbypatel@me.com

4.1 Overview of Non-surgical Root Canal Treatment

The principal aim of non-surgical root canal treatment is to prevent or cure apical periodontitis [1]. Elimination of microorganisms from within the root canal is based on sound biological and mechanical principles using antibacterial irrigation and disinfection techniques during cleaning and shaping procedures. A well-obturated root canal and final coronal restoration aims to seal this complex system entombing any remaining bacteria as well as preventing reinfection from the oral cavity (see Fig. 4.1). Our understanding of the endodontic infection continues to evolve, as cultivation methods including newer molecular techniques are refined [2]. A significant portion of the bacteria taking part in the microbiome associated with apical periodontitis still remain to be cultivated and phenotypically characterised

© Springer International Publishing Switzerland 2016
B. Patel (ed.), *Endodontic Treatment, Retreatment, and Surgery*,
DOI 10.1007/978-3-319-19476-9_4

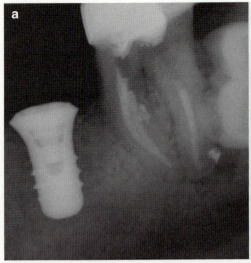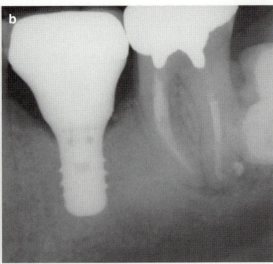

Fig. 4.1 Clinical radiographs demonstrating (**a**) immediate post-operative view of non-surgical root canal treatment of tooth 47 treated over the course of two visits using an intra-canal medicament. Preparation was carried out using ProTaper Universal files 25.06 and obturation using vertical compaction (System B and Obtura using AH Plus cement). Note adequate cleaning and shaping have allowed the lateral canal to be sealed in the mesial root. The acute apical distal curvature was maintained and apical patency confirmed with a seal puff. (**b**) Six-month post-operative view demonstrating well-placed coronal permanent cast restoration to ensure biological seal is maintained. Note the distal peri-radicular radiolucency has resolved. Nonsurgical root canal treatment has a 100 % capability of healing provided biological chemomechanical preparation and obturation have been carried out with strict adherence to common protocols. Nickel-titanium technology can produce predictable radicular preparations that can be easily obturated

[3]. The significance of these yet-to-be identified difficult-to-culture species is therefore limited and to this extent unknown to date. Further studies may provide the answers as to the biological role of these new taxa, their microbial pathogenicity and treatment strategies that may lead to future improvement in root canal treatment. To this end, the endodontic profession has benefited from numerous biological and technological advancements in an attempt to improve treatment outcomes.

However, in the last 30 years, despite these developments, there have not been any real improvements in terms of the outcome of treatment (success) and prognosis. Various cross-sectional surveys assessing root canal treatment outcome have repeatedly demonstrated a significant correlation between the presence of an apical radiolucency and a radiographically inadequate root filling. A recent systematic review confirmed a high prevalence of peri-radicular radiolucencies (PR) that vary from 0.5 to 13.9 % overall [4–7].

It is therefore obvious that certain treatment factors must potentially have an impact on treatment outcome. A recent study attempted to identify these factors and their influence on outcome measured by the periapical status of the teeth. This prospective study involved annual clinical and radiographic follow-up of non-surgical root canal treatment of 702 teeth in 534 patients carried out by endodontic postgraduate students for 2–4 years. Pre-, intra- and postoperative data was collected prospectively using customised data collection forms and investigated using multiple logistic regression models. Ten prognostic factors were identified. Four preoperative factors (the preoperative absence of a periapical lesion, in the presence of a periapical lesion the smaller the size the better the prognosis, the absence of a preoperative sinus tract and the absence of tooth/root perforation) and six intraoperative factors (achievement of patency at the canal terminus, extension of canal cleaning (and therefore filling) as close as possible to the apical terminus, abstaining from the use of 2 % chlorhexidine as an adjunct to sodium hypochlorite solution, absence of inter-appointment flare-up, the absence of root filling extrusion and the presence of a satisfactory coronal restoration) were all found to influence success based on periapical health associated with roots following non-surgical root canal treatment [8]. Interestingly the specific type of instrument utilised in mechanical preparation (stainless steel or nickel-titanium) had no direct effect on outcome. More importantly the biological factors indirectly related to preoperative and perioperative factors are what determine whether a case is successful or fails.

In order to improve the success rate of root canal treatment in general dental practice, the referral of difficult cases to dentists with advanced knowledge and training in endodontics may be appropriate. The decision to treat a case lies with the practitioner and should be based on whether the case is perceived to be treatable or beyond their abilities requiring a referral to a specialist endodontic practitioner. One can assume that, if a practitioner treats a case beyond his or her level of expertise, then there may be a greater likelihood of iatrogenic incidents that can result in an unsuccessful treatment outcome. The General Dental Council [9], the European Society of Endodontology [10] and the American Association of Endodontists [11] provide guidance for clinicians when making a referral. The American Association of Endodontists has published a form, which describes 17 areas that should be assessed when evaluating the potential difficulty of an endodontic case. Difficult cases that deserve particular attention and possibly the

need to refer include patient factors (complex medical history, difficulty with achieving anaesthesia, prominent gag reflex and significant pain and swelling), radiographic factors (difficulty obtaining radiographs, appearance of calcified canals, pulp stones and obstructions) and tooth factors (tooth type, inclination, canal curvature, canal morphology) (see Tables 4.1, 4.2 and 4.3).

Endodontic instrumentation plays an important role in the process of microbial elimination from root canal systems. Stainless steel instruments have been the principal material for fabrication of endodontic files until nickel-titanium alloy was proposed in 1989 [12]. Since its inception, nickel-titanium rotary files have become a routine part of the endodontic armamentarium enabling clinicians to treat straightforward cases in a timely and efficient manner. If one were to compare effectiveness with regard to elimination of biofilm from within the root canal system, no study to date has proved that nickel-titanium files are superior when compared to stainless steel [13]. Traditional stainless steel instruments are standardised to a taper of 0.02 mm/1.00 mm in length (2 % taper). Rotary instruments on the other hand have developed tapers ranging from 2 to 10 %. Due to the inherent inflexibility of larger-sized stainless steel instruments and to avoid canal transportation in curved canals, standardised preparation techniques proposed a final apical instrument size of #20 or #25. The clinician must be aware that nickel-titanium although inherently flexible due to the super elasticity is prone to canal transportation due to its other property of shape memory. Use of a 6 % or

Table 4.1 Patient risk factors that need to be considered when assessing case difficulty that may warrant further endodontic referral

	Moderate risk	High risk
Medical history	One or more medical problems	Complex medical history or serious illness/disability
Anaesthesia	Vasoconstrictor intolerance	Difficulty achieving anaesthesia
Patient disposition	Anxious	Uncooperative
Mouth opening ability	Slight limitation in opening	Significant limitation
Gag reflex	Gags occasionally	Severe gag reflex
Presence of swelling/pain	Moderate pain or swelling	Severe pain or swelling

Adapted from the AAE Endodontic Case Difficulty Assessment Form 2009

Table 4.2 Treatment considerations that need to be considered when assessing case difficulty that may warrant further endodontic referral

	Moderate risk	High risk
Radiographic assessment	Difficulty obtaining radiographs due to high floor of mouth, narrow or low palatal vault, presence of tori	Extreme difficulty in obtaining adequate radiographs
Tooth position in the arch	1st molar Moderate inclination (10–30°) Moderate rotation (10–30°)	2nd or 3rd molar Extreme inclination (>30°) Extreme rotation (>30°)
Tooth isolation	Pretreatment modification required for rubber dam isolation	Extensive pretreatment modification required
Crown morphology	Full coverage Bridge abutment Moderate toot/root deviation Teeth with extensive coronal destruction	Restoration does not reflect normal anatomy/alignment Significant deviation from normal tooth/root
Canal and root morphology	Moderate curvatures (10–30°) Crown axis differs from root axis Wide open apex (1–1.5 mm)	Extreme curvature (>30°) Premolars with more than two canals Lower incisors with two canals Canal division in middle/apical 1/3rd Very long teeth (>25 mm) Open apex (>1.5 mm)
Radiographic appearance of canals	Canal and chamber visible but reduced in size Pulp stones present Partial canal calcification	Indistinct canal paths Canal (s) not visible PCO present
Resorption	Apical resorption present	Extensive apical resorption Internal resorption External resorption

Adapted from the AAE Endodontic Case Difficulty Assessment Form 2009

Table 4.3 Additional considerations when assessing case difficulty that may warrant further endodontic referral

	Moderate risk	High risk
Trauma history	Complicated crown fracture Subluxation	Complicated crown fracture immature tooth Horizontal root fracture Alveolar fracture Intrusion Luxation Extrusion Avulsion
Endodontic treatment history	Previous access without complications	Previous access with complications Perforations Unlocated canal Ledging Canal transportation Instrument fracture
Periodontal-endodontic condition	Concurrent moderate periodontal disease Draining sinus	Severe periodontal disease Cracked teeth Combined perio-endo lesions Root amputation

Adapted from the AAE Endodontic Case Difficulty Assessment Form 2009

8 % tapered instrument in a curved canal can lead to either alteration in original canal anatomy or risk of file separation. Recently a proprietary method of thermo-mechanical treatment of nitinol wire was developed known as "M-wire". Vortex Blue rotary files (Dentsply, Tulsa Dental Specialities) alter the machined nitinol wire by a series of complex heating and cooling treatments resulting in a shape memory alloy that makes the instruments extremely flexible at room temperature [14]. Studies have demonstrated that rotary instruments manufactured from M-wire had significantly higher fatigue resistance, torsional strength, flexibility and higher deformation to failure when compared to conventional NiTi instruments [15, 16].

Nickel-titanium instrument development continues to strife forward in an attempt to improve flexibility and resistance using novel manufacturing processes [17, 18]. Novel instrumentation techniques such as the self-adjusting file (SAF) system (ReDent, Raanana, Israel) represent new concepts in root canal cleaning based on a hollow file that adapts itself to the shape of the canal rather than the conventional concept of shaping every canal to a round cross section and fixed taper according to the file system used [19]. Commercially available systems that have embraced the concept of reciprocation as opposed to the tried and tested rotation of files include Reciproc (VDW, Munich, Germany) and WaveOne (Dentsply Maillefer, Ballaigues, Switzerland). These systems utilise a "single file concept" through a counterclockwise cutting motion and clockwise rotation that have gained widespread appeal due to their simplicity [20]. At the same time, interest in irrigation research has not waned given the professions focus on the ease and predictability of rotary instruments to plane the canal walls efficiently. In spite of the ability to create tapered shapes of various sizes, studies have demonstrated the great extent to which canal walls remain un-instrumented. The delivery of intra-canal irrigants and its importance as well as an awareness of the biological impediments, in the form of biofilms, will no doubt lead to the introduction of new standards of irrigation in this field in the future [21].

Root canal preparation can be challenging in narrow calcified canals requiring a systematic approach for successfully negotiating canals to length. Coronally the presence of pulp stones can hinder access to the root canals and their subsequent shaping. Pulp stones have been described as compact degenerative masses of calcified tissue, which can be classified according to structure (true and false) and location (embedded, adherent or free). Embedded or adherent pulp stones within the root canal can result in significant occlusion of the canals or difficulty with negotiation if present at the curvature. Free pulp stones found in the pulp chamber may block access to canal orifices and alter the internal anatomy. Correct access cavity design, ultrasonic file use, hypochlorite irrigation and magnification should aid in the removal of pulp stones and present little difficulty during root canal treatment [22].

Pulp canal obliteration (PCO) or calcific metamorphosis occurs commonly in 4–25 % of traumatised teeth resulting in apparent loss of the pulp space radiographically and yellow discolouration of the crown. These teeth provide particular endodontic challenges with increased difficulties with location of the canal, negotiation of the canal, irretrievable instrument fracture and potential iatrogenic perforation [23, 24]. According to the American Association of Endodontist case assessment criteria [11], these cases fall into the high difficulty category.

Reactive and degenerative changes in the pulp as a direct consequence of pulpal irritants, insults and wear and tear can result in the phenomena of "calcified" or "sclerosed" canals. Pulp space diminishes throughout life by the regular deposition of secondary dentine. Pulp space can be further reduced by reactionary or reparative dentine (previously classified as tertiary or irritation dentine) as a means of reducing the porosity of dentinal tubules exposed to carious, traumatic or chemical insults. Reactionary dentine represents material laid down by existing surviving odontoblast cells. Reparative dentine,

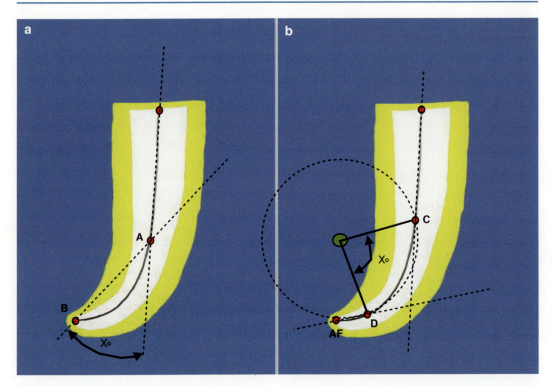

Fig. 4.2 Diagrammatic representation of the (**a**) Schneider measuring method and (**b**) Pruett et al. measuring method for determination of canal curvature. Note (**a**) a line is scribed on the radiograph parallel to the long axis of the canal. A second line was drawn from the apical foramen (Point *B*) to intersect with the first at the point where the canal begins to level the long axis of the tooth (Point *A*). These two lines intersect at an angle (*X*) as a measure of the change in direction of the canal in relation to the long axis of the tooth. Note (**b**) a straight line is drawn along the long axis of the portion of the canal. There is a point on each of these lines at which the canal deviates to the brain (Point *C*) or end (Point *D*) the canal curvature. The curved portion of the canal is represented by a circle with tangents at points *C* and *D*. The centre of the circle is thus the point at which the vertical lines intersect the tangents through *C* and *D*. This method allows calculation of the radius of curvature and angle of curvature of two independent parameters

on the other hand, is a new material laid down by new odontoblast-like cells, which have differentiated and migrated to the site of injury following the death of primary odontoblast cells. [25] In addition fibrotic changes within the root canal system can pose further challenges to canal negotiation with the increased potential of fibrotic pulp tissue compaction leading to obstructions that can be very difficult to overcome [26]. According to the American Association of Endodontist case assessment criteria [11], following radiographic assessment if the canals are obviously reduced in size or their path is indistinct or not visible, then these cases fall into the category of moderate to high difficulty.

Understanding root canal curvature is also of prime importance when carrying out instrumentation techniques in order to assess which taper will effectively shape the canal without the risk of either structural deformation of the instrument (and ultimately fracture) or iatrogenic errors including apical transportation, ledges, elbows, zips, perforations and loss of working length. Several methods have been described in the endodontic literature to determine canal curvature and more specifically the angle and radius of curvature [27]. Schneider proposed a radiographic method to determine canal curvature based on the angle that is obtained by two straight lines (Fig. 4.2). The first line is parallel to the long axis of the root canal. The second line passes through the apical foramen (point B) until it intersects with the first line at which the curvature starts (point A). The angle formed (X) allows the degree of curvature of root canals to be categorised into straight (≤5°), moderate (10–20°) or severe (25–70°) [28].

However, this method of canal curvature assessment did not consider the radius of curvature as a second independent parameter. Pruett and colleagues reported that the two root canals measured at the same angle in degrees by Schneider's method could have two very different radii or abruptness of curvatures. This radius of curvature had a significant factor on the number of cycles to failure of a NiTi engine-driven rotary instrument. As the radius of curvature decreased, instrument strain and stress increased and the fatigue life decreased. In other words, the smaller the radius of curvature, the more likely canal transportation or instrument fracture to occur. The authors graphically determined radius of curvature by drawing a straight line along the long axis of the coronal portion of the canal (see Fig. 4.2).

Along this line there lies a point at which the canal deviates to begin (point C) or end (point D) the canal curvature. A circle represents the curved portion of the canal, with tangents at points C and D. The centre of the circle is thus at the point where the vertical lines intersect the tangents through C and D. The change in direction of the long axis of the canal is described by the radius of the circle and by an angle or the arc length of this circle. The radius of curvature represents how abruptly or severely a specific angle of curvature occurs as the canal deviates from a straight line. The smaller the radius of curvature, the more abrupt is the canal deviation, which can result in file deformation and fracture [29].

Schäfer and colleagues proposed a modification of the Pruett method for measuring the angle of curvature, radius of curvature and also the length of curvature (Fig. 4.3) [30].

From a clinical standpoint, conventional radiography limits calculation on curvatures since unseen curvatures (in the bucco-lingual direction)

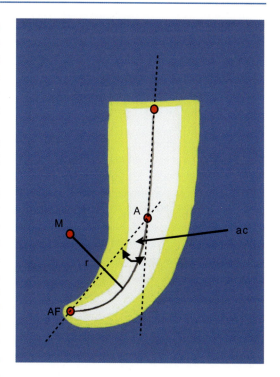

Fig. 4.3 Diagrammatic representation of the modified method proposed by Shafer et al. (2002) for measuring angle, radius and length of curvatures. A straight line is drawn along the outer side of the tooth canal in the coronal portion; this line is parallel to the long axis of the canal. The point where the canal deviates from this line to begin the canal curvature is marked (Point *A*). A second line is drawn to intersect the apical foramen (Point *AF*) with the point where the canal began to leave the long axis (Point *A*). The angle of curvature is formed between these two lines. The line between the point where the canal began to leave the long axis and the apical foramen is an arc of the hypothetical circle that defines the curved part of the canal. The curved part of the root canal between these two points *A* and *AF* is the circular arc of the hypothetical circle, which is specified by its radius (*r*). The radius of curvature can be calculated on the basis of the measured length of the arc based on geometrical principles of an isosceles triangle

can also play a significant role in the cleaning and shaping of canals. The use of cone-beam CT scanning has been advocated for determining canal curvatures, particularly in the labio-palatal direction, which cannot be seen using standardised radiographic techniques [31].

Despite the introduction of flexible nickel-titanium instruments and torque-controlled motors, root canal preparation of severely curved canals remains an endodontic challenge with risks of canal transportation, procedural errors or instrument fracture [32].

ProTaper NEXT instruments (Dentsply, Maillefer) manufactured from M-wire alloy and characterised by an innovative off-centre rectangular cross section, which gives the files a snake-like swagger movement during preparation, have been introduced specifically suited for the preparation of curved root canals [33]. ProTaper NEXT instruments have been shown to prepare severely curved canals (25–39° curved canals) up to a size 40 without an increased risk of canal straightening or canal transportation [34].

Recently, several different single file systems have been marketed with the ability to shape a canal with the use of only one instrument. WaveOne (Dentsply, Maillefer, Ballaigues, Switzerland) is manufactured from M-wire alloy, which is characterised by an increased flexibility and cyclic fatigue resistance in comparison with martensitic NiTi. These instruments are used in an alternating reciprocal motion of clockwise (CW) and counterclockwise (CCW) rotations [35]. These instruments have been shown to be safe to use even in severely curved root canals in extracted teeth [36].

4.2   Endodontic Case Assessment

Patient factors that may require endodontic referral include medical history issues, anaesthesia difficulties, uncooperative anxious patients, patients with limited mouth opening, patients with a prominent gag reflex or initial presentation of patients requiring further surgical management to alleviate acute symptoms (see Tables 4.1 and 4.2).

In routine cases such as obvious peri-radicular pathosis associated with a tooth, the diagnosis is usually straightforward. However, in certain situations such as irreversible pulpitis, where the patient cannot easily identify the offending tooth or cases where signs and symptoms are confusing as is synonymous with orofacial pain, then prompt referral may be necessary to ensure correct management and appropriate treatment is selected.

Treatment considerations warranting particular attention prior to commencing treatment include radiographic assessment of potential difficulties, tooth position in the arch, isolation problems, crown morphology, canal and root morphology, radiographic appearance of canals and extent of resorption present (see Table 4.2).

Additional considerations that should be assessed include history of trauma, previous endodontic history and periodontal-endodontic conditions that may all affect outcome if not correctly managed from the outset (see Table 4.3).

4.3   Pulp Stones and Coronal Calcifications

In order to locate calcified canal orifices, the clinician must first visualise and assess the pulp space dimensions on a two-dimensional radiographic image. Access preparation should be initiated, with this view in mind, and access burs directed towards the presumed location of the pulp chamber (see Chapter 1 for a more detailed discussion).

Accurate preoperative radiographs should be taken with a long-cone paralleling beam aiming device so that an initial measurement can be taken to ascertain depth of bur penetration (usually a distance of approximately 6.5 mm from the occlusal surface to the projected pulp chamber floor). Teeth that have undergone significant calcifications and diminished pulp volumes require particular care during access preparations. Depth of penetration to reach the underlying pulp will be less and overzealous preparation could lead to iatrogenic perforation. Teeth that have been crowned also require appropriate assessment of the crown-root orientation to ensure correct access preparation results in location of the canals (see Figs. 4.4, 4.5 and 4.6).

1. Once the pulp chamber has been located, the entire roof of the pulp chamber should be removed to facilitate straight-line access and unimpeded access to all internal anatomy. Use of a non-end cutting bur is essential, and the combination of ultrasonic, magnification and

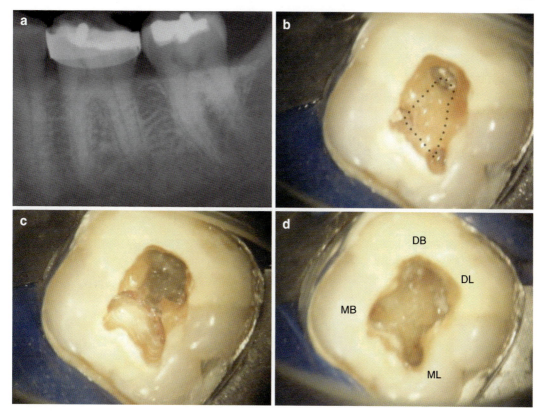

Fig. 4.4 Clinical radiograph and photographs demonstrating (**a**) pre-operative radiograph showing peri-radicular radiolucency associated with tooth 36. Referring clinician has carried out emergency pulp extirpation but had difficulties locating the 'calcified canals'. Intra-operative dental operating microscopic views show (**b**) intact root of pulp chamber and (**c, d**) unroofing and ultrasonic troughing carried out to reveal internal anatomy with straight line access of all four canals. Canals could be easily negotiated to length

illumination is invaluable (see Fig. 4.4 and Chap. 1 also for more detailed discussion).

2. Any pulp stones encountered in the coronal pulp chamber should be removed prior to initial instrumentation of any canals to avoid the risk of any stones becoming dislodged into the root canals and becoming compacted apically resulting in blockage and further difficulties with negotiation (see Fig. 4.5). If a pulp stone accidently falls into one of the root canals, then early identification is essential. Never introduce a large-sized file (#20 or more), which will further increase the chance of blockage by pushing the stone further apically. Instead small hand files (#08 and #10 Hedstroem files) should be introduced, initially bypassing the blockage, and

then used in a pull motion in an attempt to engage the stone more coronally.

3. Intermittent flushing with sodium hypochlorite solution is advised to facilitate this process. If all coronal calcifications and pulp stone remnants are removed effectively, then this minimises any risks during canal cleaning and shaping procedures.

4.4 Location of Canal Orifices

The pulpal floor should be carefully examined with prior knowledge from preoperative radiographs and likely anatomy based on tooth type to indicate probable number of canals expected. A DG-16 probe should be used with firm probing

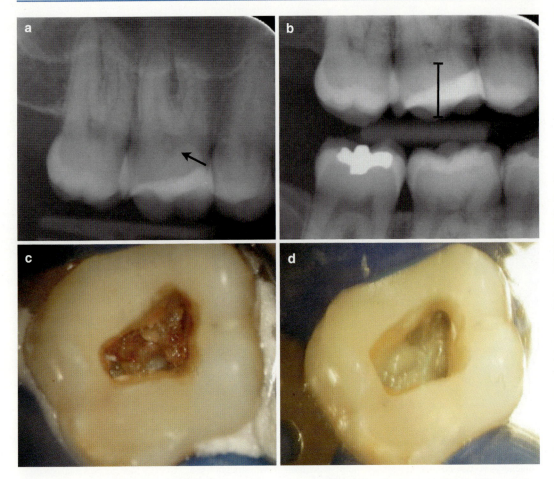

Fig. 4.5 Clinical radiographs and photographs demonstrating (**a**) pre-operative long-cone parallel radiograph demonstrating calcified coronal pulp chamber (*black arrow*). Tooth 16 presented with irreversible pulpitis and history of cracked tooth syndrome. (**b**) Parallel bitewing radiograph confirms radiopaque mass in coronal pulp chamber suggestive of pulp stones. Depth of bur penetration to roof of pulp chamber can be measured prior to access preparation. (**c**) Following access preparation pulp stones present in pulp chamber and (**d**) following use of ultrasonic refinement and troughing root canal anatomy can be seen

for signs of any "sticking" associated with the presence of a canal orifice. Once a suspected orifice is found, the canal should be checked for patency using small fine instruments such as a #08 or #10 K file. Use of a #6 file can be reserved for very fine calcified canals, but due their inherent lack of stiffness, any calcifications encountered during file penetration will result in the file bending and deflecting.

Occasionally there may be a curvature in the coronal aspect of the root canal making initial file penetration difficult. Removal of any cervical interference is mandatory to ensure straight-line access and minimal interference.

1. In cases of calcified canals, preoperative films will indicate how far the canal is calcified indicated by whether the canal is easily visible and traceable on the radiograph or not.
2. If coronal calcifications are present, then initial instrumentation will be very difficult. The first step is to identify the actual location of the orifice. Using the laws of symmetry and visualisation of the access cavity with knowledge of anatomy, the clinician should begin to get an idea as to where the suspected canal orifice lies.
3. Ultrasonic troughing in this area should help in the removal of coronal calcifications, which

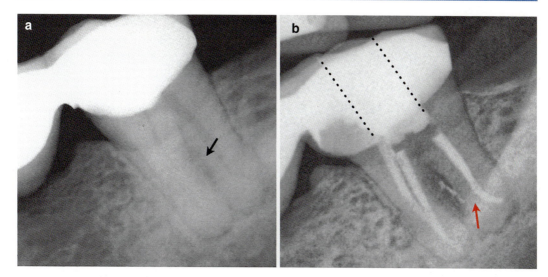

Fig. 4.6 Clinical demonstrating (**a**) pre-operative long-cone parallel radiograph demonstrating peri-radicular infection associated with distal bridge abutment tooth 47. Note inter-radicular lucency (*black arrow*). (**b**) Post operative view demonstrating final obturation following two visit non surgical endodontic therapy. Access preparation was completed through the bridge abutment. Orientation for access was made using the long axis of the tooth (*dotted lines*). Note lateral canal obturated in distal root resulting in sealer extrusion (*red arrow*). Distal apical curvature maintained to ensure patency and obturation to length

may obstruct the canal entrances. Care must be taken to avoid perforation with excessive tooth structure removal, and use of burs is not recommended.

4.5   Calcified Canal Negotiation

Once the canal orifice has been located, a 21 or 25 mm #08 K file should be selected for all calcified canals for negotiation to the apical foramen. In normal patent canals, the use of a #10 K file will be adequate. A rubber stop should be present on the shaft of the instrument with one directional point to indicate the direction of the curvature. The instrument should be advanced slowly using copious irrigation (sodium hypochlorite solution) to enhance debris removal and canal and file lubrication and ensure that debris is always flushed coronally rather than risk compaction apically resulting in further blockage. Files can be advanced in a careful watch-winding motion (see Chapter 3) until resistance is met. The instrument should always be withdrawn and flutes cleaned and inspected for signs of any unwanted unwinding requiring the file to be discarded. Once a fine instrument (#08 or 10) has reached the approximate working length, it should be verified using an apex locator and working length radiograph (initial apical file (IAF)) before withdrawing. Patency filing using a #06 file will be useful to ensure no apical blockage occurs (see Chapter 3).

1. Instruments should be pre-curved to simulate canal curvature in the apical 3–4 mm.
2. Manual or rotary glide path preparation should be carried out once working length is confirmed. At this stage, insertion of a #20 file to working length will alert you to how easy or difficult canal preparation will be. Removal of the file and inspection of curvatures will also reveal where the canal curvature begins, the length of canal curvature present and angle of curvature. Inspection of the file will also reveal the presence of any "hidden curvatures" not detected radiographically (i.e. in a bucco-lingual plane).
3. Use of rotary instruments in cases of confluent canals, moderate-severe curvatures, S-shaped curvatures, double curvatures and long teeth should be excised with care to avoid canal transportation or file separation.

4.6   Pulp Canal Obliteration

Pulp canal obliteration or calcific metamorphosis is defined as "a pulpal response to trauma that is characterized by rapid deposition of hard tissue within the canal space; the entire space may appear obliterated radiographically due to extensive deposition, even though some portion of the pulp space may remain in histological sections". This calcification process commonly occurs as a consequence of dental and occlusal trauma or orthodontic treatment. Often these types of teeth may not respond to vitality testing or exhibit delayed or diminished responses. Radiographically the diagnosis of partial or complete pulp obliteration does not indicate the need for root canal therapy. Clinical and radiographic signs and symptoms indicative of apical periodontitis or pulpal necrosis are the only indications for treatment. Root canal treatment of these cases can be fraught with difficulty if not impossible in some instances. Calcifications can partially or completely block and obscure access into the root canal system resulting in technical challenges with risk of iatrogenic perforation if care is not taken (see Figs. 4.7 and 4.8).

1. An accurate preoperative radiograph is essential to identify the pulp space, expected depth of patent pulp space if present and long axis orientation of the tooth in question.
2. Initial access preparation should be created with high-speed tapered diamond burs and outline placed more cervically in case of calcified anterior teeth (just behind the incisal edge). Orientation of bur penetration should be in relation to the long axis of the tooth to ensure correct alignment. Initial penetration should be at a level just below the cement-enamel junction. At this point, the cavity should be inspected using a clean mirror with good lighting and preferably magnification.
3. Use of a DG-16 probe can be used to assess whether any entry points or sticky spots exist

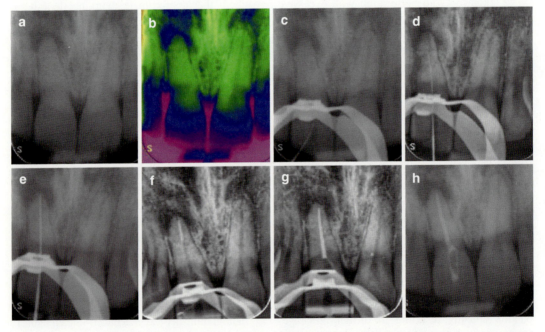

Fig. 4.7 Clinical radiographs demonstrating complete pulp canal obliteration in tooth 11. This patient had sustained trauma as a child. Note (**a**) and (**b**) preoperative long-cone parallel radiograph demonstrating no visible canal. (**c**) Following access preparation and ultrasonic troughing, 'a sticky point' was located using a small 10 K file. (**d**) Size 08 and 010 K files were slowly introduced further apically using a watch-winding motion and irrigation until apical patency was achieved. (**e**) Master apical file radiograph, (**f**) mid-fill radiograph, (**g**) backfill completed with System B and Obtura and (**h**) final obturation

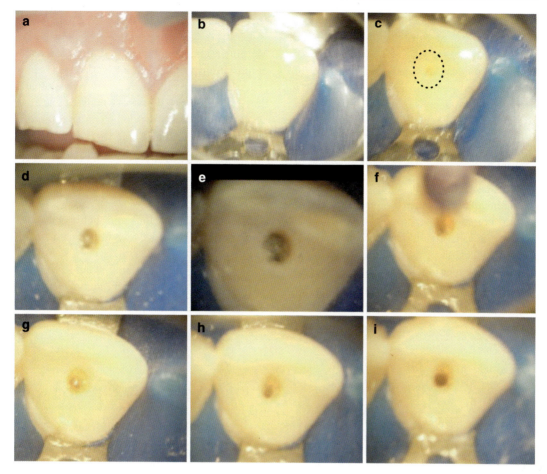

Fig. 4.8 Clinical photographs demonstrating cavity preparation pulp canal obliterated root canal of tooth 11 (as seen radiographically in Fig. 4.7). Note (**a**) and (**b**) preoperative views of labial and palatal surface, (**c**) initial bur penetration, (**d**) following bur penetration to the level of cemento-enamel junction as determined by parallel preoperative radiograph, (**e**) calcified canal system noted which was troughed using ultrasonics and (**f**) 10 K file used to locate 'sticking point' within calcifications. A check radiograph is taken at this point to verify position of file within canal, (**g**) copious irrigation with sodium hypochlorite and EDTA is used throughout, (**h**) patency achieved and (**i**) preparation and taper of canal increased to master apical size #30 with a 6 % taper

in cases of pinprick canal orifices. If no sticking is evident, then use of ultrasonic instrumentation or long-necked slow-speed burs is advisable. Care must be taken with orientation of either ultrasonic tips or burs to ensure that correct orientation is maintained. Radiographs should be periodically taken to confirm progress and whether realignment is necessary.

4. Having established a sticking point, files can now be used to attempt canal negotiation. Lubricants such as ethylenediaminetetraacetic acid (EDTA) can be useful to ease glide path entry. Use of C+ files (06, 08 and 10) is particularly beneficial due to increased rigidity. Small K files (sizes 08 and 10) can be used with the tip removed to create an end-cutting active file. Care must be taken since overzealous preparation attempts can result in canal transportation and possible perforation.

5. Files should be advanced slowly in a watch-winding motion until resistance is met. At this point, the instrument should be withdrawn. The canal should be re-irrigated

with sodium hypochlorite solution before attempting re-entry and further file advancement.

6. Files should be advanced slowly, and the clinician should feel whether a sticking sensation or tight resistance is met indicating the file is within the canal. Periodic radiographs should be taken to confirm correct canal advancement as opposed to an iatrogenic path that will lead to perforation. Heavy-handed approach to canal preparation will always be met with the incidence of either file separation or canal transportation.

7. Once apical patency has been achieved and working length established, canal shaping and cleaning can be modified with the use of larger tapered instruments.

4.7 Confluent Canals

Merging canal (confluence) requires early recognition during the cleaning and final shaping procedures to avoid unnecessary over-preparation in the apical portion, which can lead to canal transportation, stripping, root perforation or instrument fracture. One of the two canals will often reach the apex in a straighter path (main canal). The second canal (merging canal) will meet the first one at a severe angle (Fig. 4.9).

1. Using small hand files and tactile sense, the main canal should be identified and instrumented to working length.

2. The second merging canal should be instrumented to the point of merging only.

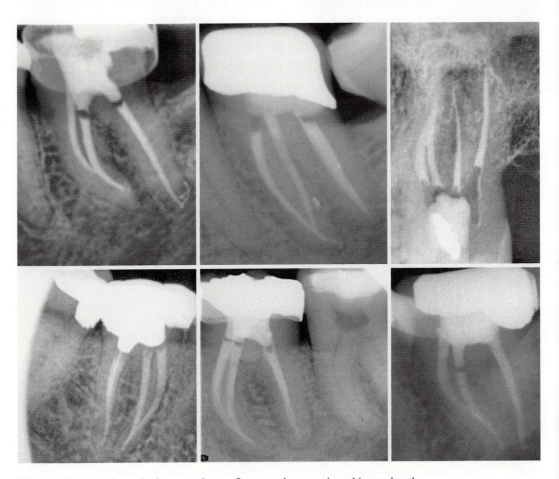

Fig. 4.9 Clinical radiographs demonstrating confluent canal systems in multi-rooted teeth

3. The main canal and merging canals should be checked for patency and recapitulated using small hand files.

4. Preparation of the main canal and merging canal to working length may lead to either file separation (at point of merging due to abrupt canal curvature) or canal transportation.

4.8   Clinical Guidelines for the Use of ProTaper NEXT Rotary Instruments

The ProTaper NEXT system (Dentsply, Maillefer) comprises of five instruments of multiple progressive tapers (increasing and decreasing) manufactured from M-wire that contributes towards greater flexibility, increased cutting efficiency and reduced contact between the dentinal wall and cutting flutes of the instrument, thereby reducing the possibility of taper lock and instrument fracture. The first instrument in the system is the ProTaper NEXT X1, with a tip size of 0.17 mm and a 4 % taper. This instrument is followed by the ProTaper NEXT $X2$ (0.25 mm tip and 6 % taper). The $X2$ can be regarded as the first finishing file in the system, and most canals could be prepared by using only these first two instruments. A further 3 finishing files X3 (0.3 mm tip and 7 % taper), X4 (0.4 mm tip and 6 % taper) and X5 (0.5 mm tip and 6 % taper) are available to increase both apical preparation size and overall canal taper.

The instruments have a bilateral symmetrical rectangular cross-sectional offset from the central axis of rotation. The exception is the X1 file which has a square cross section in the last 5 mm segment of the instrument to give it additional core strength apically. This design feature results in a rotational phenomenon known as "swagger" which further minimised contact between instrument flutes and dentinal wall during preparation. In addition to less stress on the file, the removal of debris occurs in a coronal direction due to the off-centre cross section resulting in improved cutting efficiency.

Clinical guidelines for the use of ProTaper NEXT instruments are as follows:

1. Create straight-line access and remove all coronal interferences. All triangles of dentine overlying canals should be removed using non-end cutting burs and ultrasonics to ensure no coronal interference is present.

2. Negotiate the canal to patency. Use either 08 or 10 K files until apical patency is confirmed. Confirm initial working length using apex locator and radiographs.

3. Create a reproducible glide path using either manual stainless instruments or rotary instruments. A reproducible glide path is confirmed when a minimum size 10 K file can be taken to working length, withdrawn a few mm and then lightly pushed back to working length using finger pressure. When a size 10 K file can be lightly pushed 4 mm from the working length with ease, then a reproducible glide path has been established.

4. ProTaper NEXT preparation sequence can begin. Copious use of sodium hypochlorite should be used throughout the procedure to ensure that organic and inorganic debris can be flushed from within the canals preventing apical blockage. Use of patency filing and recapitulation are essential in between files. The X1 is introduced into the canal (operating at 300 rpm and torque setting of 2.8Ncm). The file should be used in a touch and brush sequence whereby the file is allowed to passively move apically a few mm then withdrawn with an outward brushing action away from the danger zones (furcal areas and external root concavities). On removal of the file, the flutes should be inspected and debris removed before reinsertion and preparation to working length. The file may need to be inserted and removed 3–4 times before reaching working length. At this stage reconfirm patency, recapitulate to working length and irrigate.

5. The $X2$ instrument can be taken to full working length using the same protocol described in step 4. Care should be taken to ensure minimal contact at working length to minimise

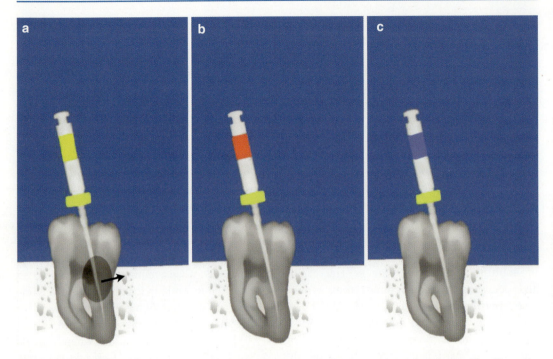

Fig. 4.10 Clinical radiographs of a mandibular molar demonstrating use of ProTaper Next files. Note (**a**) X1 tip size ProTaper Next X1, with a tip size of 0.17 mm and a 4 % taper. This instrument can be used to brush the canal walls on the outward stroke away from the danger zones (*black arrowhead*) and is followed by (**b**) The ProTaper Next *X*2 (0.25 mm tip and 6 % taper). The *X*2 can be regarded as the first finishing file in the system, and most canals can be prepared by using these first two instruments. (**c**) X3 (0.30 mm tip and 7 % taper) finishing file can be selected if the apical preparation size is deemed to be ISO size 30 at the apex

canal transportation risk. This file can also be used in a brushing action on the outward stroke, but care should be taken to prevent over-preparation and possible stripping in thin roots. Reconfirm patency, recapitulate to working length and irrigate (Fig. 4.10).

6. Apical gauging can be carried out using a 25.02 stainless steel hand file to check if the canal is adequately prepared. A light pressure should be placed on the file at working length to check whether the file moves in an apical direction indicating the apical foramen is larger than the size of preparation. If the file is snug at working length, then a master apical file (MAF) working length radiograph can be taken prior to intra-canal medicament placement and temporary seal (assuming multi-visit endodontics is being performed). If the file is not snug at the apex, then proceed to step 7.

7. Further apical gauging will be required to assess probable apical foramen size. Use of 30.02 and larger stainless steel instruments should be used to verify apical foramen size. Depending on file that is snug at length, proceed with either X3 (0.30 mm tip), X4 (0.40 mm tip) or X5 files (0.50 mm tip).

8. Care must be taken in canals with calcified canals, S-shaped curvatures, moderate-severe apical curvatures and long teeth which may require referral to a more experienced operator.

4.9   Clinical Guidelines for the Use of WaveOne Reciprocating Instruments

The WaveOne nickel-titanium file system (Dentsply, Maillefer) was first introduced into the dental market in 2010. It is a pre-sterilised single-use system that can create a continuously tapered preparation using a reciprocating file motion. The files work in a reverse "balanced force" cutting motion using a preprogrammed motor (X-Smart plus motor fitted with a 6:1 reducing handpiece)

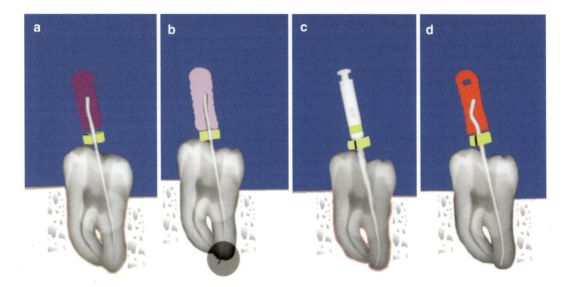

Fig. 4.11 Clinical radiographs of a mandibular molar demonstrating use of WaveOne file system. Note (**a**) initial negotiation of canal using a size 010K file to working length (**b**) patency filing using a 06K file 1 mm beyond apical foramen throughout the preparation sequence to prevent apical blockage (**c**) WaveOne Small file to length (ISO tip size 0.21 mm with a continuous taper of 6 % and (**d**) master apical file size to confirm preparation. In this instance a WaveOne Primary file would have been used to length. The MAF file is then placed in the canal and gentle pressure is applied to see whether the file is snug at the apex or moves apically indicating further apical preparation is required (apical gauging)

that is capable of moving the file in a back and forth reciprocating motion. The counterclockwise movement (CCW) of 150° allows the file to advance apically and engage and cut the dentinal wall. This is followed by a clockwise movement (CW) of 30° ensuring the instrument disengages preventing excessive torsional stress and the possibility of taper lock and instrument fracture. Three continuous reciprocating cycles will complete one complete reverse rotation allowing the instrument to advance apically.

Using a special thermal manufacturing process, the files are also made of M-wire, which has greater flexibility and resistance to cyclic fatigue. Three files are available in 21, 25 and 31 mm lengths. WaveOne Small file has an ISO tip size of 0.21 mm with a continuous fixed taper of 6 %. WaveOne Primary file has an ISO tip size of 0.25 mm with an 8 % decreasing taper from tip to shaft. WaveOne Large file has an ISO tip size of 0.40 mm with a continuously 8 % decreasing taper from tip to shaft.

Clinical guidelines for the use of WaveOne instruments are as follows:

1. Create straight-line access. Adequate access cavity preparation is essential in removing internal dentine triangles and interferences which can remove restrictive dentine.
2. Negotiate the canal to patency. Use either 08 or 10 K files until apical patency is confirmed. Confirm initial working length using apex locator and radiographs.
3. Create reproducible glide path using either manual stainless instruments or rotary instruments (as described earlier).
4. In most cases, a single file can be selected to instrument the canal. The majority of root canals (average length, mild-moderate curvatures apically or mid-root level) can be prepared using the WaveOne Primary file (25/08 red ring). If the Primary file fails to reach working length easily, then it may be necessary to prepare the canal first using a 21/06 yellow ring WaveOne Small file. If the Primary file reaches working length with minimal effort, it may be necessary to complete preparation using the WaveOne Large file (40/08 black ring) (Fig. 4.11).

5. Preparation is carried out with a progressive inward (light apical directed force) and outward circumferential brushing motion with the WaveOne instrument of choice in 3 mm cycles of apical advancement. Copious irrigation should be used throughout with checking that patency is maintained to prevent apical blockage. After each cutting cycle, whereby the file has advanced a few mm, the flutes should be inspected and cleaned. Failure to do so will result in a reduced cutting efficiency of the file and increased risk of file separation. Irrigation, check patency and recapitulate. The file should be advanced until working length has been reached.

6. Apical gauging should be carried out to ascertain whether preparation is complete or further apical refinement is necessary.

4.10   Curvatures

The majority of teeth exhibit various curvatures in multiple portions of the root canal system. Canal preparation in curved roots presents a technical challenge due to the increased risk of canal transportation related to the restoring force associated with an instrument that is used to prepare a curved canal. This can manifest itself in an increased amount of dentine removal at both the outer aspect of the apical curvature and inner aspect of the coronal curvature. The other major issue when treated curved roots is the risk of instrument fracture inside the root canal during the preparation sequence. In clinical practice, instrument fracture occurs as a result of either torsional fracture or flexural fatigue. Torsional fracture occurs when part of the instrument binds to the dentine whilst the file continues to rotate. Flexural fatigue, on the other hand, occurs when the instrument freely rotates around a curvature generating tension and compression cycles in the region of maximum flexure until inadvertent file fracture occurs.

It has been shown that there is a complex interrelationship between the degree of canal curvature and radius of curvature and length of curvature that can contribute to instrument

fracture and canal transportation. Conclusions that can be drawn are that the greater the angle of curvature, the smaller the radius of curvature and the increased length of curvature all results in increased stresses placed on endodontic instruments used for preparation. Clinical methods to assess canal curvatures are limited to single curvatures measured on a two-dimensional radiograph in the mesiodistal plane. If multiple curvatures are present or the curvature is in the bucco-lingual plane, then an accurate assessment cannot be made.

Stainless steel instruments can be used to manually prepare curved root canals, but a balanced force technique would need to be used to minimise canal transportation. Larger-sized files are inherently stiffer and more rigid resulting in a reduced ability to follow the canal curvature (greater than ISO .20 mm). Pre-curving of stainless steel files is mandatory although in severely curved canals, risks of canal transportation and strip perforations are still very high.

A vast number of nickel-titanium rotary instrumentation techniques are available for preparation of root canals with increased efficiency and speed and reduced risks of canal transportation if used correctly. Canal curvature assessment, correct access preparation, coronal orifice enlargement using a crown-down approach, reproducible glide path preparation, adherence to manufacturer recommended rotational speed and torque settings, use of irrigation, correct manipulation of instruments and operator proficiency through hands-on training and treatment carried out on extracted teeth before proceeding to clinical practice should all aim to ensure safe use with minimal iatrogenic errors.

Mild Canal Curvatures (<5°)

Case 1 A 48-year-old male patient was referred to the clinic with history of localised pain in tooth 16. Clinically tooth 16 was tender to percussion. Preoperative radiograph revealed an extensive coronal restoration overlying the pulp space. A peri-radicular radiolucency was noted with the palatal root (Fig. 4.12). A diagnosis of acute exacerbation of chronic apical periodontitis was

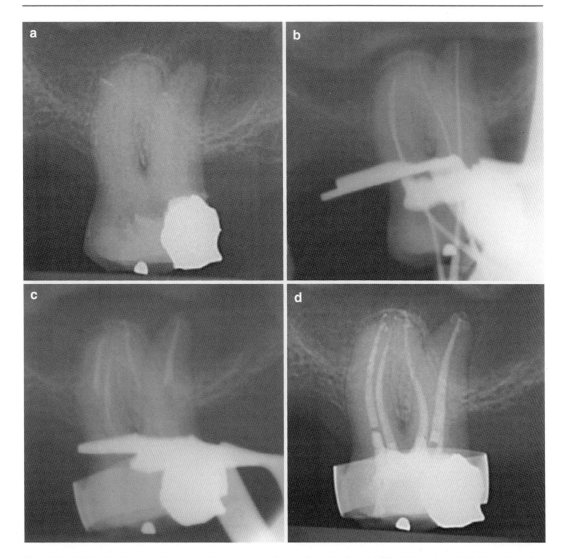

Fig. 4.12 Clinical radiographs demonstrating non-surgical root canal treatment of tooth 16 with mild canal curvatures (Case 1). Note (**a**) preoperative radiograph, (**b**) MAF radiograph, (**c**) mid-fill radiograph and (**d**) final obturation. Mild curvatures were noted in all 4 canals

made. After administration of local anaesthesia, rubber dam was placed. Initial access was made using a tapered diamond bur and access refinement carried out with the Endo Z bur (Dentsply Maillefer, Ballaigues, Switzerland). Ultrasonic troughing was carried out revealing an additional MB2 canal. Initial negotiation and scouting of all the canals was with a .010 stainless steel hand file. Working lengths were verified using the Root ZX apex locator (J. Morita Inc., Kyoto, Japan). Glide path creation was carried out using Pathfiles sizes 1–3. A crown-down instrumenta-tion technique using ProTaper Universal files was carried out using S1, S2, F1 and F2 files to working length using copious irrigation (sodium hypochlorite solution), recapitulation and patency filing. Master apical file sizes were confirmed radiographically (Fig. 4.12). An intra-canal dressing of calcium hydroxide was placed for 4 weeks. At the obturation appointment, the canals were irrigated with sodium hypochlorite solution, followed by saline and a final rinse of EDTA solution. The canals were dried, and a warm vertical compaction technique (System B and

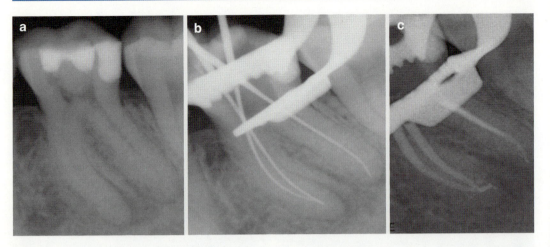

Fig. 4.13 Clinical radiographs of a mandibular left first molar demonstrating the use of WaveOne file system. Note (**a**) preoperative radiograph demonstrating mild curvatures in both mesial and distal root. (**b**) Working length radiograph following completion of preparation confirm- ing mesial confluence. (**c**) Obturation of canals with a warm vertical compaction technique. AH Plus cement using System B and Obtura. Complex apical anatomy sealed due to maintenance of patency filing throughout

Obtura) was used to obturate the canals using AH Plus cement (Fig. 4.12). The tooth was re-temporised with a double seal and the patient referred back to the general dental practitioner for further restorative work.

Case 2 A 34 year-old fit and healthy patient was referred for endodontic management of tooth 36. The general dental practitioner had carried out endodontic extirpation. Radiographic examination confirmed prior endodontic access. Mild curvatures were noted in the mesial root with periradicular radiolucencies noted (see Fig. 4.13). Access cavity was refined, working lengths were established and confluence of the mesial canals was noted. Apical patency was maintained throughout, and MB and ML canals had separate apical foramina. Chemo-mechanical preparation was completed using 1 % sodium hypochlorite solution and the WaveOne rotary system. All canals were prepared using the primary file (apical preparation size 0.25 mm). Following a 2-week dressing of calcium hydroxide, the patient was seen for obturation of the canals (see Fig. 4.13).

Moderate Canal Curvatures (10–20°)

Case 1 A fit and healthy patient underwent non-surgical root canal therapy of tooth 16. Initial scouting of the mesio-buccal root revealed multiple curvatures. Manual hand files were carefully introduced to working length to facilitate an unobstructed glide path with minimal transportation along the S-shaped curvature. Canal blockage was prevented by repeated recapitulation, and use of copious irrigation ensuring patency was maintained with a small #06 K file. Rotary preparation was completed using the ProTaper Universal system. The mesio-buccal root was prepared using the F1 finishing file only, whereas the DB and P canals were shaped using the F2 and F4, respectively (see Fig. 4.14).

Case 2 A 54-year-old well-controlled asthmatic was seen for non-surgical root canal therapy of tooth 16. A draining sinus was noted adjacent to the tooth in the alveolar mucosa. A preoperative gutta-percha sinus tracing confirmed periradicular infection associated with the complex root canal anatomy. The coronal pulp chamber appeared diminished in size with calcification of respective canals. Following careful access preparation and ultrasonic troughing, 4 canals were noted. Patency was maintained through chemomechanical preparation stages. The case was completed using ProTaper Universal files with copious irrigation and recapitulation. The acute apical curvatures were maintained with stainless

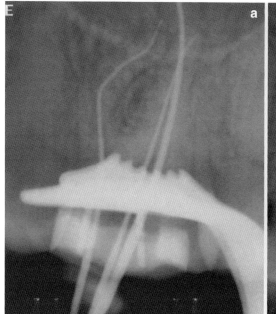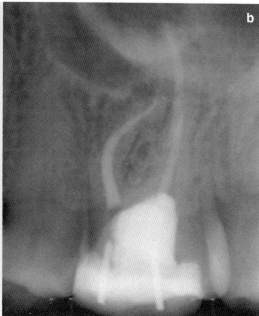

Fig. 4.14 Clinical radiographs of a maxillary left first molar demonstrating use of ProTaper Universal file system. Note (**a**) working length radiograph following completion of preparation confirming multiple curvatures in the mesiobuccal canal. This S-shaped curvature was easily prepared due to large radius of curvatures. A 25 K file could be easily placed to working length. Care was taken during the preparation procedure with manual glide path creation to a size #25. Note some straightening of the canal has taken place due to multiple curvatures, (**b**) obturation of canals with a warm vertical compaction technique and AH Plus cement using System B and Obtura

steel #10 K files. An intra-canal dressing of calcium hydroxide was placed and the patient reviewed 4 weeks later. The draining sinus had resolved and the patient remained asymptomatic. A further appointment was scheduled for obturation of the case (see Figs. 4.15 and 4.16).

Severe Canal Curvatures (25–70°)

Case 1 An anxious patient was referred for non-surgical endodontic treatment of tooth 26. Medically the patient was fit and healthy, and a decision was made to treat the patient using oral sedation (diazepam). Working length preparation confirmed multiple curvatures and an acute coronal curvature in the MB root which required particular attention to avoid instrument fracture. Canals were prepared using patency filing, recapitulation and the use of the ProTaper NEXT file system. The MB and DB roots were finished using the *X*2 file. The Palatal canal was prepared to the X3. The case was completed 4 weeks later following an intra-canal dressing of calcium hydroxide. An interim

orthodontic band was placed following completion of treatment since the patient had been aware of pain on release prior to endodontic treatment commencement. S-shaped curve preparation of the DB root canal was facilitated by unobstructive glide path creation and brushing of the X1 file to relocate the DB coronal curvature. Care must always be taken to ensure brushing of the file is carried out on withdrawal away from the danger zone where risk of strip perforation is high (Fig. 4.17).

Case 2 A fit and healthy 56-year-old female patient was referred for irreversible pulpitis associated with tooth 26. Preoperative radiograph indicated a severe acute apical curvature associated with the mesio-buccal root. The true extent of this curvature was not revealed until initial scouting with a 10 K file. Manual glide path was created with stainless steel hand files up to size #20. A decision was made to prepare the MB root to a size #20 due to risk of iatrogenic perforation. Canal shaping was completed using ProTaper Universal files following working length deter-

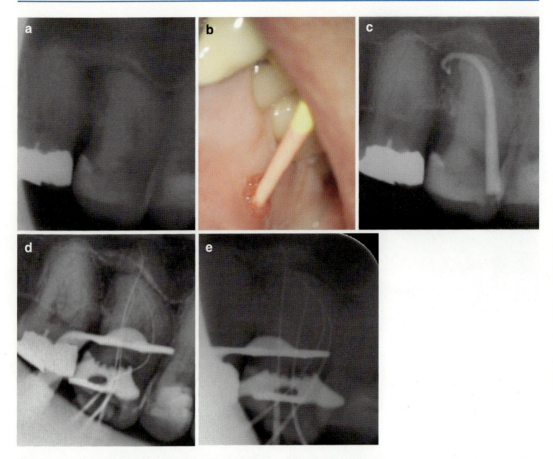

Fig. 4.15 Clinical radiographs and photographs demonstrating non-surgical root canal treatment of tooth 16. Note (**a**) preoperative radiograph demonstrating moderate curvatures and possible fused root anatomy with MB and DB apices. The root canals appeared calcified. A periradicular lesion was noted. (**b**) Gutta-percha placed in sinus tract adjacent to tooth 16, (**c**) gutta-percha sinus tracing radiograph confirming diagnosis of chronic apical periodontitis with suppuration and (**d**) initial working length radiograph confirming apical curvatures. Ultrasonic troughing revealed an additional MB2 canal. (**e**) MAF radiograph. Note preparation size to #25 and apical patency maintained to ensure access to peri-radicular infection. An intra-canal dressing of calcium hydroxide was for 4 weeks

mination. Copious irrigation was used throughout with 1 % sodium hypochlorite solution and alternate 17 % EDTA solution and saline flushes between irrigants. Recapitulation was maintained throughout to ensure apical blockage did not occur. An intra-canal dressing of calcium hydroxide was placed for a 4-week period prior to obturation of the case. The case was completed using a warm vertical compaction technique (System B and Obtura). The patient was referred to her general dental practitioner for cast restoration placement. The patient was reviewed at 6 years confirming no associated pathosis (see Figs. 4.18 and 4.19).

4.11   S-Shaped Canals

Double curvatures or S-shaped canals describe the clinical scenario where two or more curves are present in the same root canal. This type of geometry can be very challenging with high risk of anatomical deviation (canal transportation) and loss of working length. Apical curve preparation requires careful management with increased risk of file separation if careful clinical judgement is not applied during the cleaning and shaping procedure. These double curves are usually identified radiographically if they are present in the mesiodistal plane. On occasion the double

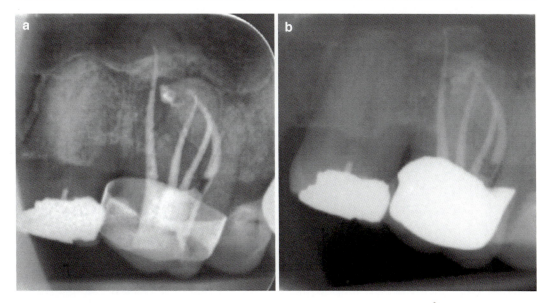

Fig. 4.16 Clinical radiographs showing (**a**) post-operative obturation and (**b**) 6-month review following placement of a cast cuspal coverage restoration. A warm vertical compaction technique and warm lateral compac-tion technique was used with AH cement. Note the sealer extrusion associated with the complex MB/DB root api-ces. At the 12-month review, appointment sealer is still present but the patient remains asymptomatic

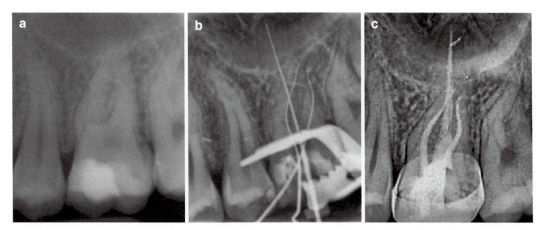

Fig. 4.17 Clinical radiographs demonstrating non-surgical root canal treatment of tooth 16. Note (**a**) preop-erative radiograph demonstrating an extensive amalgam restoration overlying a calcified pulp chamber. Note the acute coronal curvature in the mesiobuccal root. (**b**) Working length radiograph demonstrating acute coronal curvature in MB root and multiple curvatures in the DB root. (**c**) Final post-operative radiograph demonstrating cleaning and shaping procedures completed using ProTaper Next file system. A warm lateral compaction technique was used for obturation using AH Plus cement. Note lateral canal filled in palatal canal

curve may be present in the bucco-lingual plane and identified during initial preparation when the initial apical file is removed. Failure to ascertain a three-dimensional image of this curve may lead to iatrogenic preparation errors including strip-ping of the canal along the inner surface of each curve (Fig. 4.20).

1. During initial canal negotiation, scouting of the S-shaped curvature should be carried out with small .06, .08 and .10 K stainless steel files.
2. Working length should be verified using elec-tronic apex locator and radiographs.
3. Unobstructed glide path should be created using either manual or rotary files.

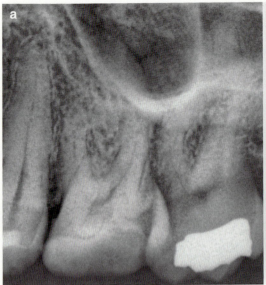
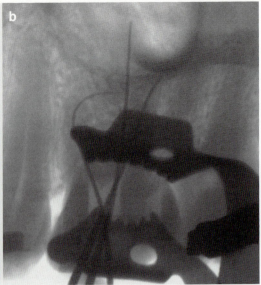

Fig. 4.18 Clinical radiograph demonstrating non-surgical root canal treatment of tooth 26. Note (a) preoperative radiograph demonstrating an extensive tooth-coloured restoration overlying a calcified pulp chamber. The mesiobuccal root apex cannot be clearly seen due to superimposition of surrounding anatomy. (b) Working length radiograph demonstrating the severe curvature in the MB root. Straight-line access was carried out and manual glide path created using stainless steel hand files

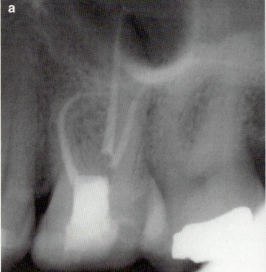
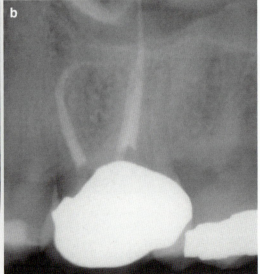

Fig. 4.19 Clinical radiographs demonstrating (a) final obturation (note straight-line access cavity preparation which helped minimize apical transportation in the MB root) and (b) 6-year recall demonstrating no apical patho-sis. The patient had remained completely asymptomatic. A cast restoration had been placed with excellent margins to ensure there is no risk of coronal leakage in the future

4. Canal enlargement can then proceed with caution using either a single rotary file system or hybrid technique (depending on suspected angle and radius of curvature).

5. Occasionally a hybrid technique may need to be employed with the use of engine-driven instruments to the first curvature and then hand file preparation in the second apical curvature.

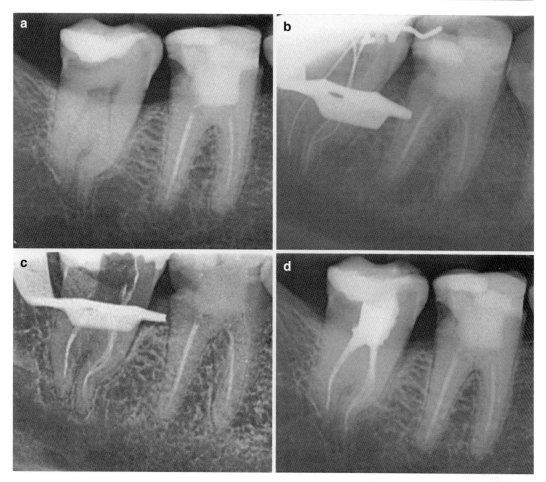

Fig. 4.20 Clinical radiographs demonstrating non-surgical root canal treatment of tooth 47. Note (**a**) pre-operative radiograph demonstrating S-shaped curvature associated with mesial root. Note also apical root anatomy is thin. (**b**) Working length determination confirming confluence of mesial canals with acute S shaped curvatures in MB and ML canals. Canal preparation was completed using 4 % Vortex Blue files (mesial preparation completed to ISO #20). Rotary glide path was created using Pathfiles. ML was prepared to point at which MB and ML canals co-join. Recapitulation and patency filing was invaluable to ensure optimal preparation was carried out. (**c–d**) Obturation of case completed using warm vertical compaction technique using AH Plus cement, System B and Obtura. Note access mesially refined to ensure straight-line access to prevent iatrogenic canal transportations

6. Blockage of the canal should be prevented by using copious irrigation (sodium hypochlorite), patency filing and recapitulation.

4.12 Extra-long Roots

Endodontic management of teeth with extra-long roots (greater than 25 mm) is no different to corresponding teeth of up to 21–25 mm in length. The critical difference is the inherent problems that can occur when establishing working length, performing instrumentation and completing obturation. From a mechanical preparation standpoint, longer instrument files sizes are available in 31 mm for both stainless steel and nickel-titanium rotary instruments. Radiographic assessments can be fraught with difficulty due to either superimposition of anatomical structures or difficulties in visualising the entire tooth during the treatment phase. Use of electronic apex locator devices is essential in collaborating radiographic findings when establishing working length determination. Canal preparation sequences do not differ although greater care may be required when managing curved canals and in particular

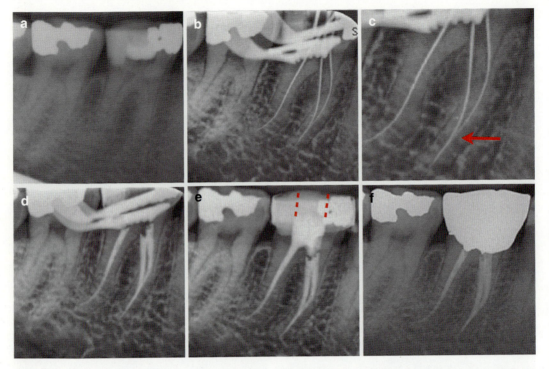

Fig. 4.21 Clinical radiographs demonstrating non-surgical root canal treatment of a mandibular right first molar with long roots. (**a**) preoperative radiograph demonstrating long roots. The case was referred due to difficulties negotiating the mesial canals to length. (**b**) Working length radiograph confirming 26.5 mm lengths mesially and 27 mm distally (**c**) presence of confluence in the mesial canals (*red arrow*). (**d**) Obturation of completed case following chemo-mechanical preparation using 1 % sodium hypochlorite solution and Protaper Universal 31 mm files. (**e**) coronal restoration replaced confirming straight-line access (*dotted red line*) and (**f**) 6-month review showing cast cuspal coverage restoration in place

reference to length of canal curvatures which can result in a greater propensity for file fracture. According to the American Association of Endodontist case criteria assessment, these teeth should be referred (see Fig. 4.21).

4.13 Hybrid Techniques

The more severe the curvature, the smaller the taper of the apical preparation should be and the more the clinician will need to reassess whether the existing file system and more specifically taper and apical file size will be adequate to accomplish treatment goals. On occasion a hybrid concept can be applied whereby the combination of instruments of different file systems can be used to manage individual clinical situations, thereby reducing procedural errors and still achieving biological treatment objectives. Risks of canal of apical enlargement in cases of severe apical curvatures may preclude the use of larger instrument sizes, although a minimum apical size of .20 will be necessary to facilitate biomechanical cleaning and shaping and final obturation (see Figs. 4.22, 4.23, and 4.24).

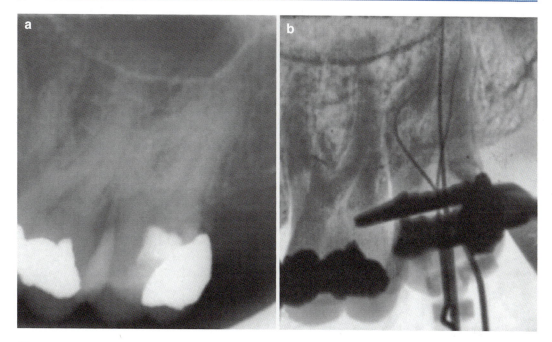

Fig. 4.22 Clinical radiographs demonstrating non-surgical root canal treatment of a maxillary left second molar (**a**) preoperative radiograph suggestive of some curvature in the mesiobuccal root. (**b**) Working length radiograph confirming multiple curvatures in the DB and MB root. The MB root has a double S-shaped curvature. This case is deemed to be extremely difficult not only due to existing root canal anatomy but also due to access difficulties often associated with upper second or third molar teeth

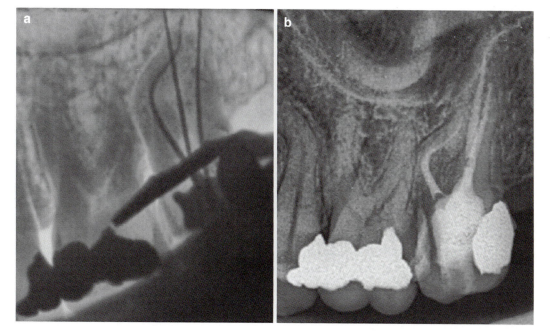

Fig. 4.23 Clinical radiographs demonstrating non-surgical root canal treatment of a maxillary left second molar (**a**) master apical file radiograph confirming preparation. The shaping was completed using a hybrid technique with ProTaper Next files and Vortex Blue. Minimal canal transportation of the MB canal. (**b**) Completed obturation using a warm vertical compaction technique with System B, Obtura and AH Plus cement

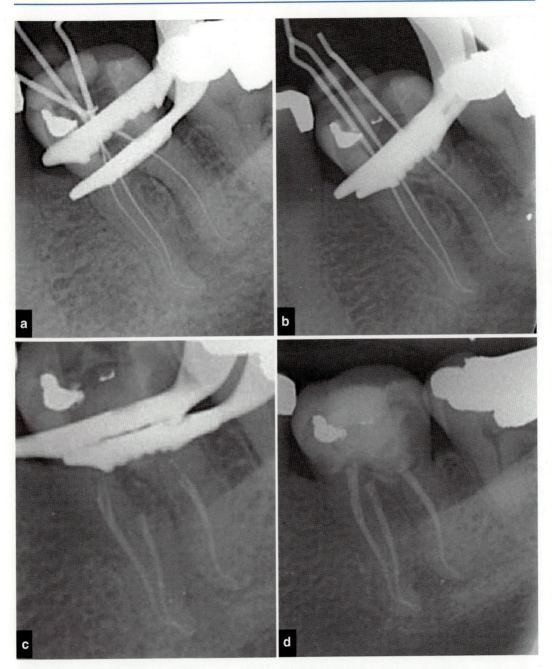

Fig. 4.24 Clinical radiographs demonstrating non-surgical root canal treatment of tooth 36 using a Hybrid technique. Files used included stainless steel hand K files and rotary Protaper Next and Vortex Blue. Note (**a**) Initial apical file, (**b**) Master apical file, (**c**) Mid-fill and (**d**) post operative radiographs. Multiple canal curvatures were maintained with apical patency

Clinical Hints and Tips for Managing Root Canal Anatomy

- **Calcified roots**

  Root canal calcifications, due to either tertiary irregular dentine deposition or dystrophic calcifications, pose negotiation challenges and increased risk of instrument separation.

- **Confluent canals**

  Canal systems that merge from two canals to one pose a special set of clinical challenges. Often an abrupt curvature exists where one canal merges with another which requires early recognition and due diligence to ensure careful negotiation and glide path preparation to prevent file separation.

- **Canal curvatures**

  Canal curvatures may not always be appreciated radiographically as often the curvature may exist in a buccal to lingual plane instead of a mesial to distal one. Occasionally a double curvature may be present in multiple planes (S-shaped canals). Management of any curvature requires the use of gentle pressure and ensuring a reproducible glide path is attainable with small tapered files (0.02) before proceeding to canal enlargement with larger files.

- **Instrument fracture**

  When an instrument is placed in a curved canal, it will undergo deformation and stress. Rotation of the instrument results in tension-compression of the instrument with greatest stress in the area of the curvature. Larger stiffer instruments will undergo greater stress compared to smaller instruments when confined to the same curved canal shape. Cyclic fatigue of any instrument is determined by specific parameters of canal radius, canal angle and instrument diameter.

References

1. Ørstavik D, Pitt-Ford TR. Apical periodontitis: microbial infection and host responses. In: Ørstavik D, Pitt-Ford TR, editors. Essential endodontology. Prevention and treatment of apical periodontitis. Oxford: Blackwell Science; 1998.
2. Sizova MV, Hohmann T, Hazen A, Paster BJ, Halem SR, Murphy CM, Panikov NS, Epstein SS. New approaches for isolation of previously uncultivated oral bacteria. Appl Environ Microbiol. 2012;78:194–203.
3. Rôças IN, Neves MAS, Provenzano JC, Siqueira Jr JF. Susceptibility of as-yet-uncultivated and difficult to culture bacteria to chemo mechanical procedures. J Endod. 2014;40(1):33–7.
4. Saunders WP, Saunders EM, Sadiq J, Cruickshank E. Technical standard of root canal treatment in an adult Scottish sub-population. Br Dent J. 1997;382–6.
5. de Moor RJG, Hommez GMG, De Boever JG, Delme KIM, Martens GEI. Periapical health related to the quality of root canal treatment in a Belgian population. Int Endod J. 2000;113–20.
6. Kirkevang LL, Òrstavik D, Horsted-Bindslev P, Wenzel A. Periapical status and quality of root fillings and coronal restorations in a Danish population. Int Endod J. 2000;509–15.
7. Pak JG, Fayazi S, White SN. Prevalence of periapical radiolucency and root canal treatment: a systematic review of cross-sectional studies. J Endod. 2012;38:1170–6.
8. Ng YL, Mann V, Gulabivala K. A prospective study of the factors affecting outcomes of nonsurgical root canal treatment: part 1:periapical health. Int Endod J. 2011;44(7):583–609.
9. GDC. Standards for dental professionals. London: General dental council; 2005.
10. European Society of Endodontology. Quality guidelines for endodontic treatment. Consensus report of the European Society of Endodontology. Int Endod J. 2006;39:921–30.
11. American Association of Endodontists. Endodontic case difficulty assessment form and guidelines. Chicago: American Association of Endodontists; 2009.
12. Walia H, Brantley WA, Gertstein H. An initial investigation of the bending and torsional properties of nitinol root canal files. J Endod. 1988;14:346–51.
13. Lin J, Shen Y, Haapasalo M. A comparative study of biofilm removal with hand, rotary nickel-titanium and self-adjusting file instrumentation using a novel in vitro biofilm model. J Endod. 2013;39:658–63.
14. Pereira ESJ, Viana ACD, Buono VTL, Peters OA, Bahia MG. Behaviour of nickel-titanium instruments manufactured with different thermal treatments. J Endod. 2015;41:67–71.
15. Campbell I, Shen Y, Zhou H, Haapasalo M. Effect of fatigue on torsional failure of nickel-titanium controlled memory instruments. J Endod. 2014;40:562–5.
16. Braga LC, Silva AC, Buono VT, Bahia MG. Impact of heat treatments on the fatigue resistance of different rotary nickel-titanium instruments. J Endod. 2014;40:1494–7.

17. Shen Y, Zhou HM, Zheng YF, Peng B, Haapasalo M. Current challenges and concepts of the thermo-mechanical treatment of nickel-titanium instruments. J Endod. 2013;39:163–72.
18. Ruddle CJ, Machtou P, West JD. Endodontic canal preparation: new innovations in glide path management and shaping canals. Dent Today. 2014; 1–7.
19. Metzger Z, Kfir A, Abramovitz I, Weissman A, Solomonov M. The self-adjusting file system. Endod Prac Today. 2013;7:189–210.
20. Yared G. Canal preparation using only one Ni-Ti rotary instrument: preliminary observations. Int Endod J. 2008;41:339–44.
21. Park E, Shen Y, Haapasalo M. Irrigation of the apical root canal. Endod Top. 2012;27:54–73.
22. Goga R, Chandler NP, Oginni AO. Pulp stones: a review. Int Endod J. 2008;41:457–68.
23. Amir FA, Gutmann JL. Calcific metamorphosis: a challenge in endodontic diagnosis and treatment. Quintessence Int. 2001;32:447–55.
24. Mcabe PS, Dummer PMH. Pulp canal obliteration: an endodontic diagnosis and treatment challenge. Int Endod J. 2012;45:177–97.
25. Smith AJ. Dentine formation and repair. In: Hargreaves KM, Goodis HE, editors. Seltzer and benders dental pulp. Berlin: Quintessence; 2002. p. 41–62.
26. Allen PF, Whitworth JM. Endodontic considerations in the elderly. Gerodontology. 2004;21:185–94.
27. Sontag D, Stachniss-Carp S, Stachniss V. Determination of root canal curvatures before and after canal preparation (part 1): a literature review. Aust Endod J. 2005;31(3):89–93.
28. Schneider SW. Comparison of canal preparation in straight and curved root canals. Oral Surg Oral Med Oral Pathol. 1971;32:271–5.
29. Pruett JP, Clement DJ, Carnes Jr DL. Cyclic fatigue testing of nickel-titanium endodontic instruments. J Endod. 1997;23:77–85.
30. Schäfer E, Diez C, Hoppe W, Tepel J. Roentgenographic investigation of frequency and degree of canal curvatures in human permanent teeth. J Endod. 2002;28:211–6.
31. Park PS, Kim KD, Perinpanayagam H, Lee JK, Chang SW, Chung SH, Kaufman B, Zhi Q, Safavi K, Kim KY. Three-dimensional analysis of root canal curvature and direction of maxillary lateral incisors using cone-beam computed tomography. J Endod. 2013;39:1124–9.
32. Bürklein S, Schäfer E. Critical evaluation of root canal transportation by instrumentation. Endod Top. 2013;29:110–24.
33. ProTaper Next: directions for use. http://www.pro-tapernext.com/benefits-concepts.html. Accessed on 26th Apr 2014.
34. Bürklein S, Mathey D, Schäfer E. Shaping ability of ProTaper NEXT and BT-RaCe nickel-titanium instruments in severely curved root canals. Int Endod J. 2014. doi:10.1111/iej12375.
35. Webber J, Machtou P, Pertot W, Kuttler S, Ruddle C, West J. The WaveOne single file reciprocating system. Roots. 2011;7:28–33.
36. Saber SEDM, Nagy MM, Schäfer E. Comparative evaluation of the shaping ability of WaveOne, Reciproc and OneShape single-file systems in severely curved root canals of extracted teeth. Int Endod J. 2015;48:109–14.

Irrigation and Disinfection

5

Mark Stenhouse and Bobby Patel

Summary

The role of microorganisms within the root canal system in causing pulp and periapical pathosis has been investigated and well documented. Bacteria that persist in biofilms show a wide range of characteristics that differ from planktonic cells including increased protection from host defence, increased antimicrobial resistance and the ability to survive and adapt despite ecological changes such as nutrient deprivation. Endodontic instruments alone have been shown to touch only 30–50 % of canal walls regardless of the instrument selected. When considering the complex anatomical irregularities (such as fins, isthmuses and recesses) within the root canal system, the emphasis on chemical disinfection and correct irrigation protocols are of paramount importance.

Clinical Relevance

The different actions and interactions of the most commonly used root canal irrigants are discussed. The clinician should be aware of the standard irrigation protocols for the management of both primary de novo infections and secondary failed cases. Common endodontic irrigants, methods of delivery and inherent risks are discussed including management of inadvertent sodium hypochlorite accidents. The clinician is also introduced to novel methods of disinfection that have been introduced in an attempt to reduce potential interactions that diminish the proteolytic and antimicrobial activity of sodium hypochlorite solution.

5.1 Overview of Endodontic Irrigation

Thorough irrigation of the root canal system is a critical step in the preparation and disinfection of the root canal system. Removal of vital and necrotic remnants of pulp tissue, microorganisms and microorganism toxins is achieved through chemomechanical debridement and is essential

M. Stenhouse, BDS, DClinDent (Endo), FRACDS
Specialist Endodontist, 1/40 Ridley St, Charlestown,
NSW 2291, Australia

B. Patel, BDS MFDS RCS MClinDent MRD MRACDS (✉)
Specialist Endodontist, Brindabella Specialist Centre,
Canberra, ACT, Australia
e-mail: bobbypatel@me.com

© Springer International Publishing Switzerland 2016
B. Patel (ed.), *Endodontic Treatment, Retreatment, and Surgery*,
DOI 10.1007/978-3-319-19476-9_5

for root canal success. While there is controversy over the antimicrobial effectiveness of intra-canal medication and its value in treatment, there is no such controversy when it comes to the importance of irrigation in reducing the microbial load within infected root canals [1–3].

Instrumentation alone is unlikely to rid the root canal system of bacteria [4, 5]. It is impossible to shape and clean the root canal system completely due to the intricate nature of the root canal anatomy. Even with the advent of modern nickel-titanium rotary systems currently available, we are only able to clean within the main body of the canal. Canal fins, isthmi and untouched avenues are often left untouched by our instrumentation techniques. However, based on current sampling techniques, antimicrobial irrigation should drastically reduce the microbial load over and above that achieved with instrumentation when applied to appropriately prepared canals and delivered in an effective way. In vivo studies have consistently found that instrumentation and irrigation consistently render 50–70 % of canals bacteria free when sampled with paper points [6–9].

Over the decades, numerous in vitro studies have been carried out to assess various irrigants and their antimicrobial effects. The interpretation of these results must be taken with due caution since the majority of studies have been carried out on single species planktonic bacteria which do not reflect the actual clinical environment in which we use these irrigants. In reality the modern understanding of root canal infections is one based on biofilms that is far more complex than previously understood [10, 11]. Biofilms are communities of bacteria that form on a surface and are embedded within protective extracellular matrix [12]. Biofilms are significant because studies have shown that when bacteria are embedded within a biofilm, they can be up to 1000 times more resistant to some antimicrobials compared to their planktonic state [13].

The ideal endodontic irrigant does not exist. This is because the ideal irrigant must fulfil a number of varying requirements, which in some instances are mutually exclusive. For example, tissue dissolution and irrigant safety are important properties for irrigation solutions but because

no solution is able to specifically dissolve pulpal tissue, it is never going to be perfectly safe if that solution is accidently extruded into the periapical tissues. The most important requirements of any irrigant include broad spectrum antimicrobial effectiveness, necrotic and vital tissue dissolution ability, smear layer prevention and removal, safety and economical for use [14].

Antimicrobial effectiveness is obviously important when treating the infected root canal system. However, it is probably less crucial when treating vital root canals where tissue dissolution is of paramount importance. Nonetheless, both these properties are still required in both infected and vital cases because tissue dissolution properties are needed for breaking down necrotic tissue and also bacterial biofilms. In addition, a degree of antimicrobial effectiveness is still needed in the treatment of vital pulps in case any residual bacteria may have contaminated a pulp after caries excavation or removal of a leaking restoration.

Smear layer is a layer of debris that is burnished to the wall of root canal by the instrumentation process. Scanning electron microscopy has shown the smear layer to be on average 1–2 μm thick on the dentine walls but can penetrate up to 40 μm into dentine tubules [15]. It is comprised of organic and inorganic material such as dentine filings and remnants of pulpal tissue and bacteria [16, 17].

There has been some controversy surrounding the removal of smear layer with one school of thought suggesting that the smear layer may actually prevent bacteria penetrating or escaping from dentinal tubules [18]. However, it is generally accepted that removal of the smear layer is desirable in order to remove potentially viable bacteria within the debris and remove necrotic tissue that may act a as nutrient source for residual bacteria left within the canal system or bacteria that may leak into the canal system in the future [19]. The smear layer may also limit the penetration of antimicrobials and sealers into tubules possibly affecting their disinfection and the seal obtained with obturation [19, 20].

Given there is no ideal irrigant that can meet all these requirements, it is more common in modern endodontics to apply an irrigation regime using two or more irrigating solutions. During the course of treatment, different solutions can be applied to the root canal system depending on the desired effect at a given time. For example, during the course of instrumentation, a practitioner may want to apply an antimicrobial irrigant in order to reduce the microbial load within the canal, but once instrumentation is complete, it is often desirable to then remove the smear layer which has no doubt been created. Alternatively, some practitioners may use a given irrigant to reduce the development of smear layer during instrumentation and then follow-up with an antimicrobial solution once instrumentation is complete.

Using two or more irrigants gives the practitioner the flexibility to choose irrigants with the most effectiveness for a given property so long as that solution is safe and economical to use. However, in so doing it is crucial they have an understanding of the properties of each irrigant and the potential interactions between irrigants.

Sodium hypochlorite (NaOCl) is the most commonly used irrigant in endodontics. It is a broad spectrum antiseptic as well as a solvent of organic tissue. In addition to being cheap and safe, when used with care, it ticks a number of boxes with regards to the previously mentioned properties of an ideal irrigant. However, its primary limitation is that it is does not effectively dissolve inorganic tissue and its ability to remove smear layer from the instrumented root canal walls has been found to be lacking [19]. It is produced industrially by passing chlorine through a solution of sodium hydroxide. In solution NaOCl dissociates into the anion OCl^- and cation Na^+ and then forms an equilibrium with hypochlorous acid (HOCl) that is pH dependent (Fig. 5.1). Pure sodium hypochlorite has a pH of around 12 at which OCl^- predominates [21]. Both OCl^- and HOCl are powerful oxidizing agents and are the active agents which exert the antimicrobial activity of sodium hypochlorite. Given it is typically used in its pure form, the high pH of sodium hypochlorite also provides additional tissue dissolving effects [22].

Sodium hypochlorite is a strong base (pH >11). The hypochlorite anion OCl^- can exert its action through non-specific degradation of proteins on cell wall, membranes and within cells. This causes the irreversible inhibition of normal cell metabolism that ultimately results in cell death and cell dissolution [22]. As this action is non-specific, sodium hypochlorite is an effective agent against bacteria, viruses and fungi but it is also active against normal healthy human tissue. This is advantageous when wanting to dissolve and remove pulp tissue but not when this irrigant is extruded beyond the confines of the canal affecting the periapical tissue.

Sodium hypochlorite is commonly used in concentrations between 0.5 and 6 %. Bryström and Sundqvist studied the effect of irrigation concentration in necrotic root canals. These investigators showed that using 0.5 % or 5 % NaOCl, with or without EDTA for irrigation, resulted in similar reductions in bacterial counts in the canals when compared to normal saline. Nevertheless, it was very difficult to render the canals completely free of bacteria, even after repeated sessions [6, 23]. In contrast Clegg and colleagues using an ex vivo biofilm study, comparing the effectiveness of 3 % and 6 % NaOCl, showed the higher concentration was more effective [24].

Higher concentrations of NaOCl have a better tissue-dissolving ability [25], although lower concentrations when used in high volumes with more frequent intervals to replenish the solution can be equally as effective [26]. The risks of toxicity increase as the concentration increases with any inadvertent extrusion beyond the confines of the root canal system risking serious irritation [27]. Furthermore, a 5.25 % solution significantly decreases the elastic modulus and flexural strength of human dentine compared to physiological saline, whilst a 0.5 % solution does not [28].

An alternative approach to increasing the effectiveness of NaOCl is to increase the temperature of

$$NaOCl + H_2O \longleftrightarrow NaOH + HOCl \longleftrightarrow Na^+ + OH^- + H^+ + OCl^-$$

Fig. 5.1 Mechanism of action of sodium hypochlorite (NaOCl)

low-concentration NaOCl solutions. The ability of 1 % NaOCl at 45 °C to dissolve human dental pulps was found to be equal to that of 5.25 % solution at 20 °C [29]. Even fast-acting biocides such as NaOCl require sufficient working time to reach their potential and the optimal time it needs to remain in the canal system is an issue yet to be resolved [14]. In summary the concentration of NaOCl is not critical, and the use of 1 % NaOCl can be recommended on the basis of less risk of tissue toxicity provided fresh hypochlorite solution is used and replenished frequently within the canal system.

As with any product used in the medical or dental field, potential toxicity is always an important consideration. Sodium hypochlorite is not genotoxic but has a non-specific cytotoxicity and can cause substantial injury if not used carefully [27, 30]. The same tissue-dissolving property that is desirable within the root canal will be equally applied if inadvertently extruded into the periapical tissues. And even though higher concentrations are more cytotoxic, lower concentrations can still cause tissue irritation and damage [31, 32].

Numerous case reports have been published in the literature of sodium hypochlorite accidents following its use as an endodontic irrigant. Symptoms include immediate severe pain, oedema of neighbouring soft tissue including possible extension to the lip and infra-orbital region, profuse bleeding within the canal, ecchymosis within the skin an mucosa of in the affected area, possible secondary infection and reversible or irreversible damage to vital structures. Inadvertent extrusion of sodium hypochlorite may be the result of open apical foramens due to incomplete root development or apical resorption, iatrogenic or pathologic perforations, lack of control of the irrigation needle depth, needle binding in the canal and use of extreme pressure when irrigating [27].

Extrusion of sodium hypochlorite can result in tissue necrosis to varying degrees depending on the volume and concentration of the irrigant extruded. It is considered to be a self-limiting process but can be extremely traumatic for patients and practitioners alike. Current treatment protocols for NaOCl accidents have been largely determined from numerous case reports. Early recognition is crucial and treatment is typically prescribed on a case-by-case basis including simple palliative care in the form of patient reassurance, pain relief and local anti-inflammatory measures. Antibiotics and steroids may be beneficial as adjunctive therapy and referral for specialist oral surgical management may be needed in severe cases [27] (Fig. 5.11 and Case 5.1).

Shelf life, storage and handling are also important factors that can affect NaOCl and its efficacy. Higher concentrations have been shown to lose their effectiveness faster than lower concentration [29, 33]. Even so they still have a very acceptable shelf life with concentrations over 3 % still easily lasting at least in the range of 3–6 months [21]. In contrast, lower concentrations of 1 % or under can remain stable at room temperature for up to 23 months [34]. This is provided they are stored are stored in appropriate conditions under 30 ° C and in their original high pH form. There is a school of thought that sodium hypochlorite buffered to a lower concentration has a superior antibacterial effectiveness, but this drastically reduces the shelf life of sodium hypochlorite [35].

The primary limitation of sodium hypochlorite is its inability to dissolve inorganic tissue. In the context of endodontic treatment, this translates to an inability to remove the smear layer that is caused during the instrumentation phase of treatment [15–19]. Ethylenediamine tetraacetic acid (EDTA) is a chelating agent used in endodontics for its ability to remove the inorganic component of smear layer (Fig. 5.2). EDTA acts by reacting with the calcium ions of hydroxyapatite to form soluble chelates that can then be rinsed from the root canal system [19]. Scanning electron microscopy has shown that with the use of EDTA, much less smear layer and thus much cleaner canals walls can be achieved than with using sodium hypochlorite alone [36].

However, EDTA alone has too many limitations to be used as a sole endodontic irrigant. It has very poor antibacterial properties. When Dunavant and colleagues tested EDTA against an *E. faecalis* biofilm it only had a 26 % kill rate compared to sodium hypochlorite's 99 % [37]. Furthermore, while EDTA is very effective at helping dissolve inorganic material it not effective at dissolving organic matter. Thus, it cannot be relied upon for tissue dissolution. For these reasons, EDTA is best considered an adjunctive

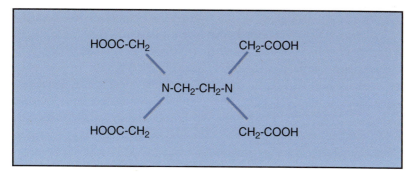

Fig. 5.2 Structural formula of EDTA (ethylenediaminetetraacetic acid)

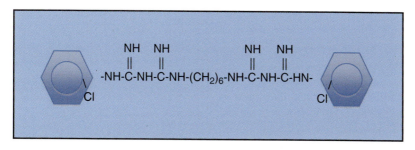

Fig. 5.3 Structural formula of chlorhexidine (CHX)

irrigant to be used in combination with other irrigants to supplement their antimicrobial and tissue dissolution properties.

EDTA is therefore most commonly used in combination with sodium hypochlorite. Indeed, smear layer removal has been shown to be most effective when both EDTA and sodium hypochlorite are used in conjunction [36, 38]. This is not surprising when considering the fact that EDTA will remove the inorganic component of the smear layer followed by NaOCl, which can then remove the exposed residual organic component. However, care must be taken when using EDTA and NaOCl together because it has been shown that NaOCl is deactivated in the presence of EDTA affecting its tissue dissolution ability and probably its antibacterial efficacy as well [39–41]. In contrast EDTA retains it chelating ability in the presence of NaOCl [42].

While it has been established that using sodium hypochlorite and EDTA in combination provides the cleanest canals, the ideal irrigation regime or sequence is a topic of some debate. A range of different combinations has been recommended. However, Goldman and colleagues found that the cleanest canals were achieved by using NaOCl throughout instrumentation and then finishing with a final rinse of EDTA followed by further NaOCl. It was surmised that the NaOCl dealt better with the larger amount of organic tissue that needed dissolving early in the instrumentation phase of treatment and thus reducing the amount of overall smear layer produced [40, 41].

Chlorhexidine digluconate (CHX) is a widely used disinfectant in dentistry because of its good antimicrobial activity. It consists of two symmetric 4-chlorophenyl rings and two biguanide groups connected by a central hexamethylene chain [42]. It is a wide-spectrum antimicrobial agent that is effective against bacteria and yeasts (*Candida albicans*) [43]. It is able to permeate the cell wall or outer membrane causing disruption of the bacterial cytoplasm, inner membrane or the yeast plasma membrane. Its low toxicity and inherent substantivity, due to its ability to bind to hard tissue [44], has led to its application in endodontics (especially re-treatment cases) as both an intra-canal medicament and irrigant (Fig. 5.3).

Numerous "in vitro" studies have evaluated the use of CHX comparing its antibacterial properties to NaOCl. Vianna and colleagues investigated the antimicrobial activity of two forms of CHX (gel and liquid) using three concentrations (0.2, 1 and 2%) against common endodontic pathogens. The results were compared to those achieved using NaOCl at five concentrations (0.5, 1, 2.5, 4 and 5.25%) [45]. Contrasting results were found when using a biofilm model. Spratt and colleagues evaluated the effectiveness of 2.25% NaOCl, 0.2% CHX, 10% povidone iodine, 5 parts per million colloidal silver and phosphate buffered solution (PBS) as a control against common monoculture biofilm isolates. They found the most effective irrigants were NaOCl, followed by iodine solution [46].

Unlike NaOCl, CHX has no tissue-dissolving capability so its sole use as an endodontic irrigant cannot be justified. Furthermore its effects on biofilm disruption have been shown to be less effective when compared to NaOCl solution [46].

The mixing of CHX with sodium hypochlorite solution has been shown to produce an orange-brown colour change and the formation of a precipitate. Basrani and colleagues used x-ray photoelectron spectroscopy (XPS) and time of flight secondary ion mass spectrometry (TOF-SIMS) to identify this precipitate. They showed the precipitate contained a significant amount of para-chloroaniline (PCA); a hydrolysis product of CHX [47]. PCA has industrial uses in pesticides and dyes and has been demonstrated to be carcinogenic. This has led to two main concerns, namely, the risk of precipitate leaching into the surrounding periapical tissues and also the occluding of dentinal tubules that could lead to reduced disinfection and/or resin penetration [48, 49]. Use of intermediate flushes of saline or distilled water and drying the canal prior to CHX irrigation may prevent the formation of PCA.

The combination of CHX and EDTA is known to produce a white precipitate. An investigation using reverse-phase high-performance chromatography analysed the precipitate formed when mixing 17% EDTA and 2% or 20% CHX. Based on the results, CHX forms a salt with EDTA rather than undergoing a chemical reaction [50].

Iodine compounds exhibit significant antimicrobial properties against both Gram-positive and Gram-negative bacteria and yeasts (*Candida albi-*

cans). Iodine potassium iodide (IKI) is the most commonly used iodine compound as an endodontic irrigant as a solution of 2% iodine in 4% potassium iodide [51]. Two percent IKI has shown less toxicity and tissue irritation compared to formocresol, camphorated monoparachlorophenol, CHX and sodium hypochlorite [52]. There is a body of opinion that has suggested the use of alternative intra-canal irrigation protocols when undergoing root canal retreatments. The school of thought has been that the causative persistent microbe responsible for failing or failed cases may be more resistant to the common endodontic irrigants used [53, 54]. Safavi and colleagues demonstrated in vitro using human teeth that 2% IKI treatment for a period of 1–2 h was sufficient to disinfect dentine. In contrast bacteria remained viable in the dentine even after relatively extended periods of calcium hydroxide treatment (24 h) [55]. IKI has no tissue-dissolving capacity, and so its use like CHX may be recommended following completion of chemomechanical preparation as an adjunctive intra-canal medicament or final antiseptic rinse. Use of iodine should be avoided in patients with known allergies.

From a historical perspective, hydrogen peroxide has been used in concentrations ranging from 3 to 5% alternating with sodium hypochlorite as part of the irrigation protocol. The release of nascent oxygen, which produces effervescence, was thought to help dislodge debris, which could drain out of the canal with the irrigant [56]. Accidental extrusion of hydrogen peroxide beyond the confines of the canal has resulted in sudden, severe pain, swelling, emphysema and crepitus, as reported in the literature [57]. Its use as an endodontic irrigant can therefore no longer be recommended.

Recently several new irrigants have been introduced to the profession in an attempt to further enhance effective debridement of the root canal system and eradicate intra-radicular infections. MTAD (Biopure, Dentsply, Tulsa Dental, Tulsa, OK) has been recommended as an alternative solution to EDTA for removing the smear layer. It is a mixture of tetracycline (3% doxycycline hyclate), acid (4.25% citric acid) and detergent (0.5% polysorbate (Tween) 80) [58]. Tetraclean (Ogna Laboratori Farmaceutici, Muggio, Italy) is another combination product containing doxycycline

(50 mg/mL compared to 150 mg/mL in MTAD), an acid and a detergent (polypropylene glycol) [59]. The combination of smear layer removal and the potential ability to exert an antibacterial effect are the main advantages when considering use of this irrigants as a final rinse following disinfection protocols. Disadvantages include tetracycline resistance amongst common root canal isolates, intrinsic staining and potential sensitivity.

The two most commonly used chelators EDTA and citric acid have been shown to react with sodium hypochlorite solution resulting in diminished antimicrobial and tissue-dissolving potential. HEBP (1-hydroxyethylidene-1,1-bisphosphonate) (etidronic acid) is a chelator that has been recommended as an alternative to EDTA that can be used in combination with sodium hypochlorite solution without affecting its proteolytic or antimicrobial properties [40].

QMiX was introduced in 2011 as a novel endodontic irrigant containing EDTA, CHX and a detergent used for smear layer removal and added disinfection [60]. This combination single solution product is available as a clear ready to use solution with no chair-side mixing involved. It has been recommended for use at the end of instrumentation as a final rinse. If NaOCl has been used then saline is used to rinse out any remaining NaOCl prior to its use to prevent potential PCA formation [47–49].

A laser is an acronym for light amplification by stimulated emission of radiation. The radiation involved in generating laser light is non-ionizing and the energy produced can be harnessed for disinfection purposes either thermally or chemically [61]. The neodymium: yttrium-aluminium-garnet (Nd: YAG), erbium: chromium: yttrium-scandium-gallium-garnet (Er: Cr: YSGG) and the erbium: yttrium-aluminium-garnet (Er: YAG) lasers have shown the most promise in endodontics. The Nd: YAG laser emits a wavelength of 1064nm close to the infrared range allowing flexible conductors to be used in narrow and curved canals yielding bactericidal effects both within the root canal walls and deeper dentine layers [62]. The Er: Cr: YSGG laser (developed by Waterlase MD, Biolase Technology, Irvine, CA, USA) is equipped with a 200 μm radially emitting laser tip equivalent to a number 20 file. It emits a wavelength of 2780 nm, which correlates close to the absorption maximum of hydroxyapatite acting through photo ablation. It can be used to remove smear layer and debris from the root canal walls thereby reducing bacterial loads [63]. The Er: YAG (developed by Powerlase, Lares research, Chico, CA, USA) has photon-induced photoacoustic streaming (PIPS) capability to create short microsecond pulse rates (50μs at a wavelength of 2940 nm). Irrigating solutions can be activated by the transfer of pulsed energy, enhancing the removal of organic tissue and microbes, resulting in improved tubular dentine disinfection [64, 65].

Photo activated disinfection (PAD) also known as light-activated disinfection, photodynamic antimicrobial chemotherapy and photodynamic therapy has been used to target microorganisms in root canals as an adjunct to current endodontic disinfection techniques. Methylene blue and toluidine blue are well-established photosensitizers that have been used in PAD for targeting both gram negative and positive microorganisms. The photosensitizer binds to the surface of the microorganism and following light activation of appropriate wavelength results in the generation of singlet oxygen and free radicals that are cytotoxic to the microbial cell wall [66, 67].

Efficient irrigation that can reach the canal terminus requires not only a suitable irrigant delivery system but one that can also work in a safe manner without causing harm to the patient. Root canal delivery irrigation systems can be broadly classified into two categories: manual and machine-assisted agitation techniques. The most common method of manual passive irrigation involves the use of a 27–30 gauge side-venting needle without binding it on the canal walls. The irrigation solution is dispensed approximately 1mm deeper than the tip of the needle. Depth of needle placement is determined by the size of the canal, canal curvature and corresponding needle size used. One must bear in mind the closer the needle tip is positioned to the apical tissues, the greater the chance of apical extrusion of the irrigant and potential for catastrophic accident (hypochlorite accident) [68, 69].

A 30-gauge irrigation needle covered with a brush (NaviTip FX; Ultradent Products Inc., South Jordan, UT) is available commercially as an adjunct for canal debridement [70]. Inherent friction created when using the brush may risk dislodgement of the radiolucent bristles in the canals.

The method of manual dynamic irrigation is well recognized as a simple method to ensure direct contact of irrigant with canal wall to enhance effectiveness of irrigant action. Gently moving a well-fitting master gutta-percha cone up and down in short 2–3 mm amplitude strokes (manual dynamic irrigation) within an instrumented canal produces a hydrodynamic effect improving irrigant displacement and exchange [71]. A recent study using a collagen "bio-molecular" ex vivo tooth model demonstrated that manual-dynamic irrigation was significantly more effective than an automated-dynamic irrigation system (RinseEndo) [72]. Despite ease of use and no costs involved the routine use of this hand-activated method has been shunned in clinical practice due to the perception of it being too labour intensive by some.

Machine assisted agitation systems have been developed to facilitate debris and smear layer removal. Rotary brushes such as CanalBrush (Coltene Whaledent, Langenau, Germany) has introduced a rotary handpiece-attached micro brush constructed from polypropylene. The micro brush is intended to rotate at 600rpm allowing and has been shown to effectively remove debris from simulated canal extensions and irregularities [73].

Sonic activation operating at low frequencies (1–6 KHz) has been shown to be an effective method for disinfecting root canals. A recently introduced sonically driven canal irrigation system known as the Endoactivator (Dentsply Tulsa Dental Specialities, Tulsa, OK) is commercially available. It consists of a plastic disposable polymer tip available in three different sizes (ISO tip 20, 25 and 30) that are easily attached to a sonic hand piece that can vibrate up to 10,000 cycles per minute [74]. A study has reported that the use of Endoactivator facilitates irrigant penetration and mechanical cleansing compared to conventional irrigation syringes and needles, with no increase in the risk of irrigant extrusion beyond the apex [75].

The use of ultrasonic energy for cleaning root canals and facilitating canal disinfection is well recognized. Ultrasonic files are oscillated at ultrasonic frequencies (25–30 kHz) resulting in characteristic patterns of antinodes and nodes along the length of the file. Passive ultrasonic irrigation whereby the ultrasonic file is vibrated within the canal following canal preparation has been advocated as a means to enhance irrigation without the adverse effect of dentine cutting and iatrogenic damage. Energy transferred from the oscillating file to the irrigant in the root canal system induces acoustic streaming and cavitation of the irrigant [76–78]. Acoustic streaming is defined as the movement of fluid, which occurs as a result of the ultrasound energy creating mechanical pressure changes within the tissues. Cavitation is defined as the formation and collapse of gas and vapour-filled bubbles or cavities in a fluid. Studies have demonstrated the effectiveness of bacterial elimination [79, 80], removal of pulpal tissue and dentine debris removal [81] and removal of smear layer when using passive ultrasonic irrigation [81, 82].

Machine assisted pressure alternation devices have been introduced in a further attempt to overcome the disadvantages of conventional syringes and needle systems. For any irrigation solution to be effective at mechanically removing root canal debris it must reach the apex, create a current, and carry the debris away [68, 69]. Furthermore air entrapment within the confines of the root canal space (apical vapour lock) can theoretically prevent both irrigation exchange and adequate flow.

EndoVac (Discus Dental, Culver City, CA, USA) was introduced as a means of concomitant irrigant delivery and aspiration using a negative pressure-approach lowering the risks of hypochlorite accident and the phenomenon of apical vapour lock [83]. It consists of a disposable syringe, a macro-cannula and a micro-cannula allowing irrigant to be placed in the pulp chamber and the ability for the irrigant to be sucked down the root canal and back up again with minimal risk of apical extrusion. A study by Brito and colleagues comparing NaviTip needles (Ultradent, South Jordon, UT, USA), EndoActivator and the EndoVac system concluded that there was no evidence of antibacterial superiority with any of the techniques used [84].

The RinseEndo system (Dürr Dental Co) is another root canal irrigant device based on a pressure-suction mechanism with approximately 100 cycles per minute [85]. 65 μL of the rinsing solution is oscillated at a frequency of 1.6 Hz and drawn from the attached syringe allowing irrigant transfer to the canal via an adapted cannula. During the suction phase, the used solution and air are extracted from the root canal and automatically merged with fresh rinsing solution thereby ensuring constant irrigant exchange and replenishment. The effectiveness of this system in cleaning canal walls has been challenged using the previously mentioned solubilized collagen-staining model that attempts to stimulate a bacterial biofilm within the canal walls. When comparing RinseEndo to manual-dynamic irrigation (using the pumping action of a master gutta-percha cone) the former proved less effective at removing the stained collagen [72]. Not enough clinical data is available to draw any firm conclusions as to the benefits of using such a system.

In summary irrigation is a key part of successful root canal treatment. It has several important functions including: reducing friction between the instrument and dentine, improving the cutting effectiveness of the files, dissolving organic tissue remnants, cooling both the file and tooth, and furthermore, it has a washing effect and an antimicrobial effect. Irrigation is also the only way to have a positive impact on areas of the root canal wall not touched by mechanical instrumentation. NaOCl is the main irrigating solution used to dissolve organic matter and kill microbes effectively. EDTA is needed as a final rinse to remove the smear layer (see Fig. 5.4). Sterile water or saline may be used between these two main irrigants, however, they must not be the only solutions used. Different means of delivery are used for root canal irrigation, from traditional syringe-needle delivery to various machine-driven systems, including automatic pumps and sonic or ultrasonic energy. In selecting any irrigant and delivery system, consideration must be given to both safety and efficacy [86].

5.2 Common Endodontic Irrigants

5.2.1 Sodium Hypochlorite

Of all the currently available choices of irrigants, NaOCl appears to be the most ideal, covering most of the requirements for endodontic irrigation. Its ability to dissolve necrotic tissue and the organic components of the smear layer as well as antimicrobial action is of paramount importance when carrying out cleaning and shaping procedures (Fig. 5.5).

The antibacterial efficacy and tissue-dissolving capability is a function of its concentration, but so too its toxicity. Typical concentrations used for irrigation purposes range from 0.5 to 6 % depending on preference. It is useful to remember that severe tissue irritations usually occur when using higher concentrations of solution, which is inadvertently forced into the periapical tissues. There is no added antimicrobial advantage when using 0.5 % NaOCl solution or 5 % solution. Replenishment of irrigant is key during treatment procedures with fresh hypochlorite solution continuously replaced.

Increasing the temperature of NaOCl solution also improves the effectiveness of irrigant solution within the canal system with respect to tissue-dissolving capacity. The ability of a 1 % NaOCl at 45 °C to dissolve human pulp tissue is equal to that of 5.25 % at 20 °C.

The most important factor to ensure optimal desired effects when using NaOCl is the factor of time. This is particularly important in regard to the concept of modern preparation techniques whereby the time taken to instrument and shape a canal has reduced significantly. The "chemo" aspect of preparation, nevertheless, requires adequate working time for the irrigant to make contact with the non-instrumented surfaces and effectively dissolve necrotic pulp tissue remnants, organic aspects of the smear layer and exerts optimal antimicrobial effects.

5.2.2 Chlorhexidine

CHX is a potent antiseptic and is commonly used in concentrations ranging from 0.1 to 2 % (the latter is the concentration of root canal irrigation commonly used in the endodontic literature). Its use has been advocated as a final irrigant owing to its substantivity, rather than the main irrigant to be used throughout the end-odontic procedure. This is due to its inability to dissolve necrotic tissue remnants. One must also bear in mind that primary endodontic cases are typically a polymicrobial infection predomi-nated by Gram-negative species. CHX has a greater effectiveness against Gram-positive bacteria.

5.2.3 Iodine Potassium Iodide

The endodontic literature has shown that 2 % IKI has been proven to be beneficial in some resistant failing cases. The use of iodine must be cautioned particularly in patients with known allergy. Like CHX it has no tissue-dissolving capability and so its use may be beneficial as part of a final irriga-

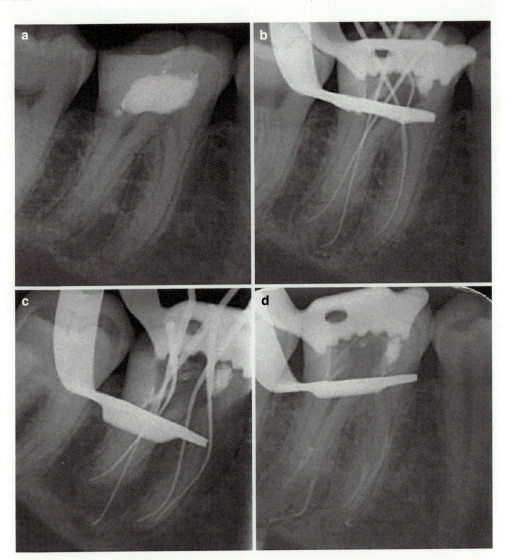

Fig. 5.4 Clinical radiographs demonstrating non-surgi-cal root canal treatment of tooth 46 using 1 % sodium hypochlorite solution and 17 % EDTA solution. Note (**a**) preoperative radiograph (**b**) initial apical file radiograph (**c**) master apical file radiograph (**d**) mid-fill (**e**) backfill and (**f**) post-operative view. Note sealer puffs in the mesial and distal root apices confirming apical patency. Sodium hypochlorite solution functions as the main bactericidal irrigant and allows dissolution of organic tissue and lubri-cation during preparation. EDTA is an organic acid, which is used to eliminate the inorganic mineral known as the "smear layer". The inability to effectively remove this layer can allow further thickening and condensing that can potentially close entrances of dentinal tubules, lateral and accessory canals and the main canal. Blockages or both organic or inorganic tissue remnants can be difficult to remove often resulting in incomplete canal preparation that can lead to failure

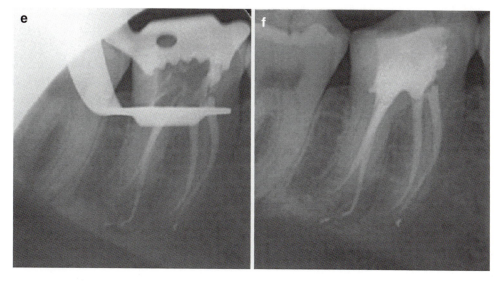

Fig. 5.4 (continued)

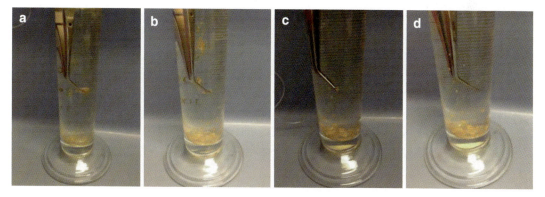

Fig. 5.5 Clinical photographs demonstrating sodium hypochlorite tissue-dissolving ability. Note experiment using organic pulp tissue immersed in 1 % NaOCl solution for (**a**) 1 min, (**b**) 10 min, (**c**) 20 min and (**d**) 30 min, respectively. This crude experiment shows that time is needed for tissue-dissolving capability. Solution replenishment and use of heat will both decrease time taken to dissolve tissue

tion protocol following chemomechanical preparation with NaOCl solution.

5.3 Removal of Smear Layer

Instrumentation procedures that make contact with the root canal walls (using hand or rotary instruments, ultrasonic tips and burs) can produce a 0.5–2 μ thick smear layer consisting of organic (pulp tissue remnants, bacteria and biofilm) and inorganic (mineralized dentine and predentine particles) components. The adjunctive use of chelating agents such as EDTA has therefore been recommended. Removal of smear layer may allow for disruption of biofilm plaques that are adherent to canal walls and opening of dentinal tubules that further optimizes either antibacterial irrigation penetration or intra-canal medicaments which may diffuse further without constraints.

The recommended protocol for smear layer removal is the use of NaOCl followed by EDTA or citric acid. One to two minutes should be sufficient working time for EDTA action prior to inactivation with saline.

EDTA should be used in liquid form and typical concentrations for endodontic use range from 15 to 17 %. The clinician must be aware of the fact that EDTA in the presence of NaOCl solution reduces the available chlorine in solution, rendering NaOCl less effective with regards to both tissue-dissolving capability and antimicrobial activity. This is the very reason why the use of chelating agents in paste form which were once recommended during the canal shaping procedure is no longer recommended.

5.4 Alcohol

The use of 95 % ethyl alcohol has been recommended as a pre-irrigation step or final irrigation step prior to intra-canal medicament placement or obturation of the canal. This is based on anecdotal practice with the assumption that the alcohol reduces the surface tension of either the irrigant fluid to be used thereafter or sealer during obturation. The evaporation of the alcohol is thought to aid either irrigant or sealer penetration. A final rinse of approximately 3–5 ml of 95 % Ethyl alcohol can be recommended in order to improve the sealing ability of the root canal filling.

5.5 Irrigant Interactions

5.5.1 Sodium Hypochlorite and EDTA

The combination of NaOCl and EDTA results in EDTA retaining its calcium-complexing ability with a reduced amount of chlorine available in solution. NaOCl on the other hand has reduced tissue-dissolving capability and antimicrobial effectiveness. When using NaOCl and EDTA, an alternating regime should be used with copious amounts of the former to ensure that any remnants of EDTA have been removed.

5.5.2 Sodium Hypochlorite and Chlorhexidine

The combination of NaOCl and CHX results in the formation of an orange-brown precipitate consisting possibly of para-chloroaniline (PCA). The amount of PCA formed is directly linked to the increasing concentration of NaOCl. Due to the potential toxicity of PCA, the ability of the precipitate to occlude the dentinal tubules and potential for the insoluble precipitate to interfere with the final seal of the root filling caution should be excised when irrigating with both of these solutions.

Clinical recommendations to avoid precipitate formation include the use of absolute alcohol, saline or distilled water following use of NaOCl and prior to the introduction of CHX within the root canal. An alternative is to use QMiX that does not appear to form any precipitate in the presence of NaOCl solution. Nevertheless manufacturers recommend use of a saline irrigation prior to QMiX use.

5.5.3 EDTA and Chlorhexidine

The combination of EDTA and CHX results in the formation of a white precipitate due to the chlorhexidine forming a salt with EDTA rather than undergoing a chemical reaction. Clinical recommendation will be to flush out the EDTA with saline after recommended working time (usually 1–3 min) prior to introduction of CHX as a final rinse (Fig. 5.6).

5.6 Methods of Delivery

5.6.1 Manual Passive Irrigation

5.6.1.1 Conventional Syringe and Needles

Plastic syringes of different sizes are available with 1 and 5 mL typically sufficient for endodontic irrigation purposes. Larger syringes (10 and 20 mL) although time saving due to their greater capacity for solution storage are more difficult to control when exerting pressure increasing the risks

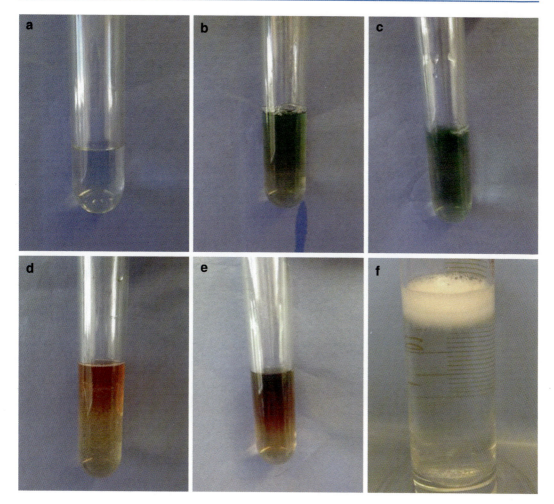

Fig. 5.6 Clinical photographs demonstrating potential irrigant interactions. Note (**a**) sodium hypochlorite solution (NaOCl) 1 %. (**b**) 1 % NaOCl solution and chlorhexidine 2 % (CHX) mix. (**c**) NaOCl and CHX after 5 min. (**d**) NaOCl and CHX after 10 min. (**e**) NaOCl and CHX after 20 min. *Orange-brown* precipitate possibly consisting of para-chloroaniline (PCA). (**f**) The combination of ethylenediaminetetraacetic acid (EDTA) and CHX results in the formation of a *white* precipitate due to the CHX forming a salt with EDTA rather than undergoing a chemical reaction

of inadvertent accidents. All endodontic syringes should have a Luer-Lok hub design, which avoids potential needle disengagement and irrigant spray, which can be harmful on skin/mucosal/eye contact and damage to clothing (Fig. 5.7).

According to the international standards organization (ISO) a 30G needle is equivalent to size 0.31 diameter at the tip and a 27G needle is 0.42 diameter at the tip. This means that the minimal master apical file size should be at least a size 30 when using a 30G needle to ensure adequate needle penetration. Smaller needles (greater than 30G) although easier to deliver irrigant to the apex are a risk of potential apical extrusion. Needle tip designs have been modified with this view in mind with side venting to minimize extrusion.

5.6.2 Manual Dynamic Irrigation

5.6.2.1 Master Cone Gutta-Percha Point

The use of an apically well-fitting master gutta-percha cone moved in an up and down motion at

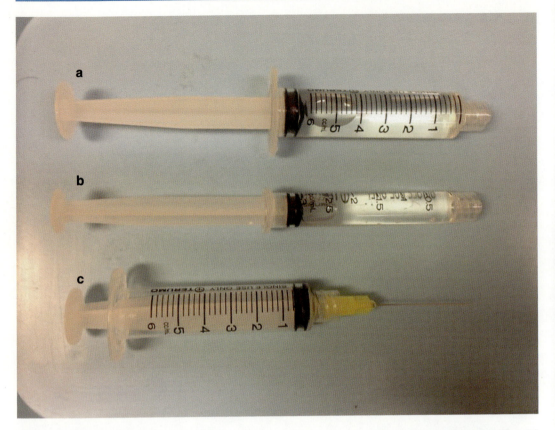

Fig. 5.7 Clinical photograph of manual passive irrigation delivery using conventional syringe and needles. Note (**a**) 5 mL and (**b**) 1 mL syringes. (**c**) Luer-Lok hub design to help prevent potential needle disengagement and spray

the working length in short amplitude motions repeatedly will facilitate irrigant exchange in the apical 1/3rd. Replenishment of fresh NaOCl solution is necessary to ensure optimal antibacterial activity. This technique has been shown to produce favourable results with minimal risk of apical extrusion (Fig. 5.8).

5.6.3 Sonic Irrigation

5.6.3.1 EndoActivator

Sonic activation has been shown to be an effective method to enhance disinfection of the root canal. The use of a battery-operated portable handpiece offers three-speed sonic motor options (high, medium and low) with the choice of three disposable medical grade polymer tips (small #15/02, medium #25/04 and large #35/04) for single use application. Manufacturers claim the

device is capable of sonic vibration up to 10,000 cycles per minute creating fluid hydrodynamics that improve both debridement and disruption of the smear layer and biofilm. The recommended protocol for use is as follows:

1. Complete canal preparation to produce a fully tapered preparation with minimal MAF size corresponding to size #25.
2. Fill the pulp chamber and root canal with choice of irrigant (NaOCl, EDTA or CHX).
3. Select the activator tip that manually fits loosely within 2 mm of the working length.
4. Attach the activator tip over the barrier protected handpiece and snap on firmly promoting a secure connection with the handpiece.
5. Place the activator tip to working length (this can be marked on the polymer tip) and use in a pumping action with short 2–3 mm vertical strokes (Fig. 5.9).

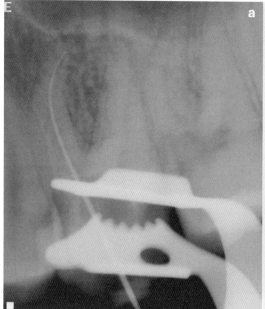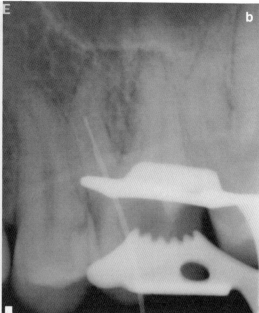

Fig. 5.8 Clinical radiographs of an upper maxillary 1st right molar showing (**a**) MAF preparation of the mesio-buccal root to a size #30 at the working length. (**b**) Placement of a 30G needle cannot be passively passed to length due to the abrupt apical curvature that is present.

Use of alternative irrigation devices such as manual-dynamic irrigation or sonic irrigation will be necessary to ensure optimal irrigant exchange in the apical 1/3rd essential for biofilm disruption, organic tissue dissolution and bacterial elimination/reduction

5.6.4 Passive Ultrasonic Irrigation

5.6.4.1 Ultrasonic Irrigation

Cleaning of the root canal system and enhancing disinfection can be achieved by the use of ultrasonics. Passive ultrasonic irrigation refers to the file being used passively with the ability to move freely within the canal without making contact that can result in ultrasonic preparation and inadvertent ledging. Cavitation and acoustic streaming of the irrigant contribute to the chemomechanical effectiveness of this procedure. The hydrodynamic response of the oscillating file with cavitation micro-streaming contributes to the cleaning of the canal (when compared to hand instrumentation alone). A proposed clinical protocol is as follows:

1. Complete canal preparation to produce a fully tapered preparation with minimal MAF size corresponding to size #25.

2. Fill the pulp chamber and root canal with choice of irrigant (NaOCl, EDTA or CHX).
3. Select a #15 Ultrasonic K file and attach to handpiece. Set ultrasonic unit to manufacturers recommended power setting.
4. Place file 2 mm short of working length and activate for 3 min. File can be moved in short vertical strokes of 2–3 mm ensuring file does not move beyond working length.
5. Replenish irrigant and repeat as necessary. Care must be taken to ensure that the file is working passively when activated with no attempt made to plane, shape or remove dentine from the canal walls.

Care must be taken since there is possible risk of file separation. This can occur if the file does not move freely within the canal or recommended manufacture power settings are not adhered to (Fig. 5.10).

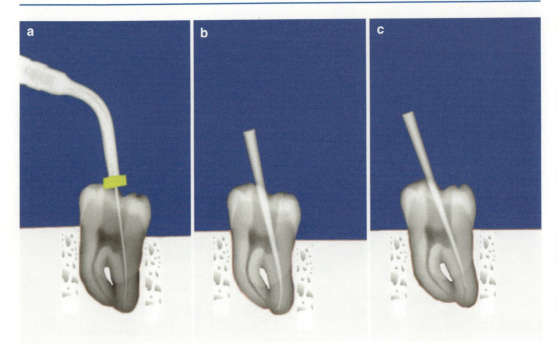

Fig. 5.9 Clinical radiographs of an extracted molar tooth where the distal canal has been prepared to a size #30 at the apex. Various methods used to facilitate irrigant exchange. Note (**a**) using passive ultrasonic irrigation using an ultrasonic #15 K file within 2 mm of working length. A low power setting is recommended to avoid inadvertent canal preparation, transportation and file separation. The file can be moved up and down using small amplitude vertical strokes. (**b**, **c**) Use of a master cone gutta-percha size #30 can be placed to length and moved in a "pumping" action to facilitate irrigant exchange

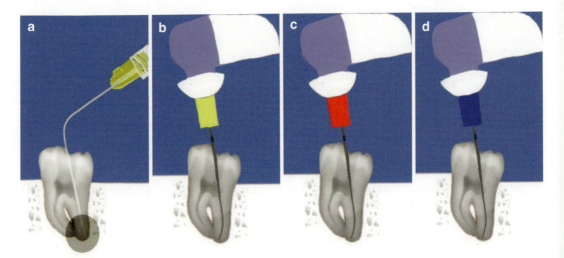

Fig. 5.10 Clinical radiographs of an extracted molar tooth where the distal canal has been prepared to a size #30 at the apex. (**a**) Using a standard 30G needle irrigant can be easily exchanged to the level of canal curvature. (**b–d**) Use of sonic irrigation using the "EndoActivator" with the choice of three disposable medical grade polymer tips (small #15/02, medium #25/04 and large #35/04) for single use application. Manufactures claim the device is capable of sonic vibration up to 10,000 cycles per minute, creating fluid hydrodynamics that improve both debridement and disruption of the smear layer and biofilm

5.6.5 Pressure Alternation Devices

5.6.5.1 EndoVac

EndoVac (Discus Dental, Culver City, CA, USA) is a proprietary product that uses negative pressure to draw irrigant within a canal and then removes it. The device is attached to a suction unit and utilizes a micro-cannula, which can be placed deep within canal. The cannula acts as a micro-suction drawing irrigant into a canal as far as its tip reaches. This imparts a degree of fluid movement although not as much as what might be achieved with ultrasonic irrigation. It does however ensure the apical extent of a canal is continuously flooded with fresh irrigant for an optimum effect. It also has the key advantage that it is not possible to extrude irrigant using this device and thus it is a very safe, almost making a hypochlorite accident impossible.

5.7 Hypochlorite Accidents

Several mishaps during root canal irrigation have been described in the dental literature ranging from damage to patient's clothing, splashing of irrigant into the patient or operator's eye and inadvertent injection beyond the apical foramen and allergic reactions.

5.7.1 Damage to Clothing

The most common incident that may occur during root canal irrigation is damage of the patient's clothing. NaOCl solution is a common household bleach whereby direct contact or spraying due to needle/syringe hub failure or ultrasonic activation and resultant aerosol spray can cause clothing to be damaged. Care must be taken when using manual irrigation with conventional needles ensuring needle and syringe are securely attached and the patient is wearing suitable protection measures (patient bib).

5.7.2 Damage to Eye

Accidental spillage of NaOCl into either the patient or operator's eye can result in immediate pain, burning and erythema. Immediate eye washing is recommended with further referral to ophthalmologist for further examination and treatment if warranted.

5.7.3 Extrusion Beyond the Apex

5.7.3.1 Sequelae of Sodium Hypochlorite Extrusion

Extrusion of NaOCl beyond the confines of the apex may occur in teeth with wide-open apices, where the apical constriction has been destroyed either during root canal preparation or due to resorption and in teeth with internal/external root resorption or perforation communications. Additionally operator factors such as extreme force during injection of irrigant, binding of the needle tip with wedging in the canal and inadequate working length determination can all lead to hypochlorite extrusion and its sequelae.

The patient may experience excruciating immediate pain during the irrigation procedure. Immediately or within a few hours the patient may exhibit swelling, ecchymosis, bleeding through the gingivae and a neurological deficit once the local anaesthetic has worn off. Within the first 24–72 h the patient may present with secondary infection, persistent pain and neurological deficit. A necrotic ulcer may form with sloughing of the gingivae surrounding the offending tooth and necrosis that may involve the bone.

Management of sodium hypochlorite accidents

The result of accidental sodium hypochlorite extrusion is unpredictable with every patient reacting differently according to the concentration and amount of extrusion and host response. Nevertheless every patient should be treated with appropriate care consisting of immediate management and follow-up with the possibility of urgent or delayed referral to an oral and maxillofacial surgeon depending severity of sequelae. Initial management should focus on alleviating swelling and controlling pain. Recommendations include use of cold compress on the first day to treat the swelling, followed by warm compress to stimulate the microcirculation. Long-acting local anaesthesia may be provided for the acute pain.

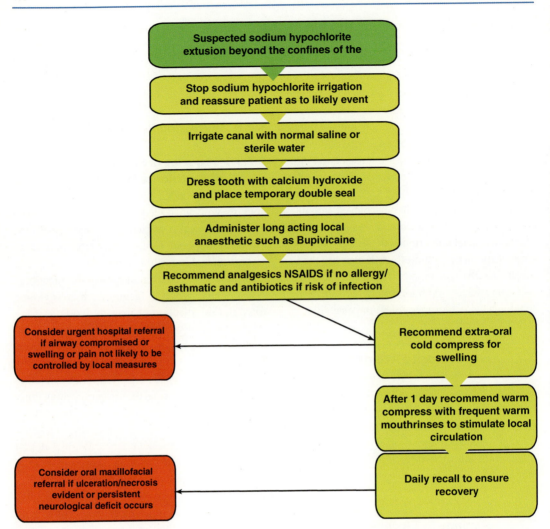

Fig. 5.11 Outpatient and in-patient management of sodium hypochlorite accidents depending on severity of symptoms. Note any acute swelling that may potentially affect the airway may require immediate urgent hospital referral. Opioid analgesics, IV antibiotics and IV steroids may be administered for up to 48 h. Consider an oral maxillofacial surgery referral if suspected ulceration, bone necrosis or persistent paraesthesia occurs

Antibiotic use may be recommended in cases where soft tissue damage could result in tissue necrosis and secondary infections. Steroids may be used for the management of the swelling although their efficacy is inconclusive.

Extensive soft tissue necrosis with or without bone involvement may require additional wound debridement and referral. Sensory neurological deficit including anaesthesia or paraesthesia will usually resolve but may take several months. All patients that develop any neurological deficit will require early follow-up with an oral maxillofacial surgeon to assess degree of severity and manage-

ment thereof. In cases of suspected or risk of upper airway obstruction, prompt referral to hospital may be indicated for in-patient management. All patients should be followed up carefully to ensure a full recovery is made (see Fig. 5.11).

5.8   Recommended Irrigation Protocol

Developing a rational irrigation protocol so that chemical disinfectants are administered in a proper manner without compromising their action is

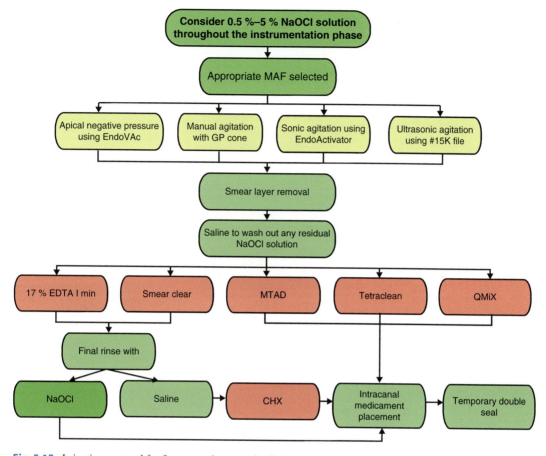

Fig. 5.12 Irrigation protocol for first stage chemomechanical cleaning and shaping procedure

imperative for the outcome of successful endodontics. For optimal irrigation, a combination of irrigants may be necessary that can differ according to whether the case is a primary endodontic "de novo" infection or a persistent secondary failing case. The clinician must keep in mind the potential precipitates that can form when irrigants are combined and care must be taken to ensure that appropriate steps are taken to reduce these risks.

The protocol is based on a multi-visit treatment wherein the clinical objective of the first appointment is appropriate chemomechanical canal shaping and intra-canal medicament placement (see Fig. 5.12) and the second appointment is the final obturation stage (see Fig. 5.13).

To remove the calcium hydroxide at the initiation of the second obturation visit, sodium hypochlorite solution is useful. In addition, it is advisable to re-enter each canal with the master apical file or rotary instrument to agitate the hypochlorite solu-

tion and thus enhance calcium hydroxide removal. Following removal of calcium hydroxide a final flush of sodium hypochlorite can be carried out prior to completion of smear layer removal using EDTA. A final flush of ethyl alcohol may be used prior to placement of sealer within the canal to ensure that following evaporation the canal is dry and to allow for optimal sealer penetration.

5.9   Clinical Case

Case 5.1 Hypochlorite accident, swelling and neurological deficit affecting the right lower lip during root canal treatment of tooth 44

A 57-year-old fit and healthy patient was referred for endodontic management of tooth 44. Four weeks earlier the patient had attended her general dental practitioner complaining of thermal sensitivity in relation to tooth 44. A provi-

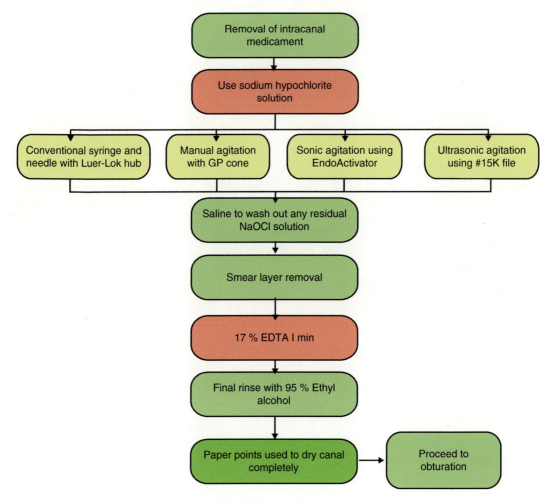

Fig. 5.13 Irrigation protocol for second stage obturation stage

sional diagnosis of irreversible pulpitis was made and endodontic treatment commenced. Following initial access preparation, the canal was irrigated with 1% sodium hypochlorite solution. Immediately the patient experienced an intense burning sensation that radiated to her lower jaw on the right hand side. A hypochlorite accident was suspected, reassurance given to the patient and saline irrigation commenced. Immediate swelling and oedema affecting the patient's lower right lip was observed with exudate noted through the access cavity in the tooth. The tooth was temporarily dressed and procedure abandoned. Due to the extent of the swelling and concern about possible airway obstruction the dentist arranged for an ambulance and the patient was subsequently seen in accident and emergency.

The patient was discharged later that evening and advised to see her general dental practitioner for further management. The dentist contacted me directly to discuss the case. I advised that the patient should be placed on oral antibiotics (amoxicillin 250 mg tds 7 days), analgesics (1 g Paracetomol qds and 400 mg ibuprofen qds alternatively at 4 hourly intervals) and oral steroids (Prednisone 5 mg tds 3 days). I also recommended prompt referral to an oral maxillofacial surgeon regarding neurological assessment and soft tissue management before completing endodontic treatment.

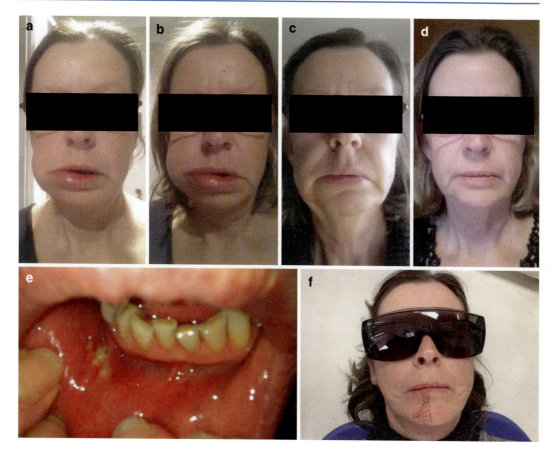

Fig. 5.14 Clinical photographs demonstrating soft tissue reaction following a sodium hypochlorite accident associated with non-surgical root canal treatment of tooth 44. Note (**a**) swelling 6 h after incident, (**b**) 24 h, (**c**) 3 days and (**d**) 5 days. (**e**) Ulceration associated with *lower right lip* 1 week after the incident. (**f**) Altered lip and chin sensation mapped out. Note also facial swelling has resolved completely after 2 weeks

At the maxillofacial consultation a week later, the swelling affecting the lower right lip had reduced significantly (Fig. 5.14). A firm swelling was noted in the buccal aspect of tooth 44. Altered sensation was evident with the right lip and chin. Although there was no obvious necrosis of soft tissues or infection, a decision was made to continue antibiotic treatment to reduce the risk of super-infection in the area of the altered tissues. The patient was reassured and further reviews were scheduled advising the patient that no further treatment could be provided other than simply a matter of waiting for the area to resolve. The patient was warned that the altered sensation affecting the right lip should improve over time although not guaranteed. A further review was recommended 2 weeks later at which time some minor ulceration was noted in the lower lip region (Fig. 5.14). The swelling had completely resolved and the some sensation had returned to the lower lip. The patient was advised to return to the endodontist for further management of tooth 44.

Following a 4-week period after the initial incident the patient was seen for endodontic assessment and treatment. Mild soft tissue scarring was noted in the lower right labial segment. Altered sensation was noted in the lower right lip and chin region. Radiographic examination confirmed previous endodontic access in tooth 44. An intact periodontal ligament space was noted. A second radiograph confirmed misaligned access with likely perforation resulting in extrusion of hypochlorite into the surrounding soft tissues

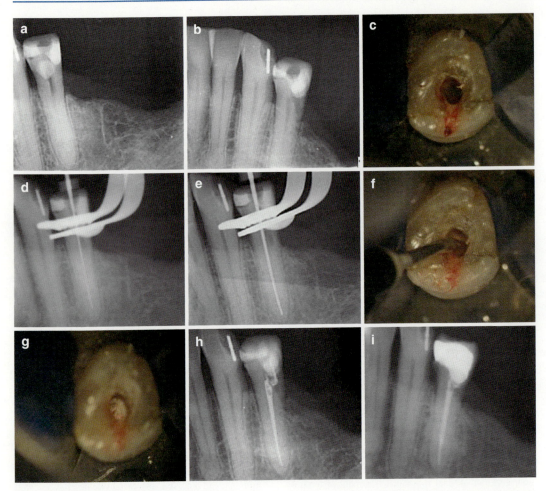

Fig. 5.15 Clinical radiographs and photographs demonstrating non-surgical management of tooth 44 and perforation repair following sodium hypochlorite extrusion injury. Note (**a**) Preoperative parallel radiograph demonstrating initial access cavity. (**b**) Horizontal tube shift radiograph demonstrated off-centre access cavity preparation which had led to extrusion of sodium hypochlorite on the labial aspect. (**c**) Initial access preparation confirmed bleeding and perforation site on the buccal aspect of the tooth. (**d**, **e**) IAF and MAF radiographs. Chlorhexidine 0.2 % solution was used for irrigation at this point to prevent any further hypochlorite extrusion and injury. Following preparation, a gutta-percha master cone was placed in the canal and sealed below the canal orifice prior to perforation repair. (**f**) Placement of bioceramic putty restoration into the perforation site. (**g**) Completed repair of the buccal perforation site. The gutta-percha cone was removed, irrigation of the canal system completed with sodium hypochlorite solution prior to intra-canal calcium hydroxide medicament placement and temporization. The patient was reviewed at 4 weeks and obturation completed. (**h**) Note completed root canal therapy, repair of perforation site and overlying Biodentine coronal restoration. (**i**) A 6-month review radiograph demonstrating asymptomatic tooth 44 restored with a cast cuspal coverage restoration

(Fig. 5.15). Options and prognosis for the tooth were discussed with the patient, who was keen to try and retain the tooth if possible. A treatment plan was formulated with the patient to non-surgically root treat the tooth with internal perforation repair if amenable. Removal of the temporary restoration revealed bleeding from within the coronal aspect of the tooth. Following irrigation with saline a buccal perforation was confirmed. Access preparation was refined and the necrotic root canal system located. Initial canal preparation was completed using 0.2 % chlorhexidine solution.

Following canal preparation gutta-percha was temporarily placed and sealed just below the canal orifice to prevent the risk of perforation repair material inadvertently sealing the canal system. Haemorrhage was controlled using a cotton wool pledget soaked in 1 % sodium hypochlorite solution and pressure. A bioceramic restoration was placed at the perforation site, gutta-percha removed, intra-canal calcium hydroxide medicament placed with an overlying double seal temporary restoration (Cavit/GIC). The patient was reviewed 4 weeks later. At the review appointment the patient had remained asymptomatic. The altered sensation in her lower lip was still present but had been improving. The patient was reassured that in all likelihood her lip sensation should return to normal over time. No abnormal periodontal probing was detected on the buccal aspect below the gingival margin.

Access was gained and the perforation site was examined under the dental operating microscope and the repair was deemed satisfactory with no further bleeding at the site. Obturation of the root canal system was completed using a warm vertical compaction technique and AH plus cement. A biodentine restoration was placed in the access cavity to provide an additional seal. The patient was advised to see her general dental practitioner for a final coronal cast cuspal coverage restoration and continue follow-up appointments with the maxillofacial surgeon with regards to her altered sensation (Fig. 5.15).

Case 5.2 Root canal treatment of tooth 45 with an acute apical curvature

A 45-year-old fit and healthy patient was referred for endodontic management of tooth 45. The patient had presented to her general dental practitioner with a draining sinus in relation to this tooth. A referral was made due to the unusual root appearance and apical curvature in the tooth. A provisional diagnosis of chronic apical periodontitis with suppuration was made. Access cavity was prepared confirming a necrotic root canal. The root canal space was initially explored using a 10K stainless steel hand file. An acute

apical curvature was confirmed with a second S-shaped curvature in the apical 3 mm. Patency was maintained throughout and chemomechanical preparation was carried out to the second curve using 1 % NaOCl solution and stainless steel hand files. The preparation was completed using rotary files. Due to the acute apical curvature, a decision was made to maintain the last 3 mm of the apical preparation using hand files only. Additional sonic irrigation was carried out using the EndoActivator. A final rinse of saline followed by 17 % EDTA was used prior to medicament placement. An intra-canal medicament of calcium hydroxide paste was placed and the patient reviewed a week later (Fig. 5.16).

At the review appointment the patient remained asymptomatic. Clinical examination confirmed the draining sinus had resolved. A further appointment was scheduled for obturation. Obturation was completed using AH plus cement and gutta-percha using System B and Obtura. Prior to obturation the canal system was washed with 1 % NaOCl, normal saline and then 17 % EDTA. The canal space was dried using paper points prior to cone-fit placement and radiographic verification. Following the down-packing sealer extrusion was noted confirming patency. The obturation was back-filled using Obtura. A double temporary seal of IRM and glass ionomer cement was placed as an interim restoration. The patient was scheduled to see her general dental practitioner for placement of a cast cuspal coverage restoration (Fig. 5.17).

Anatomical complexities such as S-shaped or bayonet-shaped canals can be challenging due to the presence of two curves, with the apical curve being subjected to anatomical deviation and loss of working length. Constant recapitulation with small files and frequent irrigation is necessary to prevent both blockage and ledging in the apical curve. Use of master apical file sizes larger than 25 should be avoided in most cases to prevent stripping and ledging in the apical curvature. Copious irrigation must always be used during canal penetration, debridement, cleaning and shaping. Use of small files with short amplitude strokes can be useful to ensure irrigant is introduced into the

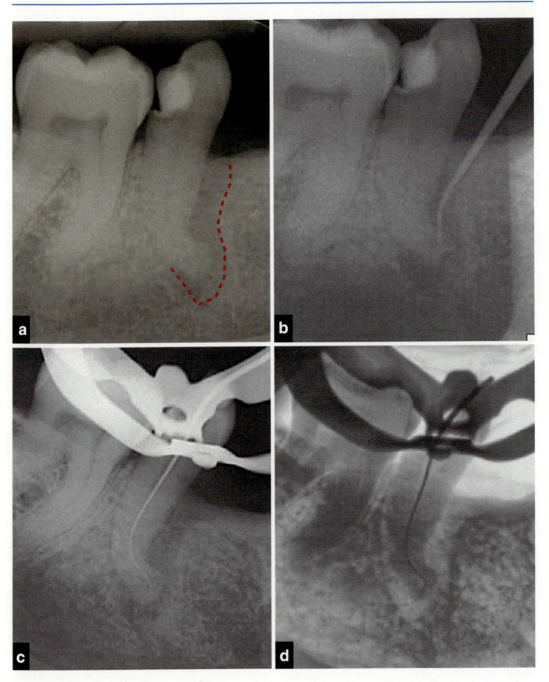

Fig. 5.16 Clinical radiographs demonstrating non-surgical root canal treatment of tooth 45. Note (**a**) preoperative radiograph demonstrating large peri-radicular radiolucent lesion with the periapex of tooth 45 (*dotted red line*). An acute apical curvature is noted. (**b**) A gutta-percha sinus tracing radiograph was tracked to this lesion. A diagnosis of chronic apical periodontitis with suppura-tion 45 was made. (**c**, **d**) Initial apical file x-rays showing working length and acute apical curvature. The last 3 mm of the root canal space could only be negotiated with a stainless steel K file #10. Patency was maintained and copious irrigation was used with 1 % NaOCl solution. It was vital for the irrigation to penetrate this area and debride adequately to ensure the sinus resolves

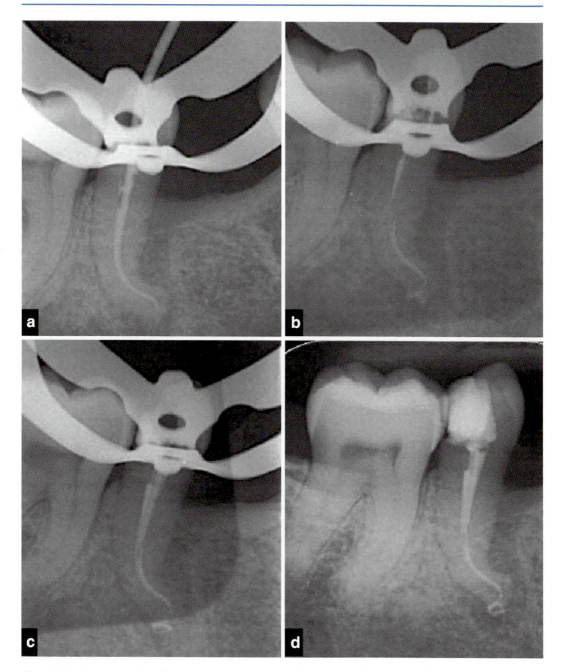

Fig. 5.17 Clinical radiographs demonstrating non-surgical root canal treatment of tooth 45. Following completion of chemomechanical preparation using rotary files an intra-canal medicament of calcium hydroxide was placed. The patient was reviewed 1 week later and the sinus had healed. A further appointment was scheduled for obturation of the case. Note (**a**) cone-fit radiograph, (**b**) mid-fill radiograph, (**c**) back fill and (**d**) post-operative view. The final obturation is a mirror-image of the preparation technique and irrigation protocol that not only serves to reduce the bacterial load but also penetrate areas of canal space that instruments are not capable of reaching

apical curvature where conventional mechanical preparation may be limited.

Clinical Hints and Tips for Endodontic Irrigation

- In primary root canal treatments, the use of 1–5.25 % sodium hypochlorite solution (NaOCl) is the first choice endodontic irrigant primarily due to its tissue-dissolving ability and antimicrobial activity.
- In the context of re-treatment, use of either or both 2 % chlorhexidine and 2 % iodine 4 % potassium iodide may be indicated.
- When using a combination of irrigants, the clinician must be aware of the possible precipitates that can form. Thorough washing out of the irrigant previously used with saline should avoid this occurrence.
- Smear layer removal is carried out with a combination of NaOCl and EDTA to remove both organic and inorganic products.
- Manual agitation with a gutta-percha cone is the simplest step that should be undertaken during irrigation procedures. Use of sonic, ultrasonic or negative pressure devices are useful adjuncts to ensure optimal disinfection.
- Extrusion of NaOCl into the periapical tissues can cause severe injury the patient. Steps to minimize NaOCl accidents include needle placement short of working length, needle placement to fit loosely within the canal and not wedged in, irrigation flow rate with gentle pressure (do not use thumb to inject but palm of hand), constant moving of the needle in an up and down motion to ensure wedging does not occur, use of side-venting needles to reduce the possibility of forcing irrigant beyond the apex and using negative pressure devices such as EndoVac.
- Treatment of NaOCl accidents is palliative and consists of observation of the patient as well as prescribing antibiotics and analgesics. Prompt referral may be necessary in cases of bone necrosis or swelling which can compromise the airway.

References

1. Peters LB, van Winkelhoff AJ, Buijs JF, Wesselink PR. Effects of instrumentation, irrigation and dressing with calcium hydroxide on infection in pulpless teeth with periapical bone lesions. Int Endod J. 2002; 35:13–21.
2. Trope M, Delano E, Ørstavik D. Endodontic treatment of teeth with apical periodontitis: single vs. multivisit treatment. J Endod. 1999;25:345.
3. Weiger R, Rosendahl R, Löst C. Influence of calcium hydroxide intracanal dressings on the prognosis of teeth with endodontically induced periapical lesions. Int Endod J. 2000;33:219–26.
4. Byström A, Sundqvist G. Bacteriologic evaluation of the efficacy of mechanical root canal instrumentation in endodontic therapy. Eur J Oral Sci. 1981;1981(89):321–8.
5. Dalton BC, Ørstavik D, Phillips C, Pettiette M, Trope M. Bacterial reduction with nickel-titanium rotary instrumentation. J Endod. 1998;24:763–7.
6. Byström A, Sundqvist G. Bacteriologic evaluation of the effect of 0.5 percent sodium hypochlorite in endodontic therapy. Oral Surg Oral Med Oral Pathol. 1983;55:307–12.
7. Shuping GB, Ørstavik D, Sigurdsson A, Trope M. Reduction of intracanal bacteria using nickel-titanium rotary instrumentation and various medications. J Endod. 2000;26:751–5.
8. Sjögren U, Figdor D, Persson S, Sundqvist G. Influence of infection at the time of root filling on the outcome of endodontic treatment of teeth with apical periodontitis. Int Endod J. 1997;30:297–306.
9. Sjögren U, Figdor D, Spandberg L, Sundqvis G. The antimicrobial effect of calcium hydroxide as a short-term intracanal dressing. Int Endod J. 1991;24:119–25.
10. Nair P, Henry S, Cano V, Vera J. Microbial status of apical root canal system of human mandibular first molars with primary apical periodontitis after "one visit" endodontic treatment. Oral Surg Oral Med Oral Pathol Oral Radiol Endod. 2005;99:231–52.
11. Riccuci D, Siqueira J. Biofilms and apical periodontitis: study of prevalence and association with clinical and histopathologic findings. J Endod. 2010;36:1277–88.
12. Hall-Stoodley L, Costerton J, Stoodley P. Bacterial biofilms: from the natural environment to infectious diseases. Nat Rev Microbiol. 2004;2:95–108.
13. Stewart P, Costerton J. Antibiotic resistance of bacteria in biofilms. Lancet. 2001;358:135–8.
14. Zehnder M. Root canal irrigants. J Endod. 2006;32:389–98.
15. Mader CL, Baumgartner JC, Peters DD. Scanning electron microscopic investigation of the smeared layer on root canal walls. J Endod. 1984;10:477–83.
16. McComb D, Smith DC. A preliminary scanning electron microscopic study of root canals after endodontic procedures. J Endod. 1975;1(7):238–42.
17. Pashley DH. Smear layer: physiological considerations. Oper Dent. 1984;3 Suppl 3:35–42.

18. Sen BH, Wesselink PR, Türkün M. The smear layer: a phenomenon in root canal therapy. Int Endod J. 1995;1995(28):141–8.
19. Violich DR, Chandler NP. The smear layer in endodontics – a review. Int Endod J. 2010;43:2–15.
20. Moon Y, Shon W, Baek S, Bae K, Kum K. Effect of final irrigation regimen on sealer penetration in curved root canals. J Endod. 2010;36(4):732–6.
21. Frais S, Ng YL, Gulabivala K. Some factors affecting the concentration of available chlorine in commercial sources of sodium hypochlorite. Int Endod J. 2001;34:206–15.
22. Estrela C, Barbin E, Spanó J, Maarchesan M, Pécora J. Mechanism of action of sodium hypochlorite. Braz Dent J. 2002;13:113–7.
23. Byström A, Sundqvist G. The antibacterial action of sodium hypochlorite and EDTA in 60 cases of endodontic therapy. Int Endod J. 1985;18:35–40.
24. Clegg MS, Vertucci FJ, Walker C, Belanger M, Britto LR. The effect of exposure to irrigant solutions on apical dentin biofilms in vitro. J Endod. 2006;32(5):434–7.
25. Hand RE, Smith ML, Harrison JW. Analysis of the effect of dilution on the necrotic tissue dissolution property of sodium hypochlorite. J Endod. 1978;4(2):60–4.
26. Moorer W, Wesselink P. Factors promoting the tissue dissolving capability of sodium hypochlorite. Int Endod J. 1982;15:187–96.
27. Hülsmann M, Hahn W. Complications during root canal irrigation – literature review and case reports. Int Endod J. 2000;33:186–93.
28. Sim TP, Knowles JC, Ng YL, Shelton J, Gulabivala K. Effect of sodium hypochlorite on mechanical properties of dentine and tooth surface strain. Int Endod J. 2001;34:120–32.
29. Sirtes G, Waltimo T, Schaetzle M, Zehnder M. The effects of temperature on sodium hypochlorite short-term stability, pulp dissolution capacity, and antimicrobial efficacy. J Endod. 2005;31:669–71.
30. Aubut V, Pommel L, Verhille B, Orsière T, Garcia S, About I, Jean Camps J. Biological properties of a neutralized 2.5% sodium hypochlorite solution. Oral Surg Oral Med Oral Pathol Oral Radiol Endod. 2010;109:120–5.
31. Pashley EL, Bridsong NL, Bowman K, Pashley DH. Cytotoxic effects of sodium hypochlorite on vital tissue. J Endod. 1985;11:525–8.
32. Spangberg L, Engstrom B, Langeland K. Biological effects of dental materials. 3. Toxicity and antimicrobial effect of endodontic antiseptics in vitro. Oral Surg. 1973;36:856–71.
33. Piskin B, Turkun M. Stability of various sodium hypochlorite solutions. J Endod. 1995;21:253–5.
34. Fabian TM, Walker SE. Stability of sodium hypochlorite solutions. Am J Hosp Pharm. 1982;39(6):1016–7.
35. Cotter JL, Fader RC, Lilley C, Herndon DN. Chemical parameters, antimicrobial activities, and tissue toxicity of 0.1 and 0.5% sodium hypochlorite solutions. Antimicrob Agents Chemother. 1985;28:118–22.
36. Yamada R, Armas A, Goldman M, Lin P. A scanning electron microscopic comparison of a high-volume final flush with several irrigation solutions. Part 3. J Endod. 1983;9:137–42.
37. Dunavant TR, Regan JD, Glickman GN, Solomon ES, Honeyman AL. Comparative evaluation of endodontic irrigants against Enterococcus faecalis biofilms. J Endod. 2006;32(6):527–31.
38. Niu W, Yoshioka T, Kobayashi C, Suda H. A scanning electron microscopic study of dentinal erosion by final irrigation with EDTA and NaOCl solutions. Int Endod J. 2002;35(11):934–9.
39. Grawehr M, Sener B, Waltimo T, Zehnder M. Interactions of ethylenediamine tetraacetic acid with sodium hypochlorite in aqueous solutions. Int Endod J. 2003;36:411–5.
40. Zehnder M, Schmidlin P, Sener B, Waltimo T. Chelation in root canal therapy reconsidered. J Endod. 2005;31(11):817–20.
41. Goldman M, Goldman LB, Cavaleri R, Bogis J, Lin PS. The efficacy of several endodontic irrigating solutions: a scanning electron micrograph study: part 2. J Endod. 1982;8:487–92.
42. Greenstein G, Berman C, Jaffin R. Chlorhexidine: an adjunct to periodontal therapy. J Periodontol. 1986;57:370–6.
43. Russel AD, Day MJ. Antibacterial activity of chlorhexidine. J Hosp Infect. 1993;25:229–38.
44. Komorowski R, Grad H, Wu XY, Friedman S. Antimicrobial substantivity of chlorhexidine-treated bovine root dentin. J Endod. 2000;26:315–7.
45. Vianna ME, Gomez BP, Berber VB, Zaia AA, Ferraz CCR, Souza-Filho FJ. In vitro-evaluation of the antimicrobial activity of chlorhexidine and sodium hypochlorite. Oral Surg Oral Med Oral Pathol Oral Radiol Endod. 2004;97:79–84.
46. Spratt DA, Pratten J, Wilson M, Gulabivala K. An in-vitro evaluation of the antimicrobial efficacy of irrigants on biofilm of root canal isolates. Int Endod J. 2001;34:300–7.
47. Basrani B, Manek S, Sodhi R, Fillery E, Manzur A. Interaction between sodium hypochlorite and chlorhexidine gluconate. J Endod. 2007;33:966–9.
48. Bui TB, Baumgartner JC, Mitchell JC. Evaluation of the interaction between sodium hypochlorite and chlorhexidine gluconate and its effect on root dentine. J Endod. 2008;34:181–5.
49. Vivacqua-Gomes N, Ferraz CC, Gomes BP, Zaia AA, Teixeira FB, Souza-Filho FJ. Influence of irrigants on the coronal micro-leakage of laterally condensed gutta-percha root fillings. Int Endod J. 2002;35:791–5.
50. Rasimick BJ, Nekich M, Hladek MM, Musikant BL, Deutsch AS. Interaction between chlorhexidine digluconate and EDTA. J Endod. 2008;34(12):1521–3.
51. Siren EK, Haapasalo MPP, Waltimo TMT, Orstavik D. In vitro antibacterial effect of calcium hydroxide combined with chlorhexidine or iodine potassium iodide on Enterococcus faecalis. Eur J Oral Sci. 2004;112:326–31.

52. Spangberg L, Engstrom B, Langeland K. Biologic effects of dental materials. 3. Toxicity and antimicrobial effect of endodontic antiseptics in vitro. Oral Surg Oral Med Oral Pathol. 1973;36:856–71.

53. Hancock HH, Sigurdsson A, Trope M, Moiseiwitsch J. Bacteria isolated after unsuccessful endodontic treatment in a North American population. Oral Surg Oral Med Oral Pathol Oral Radiol Endod. 2001;91:579–86.

54. Peciuliene V, Reynaud AH, Balciuniene I, Haapasalo M. Isolation of yeasts and enteric bacteria in root-filled teeth with chronic apical periodontitis. Int Endod J. 2001;34:429–34.

55. Safavi KE, Spångberg LSW, Langeland K. Root canal dentinal tubule disinfection. J Endod. 1990;16:207–10.

56. Grossman LI. Endodontic practice. 9th ed. Philadelphia: Lea & Febiger; 1978. p. 232–4.

57. Hülsmann M, Rödig T, Nordmeyer S. Complications during root canal irrigation. Endod Top. 2009;16:27–63.

58. Torabinejad M, Shabahang S, Aprecio RM, Kettering JD. The antimicrobial effect of MTAD: an in vitro investigation. J Endod. 2003;29:400–3.

59. Giardino L, Pecora G, Ambu E, Savoldi E. A new irrigant in the treatment of apical periodontitis from research to clinic. 12th Biennial Congress European Society of Endodontology, Dublin, 2005. p. 15–7.

60. Stojicic S, Shen Y, Qian W, Johnson B, Haapasalo M. Antibacterial and smear layer removal ability of a novel irrigant, QMiX. Int Endod J 2012;45:363–71.

61. Stabholz A, Zeltser R, Sela M, Peretz B, Moshonov J, Ziskind D, Stabholz A. The use of lasers in dentistry: principles of operation and clinical applications. Compend Contin Educ Dent 2003;24:935–48.

62. Rooney J, Midda M, Leeming J. A laboratory investigation of the bactericidal effect of a Nd: YAG laser. Br Dent J 1994;176(2):61–4.

63. Yavari HR, Rahimi S, Shahi S, Lotfi M, Barhaghi MH, Fatemi A, Abdolrahimi M. Effect of Er, Cr: YSGG laser irradiation on Enterococcus faecalis in infected root canals. Photomed Laser Surg 2010;28:S91–S96.

64. Dostálová T, Jelínková H, Housová D, Sulc J, Nemeć M, Dusková J, Miyagi M, Krátky M. Endodontic treatment with application of Er: YAG laser waveguide radiation disinfection. J Clin Laser Med Surg. 2002;20:135–9.

65. Peters OA, Bardsley S, Fong J, Pandher G, DiVito E. Disinfection of root canals with photon-initiated photo acoustic streaming. J Endod. 2011;37:1008–12.

66. Bonsor SJ, Nichol R, Reid TM, Pearson GJ. An alternative regimen for root canal disinfection. Br Dent J 2006;201:101–5.

67. Ng R, Singh F, Papamanou DA, Song X, Patel C, Holewa C, Patel N, Klepac-Ceraj V, Fontana CR, Kent R, Pagonis TC, Stashenko PP, Soukos NS. Endodontic photodynamic therapy ex vivo. J Endod. 2011;37(2):217–22.

68. Ram Z. Effectiveness of root canal irrigation. Oral Surg Oral Med Oral Pathol 1977;44:306–12.

69. Chow TW. Mechanical effectiveness of root canal irrigation. J Endod. 1983;9:475–9.

70. Al-Hadlaq SM, Al-Turaiki SA, Al-Sulami U, Saad AY. Efficacy of a new-brush covered irrigation needle in removing root canal debris: a scanning electron microscopic study. J Endod. 2006;32:1181–4.

71. Machtou P. Irrigation investigation in endodontics. Master thesis. Paris: Paris VII University; 1980.

72. McGill S, Gulabivala K, Morden N, Ng YL. The efficacy of dynamic irrigation using a commercially available system (RinseEndo) determined by removal of a collagen "bio-molecular film" from an ex vivo model. Int Endod J. 2008;41:602–8.

73. Weise M, Roggendorf MJ, Ebert J, Petschelt A, Frankenberger R. Four methods for cleaning simulated lateral extensions of curved root canals: a SEM evaluation. Int Endod J. 2007;40:991–2.

74. Ruddle CJ. Endodontic disinfection: tsunami irrigation. Endod Pract. 2008;11:7–15.

75. Desai P, Himel V. Comparative safety of various intracanal irrigation systems. J Endod. 2009;35:545–9.

76. Ahmad M, Pitt Ford TR, Crum LA. Ultrasonic debridement of root canals: an insight into the mechanisms involved. J Endod. 1987;13:93–101.

77. Ahmad M, Pitt Ford TR, Crum LA. Ultrasonic debridement of root canals: acoustic streaming and its possible role. J Endod. 1987;13:490–9.

78. Ahmad M, Pitt Ford TR, Crum LA, Walton AJ. Ultrasonic debridement of root canals: acoustic cavitation and its relevance. J Endod. 1988;14:486–93.

79. Burleson A, Nusstein J, Reader A, Beck M. The in vivo evaluation of hand/rotary/ultrasonic instrumentation in necrotic, human mandibular molars. J Endod. 2007;33:782–7.

80. Spoleti P, Siragusa M, Spoleti MJ. Bacteriological evaluation of passive ultrasonic activation. J Endod. 2003;298:12–4.

81. Cameron JA. The synergistic relationship between ultrasound and sodium hypochlorite: a scanning electron microscope evaluation. J Endod. 1987;13:541–5.

82. Guerisoli DM, Marchesan MA, Wamsley AD, Lumley PJ, Pecora JD. Evaluation of smear layer removal by EDTAC and sodium hypochlorite with ultrasonic agitation. Int Endod J. 2002;35:418–21.

83. Mitchell RP, Yang SE, Baumgartner JC. Comparison of apical extrusion of NaOCl using the EndoVac or needle irrigation of root canal. J Endod. 2010;36(2): 338–41.

84. Brito PR, Souza LC, Machado de Oliveira JC, Alves FR, De-Deus G, Lopes HP, Siqueira Jr JF. Comparison of the effectiveness of three irrigation techniques in reducing intra-canal Enterococcus faecalis populations: an in vitro study. J Endod. 2009;35(10): 1422–7.

85. Hauser V, Braun A, Frentzen M. Penetration depth of dye marker into dentine using a novel hydrodynamic system (RinseEndo). Int Endod J. 2007;40:644–52.

86. Haapasalo M, Shen Y, Wang Z, Gao Y. Irrigation in endodontics. Br Dent J. 2014;216(6):299–303.

Medicated Intra-pulpal Dressings

6

Bobby Patel

Summary

Disinfection of the root canal system in primary root canal treatments and retreatments is restricted due to the anatomical complexities, dentinal structure and limitations associated with chemical disinfection. Furthermore resident endodontic microorganisms form complex biofilm structures that afford therapeutic resilience to conventional chemical, mechanical and antimicrobial treatments. The use of an intra-canal medicament is an indispensable adjunct after completion of chemo-mechanical instrumentation of the infected pulp space. It primarily serves to augment disinfection of the root canal system further reducing the intra-canal biofilm load. To date no current method of disinfection can reliably remove or inactivate all microorganisms from within the root canal. Novel methods of disinfection continue to evolve including the recent investigation of using various antibacterial nanoparticles. These potential therapeutic treatment strategies are aimed at further improvements and ultimate elimination of biofilm that is responsible for sustaining peri-radicular disease.

Clinical Relevance

Placement of antimicrobial agents in the pulp space following chemomechanical preparation has long been a practised technique in an effort to reduce the bacterial content of the root canal system. Common intra-canal dressings include calcium hydroxide, Ledermix, chlorhexidine and iodine potassium iodide. Direct contact with the root canal walls in the very apical portion of the pulp space is critical for the effectiveness of the chosen antiseptic. Controversy remains with regard to single- or multiple-visit treatment, but the additional use of appropriate antimicrobial inter-appointment dressings appears to support the notion of multi-treatment visits particularly in cases of endodontic revision (retreatment).

B. Patel, BDS MFDS MClinDent MRD MRACDS
Specialist Endodontist, Brindabella Specialist Centre,
Canberra, ACT, Australia
e-mail: bobbypatel@me.com

© Springer International Publishing Switzerland 2016
B. Patel (ed.), *Endodontic Treatment, Retreatment, and Surgery*,
DOI 10.1007/978-3-319-19476-9_6

6.1 Overview of Medicated Intra-pulpal Dressings

Intra-canal medicaments should only be used for root canal disinfection as part of controlled asepsis in infected root canals, and their role is secondary to cleaning and shaping of the root canal [1]. Mechanical removal of infectious debris using hand or rotary instrumentation and chemical cleansing with a bactericidal solution (sodium hypochlorite) destroys and reduces the numbers of microbes present in an infected root canal. Further use of antimicrobial inter-appointment dressings serves to reduce microbial numbers further and prevents recolonisation during the interim period prior to obturation. Although no treatment strategy is currently 100 % effective at eliminating all bacteria, careful adherence to these steps is key to ensuring success and reducing microbial numbers to levels conducive to healing. Traditionally endodontic treatment has therefore been divided into two or more appointments before completion of treatment and placement of a permanent root filling.

Single-visit treatments are however regarded as an accepted approach to root canal treatment, where no intra-canal medicaments are included in the treatment protocol. Two systematic reviews have corroborated the findings that there is no statistical difference in success rates between single- and multiple-visit endodontics [2, 3]. Proponents of single-visit therapies claim many advantages including no difference in treatment outcomes when compared to multi-visit treatments, less time-consuming, less cost to the patient, less postoperative pain and potentially more profit for the dentist [4–9]. Often the advocates for providing such treatments are based on exclusion criteria that have no scientific basis including suggestions, single-visit treatments are provided on the time available for treatment [7] and that multi-rooted teeth should be excluded and reserved for "teeth in my practice, which could be conveniently treated in a single visit" [10].

Strict selection criteria for whether teeth are amenable to single- or multiple-visit treatment should be based on underlying pathology and whether the tooth is vital with sterile necrosis or necrotic and often infected. The argument for completing the endodontic case in a single visit appears to favour the former where the goal of treatment is to prevent bacterial invasion of the sterile root canal space and avoid the unnecessary use of additional inter-appointment dressings to eliminate bacteria that are not present. Currently there is no diagnostic tool available that is 100 % reliable, sensitive and specific in confirming the true pulpal status and whether bacteria are present prior to treatment. Even the gold standard of histopathological examination of the pulp lends itself to critique depending on the number and type of sections examined. It may therefore be sensible to reserve single-visit treatments to those cases where elective root canal procedures are undertaken. The prerequisite for success is based solely on an aseptic vital pulp extirpation and subsequent obturation with the goal of contamination prevention of the root canal space as a priority.

The aims of treating an infected pulp are the goal of either prevention or treatment of apical periodontitis and more specifically prevention or elimination of a microbial infection in the root canal system. Technically this is achieved by instrumentation and irrigation to remove all necrotic and vital organic tissue giving the canal system a shape that allows easy debridement and predictable placement of locally used medicaments and a permanent root filling of high quality. Microbiologically instrumentation and irrigation is aimed at removing and/or killing all microorganisms within the root canal system. If this goal could be predictably achieved at the first appointment, then time permitting, all cases could be completed in a single visit appointment. Mechanical instrumentation and irrigation alone cannot ensure complete bacterial reduction in the infected root canal. Byström and Sundqvist measured the reduction in bacterial counts cultured from infected root canals following hand stainless steel instrumentation under irrigation with physiological sterile saline solution. Fifteen necrotic root canals with periapical lesions were instrumented at five sequential appointments. The access cavities were sealed between appointments with a bacteria-tight temporary restoration, but the canals were left empty with no antibacterial dressing. A substantial reduction in bacterial numbers occurred (1000-fold) but achieving bacteria-free root canals proved difficult. After five appointments, seven of the 15 canals still had cultivable bacteria [11]. The persistence of bacteria despite the use of chemomechanical techniques (rotary or stainless steel instrumentation) was supported by the findings from a microscopic study which revealed the presence of residual bacteria in 14 out of 16 amputated mesial roots of molar teeth immediately following single-visit treatment using stringent canal decontamination protocol with sodium hypochlorite and EDTA as the canal irrigants [12]. The fate of these persistent bacteria following obturation of the canal system and provision of coronal restoration has not been followed. Additional use of an antimicrobial irrigant further reduces but does not completely eliminate bacterial loads [13, 14]. Since complete eradication of root canal microorganisms cannot be predictably achieved, the placement of an antibacterial inter-appointment dressing is aimed at enhancing the disinfection of the root canal system further [15].

A medicament is an antimicrobial agent that is placed inside the root canal system between treatment appointments in an attempt to destroy remaining microorganisms and prevent reinfection. Medicaments used for inter-appointment intra-canal disinfection include calcium hydroxide, phenolic and non-phenolic biocide compounds (phenol, paraphenol, camphorated parachlorophenol, cresol, formocresol, creosote, cresatin and cresonol), halogens (iodine solution), corticosteroids, antibiotics, sulphonamides, eugenol, chlorhexidine, a mixture of calcium hydroxide and chlorhexidine, medicated gutta-percha and bioactive glass [16].

Several disinfecting agents used in endodontics that are rapidly able to kill microbes when tested in vitro are clearly weaker and less effective in the in vivo situation. Studies have used dentin powder, chips and blocks and have also used components of dentine, such as hydroxyapatite and serum albumin to test the antibacterial effectiveness against common intra-canal irrigants and medicaments. Most results indicate that interactions between medicaments and dentine seem to have a negative impact on the medicament performance. This is speculated to be a result of both the organic and inorganic components of dentine: the presence of a hydration layer in the hydroxyapatite allows changes in the chemical microenvironment with the exchange and absorption of ions, and dentinal collagen is relatively insoluble in acid and neutral solutions compared to collagen from other sources [17, 18].

Calcium hydroxide has been included within several materials and antimicrobial formulations that are used in a number of treatment modalities in endodontics including intra-canal medicaments. Pure calcium hydroxide paste has a high pH (approximately 12.5–12.8) and is classified as a strong base, which prevents the growth and survival of bacteria. Its main antibacterial actions are achieved through the ionic dissociation of Ca^{2+} and OH^- ions resulting in bacterial cell protein denaturation and damage to DNA and cytoplasmic membranes. It has a wide range of antimicrobial activity against common endodontic pathogens but is less effective against *Enterococcus faecalis* and *Candida albicans* [19–21]. *E. faecalis* has been reported to withstand the high pH of calcium hydroxide due to a functioning proton pump with the ability to acidify the cytoplasm increasing it chances of survival [22]. A 10-minute application of calcium hydroxide does not reduce viable bacterial counts in infected root canals, whilst a 1-week application has a major effect [23]. Ideally calcium hydroxide suspension should be applied for the interim and administered as thin slurries using a spiral-type filler [24]. Thin slurries enable ionic (calcium and hydroxyl ions) flow, which is only possible in an aqueous environment responsible for the calcium hydroxide effect. To remove the calcium hydroxide at the initiation of the second visit, calcium-chelating agents can be used (see Fig. 6.1). Agitation of the chelating agent using the master apical file size or an ultrasonic or sonic instrument can further enhance the removal of calcium hydroxide deposits within the canal system [25].

Intra-canal medicaments and the use of phenolic and non-phenolic biocide compounds have been used for chemical fixation of tissue remnants remaining after canal preparation. The concept of using chemical fixatives was the treatment modality when endodontic instruments and techniques were less well developed. Due to anatomical ramifications of the root canal system, poor penetration of fixatives, irritation and toxicity and carcinogenic potential, these types of medicaments should not be used [1].

Iodine has been used for many years and is known for its bactericidal and fungicidal properties. The two most common preparations used in dentistry are iodine tincture (5 % in alcohol) and iodine potassium iodide (2 % iodine, potassium iodide 4 % and distilled water 94 % (2 % IPI 4 %)). The former solution is used for the disinfection of endodontic surgical fields,

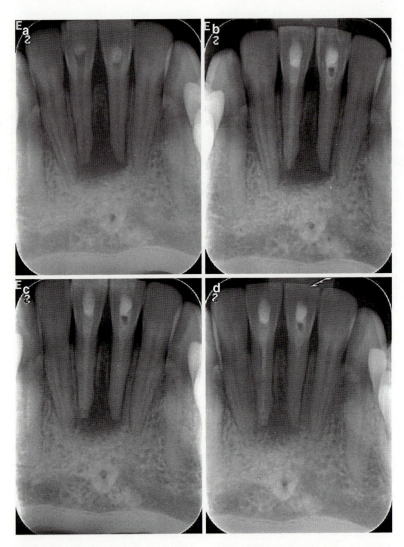

Fig. 6.1 Clinical radiographs demonstrating long-term calcium hydroxide dressing placement in teeth 31 and 41. A fit and healthy 27-year-old female patient was seen for endodontic consultation regarding management of teeth 31 and 41. The patient had previously seen her general dental practitioner who had started root canal therapy but was unable to achieve dry canals. The patient was then referred to an oral maxillofacial surgeon regarding apicectomy procedures. The patient was not keen on a surgical approach and decided to seek a second opinion. At time of consultation, the patient was asymptomatic. Clinical examination confirmed both teeth 31 and 41 had intact lingual access cavities. Radiographic examination revealed a periradicular radiolucent lesion associated with the periapices of teeth 31 and 41. Nonsurgical root canal treatment was commenced, and a decision was made to place long-term calcium hydroxide dressings that were replaced at 3 monthly intervals. Note (**a**) preoperative view. (**b**) Following chemomechanical debridement and intra-canal dressing, calcium hydroxide was placed. (**c**) Three-month review demonstrating periapical healing. The dressing was replaced in both teeth. (**d**) Six-month review demonstrating further healing. Calcium hydroxide was placed in a thin slurry using Lentulo spiral fillers. At the redress appointment, the calcium hydroxide was removed using ultrasonic agitation and 17 % EDTA

whilst the latter has proven useful as an intra-canal medicament. 2 % IPI 4 % has been used in re-treatment cases for its effectiveness in killing *E. faecalis* [26] and *C. albicans* [27].

Antibiotic pastes have been used as intra-canal medicaments, and the two commonest antibiotic-corticosteroid-containing commercial preparations include Ledermix™ paste and Septomixine Forte™. Ledermix paste is a glucocorticoid antibiotic compound that was developed by Schroeder and Triadon in 1960. It is used to control pain and inflammation. The sole reason for adding the antibiotic component to Ledermix was to compensate for what was perceived to be a possible corticoid-induced reduction in the host immune response. Today Ledermix paste remains a combination of the tetracycline antibiotics, demeclocycline, HCL (at a concentration of 3.2 %) and a corticosteroid triamcinolone acetonide (concentration 1 %) in a polyethylene glycol base. A 50:50 mixture of Ledermix paste with calcium hydroxide has also been advocated as an intra-canal medicament in cases of infected root canals and pulpal necrosis (see Fig. 6.2) [28].

Chlorhexidine digluconate (CHX) has been recommended as an intra-canal medicament used as either CHX gel (2 % weight/volume) or a mixture of CHX and calcium hydroxide. CHX has a wide range of antibacterial activity (both anaerobes and aerobes), antifungal activity (candida species) and substantive properties. Its ability to absorb onto dentine, preventing microbial colonisation for some time beyond the actual medication period is an obvious advantage. The basis for mixing chlorhexidine with calcium hydroxide was on the speculation that it would be more effective against *E. faecalis* and *C. albicans* and in particular as a disinfectant during retreatment of failed endodontic cases [26, 27, 29–31].

Bioactive glass (BAG) contains calcium, phosphorus, sodium and silicon in a proportion that provides the material with surface activity and the ability to bond with mineralised hard tissue such as the bone or dentine. In an aqueous environment, BAG liberates Ca, Na, PO4 and Si, causing an increase in pH and osmotic pressure that results in an indirect antimicrobial effect. It has also been reported to chemically bond with mineralised tissues giving rise to a Si-rich layer that acts as a template for calcium phosphate precipitations. Due to its biocompatibility and antimicrobial activity (enhanced when in direct contact with dentine) makes BAG a possible alternative to calcium hydroxide inter-appointment dressings in the future [17, 32].

Application of nanoscaled antimicrobials to control oral infections, as a function of their biocidal, anti-adhesive and delivery capabilities, is of increasing interest. Future developments are likely to concentrate on those nanoparticles with maximal antimicrobial activity and minimal host toxicity. Although certain nanoparticles may be toxic to oral and other tissues, the surface characteristics of a given particle will help to determine whether or not it will have potential for oral applications with particular respect to biofilm formation [33].

6.2 Inter-appointment Application and Removal of Medicaments

Antibacterial intra-canal medicament is used to help eliminate any residual bacteria that have not been removed following canal preparation. Furthermore studies have shown that during the period between appointments, bacteria that survive instrumentation and irrigation have been shown to rapidly increase in numbers in empty root canals. A number of techniques have been proposed for the placement of intra-canal medicament with varying results in terms of effectiveness in filling the root canals (Table 6.1).

Placement of the intra-canal medicament such as calcium hydroxide within the root canal system requires special attention in order to completely fill the root canal space with minimal apical extrusion. The material needs to be placed in direct contact with the dentinal walls to ensure both direct and indirect modes of action. The following protocols are recommended to ensure safe and optimal placement of any intra-canal medicament (see Figs. 6.3, 6.4 and 6.5):

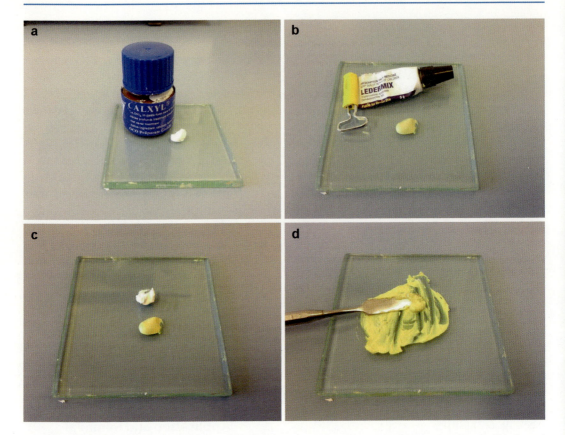

Fig. 6.2 Clinical photographs showing (**a**) calcium hydroxide dressing, (**b**) Ledermix dressing (antibiotic and corticosteroid), and (**c–d**) 50:50 mixture of calcium hydroxide/Ledermix

Table 6.1 Methods for placement of intra-canal medicament

K files/reamers
Absorbent paper points
Gutta-percha cones
Amalgam carriers
McSpadden compactors
Lentulo spiral fillers
Ultrasonic files
Syringe and needles

1. Chemomechanical preparation of the root canal system needs to be completed. If the root canal system is not well instrumented or irrigated, then the dressing will not be effective.
2. Optimal canal enlargement is a prerequisite for intra-canal medicament placement ensuring.
3. A lentulo #25 or #40 depending on master apical file size can be selected and coated with either calcium hydroxide paste or other medicament of choice.
4. The lentulo paste carrier is then passed to either 1 mm short of the binding point or 3 mm short of the working length at 800–1000 rpm. The file can be passed up to three times or until extrusion of calcium hydroxide paste is evident through the coronal canal orifice. Care must be taken in cases with extensive apical resorption or large open apices to avoid apical extrusion. Extremely curved canals or narrow canals require particular attention and care to avoid inadvert file separation.
5. A radiographic film can be taken to assess quality of fill and whether any extrusion has occurred. In the latter the patient should be warned of possible post-operative pain and sequelae.

Prior to obturation of the root canal system, intra-canal medicament such as calcium hydroxide must be removed, since the presence of any remnants of dressing can impede the penetration of root canal sealers into the dentinal

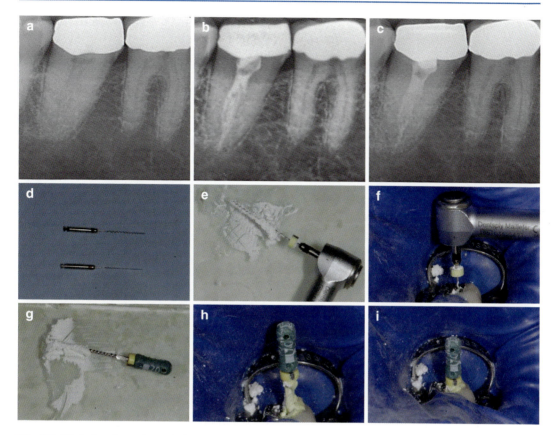

Fig. 6.3 Clinical radiographs and photographs demonstrating methods of placing intra-canal inter-appointment medication. Note (**a**) preoperative radiograph showing C-shaped canal anatomy associated with tooth 47 which required endodontic treatment following recent crown placement, (**b**) intra-canal medication using K-file, (**c**) intra-canal medication using spiral fillers, (**d–f**) spiral fillers #40 and #25 in 21 mm. The spiral filler is used 1 mm short of working length to minimize extrusion apically. (**g–i**) Method using K-files. The K-file is inserted into the canal in an anticlockwise direction to working length

tubules and obstruct the bonding of resin sealers to dentine (Fig. 6.4). Effectiveness of removal relies on the use of a combination of irrigation (sodium hypochlorite and EDTA) with the use of hand, rotary or ultrasonic instrumentation. Furthermore, the use of patency filing improves the efficacy of calcium hydroxide paste removal.

6.3   Recommended Medicament Regimens

Intra-canal medicaments are used for root canal disinfection and their role is secondary to cleaning and shaping procedures. Intra-canal medicaments have been used for a variety of purposes including elimination of remaining bacteria after root canal instrumentation, an aid to reducing inflammation of the periapical tissues, an aid to rendering root canals inert and further neutralising any remaining tissue debris within the canals, to act as a barrier to further bacterial ingress that may arise from the temporary restoration and to help dry wet, purulent canals. No ideal root canal material exists to date, which can fulfil all the desired properties a medicament should fulfil (see Table 6.2).

Calcium Hydroxide

This material has been well accepted as an effective intra-canal medicament that is not only effective against most root-canal bacteria but also has the ability to degrade residual organic tissue remnants not removed from initial chemomechanical preparation procedures.

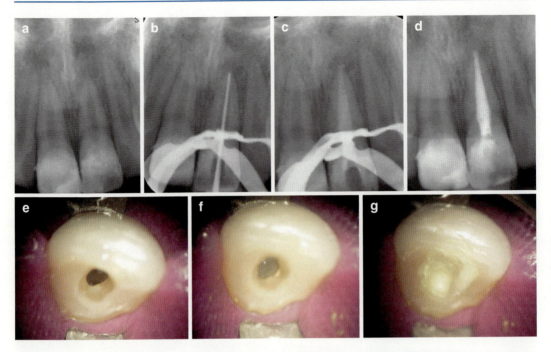

Fig. 6.4 Clinical radiographs and photographs demonstrating multi-visit root canal treatment (two visits) using an intra-canal calcium hydroxide medicament for 3 weeks duration. Note (**a**) preoperative film, (**b**) master apical file, (**c**) intra-canal medicament placed using spiral filler technique, (**d**) postoperative film using chloroform dip/warm vertical compaction using AH Plus cement and Obtura. Remnants of calcium hydroxide medicament were removed using a combination of irrigation using NaOCl and EDTA and mechanical re-instrumentation. (**e**) Access preparation, (**f**) chemomechanical preparation using 1 % NaOCl solution, and (**g**) intra-canal medicament placement

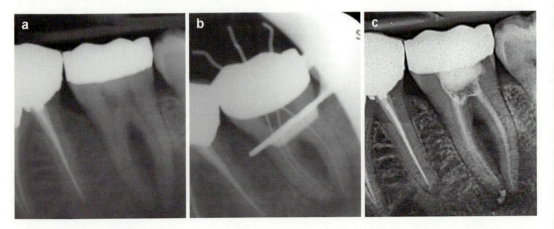

Fig. 6.5 Clinical radiographs showing (**a**) preoperative view of tooth 36. (**b**) Working length radiograph and (**c**) intra-canal inter-appointment medicament of calcium hydroxide. Note medication was placed using a spiral filler. Some extrusion has occurred confirming apical patency. The medication will be resorbed over time. Excessive extrusion should be avoided since there is potential risk of tissue reaction

Furthermore, calcium hydroxide inhibits microbial growth from within canals. Its antibacterial effect is due to its alkaline pH.

It can be placed as either a dry powder, a powder mixed with liquid such as water, saline, local anaesthetic, a sodium hypochlorite solution or as a proprietary paste in a syringe. Due to its low solubility, it can exert a lasting effect with slow dissolution over time. Advantages of using this material include its relative in

Table 6.2 Ideal properties of an inter-appointment medicament used in either non-surgical treatment or retreatment cases

The ability to eradicate all intra-canal bacteria with a long-lasting antibacterial affect
Not inactivated when in the presence of organic material
Ability to degrade residual organic material including necrotic pulp tissue remnants and microbial biofilm
Well tolerated and no toxicity or irritation if extruded beyond the confines of the canal
Ability to induce regeneration of the periapical tissues
No effect on the physical properties of the temporary access restoration or subsequent root canal sealer used within the tooth
Ease of placement
Ease of removal
Radiopaque so easily discernible on radiographs
Inability to stain the tooth
Inability to weaken the tooth
Ability to suppress pain if present

expense, simplicity in placement and nonstaining of teeth. It has also been cited as a method to control "weeping canals" resulting in the drying out of any exudate that may arise from the periapical tissues. A major disadvantage is related to extrusion of the material into the periapical tissues that can result in severe pain and localised tissue necrosis (especially if large amounts have been extruded). Small amounts that are extruded are of no real concern and it should resorb over time (Fig. 6.6). Some clinicians prefer to mix it with a steroid paste to reduce any post-operative discomfort (Fig. 6.7).

Its use is not only confined to treating necrotic infected cases but also utilised as an aid to forming a hard tissue calcific barrier. Teeth with immature apices, apexogenesis, perforation repairs and horizontal root fractures have all benefited from its use. In infected cases, thin slurries are preferred which enable ionic flow (calcium and hydroxyl ions), which is only possible in an aqueous environment. In cases where the primary aim is to create a hard tissue barrier as opposed to disinfection, then thicker pastes are preferred whereby the material can be compacted against the periapical tissue thereby increasing its effectiveness to induce localised necrosis rather than being washed away.

In endodontic re-treatment cases, there has been some concern in the literature as to its resistance to *Enterococcus faecalis* directly related to a proton pump mechanism, which inactivates the alkaline medicament.

As a routine intra-canal medicament, its duration of use should be a minimum of 14 days that can be extended depending on the case. Research has shown that calcium hydroxide takes 3–4 weeks to increase the pH of outer dentine. The maximum time of use will be depending on the pathological condition being treated and the medicament being used. Long-term calcium hydroxide dressings have fallen out of favour, particularly in the treatment of immature teeth, where there is a risk that the underlying mechanical properties of dentine can be changed rendering the tooth weaker and more susceptible to fracture. In addition, the advent of single-visit mineral trioxide aggregate (MTA) apexification procedures has meant that a predictable result can be gained without prolonged treatment appointments – a benefit for both clinician and patient.

Calcium hydroxide can be removed from the canal using irrigants such as saline, sodium hypochlorite solution and EDTA. As discussed previously, the use of patency filing, ultrasonic activation and irrigation are highly effective at removing any traces of the dressing from within the tooth.

Corticosteroids

Steroid preparations have been advocated for the use as intra-canal medicaments mainly due to their ability to provide pain relief and anti-inflammatory actions. Reduction of post-operative pain may be particularly useful when treating irreversible pulpitis or symptomatic apical periodontitis. Its use has also been advocated in the field of dental traumatology, whereby the corticosteroid component has been found to inhibit external root resorption. Nevertheless, it does not possess any antibacterial effects and so has been commonly mixed with calcium hydroxide in a 50:50 ratio. Commercially available steroid pastes include Ledermix (3.21 % demeclocycline and triamcinolone). Recently due to the concerns of potential tooth staining associated with the tetracycline component of

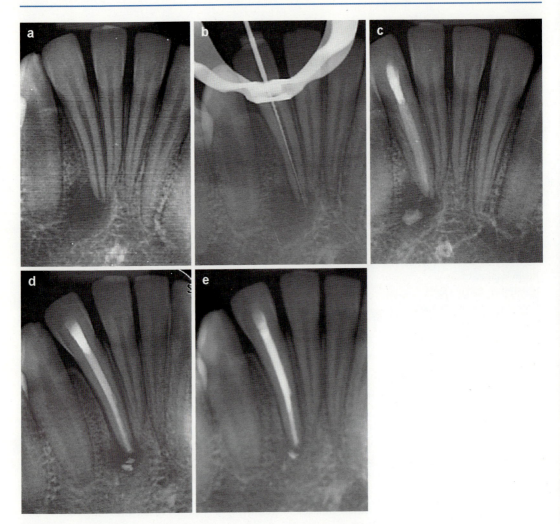

Fig. 6.6 Clinical radiographs demonstrating nonsurgical root canal multi-visit treatment of tooth 42. Note (**a**) preoperative radiograph demonstrating large periradicular radiolucent lesion associated with the periapex of tooth 42. (**b**) Working length radiograph prior to carrying out chemomechanical debridement of the root canal system. (**c**) Radiograph demonstrating homogenous well-condensed inter-appointment calcium hydroxide dressing with temporary double seal coronally. Note extrusion of calcium hydroxide into the surrounding periapex of the tooth. (**d**) Following an interim period of 3 months, the case was obturated using a warm vertical compaction technique. Note there has been some resorption of the extruded calcium hydroxide with obvious reduction in the size of the periapical lesion. There appears to be some sealer extrusion at the periapex; (**e**) 6-month follow-up radiograph showing complete resolution of the periapical radiolucent lesion. Note extruded sealer still present

Ledermix when exposed to light has led to the development of an alternative medicament called Odontopaste (Australian Dental Manufacturing, Kenmore Hills, Australia) that has become commercially available. It is a zinc oxide-based root canal paste that contains 5 % clindamycin hydrochloride and 1 % triamcinolone acetonide. The antibiotic clindamycin provides a bacteriostatic activity in addition to the benefits of a zinc oxide paste. When used as intra-canal medicament, it prevents bacteria and temporarily reduces inflammation. It is useful for transient reduction of post-operative pain. Mixing of additional calcium hydroxide in a 50:50 combination with Odontopaste is not recommended because the steroid component becomes ineffective, thereby

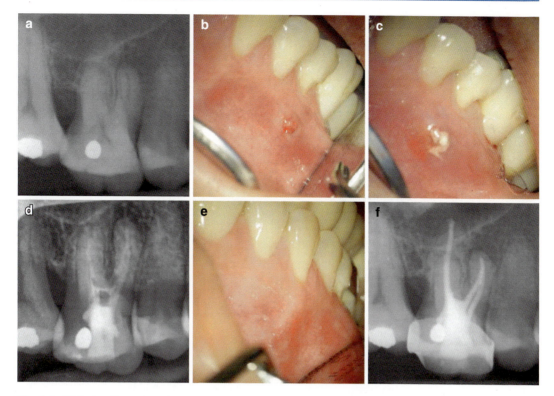

Fig. 6.7 Clinical radiographs and photographs demonstrating nonsurgical endodontic treatment of tooth 16 diagnosed as chronic apical periodontitis with suppuration. Note (**a**) preoperative radiograph showing a periradicular radiolucency associated with the mesial root. (**b**) Intraoral view of adjacent buccal alveolar mucosa where a draining sinus is present. (**c**) Following chemomechanical preparation, a well-placed intra-canal medicament of Ledermix/calcium hydroxide 50:50 ratio was placed. Dressing material can be seen extruding through the draining sinus. (**d**) Radiographic view confirming MB1 and MB2 intra-canal dressing placement. (**e**) Four-week follow-up demonstrating complete healing of the preoperative sinus. (**f**) Completion of endodontic treatment with a well-obturated canal system and overlying semipermanent coronal restoration

offering only minimal benefits over the use of calcium hydroxide alone.

6.4 Clinical Cases

Case 1 Endodontic treatment of tooth 12 with long-term calcium hydroxide dressings

A 19-year-old fit and healthy female patient was referred for endodontic management of tooth 12. The patient had initially presented to her general dental practitioner with severe pain and swelling in relation to tooth 12. The patient lived interstate with the nearest specialist endodontist (myself) being over 4-h drive away. The general dental practitioner therefore attempted to manage

the case, and the patient was seen for three appointments with repeated dressing placements. The dentist had found that the canal had a persistent exudate of pus upon entry at each subsequent visit, and the patient continued to remain symptomatic. At the endodontic consultation/treatment appointment, obvious pain and tenderness were noted in the overlying alveolar mucosa. Tooth 12 had an intact palatal restoration. Radiographic examination confirmed prior endodontic access with a lucent material noted in the canal space (medicament). An extensive peri-radicular radiolucency was noted (see Fig. 6.8). After a lengthy discussion in relation to treatment options, a decision was made to embark upon non-surgical root canal

Fig. 6.8 Clinical radiographs demonstrating nonsurgical management of tooth 12 with a calcium hydroxide long-term dressing. Note (**a**) preoperative view demonstrating prior endodontic access and root canal treatment initiated by the patient's general dental practitioner. The patient had been seen on three consecutive appointments, but the treatment could not be completed due to persistent intra-canal exudate (pus). Note the extensive periradicular radiolucent lesion in relation to tooth 12. (**b**) Following chemomechanical preparation, an intra-canal interim calcium hydroxide dressing was placed using a Lentulo spiral filler. Note the overfill. (**c**) Three-month review radiograph demonstrating significant resorption of extruded medicament and periapical healing. (**d**) Nine-month review appointment showing further reduction in apical lucency and the patient was finally asymptomatic

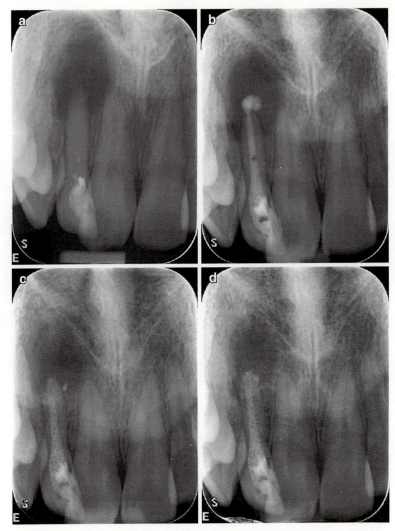

treatment. The patient was warned that if the tooth remained symptomatic, then a surgical approach would be recommended.

The access restoration was dismantled and initial working length established using a conventional electronic apex locator and radiographic verification. An exudate of pus was noted at the peri-apex. Chemomechanical debridement was carried out using stainless steel hand files, and the master apical file (MAF) size was determined to be #90. A 0.5 mm step-back preparation was carried out and 1 % sodium hypochlorite (NaOCl) irrigation used throughout. At the end of chemomechanical preparation and following drying of the canal lumen, a persistent exudate was still present. The canal was re-irrigated and dried followed by an intra-canal calcium hydroxide medicament placement. A size #40 lentulo spiral filler was used for placement of the medicament and intentionally placed 3 mm short of the working length. Despite this precaution and in an aim to ensure that the entire canal lumen was filled with medicament, an overfill was noted on radiographic examination. The patient was warned of the possible risk of post-operative pain and discomfort, but the calcium hydroxide should resorb over time. The patient informed me that she would be moving to Canberra for university studies, and I advised her that 3 monthly reviews would be arranged to monitor signs of clinical and radiographic healing.

At the 3-month review appointment, the patient informed me that she was still aware of occasional percussion and palpation tenderness in relation to this tooth. Clinical examination revealed minor tenderness in the overlying alveolar mucosa on palpation. Radiographic examination revealed significant resorption of the overfilled calcium hydroxide dressing with some medicament still present. The periapical radiolucency had diminished in size considerably (Fig. 6.8). A further follow-up was arranged in a further 3 months. Unfortunately the patient was unable to return until a further 6 months later. At this second review appointment, the patient was not aware of any clinical symptoms. Clinical examination revealed the tooth was asymptomatic with no pain or tenderness on percussion and palpation. Radiographic examination revealed further evidence of periapical healing and bony infilling (Fig. 6.8). The patient was advised to return for a further treatment appointment to complete the endodontic treatment.

Case 2 Endodontic retreatment of tooth 22 with long-term calcium hydroxide dressing and surgical decompression

A fit and healthy 34-year-old female patient with a peanut allergy was referred for endodontic retreatment of tooth 22. At the initial endodontic consultation appointment, the patient reported that this tooth had undergone conventional root canal treatment 6 months earlier but had failed to settle down. She was aware of pain and discomfort particularly when pressing the left alar region of her nose. Clinical examination confirmed tooth 23 responded positively to both electric pulp testing and thermal stimulus (CO2 snow). Radiographic examination confirmed previous endodontic treatment in tooth

22. An extensive periapical radiolucency was noted at the peri-apex of tooth 22. After a lengthy discussion of treatment options, a decision was made to embark upon root canal retreatment of tooth 22.

At the first treatment appointment, palatal access was gained and refined using ultrasonic burrs. Gutta-percha root filling material was removed using a chloroform wicking technique. Apical patency was achieved and working lengths verified using both electronic and radiographic confirmation. Chemomechanical preparation was completed using stainless steel hand files and 1 % NaOCl solution to an MAF size #80. An intra-canal dressing of calcium hydroxide was placed using a combination of hand files and paper points. Radiographic examination was carried out to assess dressing placement revealing the canal lumen was completely filled. An overfill was also noted beyond the confines of the canal. The patient was warned of the possible risk of post-treatment pain and discomfort but reassured that the dressing should dissipate over time. No post-operative complications occurred (Fig. 6.9).

At the 3-month review period, the patient was still aware of pain and tenderness in relation to her left alar region. A decision was made to refer the patient for a cone beam CT (CBCT) scan to determine the extent of the pathology and whether a surgical approach would be feasible. The patient was referred to a local imaging centre for a dental CBCT of the maxillary jaw only to reduce the amount of radiation exposure for the patient. The CBCT report presented by a radiologist stated that a "periapical lucency had caused marked thinning of both buccal and palatal cortical plates and was in close proximity to the floor of the left nasal fossa". The scan also confirmed extruded calcium hydroxide medicament within the lesion as seen 3 months earlier following medicament placement (Fig. 6.10).

After a further discussion with the patient, a decision was made to consider surgical decompression of the lesion in order to relieve the patient's symptoms and also allow the lesion

Fig. 6.9 Clinical radiographs demonstrating nonsurgical root canal re-treatment of tooth 22 and surgical decompression. Note (**a**) preoperative film showing previous root filling with persistent periapical lucency. The patient had undergone root canal treatment 6 months earlier, but symptoms related to pain and tenderness in the left alar region persisted. (**b**) MAF radiograph following removal of previous gutta-percha and chemomechanical preparation using stainless steel hand files using a step-back preparation. (**c**) Immediate postoperative radiograph following placement of calcium hydroxide medicament. (**d**) Radiograph taken immediately following surgical decompression procedure and irrigation of the periapical lesion using sterile saline. Note all the previous medicament overfilling has been removed

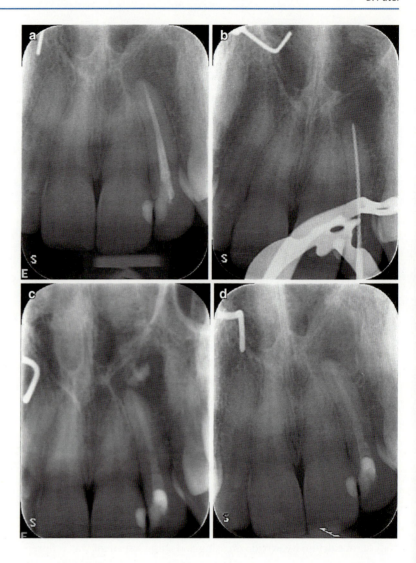

to diminish in size such that any further planned surgical intervention may be permissible with less associated risks. A further appointment was then scheduled for the patient.

After infiltration anaesthesia, a vertical incision of approximately 5 mm was made in the alveolar mucosa above teeth 22 and 23. Blunt dissection was carried out to the underlying cortical buccal plate, and the exact position of the underlying defect was determined. A pre-fitted 1 cm long segment of a nasal oxygen cannula was

adapted, inserted into the incision to the level of the underlying bony crypt and stabilised with two silk 5.0 sutures (Fig. 6.10). The cavity was then copiously rinsed with saline and a radiographic film taken to check. The radiograph showed that the overfilling of calcium hydroxide medicament had been removed (Fig. 6.9). The patient was advised to irrigate the lesion using sterile saline herself, and further reviews were scheduled to ensure that continued healing occurred without further complications.

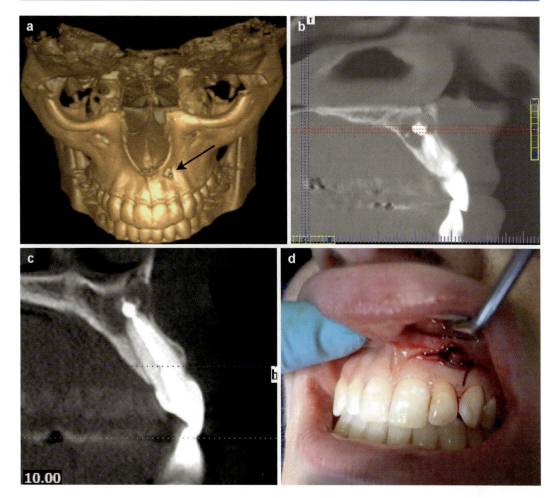

Fig. 6.10 Cone beam CT (CBCT) scans and clinical photographs demonstrating extent of apical lesion, medicament overfilling, and surgical decompression procedure. Note (**a**) reformatted image of the maxilla using CBCT slices showing cortical buccal plate defect (*black arrow*). (**b, c**) CBCT slices demonstrating intra-canal medicament in tooth 22 and overfilling following root canal re-treatment procedure and medicament placement. (**d**) Clinical photograph following surgical decompression showing adapted nasal cannula tubing sutured in place

---

Clinical Hints and Tips Regarding Intra-canal Medicaments

- **Rationale for using intra-canal medicaments**

  The use of antimicrobial intra-canal medicaments has been advocated to disinfect the root canal system. The primary aim of root canal therapy is to reduce or eliminate microorganisms and their by-products from the root canal system. Thorough chemomechanical debridement using a number of instrumentation and irrigation techniques aids removal but does not ensure elimination due to the complex anatomy and limitations of techniques used. Therefore, adjunctive intra-canal medicaments are aimed to further reduce this load, whereby bacterial loads are further reduced below a critical threshold that is conducive to healing.

- **Calcium hydroxide pastes**

  Calcium hydroxide is recognised as one of the most effective intra-canal medicaments used in endodontics due to its bactericidal properties. Although its specific mechanism of action is debatable, some researchers suggest that its antimicrobial effects are due to the release and diffusion of hydroxyl (OH^-) ions leading to a highly alkaline environment (pH 12.5–12.8), which is unfavourable to the survival of microorganisms. Effects can be limited by buffering effect of dentine particularly in the apical one third and limited penetration of dentinal tubules. Ineffective against *Enterococcus faecalis* microorganism associated with re-treatment cases.

- **Corticosteroids**

  Ledermix, a glucocorticosteroid-antibiotic compound, has anti-inflammatory, antibacterial and anti-resorptive properties. These properties help dampen the periapical inflammatory process including clastic-cell-mediated resorption (replacement resorption). Its use has been advocated in reducing pain and inflammation as well as the promotion of more favourable healing in replanted teeth. Potential staining of teeth.

- **50:50 mixture of Ledermix paste and calcium hydroxide**

  This combination has been advocated as an intra-canal medicament in cases of pulpless infected root canals, pulp necrosis, teeth with incomplete root formation undergoing apexification procedures, perforations, inflammatory root resorption and inflammatory peri-radicular bone resorption.

- **Iodine**

  Iodine has been advocated in retreatment cases due to possible *Enterococcus faecalis* bacteria and their inherent resistance to calcium hydroxide medicament by virtue of their proton-pump inhibitor. Care must be excised in patients with known allergy.

- **Techniques for placement of medicaments**

  The use of syringe, rotary instruments (lentulo spiral filler) and hand instruments such as files, spreaders and pluggers has been advocated for placement of intra-canal medicaments. Care must be taken when extensive apical root resorption is evident or wide-open apices are noted due to higher risk of extrusion beyond the confines of the canal.

References

1. Chong BS, Pitt Ford TR. The role of intracanal medication in root canal treatment. Int Endod J. 1992;25:92–106.
2. Sathorn C, Parashos P, Messer HH. Effectiveness of single verses multiple visit endodontic treatment of teeth with apical periodontitis: a systematic review and meta analysis. Int Endod J. 2005;38:347–55.
3. Figini L, Lodi G, Gorni F, Gagliani M. Single verses multiple visits for endodontic treatment of permanent teeth: a Cochrane systematic review. J Endod. 2008;34:1041–7.
4. Soltanoff W. A comparative study of the single-visit and the multiple-visit endodontic procedure. J Endod. 1978;4:278–81.
5. Mulhern JM, Patterson SS, Newton CW, Ringel AM. Incidence of postoperative pain after one-appointment endodontic treatment of asymptomatic pulpal necrosis in single-rooted teeth. J Endod. 1982;8:370–5.
6. Oliet S. Single visit endodontics: a clinical study. J Endod. 1983;9:147–53.
7. Roane JB, Dryden JA, Grimes EW. Incidence of postoperative pain after single- and multiple-visit endodontic procedures. Oral Surg Oral Med Oral Pathol. 1983;55:68–72.
8. Southard DW, Rooney TP. Effective one-visit therapy for the acute apical abscess. J Endod. 1984;10:580–3.
9. Ashkenaz PJ. One-visit endodontics. Dent Clin N Am. 1984;28:853–63.
10. Pekruhn RB. The incidence and failure following single visit endodontic therapy. J Endod. 1986;12:68–72.
11. Byström A, Sundqvist G. Bacteriological evaluation of the efficacy of mechanical root canal instrumentation in endodontic therapy. Scand J Dent Res. 1981;89:321–8.
12. Nair PN, Henry S, Cano V, Vera J. Microbial status of apical root canal system of human mandibular first, molars with primary apical periodontitis after "one-visit" endodontic treatment. Oral Surg Oral Med Oral Pathol Oral Radiol Endod. 2005;99:231–52.
13. Byström A, Sundqvist G. Bacteriological evaluation of the effect of 0.5 per cent sodium hypochlorite solution in endodontic therapy. Oral Surg Oral Med Oral Pathol. 1983;55(3):307–12.
14. Byström A, Sundqvist G. The antibacterial action of sodium hypochlorite and EDTA in 60 cases of endodontic therapy. Int Endod J. 1985;18:35–40.

15. Sjögren U, Figdor D, Persson S, Sundqvist G. Influence of infection at the time of root filling on the outcome of endodontic treatment of teeth with apical periodontitis. Int Endod J. 1997;30:297–306.
16. Weine FS. Endodontic therapy. 6th ed. St. Louis: Mosby; 2004. p. 226–8.
17. Haapasalo HK, Siren EK, Waltimo TM, Ørstavik D, Haapasalo MP. Inactivation of local root canal medicaments by dentine: an in vitro study. Int Endod J. 2000;33:126–31.
18. Haapasalo M, Qian W, Portenier I, Waltimo T. Effects of dentin on the antimicrobial properties of endodontic medicaments. J Endod. 2007;33(8):917–21.
19. Fava LR, Saunders WP. Calcium hydroxide pastes: classification and clinical indications. Int Endod J. 1999;32:257–82.
20. Athanassiadis B, Abbott PV, Walsh LJ. The use of calcium hydroxide, antibiotics and biocides as antimicrobial medicaments in endodontics. Aust Dent J. 2007;52(1):S64–82.
21. Mohammadi Z, Dummer PM. Properties and applications of calcium hydroxide in endodontics and dental traumatology. Int Endod J. 2011;44:697–730.
22. Evans M, Davies JK, Sundqvist G, Figdor D. Mechanisms involved in the resistance of Enterococcus faecalis to calcium hydroxide. Int Endod J. 2002;35:221–8.
23. Sjögren U, Figdor D, Spangberg L, Sundqvist G. The antimicrobial effect of calcium hydroxide as a short-term intracanal dressing. Int Endod J. 1991;24:119–25.
24. Peters CI, Koka RS, Highsmith S, Peters OA. Calcium hydroxide dressings using different preparation and application modes: density and dissolution by stimulated time pressure. Int Endod J. 2005;38:889–95.
25. Salgado RJ, Moura-Netto C, Yamazaki AK, Cardoso LN, de Moura AA, Prokopowitsch I. Comparison of different irrigants on calcium hydroxide medication removal: microscopic cleanliness evaluation. Oral Surg Oral Med Oral Pathol Oral Radiol Endod. 2009;107:580–4.
26. Siren EK, Haapasalo MP, Waltimo TM, Ørstavik D. In vitro antibacterial effect of calcium hydroxide combined with chlorhexidine or iodine potassium iodide on Enterococcus faecalis. Eur J Oral Sci. 2004;112:326–31.
27. Waltimo TM, Ørstavik D, Siren EK, Haapasalo MP. In vitro susceptibility of Candida Albicans to four disinfectants and their combinations. Int Endod J. 1999;32:421–9.
28. Abbott PV. Medicaments: aids to success in endodontics. Part 1. A review of the literature. Aust Dent J. 1990;35(4):438–48.
29. Rosenthal S, Spangberg LS, Safavi K. Chlorhexidine substantivity in root canal dentine. Oral Surg Oral Med Oral Pathol Oral Radiol Endod. 2004;98: 488–92.
30. Zerella JA, Fouad AF, Spangberg LS. Effectiveness of a calcium hydroxide and chlorhexidine digluconate mixture as a disinfectant during re-treatment of failed endodontic cases. Oral Surg Oral Med Oral Pathol Oral Radiol Endod. 2005;100:756–61.
31. Mohammadi Z, Abbott PV. The properties and applications of chlorhexidine in endodontics. Int Endod J. 2009;42:288–302.
32. Gubler M, Brunner TJ, Zehnder M, Waltimo T, Sener B, Stark WJ. Do bioactive glasses convey a disinfecting mechanism beyond a mere increase in pH? Int Endod J. 2008;41:670–8.
33. Allaker RP, Memarzadeh K. Nanoparticles and the control of oral infections. Int J Antimicrob Agents. 2014;43:95–104.

Root Canal Obturation

7

Bobby Patel

Summary

Several obturation techniques are available for root canal treatment. Selection of any technique is determined not only by operator preference but also key factors including canal anatomy, preparation technique used and the unique treatment objectives of each case. The two basic obturation procedures are lateral condensation and warm vertical condensation. Gutta-percha root fillings remain the ideal filling material despite the advent of new devices and techniques, such as synthetic resin-based polycaprolactone polymer (Resilon). Paste fills utilising highly toxic resin cements such as 'SPAD' and formaldehyde-containing Endomethasone and silver point fillings have a poor reputation and cannot be recommended. However, the use of mineral trioxide aggregate has been advocated in the management of large open apices that may not be easily customised with traditional gutta-percha techniques. Obturation is the final treatment objective that ensures that the canal remains cleaned, disinfected and sealed from the apical minor constriction of the root canal system to the orifice.

Clinical Relevance

Success or failure in endodontics does not necessarily relate to the radiographic white lines that we produced at the end of endodontic treatment unless follow-up images demonstrate biological healing. The final obturation is simply a mirror image of our cleaning and shaping goals and provides a partial indication of whether our treatment objectives were met. The final obturation and material used can be seen as a penultimate step in the reduction and prevention of microbial contamination of the root canal system. The quality of obturation has been associated with endodontic treatment success and the method employed relies on using materials and methods capable of densely filling the entire root canal system. The clinician should be aware of the various techniques available that can be utilised according to individual case requirements and anatomical constraints. One must also bear in mind the inherent risks associated with overextension of root filling materials including neural, sinus and alveolar bone complications that should be avoided when seeking the 'thrill of the fill'.

B. Patel, BDS MFDS MClinDent MRD MRACDS
Specialist Endodontist, Brindabella Specialist Centre, Canberra, ACT, Australia
e-mail: bobbypatel@me.com

© Springer International Publishing Switzerland 2016
B. Patel (ed.), *Endodontic Treatment, Retreatment, and Surgery*,
DOI 10.1007/978-3-319-19476-9_7

7.1 Overview of Material, Methods and Risks Associated with Root Canal Obturation

Microorganisms and their by-products are the major cause of pulpal and periapical disease and we are unable to totally disinfect the residual biofilm within the instrumented and un-instrumented root canal system (30–50 % of the root canal wall) despite the revolution of newer materials and methods over the last century. Therefore, the goal of three-dimensional obturation is to provide an impermeable fluid tight seal within the entire root canal system, to prevent oral and apical micro-leakage, successfully entombing persistent or resistant bacteria and their by-products [1–3].

Prior to the obturation phase, the clinician must establish proper canal preparation of the root canal to provide an apical resistance form for the adequate adaptation of filling materials and the prevention of excessive apical extrusion of these materials. The importance of maintaining the original shape of a root canal during and after cleaning and shaping and avoiding iatrogenic errors such as ledges and perforations is primary in the pursuit of promoting periapical healing in endodontic cases. Poor obturation quality (over-filling or underfilling) as judged by radiographs has been correlated with a decreased prognosis for healing [4–6].

The radiographic appearance of a completed case should demonstrate the obturation material at the apical terminus without excessive material overextending into periapical tissues, completely filling the root canal system in three dimensions and appearing as a dense radiopaque filling of the root canal system [7].

Many materials and techniques for obturation are available on the market. Dr. Louis I. Grossman, one of the founders of the specialty of endodontics, determined the ideal properties of obturation materials (Table 7.1) [8]. These materials are divided into two basic groups—core materials and sealers—each of which can be found in a large variety of materials and brands (Table 7.2 and 7.3). Materials approved by the International

Table 7.1 Ideal properties of a root canal filling material

Easily manipulated with ample working time
Radiopaque and easily discernible on radiographs
Dimensionally stable with no shrinkage once inserted
Seals the canals laterally and apically conforming to the canal anatomy
Impervious to moisture and non-porous
Inhibits bacterial growth
Non-irritating to periapical tissues
Unaffected by tissue fluids (no corrosion or oxidation)
Does not stain tooth structure
Easily removed from canal if necessary
Sterile

Adapted from Grossman

Table 7.2 Overview of core materials and chemical composition

Function	Material	Main composition
Core materials	Gutta-percha	Gutta-percha, zinc oxide, metallic salts, waxes, colouring agents antioxidants
	Silver point	Silver, nickel
	Resin-coated gutta-percha	Resin, gutta-percha, zinc oxide
	Thermoplastic polymer	Polyester, bioactive glass, bismuth oxychloride, barium sulphate
	Mineral trioxide aggregate (MTA)	Tricalcium silicate Dicalcium silicate Bismuth oxide Calcium sulphate Tetracalcium aluminoferrite

Standards Organization and the relevant Dental Association within your jurisdiction should be used.

Jasper introduced silver cones and due to their inherent rigidity made them easy to place. However, their inability to fill the irregularly shaped root canal system permitted leakage and resulted in corrosion products that were found to be highly cytotoxic. Silver cones are no longer utilised for root canal obturation [9, 10].

Sargenti and Richter proposed the principle of mummification and fixation of pulp tissues using highly toxic paraformaldehyde pastes (N2) in

Table 7.3 Overview of sealers, chemical composition and various brands

Type	Brand	Main composition
Zinc oxide eugenol	Roth	Zinc oxide eugenol, colophony, bismuth and barium
	Kerr PCS	Zinc oxide eugenol, thymol, silver
	ProcoSol	Zinc oxide eugenol, colophony, bismuth and barium
	Endomethasone	Zinc oxide eugenol, paraformaldehyde
Resin	AH Plus	Epoxy-bis-phenol resin, adamantine
	Epiphany	BisGMA, UDMA and hydrophilic methacrylates
	EndoREZ	UDMA
	Russian Red	Recorcin-formaldehyde
Calcium hydroxide	Sealapex	Toluene salicylate, calcium oxide
	Apexit	Salicylates, calcium hydroxide
Silicone	RoekoSeal	Polydimethylsiloxane, silicone oil, zirconium oxide, catalyst
	GuttaFlow	Polydimethylsiloxane, silicone oil, zirconium oxide, gutta-percha
Glass ionomer	Ketac Endo	Polyalkenoate cement
Calcium silicate	iRoot SP	Calcium phosphate, calcium silicate, zirconium oxide, calcium hydroxide

view of its antimicrobial activity. Other paste fills containing formaldehyde include SPAD and Endomethasone. Inadvertent overextension often resulted in biologically unacceptable outcomes or worse still with accompanying neural damage. Coupled with treatment difficulties encountered when attempting to retreat such cases, their use is frowned upon within the endodontic community [11–15].

Gutta-percha has proven to be the material of choice worldwide for successful obturation when used in combination with a root canal sealer. Gutta-percha points alone cannot completely seal the space between the dentinal walls, root canal irregularities, lateral and accessory canals and spaces between gutta-percha points used in lateral condensation. So a sealer is necessary and volumes should be minimal to counteract possible shrinkage and dissolution over time. Gutta-percha can be made to flow using heat or using solvents, such as chloroform or eucalyptus, as well as by ultrasonics and vibration. It is a trans-isomer of polyisoprene and exists in two crystalline forms alpha and beta, with differing properties. The use of alpha phase gutta-percha has increased as thermoplastic techniques have become more popular [16–18].

Gutta-percha cones consist of approximately 20 % gutta-percha, 65 % zinc oxide, 10 % radiopacifiers and 5 % plasticisers. Gutta-percha points are manufactured in various forms including standardised points that match the ISO sizes and have a 2 % taper. Accessory points have fine tips and variable taper to facilitate and improve lateral compaction. Greater taper points are available in 4 % and 6 % taper to match modern rotary preparation techniques. Feather-tipped points permit individual and specific cone fitting to the prepared root canal. As clinicians we expect that the diameter and tapers of GP cones to be accurate with no variability. However, even if the manufacturers are following the current standards, the accepted diameter tolerance levels vary from 0.05 to 0.07 mm, depending on the cone size. Such tolerance means that cones of one size can theoretically span more than one size above and/or below the stated size. For example, a size #30 cone has an allowable tip diameter of 0.23–0.37 mm. Therefore, the nominal diameter and taper values as listed by the manufacturer may vary greatly and still be in accordance with the 'standards'. Gutta-percha points cannot be sterilised by traditional means, but rapid disinfection before use by placing the cones with 70 % isopropyl alcohol, 2 % chlorhexidine or 1–5 % NaOCl is effective [16, 19, 20].

Several techniques have been developed for placing gutta-percha into root canals including single-cone techniques [21, 22], cold lateral compaction [23], warm lateral compaction using ultrasonics (energised spreading) [24], chloroform customization of gutta-percha [25],

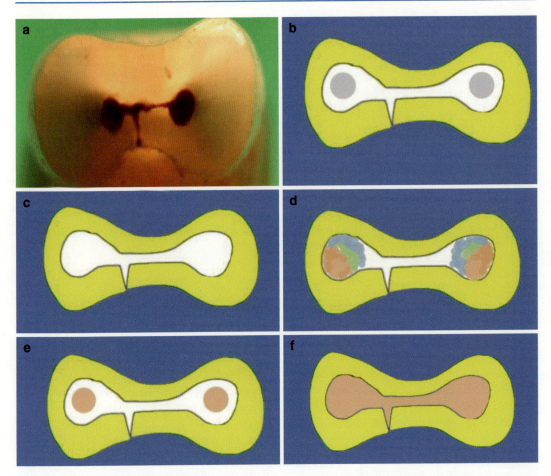

Fig. 7.1 Diagrams representing different methods of obturation used and how these techniques fill the apical portion of the tooth. Note (**a**) sectioned mesial root of a lower first molar demonstrating apical anatomy 1 mm from the apex. Obturation methods using (**b**) silver points, (**c**) paste fill, (**d**) single-cone obturation, (**e**) cold lateral compaction, and (**f**) warm lateral compaction, and warm vertical compaction, thermomechanical compaction, and injection techniques (Adapted from Professor John Whitworth)

thermomechanical compaction technique [26], hybrid thermomechanical compaction technique [27], warm vertical compaction [28], continuous wave compaction [29], thermoplasticised injectable gutta-percha obturation [30] and solid-core carry insertion techniques [31, 32] (see Figs. 7.1 and 7.2).

As no single approach can unequivocally boast superior evidence of healing success, the choice depends on the canal anatomy, unique objectives of treatment in each case and other factors such as speed, simplicity and economics [33].

A shortcoming of gutta-percha-based root filling materials is their lack of adhesiveness to the canal walls relying on a sealer or cement interface to fill the voids and irregularities in the root canal, lateral and accessory canals and spaces between gutta-percha and dentinal walls and within the homogenous mass of gutta-percha created using lateral condensation techniques. A number of different type of sealers are commercially available including zinc oxide eugenol [34, 35] and non-eugenol paraformaldehyde-containing sealers [15, 36], calcium hydroxide sealers [37], methacrylate resin-based sealers [38, 39], silicone sealers [40, 41] and calcium silicate sealers [42] (Table 7.3).

Resin-based obturation systems have been introduced as an alternative to gutta-percha in an attempt to seal the root canal system more

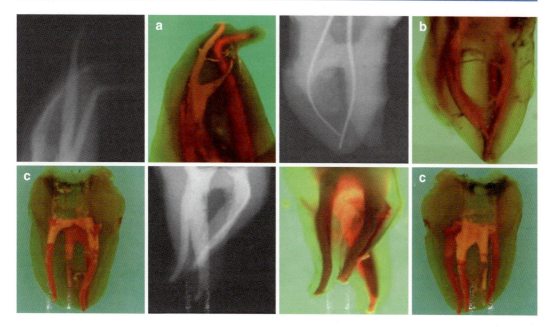

Fig. 7.2 Clinical radiographs and photographs demonstrating different methods of obturating root canals. Extracted teeth were obturated using different techniques and cleared. Note (**a**) obturation using McSpadden technique resulting in filling of MB2 canal and lateral anatomy. (**b**) Extracted upper first molar tooth with two palatal canals. Obturation technique using warm vertical compaction. (**b, c**) The importance of disinfection is highlighted by the fins and isthmuses between the two roots that cannot be prepared using mechanical preparation alone

effectively by creating an intra-canal adhesive monoblock and perhaps strengthening the root. Resilon is a biodegradable polycaprolactone-based thermoplastic root filling material bondable to self-etch or self-adhesive root canal sealer. It resembles gutta-percha and can be manipulated similarly, consisting of a resin core material, available in conventional/standardised cones or pellets, and a resin sealer. However, the desire to create a three-dimensional impervious seal has been unattainable due to ineffective bonding challenges due to root canal anatomy and limitations in the physical and mechanical properties of current adhesive materials [43, 44].

Calcium hydroxide, dentine plugs and hydroxyapatite have been advocated for placement as barriers in canals exhibiting an open apex to permit obturation, whilst minimising extrusion of traditional materials such as gutta-percha into the periradicular tissues. Placement of an apical barrier and immediate obturation is an alternative to apexification. Mineral trioxide aggregate (MTA) has been suggested as an apical barrier material. MTA is sterile, biocompatible and capable of inducing hard tissue formation. The material is compacted into the apical portion of the root and allowed to be set, and then gutta-percha can be compacted without extrusion. The technique is quick and clinically successful and eliminates the need for numerous visits and possible recontamination during apexification or theoretical root fracture [45, 46].

The apical limit of root canal instrumentation and obturation has been contested with most clinicians preferring to end biomechanical preparation at the apical constriction. All endodontic materials including relatively inert gutta-percha can induce a foreign body-type reaction when extruded beyond the confines of the root canal system. A small puff of sealer through apical ramifications or lateral canals, although viewed by some clinicians as a sign of optimal cleaning and shaping, can elicit an inflammatory response resulting in on-going pain for the patient [47].

Overfilling of root canals (beyond the radiographic apex) can occur as a result of inflammatory apical root resorption, an incompletely formed root apex or over-instrumentation through the apical foramen resulting from inaccurate measurement of the working length. In such cases, creating an apical stop becomes more difficult, thus leading to overfilling. There is evidence to suggest that overfilling has a negative effect on the long-term prognosis for endodontic therapy whereby the filling material might act as a foreign body, causing irritation of the periradicular tissues, localised inflammation and a delay in periradicular healing [48].

Gross overextension of root canal filling material and/or sealer is potentially harmful, particularly when in contact with vital structures such as the inferior alveolar nerve or maxillary sinuses. The use of toxic materials should be avoided, and even common sealers that do not release formaldehyde can result in paraesthesia when in contact with surrounding neural tissues. Mechanical compression, chemical neurotoxicity and local infection as a direct result of overfilling may cause irreversible nerve damage. Neural injuries, most commonly classified using the Seddon classification, include neurotmesis (the most severe), axonotmesis or neuropraxia. If neurological complaints appear after root filling in the lower jaw, a nerve injury due to root filling material should be ruled out. In cases of overfilling, an urgent referral may be warranted to consider immediate apicectomy and decompression of the nerve with conservation of the tooth if possible, thereby providing the best chance of avoiding permanent nerve damage. Even if nerve damage is not suspected, the clinician must bear in mind that the worst prognosis for endodontics is instrumentation and filling beyond the confines of the canal and this should be avoided in every case [4, 6, 7, 11, 13, 14, 49–51].

Root canal-treated teeth with overextension of the root canal sealer or solid materials such as gutta-percha or silver points into the sinus may be the main aetiological factor for aspergillosis of the maxillary sinus in healthy patients. Root filling materials such as zinc oxide eugenol are considered to be a growth factor for *Aspergillus*.

Aspergillus fumigatus need heavy metals such as zinc oxide for proliferation and metabolism. If the sinus has been breached with extrusion of either sealer or solid materials, then mechanical irritation can ensue resulting in an inflammatory reaction. Management of extruded obturation material into the maxillary sinus may require surgical endodontic therapy with the need for a subsequent Caldwell-Luc approach to remove the foreign material from within the sinus cavity [52–54].

Underfilling or incomplete filling of the root canals (more than 2 mm short of the radiographic apex) often occurs as the result of incomplete instrumentation, ledge formation or loss of working length due to inadequate irrigation and recapitulation of canal patency. The latter leads to the accumulation of dentine filings and debris resulting in canal blockage. Consequently, the clinician does not remove the infected necrotic tissue remaining in the apical portion of the root canal leading to persistent bacterial infection that may initiate or perpetuate periradicular inflammation after endodontic therapy. There is evidence to suggest that instrumentation and filling canals as near to the apical terminus as possible ('canal terminus patency' and 'extension of canal cleaning as close as possible to its apical terminus') and prevention of overfilling ('extruded root filling') are important prognostic factors for the long-term survival of endodontically treated teeth [55–59].

The life of an endodontically treated tooth depends on the accuracy of the diagnosis and planning, excellence of disinfection, instrumentation and filling procedures (antimicrobial strategies, root canal shaping and coronal and apical seal) and finally the rehabilitation management [60].

The final obturation is a culmination of all these factors giving us an insight into the likely success of treatment provided where due diligence and optimal treatment were performed at all stages. Choice of obturation technique and materials used is based both on sound scientific evidence and also the concept of what works best in your hands. No single approach can unquestionably be relied upon to successfully

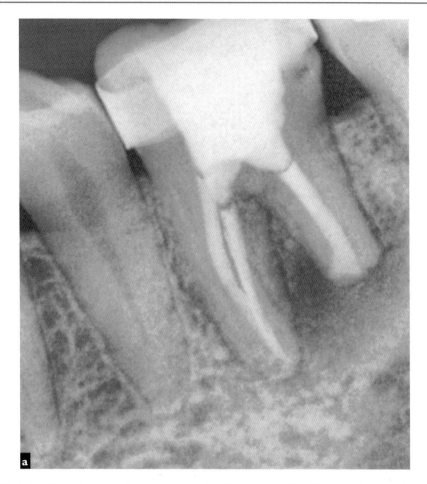

Fig. 7.3 Clinical radiograph demonstrating the use of different obturation techniques in a single case to achieve the desired outcome of a correctly cleaned, shaped, and obturated case. The distal canal had a very unusual apical irregular shape as a result of extensive apical root resorption that had occurred. The mesial canals were obturated using a warm vertical compaction technique. The distal canal was filled using MTA in the apical 1/3 followed by Obtura back fill. The use of conventional techniques would have increased the risk of a gross overfill which may only have been rectified by further surgery. This was avoided due to an understanding of techniques available including inherent limitations, thereby selecting the most appropriate technique which would achieve the necessary result with minimal complications

manage all cases. Instead the clinician should be aware of several different approaches that can be applied according to individual tooth requirements (see Fig. 7.3).

7.2   Sealers

Sealers are used between dentine surfaces and core materials to seal the space, between core and filling materials in lateral condensation techniques, to seal complex canal anatomical irregularities such as lateral canals and dentinal tubules, to lubricate and facilitate seating of the master cone and provide antimicrobial properties within the final obturation material. Traditionally desirable characteristics were to adhere to dentine and the core material as well as to have adequate cohesive strength. Newer-generation sealers are being engineered to improve their ability to penetrate into dentinal tubules and bond to, instead of just adhering to, both the dentine and core material surfaces. Although no sealer meets all the properties of Grossman's ideal sealer (Table 7.1), there are many sealers available that are clinically acceptable and widely used.

Zinc oxide eugenol based

The materials are produced in a powder and liquid form (e.g. Roth Root Canal cement, Roth International Ltd., Chicago, USA) or a two-paste preparation (e.g. Tubli-Seal Kerr, Orange, USA). The components of the powder, consisting of zinc oxide, bismuth subcarbonate, barium sulphate and sodium borate, are mixed with the eugenol to form the sealer. These sealers are radiopaque (due to the addition of silver, bismuth and barium), antimicrobial and toxic to vital tissues. The setting reaction of the sealer is due to the formation of zinc eugenolate crystals embedded with zinc oxide. Free eugenol is present as the material sets, decreasing over setting time and is responsible for most of the cytotoxicity when unset. Setting time and working time are dependent on the proportion of bismuth subcarbonate to sodium borate and are affected by temperature and humidity. Paraformaldehyde was added to the controversial N2 paste and in Endomethasone for added antibacterial activity.

Resin based

AH Plus (Dentsply Detrey, GmbH, Konstanz, Germany) is an epoxy resin-based sealer, which was produced as an alternative to its predecessor AH26 that released formaldehyde during the setting reaction. AH Plus exhibits acceptable biocompatibility, dimensional stability and insolubility.

Epiphany (Pentron Clinical Technologies, Wallingford, Conn.) consists of a dual cured sealer based on BisGMA, UDMA (urethane dimethacrylate) and hydrophilic methacrylates with radiopaque fillers that can coat the dentinal walls. Prior to application of the sealer, a primer must be applied to the dentine surface after a chelator such as EDTA has removed the smear layer. The sealer may then form a secondary monoblock bonding effectively to both dentines via the primer and with a chemical integration with the core material (Resilon).

EndoREZ is a hydrophilic UMDA resin capable of flowing into dentinal tubules with good biocompatibility. The sealer is used in combination with resin-coated gutta-percha points allowing the possibility of dual curing with both dentine and core material even in the presence of moisture.

Russian Red sealer is a variant of the phenol-formaldehyde resin, which sets very hard resulting in an insoluble mass within the root canal system. The sealer is strongly antibacterial and on setting results in shrinkage that leaves a reddish hue in the surrounding tooth structure. This type of paste filling is not advocated and can be very difficult to retreat.

Calcium hydroxide based

Sealapex (SybronEndo, Orange, USA) and Apexit (Ivoclar Vivadent, Schaan, Liechtenstein) are well-known sealers based on calcium hydroxide that when used in conjunction with gutta-percha core material provides biocompatibility with the possible advantage of bioactivity of calcium hydroxide when placed adjacent to vital tissue. However, for this to occur, calcium hydroxide must dissociate into calcium and hydroxyl ions requiring the sealer to break down or dissolve compromising the seal. Questions remain regarding the long-term stability of these sealers.

Silicone based

Roekoseal (Coltene Whaledent, Altstätten, Switzerland) is a polydimethylsiloxane-based root canal sealer that polymerises with minimal shrinkage and shows good biocompatibility. The material is mixed with auto-mix tips similar to impression materials producing a white fluid paste that has low viscosity to flow within the root canal system. GuttaFlow (Coltene Whaledent Ltd., Sussex, UK) is a cold gutta-percha filling system that utilises a silicone matrix and powdered gutta-percha that is triturated before carriage to the canal on either a gutta-percha cone or by passive injection using a plastic cannula.

Glass ionomer based

Ketac Endo (3M ESPE, St. Paul, MN, USA) is an adhesive root canal sealer with good biocompatibility and claims of root reinforcement due to adhesion to dentine. These sealers have been found to be more soluble and less antimicrobial with in vitro findings of leakage and disintegration over time. Due to its potential chemical bonding with dentine, issues about insolubility when using traditional gutta-percha solvents potentially make retreatment difficult.

Calcium silicate based

A new category of root canal sealers based on MTA such as iRoot SP (Innovative BioCeramix, Vancouver, Canada) has been introduced in an attempt to address the inherent problems with existing sealers and biocompatibility particularly when extruded beyond the confines of the root canal. Calcium silicate sealers include some of the same hydraulic compounds found in Portland cement including tricalcium silicate and dicalcium silicate powder that reacts with water to form a highly alkaline cement (pH 12) to create a rigid matrix of calcium silicate hydrates and calcium hydroxide. When these sealers set, the dimensional change is less than 0.1 % expansion, which helps create a barrier that has superior sealing ability. The combination of a hydrophilic sealer that is biocompatible with excellent dimensional stability seems ideal, particularly with the potential of obturation materials coming into contact with fluid either apically or coronally potentially salvaging a compromised seal.

7.3   Core Materials Used for Obturation

Gutta-percha

Gutta-percha has been the most popular core material used for obturation. It is derived from the Taban tree (*Isonandra perchas*) and has been used for various purposes such as coating the first trans-Atlantic cable and for the cores of golf balls. It can be made to flow using heat or using solvents, such as chloroform or eucalyptus, as well as by ultrasonics and vibration. It is a trans-isomer of polyisoprene and exists in two crystalline forms (alpha and beta) with differing properties. Gutta-percha undergoes phase transitions when heated from beta to alpha phase at around 115 °F (46 °C). At a range between 130 and 140 °F (54–60 °C), an amorphous phase is reached. When cooled at an extremely slow rate, the material will recrystallise to the alpha phase.

Traditional gutta-percha points or cones are produced in the beta phase and contains a mixture of zinc oxide, gutta-percha, radiopacifiers and plasticisers. Cones are manufactured as standardised 0.02 taper ISO cones and non-standardised 0.04, 0.06, 0.10 and 0.12 taper with specified tips or feathered tips according to manufacturing brand. Accessory points are also available from various manufacturers sized according to specified matched spreaders (e.g. SybronEndo system, SybronEndo, Orange, USA - XF, FF, MF, F, FM and M) (see Fig. 7.4).

An important characteristic of gutta-percha and of clinical importance is the fact that when it is exposed to air and light over time it becomes more brittle. Storage of gutta-percha in a refrigerator extends the shelf life of the material.

Gutta-percha is unable to provide a hermetic seal on its own and requires the use of an appropriate sealer. Gutta-percha is often applied to the canal using either a lateral condensing and/or vertical condensing force using spreader or pluggers to ensure adaptation occurs within the anatomical intricacies of the root canal system.

Cones can be sterilised chair side by immersion in sodium hypochlorite solution for 1 min. Gutta-percha is easily dissolvable by organic solvents such as chloroform, halothane or xylene making retreatment possible. The biocompatibility of gutta-percha has been tested thoroughly using cytotoxic, implantation, mutagenicity and usage tests.

Resilon

Resilon, a new, synthetic resin-based polycaprolactone polymer has been developed as a gutta-percha substitute to be used with Epiphany, a new resin sealer in an attempt to form an adhesive bond at the interface of the synthetic polymer-based core material, the canal wall and the sealer, otherwise known as a secondary 'monoblock'. It is manufactured in standardised ISO sizes and shapes, conforms to the configuration of the various nickel-titanium rotary instruments and is available in pellet form for injection devices. The manufacturer states that its handling properties are similar to those of gutta-percha, and therefore it can be used with any obturation technique. Resilon contains polymers of polyester, bioactive

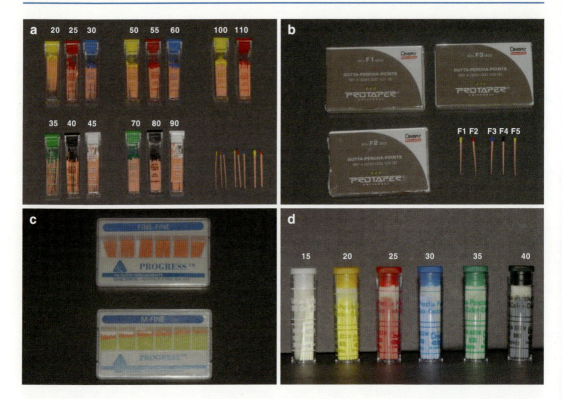

Fig. 7.4 Clinical photographs demonstrating a variety of tapered gutta-percha cones available for obturation. Selection of cone is dependent on preparation technique and canal anatomy. Note (**a**) standardized 2 % gutta-percha cones available in corresponding sizes to match 2 % stainless steel files. (**b**) ProTaper-matched gutta-percha cones corresponding to final master apical size (F1, F2, F3, F4, or F5). (**c**) Accessory gutta-percha cones selected to match corresponding finger spreaders. (**d**) Four percent gutta-percha cones specific to rotary file system selected

glass and radiopaque fillers (bismuth oxychloride and barium sulphate) with a filler content of approximately 65 %. It can be softened with heat or dissolved with solvents like chloroform.

Like traditional dentine bonding systems, etching and priming of the dentine surface is required to achieve a chemical bond. The root canal system must first be rinsed with 17 % ethylene-diamine-tetra-acetic acid (EDTA) to remove the smear layer. The Epiphany, a self-etch primer, is then applied to the canal and Resilon core material used to fill the root canal system. Light curing for 40 s will cure the coronal 2 mm of the canal, and self-curing of the remainder of the canal will occur within 15–30 min. This creates a secondary 'monoblock' in which the Resilon bonds to the Epiphany sealer, which in turn bonds to the dentine wall.

The ability of Resilon to effectively bond to tooth structure and thereby preventing leakage has been unproven to date. The reality of achieving an adhesive 'monoblock' in the apical portion of the canal is unpredictable with current available materials. The literature also suggests that Resilon is not stiff enough to strengthen residual root structure. Concerns remain regarding the biocompatibility and cytotoxicity of the Epiphany sealer. Evidence-based randomised controlled trials are lacking comparing Resilon to current gold standard gutta-percha techniques that have a proven track record at this time.

Coated cones

Another strategy to achieve an intra-canal monoblock utilising traditional gutta-percha was to chemically bind or mechanically impregnate a coating over the surface of gutta-percha cones creating a similar chemistry to the sealer.

Ultradent Corporation has surface coated their gutta-percha cones with a resin (functional methacrylate groups) in attempt to create a bond between the canal wall, the core material and sealer (hydrophilic self-priming methacrylate-resin based) (Ultradent, South Jordan, Utah). A bond is formed when the resin sealer (EndoREZ) contacts the resin-coated gutta-percha cone creating a hypothetical tertiary 'monoblock' within the root canal system with three adhesive interfaces (dentine-sealer, sealer-coating and coating-gutta-percha).

Paste fills

Since the inception of the cement material generally known by its trade name 'Mineral Trioxide Aggregate' in 1993 by Torabinejad, it has found many applications in dentistry including direct pulp capping, pulpotomy, root-end filling, apexification and apexogenesis, treatment of horizontal root fractures, repair of internal and external resorption defects, perforation repair and obturation of the root canal system. It is a hydraulic cement (e.g. sets and is stable under water) relying primarily on a hydration reaction for setting to occur. Apical barriers are important for the obturation of canals with immature roots with large open apices. Traditional techniques employed have been to use chloroform customization of gutta-percha that can result in extrusion with either long-term biocompatibility issues or the need for surgical revision. Alternative barriers to prevent extrusion of material have included the use of calcium hydroxide, dentine plugs and hydroxyapatite, which permit obturation, whilst minimising potential extrusion of material beyond the confines of the canal. Calcium hydroxide apical barriers are often time-consuming repeated treatments that have been associated with the potential of root fractures when used for prolonged periods of time. Placement of an apical barrier and immediate obturation is an alternative to apexification using MTA. The material is compacted into the apical portion of the root canal and allowed to set. Gutta-percha is then compacted against this apical barrier without risk of extrusion. The technique is quick, reliable and clinically successful, eliminating the need for numerous visits and possible recontamination during traditional calcium hydroxide-based apexification procedures. It is worth noting that when a root canal system is fully obturated with MTA, re-entry for retreatment or the ability to create a post space can be very difficult using ultrasonic or rotary nickel-titanium instruments due to the inherent hardness and strength of the material.

Silver points

Silver points were historically introduced as root canal obturation materials that were easily placed due to their inherent rigidity. However, their inability to three-dimensionally flow and conform to irregularly shaped root canal systems permitted leakage and the potential for corrosion. Corrosion by-products can cause irreversible staining and the potential for cytotoxicity inducing persistent periapical inflammation. Other potential shortcomings including complications encountered during apical surgery and the difficulties when needing to create a post space have made these materials redundant, particularly in the face of modern techniques and improved materials that are available today (Fig. 7.5).

7.4   Cold Lateral Compaction

A master cone corresponding to the final instrumentation size and length of the canal is coated with sealer, inserted into the canal, laterally compacted with spreaders and filled with additional accessory cones (see Figs. 7.6, 7.7 and 7.8). This technique has been the 'gold standard' to which other techniques have been compared. Lateral cold condensation has the advantage of excellent length control and can be accomplished with any of the acceptable sealers. The disadvantage of this technique is that it may not fill canal irregularities as well as the warm vertical compaction technique. The technique is as follows:

1. A standardised gutta-percha cone is selected with a diameter consistent with the largest file used at working length. Standardised

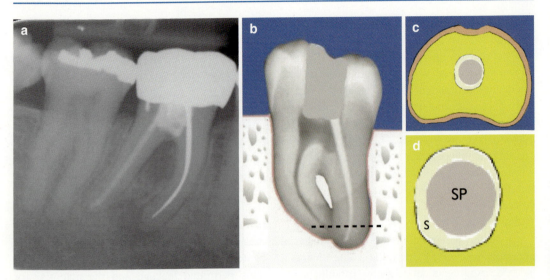

Fig. 7.5 Clinical radiograph and diagrams demonstrating silver cone obturation of a tooth. Note (**a**) tooth 46 with silver cone root filling in mesial root with obvious periradicular infection. (**b**) Silver cone placement in a prepared canal resulting in voids which are filled using sealer (*dashed line* represents cross-section of root taken at this level. (**c, d**) Apical cross section demonstrating silver cone (*SP*) and sealer (*S*) obturation. Over time, the sealer is likely to wash away, and in combination with silver cone corrosion products increase the probability of leakage and failure

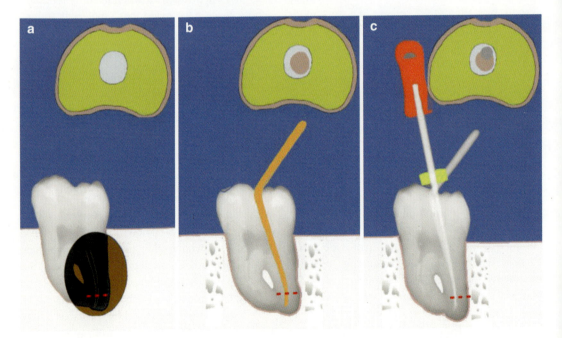

Fig. 7.6 Clinical diagrams demonstrating cold lateral obturation technique. Note (**a**) preoperative view, (**b**) master gutta-percha cone matching master apical file size placed to length with sealer, and (**c**) finger spreader placed to within 1 mm of working length. Cross sections of the distal canal taken at 1 mm from the working length (*red dashed line*) have been diagrammatically represented showing unfilled/filled canal space in relation to each step

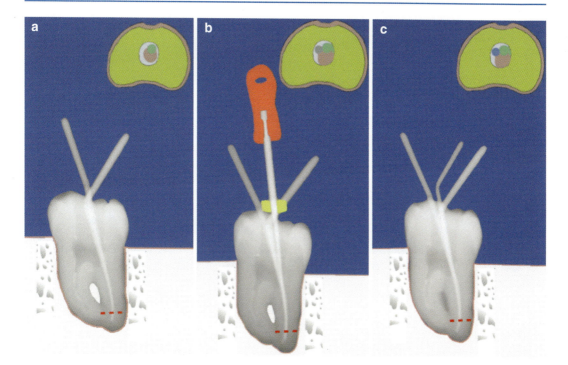

Fig. 7.7 Clinical diagrams demonstrating cold lateral obturation technique. Note (**a**) matched accessory cone (*green*) placed in space created by finger spreader. (**b**) Process of placing finger spreader repeated to create space for placement of (**c**) another accessory cone (*blue*). The process is repeated until no more cones can be placed. The key is to select a finger spreader that reaches to within 1 mm of the working length and select matched accessory cones that are repeatedly placed to the level of where the finger spreader has been placed. Cross sections of the distal canal taken in the apical 1/3 (*red dashed line*) have been diagrammatically represented showing unfilled/filled canal space in relation to each step

cones (0.02) generally have less taper than conventional cones and permit deeper spreader penetration. This 'master cone' is measured and grasped with a forceps so that the distance from cone tip to forceps is equal to the prepared length. The cone is placed in the canal to working length, and if an appropriate size has been selected, there will be resistance to displacement or 'tug back'. If there is no resistance, modifications are required.

2. Master cone placement can be confirmed with a periapical radiograph. Sealer is applied to the canal walls via the last-sized file used at working length. A finger spreader is selected that matches the taper of the canal. Appropriate accessory points are selected according to the

taper of the spreader. The spreader should fit within 1–2 mm of the prepared length, and when introduced into the canal with the master cone in place, it should be within 2 mm of the working length.

3. After placement, the spreader is removed by rotating it back and forth as it is withdrawn, whilst being careful not to spear the master point. An accessory cone is placed in the space made by the instrument, and the process is repeated until the spreader no longer penetrates beyond the coronal third of the canal. Excessive forces should be avoided to prevent potential root fracture.

4. Excess gutta-percha in the chamber is then seared off and vertically compacted with a heated plugger at the canal orifice.

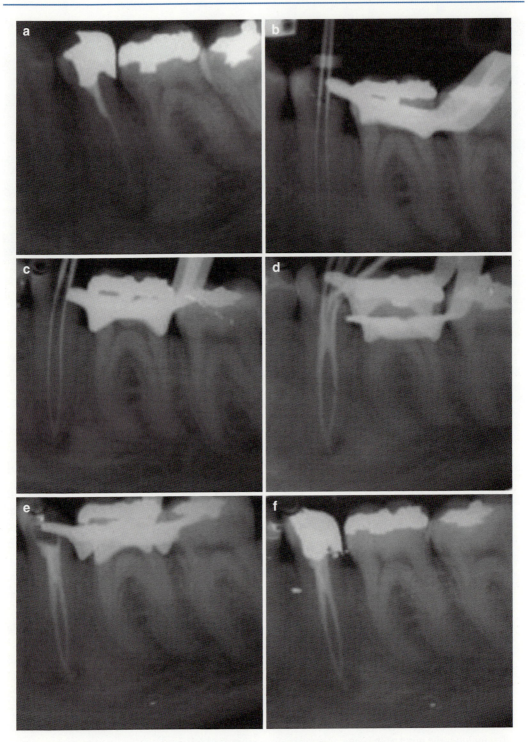

Fig. 7.8 Clinical radiographs demonstrating nonsurgical root canal re-treatment of tooth 35. Note (**a**) preoperative view demonstrating off-centered root filling with untreated additional anatomy. (**b**) Following removal of previous gutta-percha, two canals were located and working lengths established. (**c**) Master apical file radiograph demonstrating confluence of canals. Preparation completed using 2 % stainless steel files using a 1 mm step-back technique. (**d**) Cold lateral compaction using ZnOE sealer. Note the "Christmas tree" effect with placement of additional accessory cones (**e, f**) posttreatment completed case

7.5   Chloroform Customization

Solvents such as chloroform, eucalyptol or halothane are used to soften the outer surface of the cone as if making an impression of the apical portion of the canal. The canal must be wet with sodium hypochlorite solution prior to 'impression' taking to ensure that the gutta-percha master cone does not stick to the canal walls. The chloroform cone-dipped master gutta-percha cone is then removed from the canal and allowed to dry for 1 min to ensure that all solvent has evaporated and shrinkage is minimal. The cone is reinserted into the canal ensuring it follows the same path of insertion as withdrawal previously. The cone must be coated with sealer and laterally condensed with spreaders and accessory cones (same as cold lateral compaction) (Fig. 7.9).

7.6   Warm Lateral Compaction

Ultrasonics has also been advocated for obturation of the root canal system using a warm lateral condensation technique. Lateral condensation can be used by alternating heat after the placement of an accessory gutta-percha cone. Heat is transferred to the gutta-percha using an ultrasonically vibrated K-file, which softens the mass of gutta-percha allowing penetration of the finger spreader and matched accessory cone. This technique allows for better condensation and homogeneity of both sealer and gutta-percha (see Figs. 7.10, 7.11, 7.12 and 7.13).

A master cone corresponding to the final instrumentation size of the canal is coated with sealer, inserted into the canal, heated with a warm spreader (using warm lateral sterilisation beads) or ultrasonics (energised spreading), laterally compacted with spreaders and filled with additional accessory cones.

Energised spreading follows the same protocol for cold lateral sterilisation with a modification. A piezoelectric ultrasonic unit is required, as well as a file adaptor and a 15 K-type file. The ultrasonic unit is set to a high power setting and is activated only when the file comes into contact with gutta-percha. The file is gradually introduced into the gutta-percha and moved apically to within 1 mm of the working length. A finger

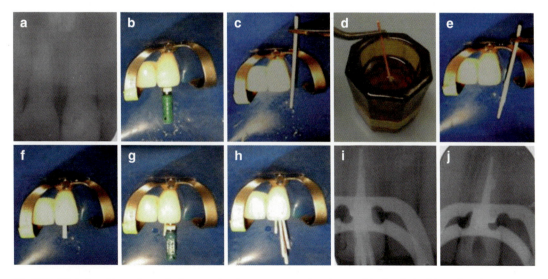

Fig. 7.9 Clinical radiographs and photographs demonstrating nonsurgical root canal treatment of tooth 21 using cold lateral compaction and chloroform dip technique. Note (**a**) preoperative view of tooth 21. No obvious external root resorption is noted. (**b**) Master apical file size verified to working length. (**c**) Trial insertion of master gutta-percha cone. (**d**) Cone is dipped in chloroform to soften apical 1/3. (**e**) Cone is placed in the canal making sure that the canal is flooded with sodium hypochlorite solution. The cone is then removed with an impression of the apical anatomy. The canal is subsequently dried before seating of the master cone. (**f**) Placement of dipped cone coated with sealer to length. (**g**) Placement of finger spreader. (**h**) Cold lateral compaction technique. (**i**, **j**) Radiograph demonstrating obturated canal space. Note lateral defect has been obturated with sealer

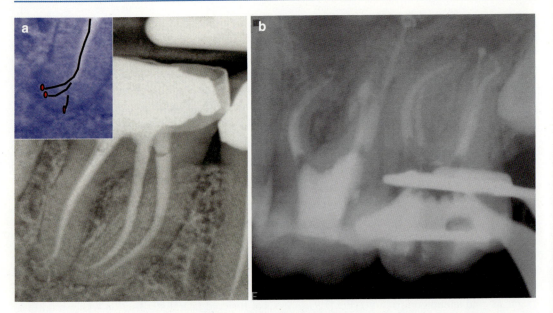

Fig. 7.10 Clinical radiographs demonstrating warm lateral compaction technique. Note (**a**) multiple apical foramina have been obturated in the distal root. (**b**) Complex anatomy both apically and internally obturated in both the upper first and second molar teeth

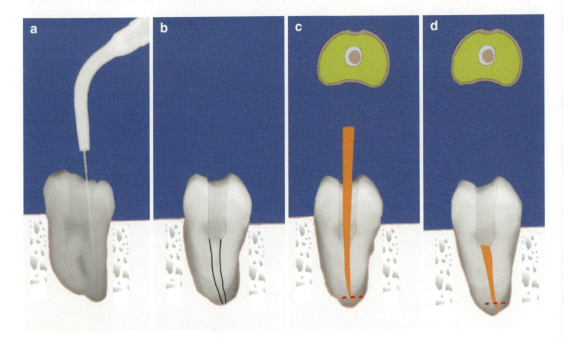

Fig. 7.11 Diagrammatic representation of the energized spreading technique. Note (**a**) the use of ultrasonic K-file #15 that can pass easily to working length provided canal curvature is not excessive and master apical file size is at least 0.25 mm. (**b**) Preoperative view of the canal. (**c**) Placement of the master gutta-percha cone to length coated with sealer. (**d**) Single cone sealed to orifice prior to warm lateral compaction technique. Cross sections of the distal canal taken in the apical 1/3 (*red dashed line*) have been diagrammatically represented showing unfilled/filled canal space in relation to each step

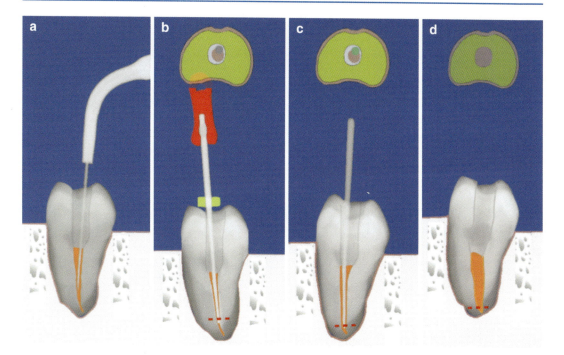

Fig. 7.12 Diagrammatic representation of the energized spreading technique. Note (**a**) Following placement of master gutta-percha cone, an ultrasonic K-file #15 is gradually introduced into the gutta-percha and moved apically to within 1 mm of the working length. (**b**) A finger spread is then placed in this tract within the gutta-percha to working length. (**c**) A corresponding matched gutta-percha cone is then inserted. This process can be continued a few times depending on the canal anatomy. Care must be taken since repeated placement of cones to working length can result in apical movement of gutta-percha with risk of overfilling. (**d**) Final completed obturation showing homogenous mass of gutta-percha three dimensionally obturated. Cross sections of the distal canal taken in the apical 1/3 (*red dashed line*) have been diagrammatically represented showing unfilled/filled canal space in relation to each step

spreader is then placed in this tract within the gutta-percha, followed by a corresponding accessory point. This can be repeated two or three times depending on the case selected. The risk of apical extrusion of both gutta-percha and cement is greater when compared to cold lateral compaction, and ultrasonic file placement will be dependent on the pre-existing canal anatomy. Canals with acute curvatures may risk file separation and canal transportation may occur if the file fails to follow gutta-percha.

7.7 Warm Vertical Compaction

Introduced by Schilder, the technique is associated with placement of a master cone, coated with sealer, corresponding to the final instrumentation size and length of the canal and then heated and compacted vertically with pluggers until the apical 3–4 mm segment of the canal is filled. Then the remaining root canal is backfilled using warm pieces of core material. Advantages of the warm vertical compaction technique include movement of the plasticised gutta-percha and filling of canal irregularities and accessory canals. Disadvantages include the risk of extrusion of material into the periradicular tissues and difficulties encountered in curved canals where rigid pluggers are unable to penetrate to the necessary depth. Traditionally, the pluggers were heated using an open flame.

The System B (SybronEndo) device is an alternative to applying heat with a flame-heated instrument, which permits temperature control. The continuous wave compaction technique is a

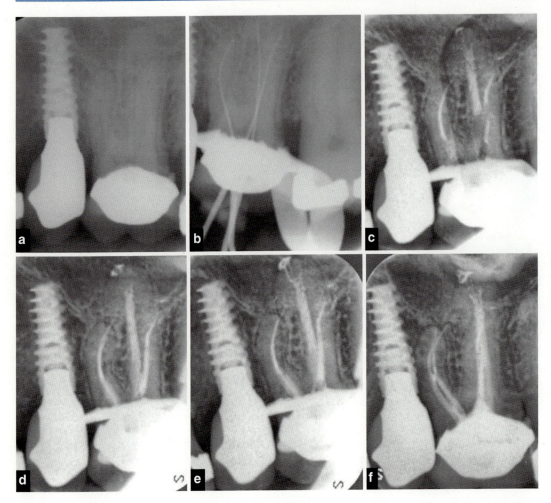

Fig. 7.13 Clinical radiographs demonstrating root canal treatment of tooth 26. Note (**a**) preoperative view. Patient was experiencing irreversible pulpitis. (**b**) Initial apical file radiograph demonstrating MB1, DB, and P canals. An MB2 canal was also located with separate apical foramina. (**c**) Mid-fill radiograph using a warm vertical compaction technique and AH Plus cement. Multiple foramina appear to be evident in the P canal. (**d**) Following backfill using Obtura. The P canal appears underfilled in the apical 1/3. A warm lateral compaction technique is used in the P canal only. (**e**) After introducing the energized file to working length at a suitable power setting on the ultrasonic unit for 10–12 strokes, a finger spreader is taken to length and then a matched accessory cone is placed using minimal sealer. Note the apical portion of the canal and further sealer puffs. (**f**) Final postoperative view of tooth 26 with complex apical anatomy in the P canal. Note also the isthmus that has been obturated between MB1 and MB2 canals

variation of Schilder's warm vertical compaction. The Elements Obturation Unit (SybronEndo) contains a System B device and a gutta-percha extruder in a motorised handpiece. The extruder tips are sized 20, 23, and 25 gauge and are pre-bent. The disposable cartridges of gutta-percha are heated quickly and the unit shuts off automatically to prevent overheating of the material. Various tapered stainless-steel pluggers (each with a tip diameter of 0.5 mm) are available depending on canal taper and diameter. The technique is as follows:

1. Once master cone-fit has been accomplished and verified, a plugger is sized to fit within 5–7 mm of the canal length. The point of plugger binding should be noted, as once the instrument reaches this point, the hydraulic

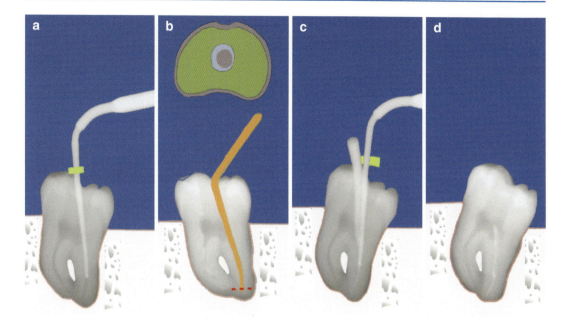

Fig. 7.14 Clinical diagrams representing the warm vertical compaction technique. Note (**a**) the appropriate size of System B plugger checked for fit to within 5–7 mm of working length and (**b**) insertion of master gutta-percha cone coated with sealer and seated to length. Note insert showing cross-sectional view taken at 1 mm from working length (*red dashed line*) verifying space around cone (**c**) System B plugger heated to within 5–7 mm of working length and (**d**) excess gutta-percha removed

forces on the gutta-percha will decrease and forces on the root increase. The canal is dried and the master cone is coated with sealer and cemented in the canal.

2. The System B unit is set to 200 °C in touch mode. The master cone is seared at the orifice using the pre-heated system B plugger previously sized. Further compaction is initiated by placing a hand plugger against the gutta-percha in the canal orifice.

3. The System B plugger is moved rapidly (for 1–2 s) to within 3 mm of the binding point. The heat is inactivated whilst firm pressure is being maintained on the plugger for 5–10 s to take up any shrinkage that occurs upon cooling of the softened gutta-percha. After the gutta-percha has cooled, a 1-s application of heat separates the plugger, and it is slowly removed (Figs. 7.14 and 7.15).

4. The canal is now ready for the backfill by using the extruder function of the System B/Elements unit. If post space is required, then this has already been achieved. The speed of extrusion is set on the control panel. The needle is primed, after preheating is complete (45 s), by the forward toggle switch on the handpiece, which is pressed until material extrudes out. The heated needle is then placed into the canal, and after a few seconds, the handpiece toggle switch is activated in order to extrude gutta-percha material within the canal. The gutta-percha is then compacted one final time using a hand plugger to either the level of the orifice or 2–4 mm below depending on core material to be used (Figs. 7.16, 7.17 and 7.18).

7.8 Solid Core Carrier Techniques

Carrier-based thermoplasticised techniques are based on warm gutta-percha on a plastic carrier, which is delivered directly into the canal as a root canal filling. Thermafil consists of a plastic core coated with alpha phase gutta-percha and a heating device that controls the temperature. A verifier is used to check which

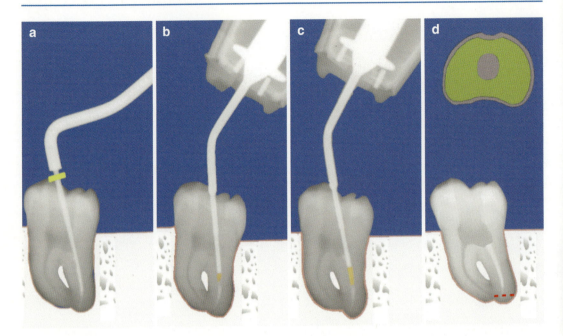

Fig. 7.15 Clinical diagrams representing the warm vertical compaction technique. Note (**a**) following "downpack," a pre-fitted plugger is placed to level of previous System B plugger and warm gutta-percha is apically compacted. (**b, c**) Following compaction the system B extruder is used to "backfill" the remaining middle and coronal 1/3 of the canal.

Each segment of gutta-percha can be further vertically compacted to prevent any voids. (**d**) The final obturation should result in a homogenous three-dimensional mass of gutta-percha from the apex to coronal orifice. Note the insert showing diagrammatic representation of the cross section taken at 1 mm from the working length (*red dashed line*)

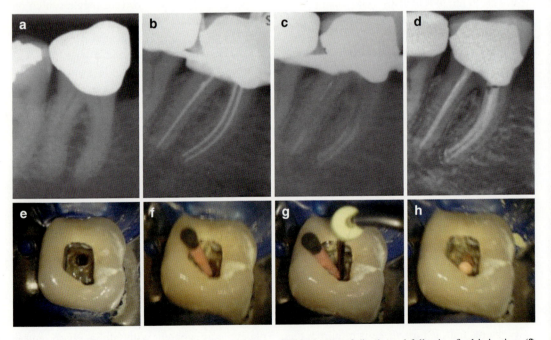

Fig. 7.16 Clinical radiographs and photographs demonstrating nonsurgical root canal treatment of tooth 46 through a cast restoration. Note (**a**) preoperative view of tooth 46, (**b**) master apical file sizes confirming working lengths, (**c**) downpack, and (**d**) postoperative view. (**e**)

Clinical view of distal canal following final irrigation, (**f**) placement of master gutta-percha cone with sealer to length, (**g**) downpack using System B plugger to within 4 mm of working length, and (**h**) backfill completed using Obtura

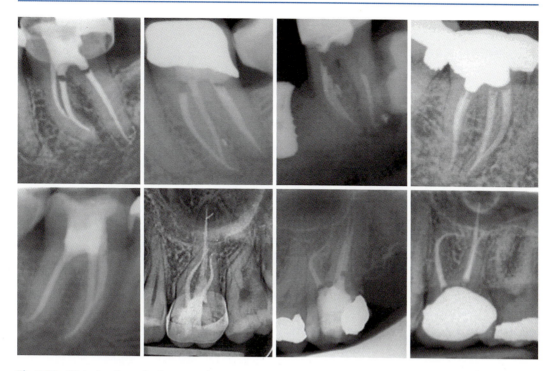

Fig. 7.17 Clinical radiographs demonstrating cases treated with the warm vertical compaction technique

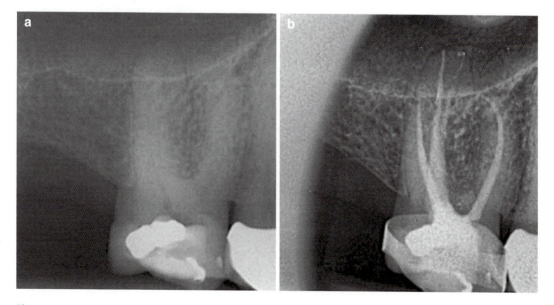

Fig. 7.18 Clinical radiographs demonstrating unusual anatomy in an upper right first molar obturated using a warm vertical compaction technique using AH Plus cement. Note (**a**) preoperative view showing a bulbous palatal root. (**b**) Postoperative view demonstrating two independent palatal canals

size carrier should be employed. The carrier is set to the predetermined length using the millimetre calibration markings on the carrier shaft. The canal walls are coated with the appropriate sealer. After heating the carrier in a purpose-designed oven for a specified time, the clinician must then insert it into the canal, without rotating or twisting it (see Figs. 7.19

Fig. 7.19 Clinical photographs showing Thermafil carrier-based system

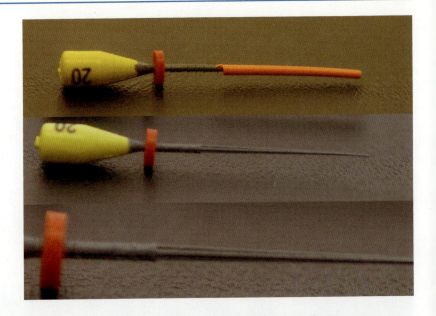

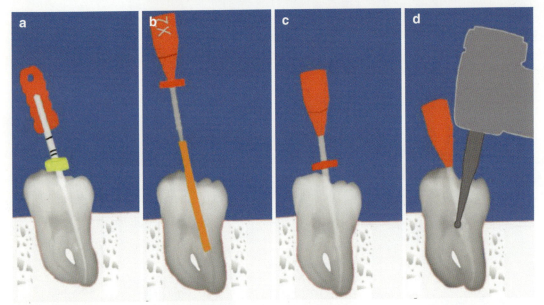

Fig. 7.20 Clinical diagrams showing carrier-based thermoplasticized compaction technique. Chemomechanical preparation must be completed to adequate taper and size prior to obturation. Note (**a**) verifier used to confirm appropriate size carrier is selected. (**b**, **c**) The canal walls are lightly coated with sealer. A matched carrier is heated in the oven according to specific time and temperature before insertion to working length. (**d**) Plastic carrier is sectioned at coronal level prior to final coronal restoration. The plastic carrier-type system has now been superseded with a Gutta-Core which enables re-treatment to be easier according to the manufacturers

and 7.20). An advantage of this technique is the movement of gutta-percha into lateral and accessory canals. The main disadvantage however is the risk of extrusion of material beyond the apical extent of the preparation. Matched carriers are available depending on the preparation system employed (e.g. ProTaper, Reciproc, WaveOne).

7.9   Thermomechanical Compaction Techniques

Introduced by McSpadden, this method utilises a compactor with flutes similar to a Hedstrom file, but reversed. The appropriate compactor is selected depending on the size of canal preparation and inserted using a handpiece alongside the gutta-percha cone to within 3–4 mm of the working length. The gutta-percha is heated using friction of the rotating bur resulting in gutta-percha compaction both laterally and apically as the device is slowly withdrawn from the canal. The advantages of using such a system included speed, simplicity and the ability to fill irregular canal anatomy. Disadvantages include the possibility of extrusion of filling material beyond the apex, the potential for instrument separation and inherent problems associated with curved canals.

7.10   Injection Techniques

The Obtura system (Obtura Spartan) consists of a handheld 'gun' with a chamber into which pellets of gutta-percha are loaded, along with needles of varying gauges used to deliver the thermoplasticised material into the canal. The temperature, and thus the viscosity, of the gutta-percha can be adjusted. A hybrid technique can be employed to ensure minimal extrusion of material beyond the confines of the canal apically by filling the canal to approximately 4–5 mm from the apex using the cold lateral compaction technique before gradually filling the coronal portion with thermoplasticised gutta-percha. The needle backs out of the canal as it is filled, and hand pluggers are used to compact the gutta-percha until the gutta-percha cools and solidifies to compensate for the contraction or shrinkage that occurs upon cooling.

The Calamus Flow Obturation Delivery System (Dentsply-Tulsa Dental, Tulsa, OK, USA) has a calamus pack and flow handpiece with an activation cuff to enable control of the flow and temperature of the gutta-percha into the canal. The activation cuff is released to stop the flow. The calamus pack handpiece utilises an appropriately sized heat plugger (available in ISO colours black, yellow and blue corresponding to working length diameters and tapers of 40/03, 50/05 and 60/06, respectively). The calamus flow handpiece is utilised in conjunction with a one-piece gutta-percha cartridge (available in 20- and 23-gauge sizes) to dispense warm gutta-percha into the canals.

GuttaFlow (Coltene Whaledent, Cuyahoga Falls, Ohio) is a cold, flowable technique that combines a polydimethylsiloxane sealer (RoekoSeal), powdered gutta-percha with a particle size of less than 30 µm and nanosilver particles contained in a plastic capsule that is triturated prior to use. The apical preparation should be as small as possible to prevent extrusion, and the canal is filled in combination with a single master gutta-percha cone.

7.11   Obturation Mishaps

Obturation mishaps including underfilling, suboptimal obturation, overextension and overfilling can arise as a result of inadequate cleaning and shaping (ledges, perforations, inaccurate working lengths and underprepared or overprepared canals) (Fig. 7.21). If inadequate obturation is not a result of an instrumentation error, the clinician should recognise this reversible procedural error on the obturation check film. The obturation material should then be removed and the canal re-obturated prior to placement of the coronal restoration (see Figs. 7.22 and 7.23). If the procedural error is gross overextension of material into the periapical tissues, removal by conventional means may not be possible and periapical surgery may be necessary. If a clinician is having difficulty with the obturation phase of endodontic therapy, their cleaning and shaping technique should be re-evaluated prior to consideration of changing obturation techniques.

Using conventional techniques employing the use of gutta-percha and sealer, warm lateral and vertical compaction techniques will lead to

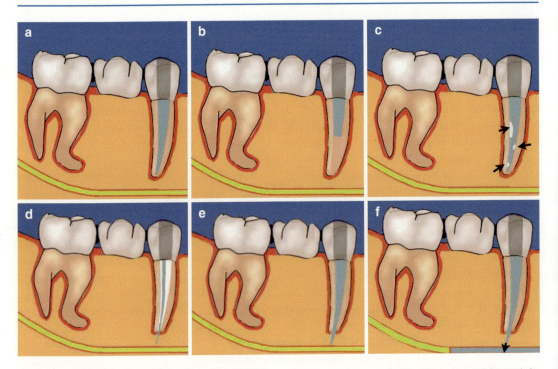

Fig. 7.21 Clinical diagrams showing obturation mishaps. Note (**a**) well-obturated canal space with no evidence of voids. (**b**) Underfilled case. (**c**) Suboptimal obturation with voids. (**d**) Overextension Note this type of filling is not well filled in three-dimensions. (**e**) Over-filled whereby surplus material has been extruded beyond the confines of the canal. Retrieval of the overfilled gutta-percha will be very difficult. (**f**) Risk of overfilling in the mandibular arch is neural damage

greater risk in both sealer and gutta-percha extrusion. Correctly shaped canals result in tapered preparations that serve to control and limit the movement of warm gutta-percha during obturation techniques. An ultra-thin film of sealer is desirable to fill remaining canal space between master cone and dentine walls ensuring that minimal shrinkage and predisposition to dissolution over time occur. More importantly, the objective of warm vertical condensation techniques to continuously carry a wave of warm gutta-percha and sealer along the length of the canal will inadvertently result in some sort of sealer puff laterally or apically. Extrusion of small amounts of sealer is of no concern and although may result in mild inflammation initially is usually well tolerated over time. On the other hand, extrusion of large amounts of sealer from beyond the confines of the canal will inadvertently lead to persistent inflammation, pain and risk of damage to surrounding structures (such as the maxillary sinus

and neurovascular bundles) (Figs. 7.24, 7.25 and 7.26). Generally, gutta-percha in bulk forms of sterile material with smooth surfaces placed within the bone or soft tissue evokes a fibrous tissue encapsulation. Particulate materials on the other hand have the capacity to invoke a foreign body and chronic inflammatory reaction. It is therefore the sealer and components of sealers that are recognised by scientific literature as highly irritating or neurotoxic that warrants attention, recognition and early management thereof.

Nerve recovery subsequent to an endodontic mishap is unpredictable, and so the clinician's timely response is important both from careful follow-up and appropriate referral where necessary. Neurosensory perception can be divided into mechanoreception and nociception. Mechanoreception can further be divided into two-point discrimination and brush directional stroke. Nociception can be subdivided into pin-prick and thermal discrimination. Neural injuries

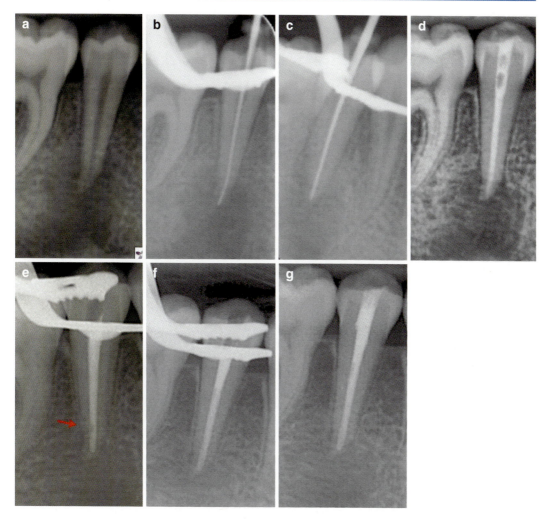

Fig. 7.22 Clinical radiographs demonstrating nonsurgical root canal re-treatment of tooth 45. Note (**a**) preoperative view demonstrating large periradicular radiolucent lesion associated with the periapex of tooth 45. (**b**) IAF and (**c**) MAF working length radiographs. (**d**) Placement of intracanal calcium hydroxide dressing for 3 months. (**e**) Obturation completed using a warm vertical compaction technique. Note apical 1/3 void (*red arrow*). (**f**) Additional ultrasonic energized spreading was carried out to this level with accessory gutta-percha placed to length. (**g**) Completed obturation with no obvious voids and coronal double seal restoration

are most commonly classified using Seddon's classification depending on the extent of injury. Neurotmesis is the most severe nerve injury where nerve conduction is completely disrupted resulting in complete anaesthesia and loss of feeling or sensation. It can produce dysaesthesia (an abnormal unpleasant sensation often burning in character) and recovery can be limited. Axonotmesis is when an injury occurs to the underlying axons resulting in paraesthesia or abnormal altered sensation. These types of injuries may show some degree of sensory nerve recovery after several months. Neuropraxia occurs when the nerve is injured leading to conduction blockage with no Wallerian degeneration. This will result in transient paraesthesia that has the possibility of recovery within a few days to weeks. Where anaesthesia or painful dysaesthesia is a direct result of overfilling, the clinician must consider prompt referral to an oral-maxillofacial surgeon who can provide an appropriate and timely surgical intervention if

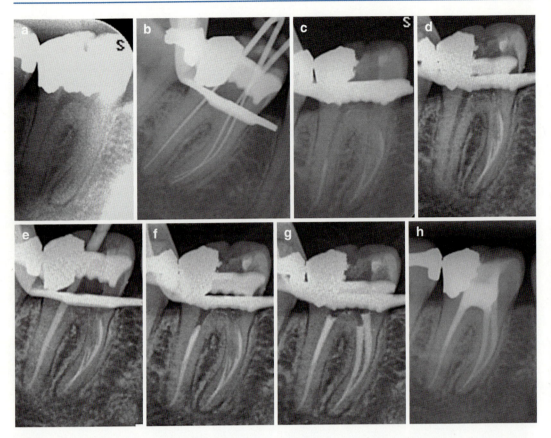

Fig. 7.23 Clinical radiographs demonstrating non-surgical root canal treatment of tooth 46 with obturation problems that were addressed at the mid-fill stage. Note (**a**) preoperative film, (**b**) master apical file (MAF) working lengths, and (**c**) warm vertical compaction following downpack using System B and Obtura (midfill radiograph). Obvious extrusion can be seen in the distal canal. (**d**) The distal root filling was completely removed using H files. (**e**) Master gutta-percha cone film in the distal root to verify length prior to proceeding with warm vertical compaction. (**f**) Second downpack. Note no overfilling noted. (**g**) Obtura backfill, and (**h**) final completed obturation. All canals were obturated to length according to respective MAF lengths and radiograph

indicated to allow for nerve recovery. Extrusion of material into the maxillary division of the trigeminal nerve or into the sinus can also lead to potential neural injuries and sinus complications that may need further surgical intervention (see Figs. 7.24, 7.25 and 7.26).

7.12 Clinical Cases

Case 1 Non-surgical root canal treatment of tooth 17 and non-surgical root canal retreatment of tooth 16 using a warm vertical compaction technique

A fit and healthy 22-year-old male patient was referred for endodontic management of teeth 16 and 17. He had recently been seen for emergency pulp extirpation in tooth 17 following severe localised pain and tenderness to percussion. At the consultation appointment, the patient was still aware of pain and tenderness in the area. Clinical examination confirmed previous endodontic access cavity in tooth 17. Tooth 16 was restored with an extensive tooth-coloured restoration. This tooth had undergone root canal treatment a few years earlier. Obvious percussion tenderness was noted in relation to both these teeth. Radiographic examination confirmed previous endodontic access in tooth 17. A periradicular radiolucency was noted with the MB root. Tooth 16 had evidence of previous root canal treatment.

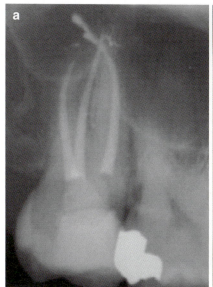
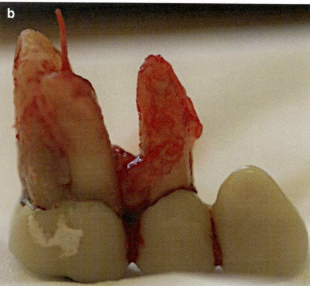

Fig. 7.24 (**a**) Clinical radiograph demonstrating overfilling in an upper right second molar resulting in extrusion (overfill) of material into the maxillary sinus (not treated by author). The patient reported ongoing pain in the region following endodontic treatment with her general dental practitioner. An endodontic referral was sought for a second opinion from the patient who was a healthcare professional. A cone beam CT scan (see Fig. 7.25) was organized to assess the extent of overfill and its relationship to the maxillary sinus. Nonsurgical re-treatment is unlikely to retrieve the excess material beyond the confines of the canal. Surgical apicectomy or extraction with additional removal of material from the maxillary sinus will be the only options to manage this case. (**b**) An example of an overextended root filling. Note the single point gutta-percha with canal transportation and perforation. Surgery would have been the only option to rectify this situation

Gutta-percha root fillings were noted in the P, MB1 and DB canals. Periradicular radiolucencies were noted with the MB and P apices. Previous gutta-percha root filling material was underfilled in the P canal and significantly short in the MB canal.

After a lengthy discussion with the patient, a decision was made to complete non-surgical endodontic treatment in tooth 17 and consider retreatment of tooth 16 (see Fig. 7.27).

Access cavity preparation was refined in tooth 17, and following ultrasonic troughing mesially, four canals were identified. The MB1 and MB2 canals had separate apical foramina. Patency was maintained and chemomechanical preparation was completed using rotary Ni-Ti files (ProTaper Next) and sodium hypochlorite solution. An intra-canal dressing of calcium hydroxide was placed. The patient was seen a week later to commence endodontic retreatment of tooth 16. An initial access cavity was prepared and ultrasonic troughing used to refine access cavity design and aid dismantling of the composite core. Gutta-percha root fillings were identified. Further troughing mesially revealed an untreated MB2 canal. Gutta-percha root fillings were removed using a combination of chloroform wicking and retreatment rotary files. Patency was achieved in all canals. Chemomechanical preparation was completed using sodium hypochlorite solution and rotary Ni-Ti instruments (ProTaper Next). An intra-canal dressing of calcium hydroxide was placed and a final obturation appointment scheduled for both teeth in a further 4 weeks. At time of obturation, the patient remained asymptomatic. Obturation of both cases was completed using a warm vertical compaction technique using AH plus cement and gutta-percha using System B and Obtura backfill. Both teeth had temporary IRM/GIC cores placed, and the patient was advised to see his general dental practitioner for placement of cores and cast restorations when convenient (Figs. 7.27 and 7.28).

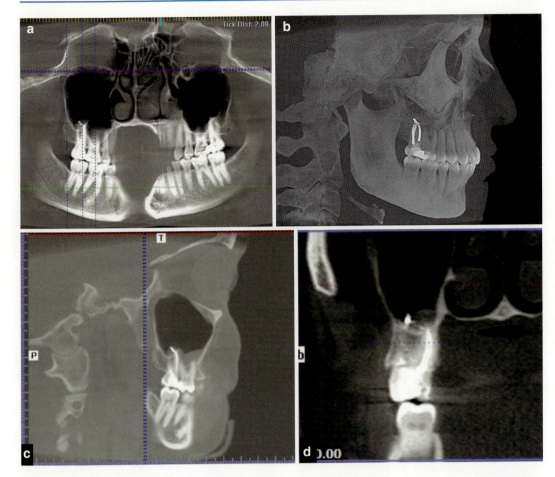

Fig. 7.25 (a–d) Conebeam CT scan images demonstrating overfill case of tooth 17 with surplus material beyond the confines of the root canal within the maxillary sinus. A number of cases of aspergillosis of the maxillary sinus have been reported in association with overextension of root canal fillings with certain root canal cements. It has been suggested that zinc oxide-based root canal cements might promote the infection with the Aspergillus species. In particular, *Aspergillus fumigatus* has been found to be associated with the maxillary sinus infection. Radiographically, the unique appearance of a dense opacity foreign body reaction in the maxillary sinus was considered a characteristic finding in maxillary sinus aspergillosis. A surgical approach and referral to OMFS was discussed with the patient

Case 2 Non-surgical root canal treatment of tooth 37 with C-shaped anatomy using a combination of warm vertical compaction and warm lateral compaction

A fit and healthy 48-year-old female patient was referred for endodontic management of tooth 37. The patient had previously attended her general dental practitioner with regards to severe localised pain. A pulpotomy was performed and referral sought. At time of consultation, tooth 37 was asymptomatic. Radiographic examination revealed a single fused root system (Fig. 7.29).

The patient was warned of the risks associated with treating a C-shaped canal system, and a decision was made to complete non-surgical root canal treatment. Access preparation was refined confirming a C-shaped canal system. MB, ML and D canals were initially prepared using hand files and rotary Ni-Ti files (ProTaper Next). The isthmus between the canals was further prepared using ultrasonic troughing. MB and ML canals were confluent. The distal C-shaped canal system was also confluent with the ML canal. Supplementary sonic irrigation using sodium

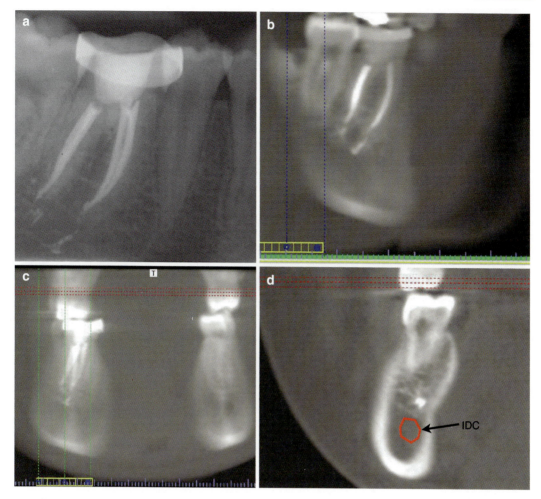

Fig. 7.26 Clinical radiographs and cone beam CT scan of tooth 46 which had been referred for an endodontic opinion following extrusion of root filling material. Note (**a**) posttreatment parallel periapical radiograph showing extruded material associated with mesial and distal apices. (**b–d**) Multiplanar cone beam images showing relationship between extruded material and inferior dental canal (IDC). The case had been obturated using Thermafil and AH Plus cement. During posttreatment, the patient experienced ongoing pain in relation to this tooth. The patient was referred for a cone beam CT scan which confirmed extruded root filling material inferior to the mesial root of tooth 46 and in close proximity to the superior margin of the right inferior dental canal. The patient's symptoms were improving and there were no signs of anesthesia or paresthesia in the area. A decision was made to continue monitoring and eventually her symptoms subsided. This case highlights the obvious risks when obturating canals, and in cases where there is obvious neural deficit, a prompt referral and timely management will dictate whether long-term paresthesia/anesthesia may persist

hypochlorite was performed to further debride the complex canal system and isthmuses. An intracanal medicament of calcium hydroxide was placed for a 4-week period prior to obturation.

Obturation was completed using a warm vertical compaction technique using AH plus cement and Obtura. Following backfill, voids were noted in the C-shaped canal system. Further use of ultrasonic energised warm lateral compaction was carried out using a 15K file to working lengths in all three canals. A fine finger spreader was placed to length and accessory fine cones used with AH plus cement. A temporary IRM/GIC coronal restoration was placed and the patient was advised to see her general dental practitioner for definitive cast restoration (Fig. 7.30).

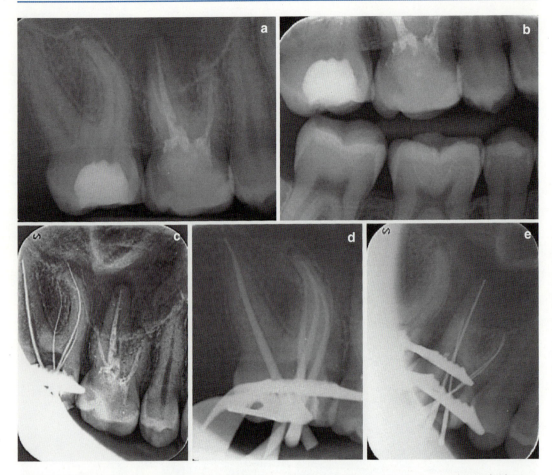

Fig. 7.27 Clinical radiographs demonstrating nonsurgical root canal treatment and re-treatment of teeth 16 and 17 obturated using a warm vertical compaction technique. Note (**a**) preoperative view of teeth 16 and 17. Note periradicular radiolucencies associated with MB root of tooth 17 and P root of tooth 16. Previous root treatment in tooth 16 short in MB root with only one canal treated. Also note underfilled P canal with internal root resorption lesion in apical 1/3 of canal. (**b**) Right bitewing radiograph. (**c**) IAF and (**d**) master gutta-percha points in tooth 17. (**e**) Master apical files in tooth 16 following removal of previous root filling material and chemomechanical preparation

Case 3 Surgical apicectomy of tooth 25 with persistent apical pathology due to overfilling

A fit and healthy 45-year-old female patient was referred for management of tooth 25. The patient recalled endodontic treatment had been carried out 5 years previously. For the past 5 months, the patient had been aware of localised gum swelling and pus in the overlying buccal mucosa. Clinical examination revealed tooth 25 had been restored with an intact coronal tooth-coloured restoration. A draining sinus was noted in the overlying buccal mucosa. Radiographic examination revealed a satisfactory root filling with surplus material beyond the confines of the canal. A periradicular radiolucency was noted. A gutta-percha sinus-tracing radiograph was tracked to the periapex of tooth 25 (Fig. 7.33). Treatment options were discussed including non-surgical root canal retreatment, surgical apicectomy and retrograde filling and extraction and prosthodontics replacement. The patient was referred for a cone-beam CT scan for further assessment. The cone-beam report confirmed an extensive periradicular radiolucent lesion with loss of cortical buccal bone. Two canals were seen obturated to length with an overfill confirmed (Fig. 7.31).

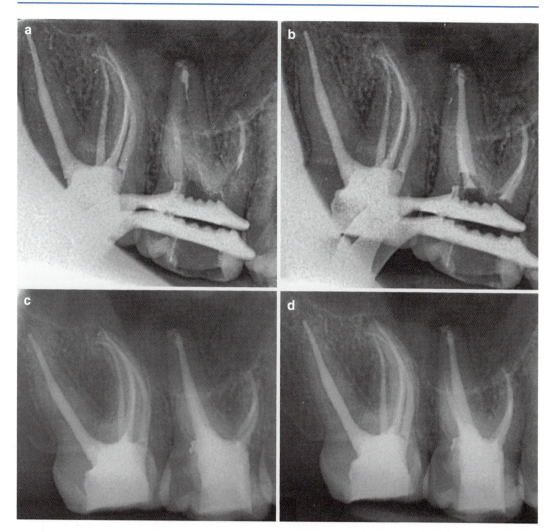

Fig. 7.28 Clinical radiographs demonstrating obturation of teeth 16 and 17 using warm vertical compaction technique and AH Plus cement. Note (**a**) completed RCT in tooth 17 and downpack in tooth 16. Palatal canal working length 23.5 mm and downpack performed to 20 mm to ensure internal root resorption defect is obturated. (**b**) Backfill using Obtura. Note (**c**, **d**) completed obturation of the case with IRM/GIC temporary coronal restorations. The patient was warned about possible postoperative sensitivity as a result of the sealer puffs

After a lengthy discussion with the patient, a decision was made to proceed with surgical apicectomy of tooth 25. A papillary preservation flap was raised with a mesial relieving incision. Following mucoperiosteal flap reflection, the bony crypt was identified with extensive erosion of the buccal cortical plate (Fig. 7.32).

Soft tissue excision was carried out and granulation tissue removed ensuring all endodontic overfilling material had been removed. Root-end resection was carried out and retrograde preparation completed using ultrasonics. A bioceramic retrograde filling was placed (Biodentine) (Fig. 7.33). The bony crypt was irrigated with saline and closure achieved using 5.0 Vicryl sutures. The patient was reviewed at 1 week for suture removal and followed up 4 weeks later to ensure soft tissues were healing. At the 4-week review, the patient remained asymptomatic and the buccal sinus had resolved. A further review was scheduled to assess bony healing in a further 6 months.

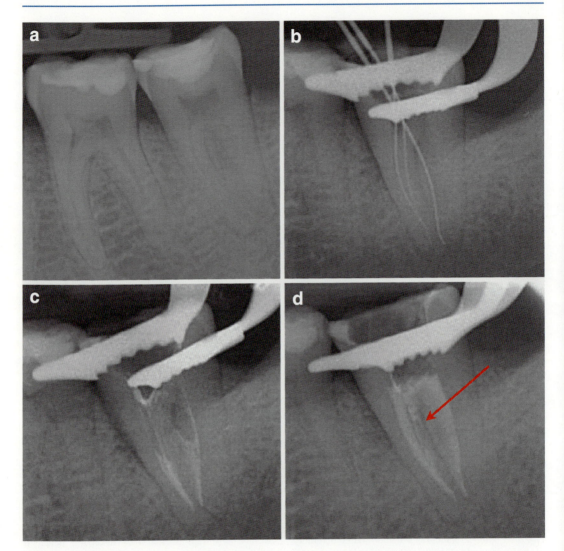

Fig. 7.29 Clinical radiographs demonstrating nonsurgical root canal treatment of tooth 37. Obturation was completed using a combination of warm vertical compaction and warm lateral compaction using the energized spreading technique using gutta-percha and AH Plus cement. Note (**a**) preoperative view of tooth 37 showing a fused root. (**b**) Master apical file radiograph with confluence of the mesial canals. A C-shaped root canal system was confirmed. Following initial chemomechanical preparation, additional sonic irrigation was used to debride the complex root canal system. An intracanal calcium hydroxide medicament was placed for 4 weeks prior to obturation. (**c**) Downpack radiograph using gutta-percha master cones and AH Plus cement. (**d**) Backfill radiograph using Obtura. Note underfilled canal system with voids (*red arrow*)

Case 4 Non-surgical root canal treatment of tooth 36 with confluent canals obturated with combination of warm vertical and warm lateral compaction techniques

A 45-year-old gentleman was referred for endodontic management of tooth 36. The referring dentist had previously seen the patient and started root canal therapy through a ceramic crown restoration following symptoms of pulpitis. Due to difficulties negotiating the mesial canals, a referral was sought. At time of consultation, the patient had been asymptomatic. Clinical examination revealed tooth 36 had been restored with a ceramic crown restoration with good marginal integrity. An occlusal access was confirmed. Radiographic examination confirmed prior endodontic access.

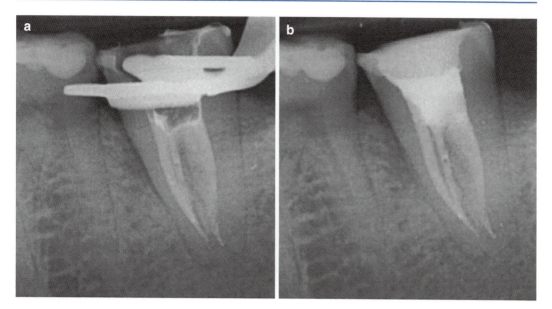

Fig. 7.30 Clinical radiographs demonstrating completed obturation of tooth 37 with C-shaped canal system. Note (**a**) completed obturation following warm vertical compaction and warm lateral compaction using gutta-percha and AH Plus cement. (**b**) Final radiograph showing IRM and GIC coronal temporary restoration

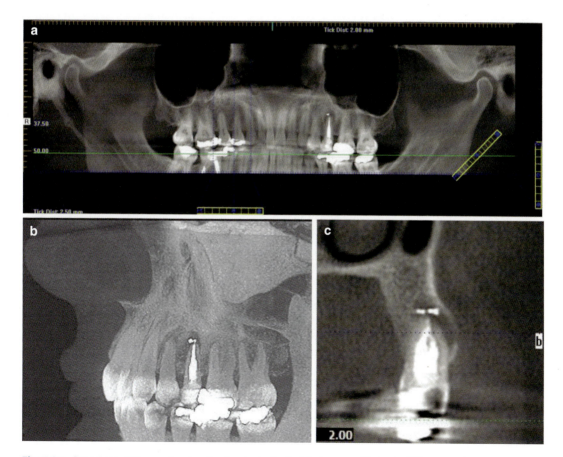

Fig. 7.31 Cone beam CT scan showing (**a–c**) extent of apical lesion, overfilled root filling material, and erosion of buccal cortical plate

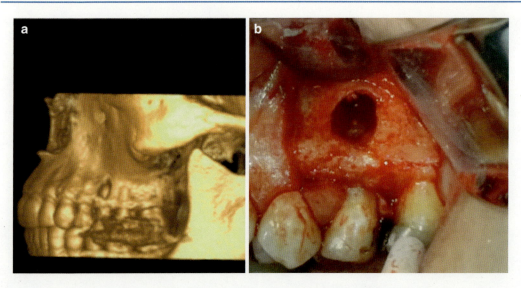

Fig. 7.32 (**a**) Cone beam CT reformatted demonstrating buccal cortical plate erosion with tooth 25. (**b**) Following papillary preservation flap elevation the bony crypt could be visualized with obvious cortical plate erosion

The roof of the pulp chamber was still intact distally. A periradicular radiolucency was noted with the mesial root apex. Treatment options were discussed and the patient was keen to continue with non-surgical root canal therapy.

Access cavity was refined and the roof of the pulp chamber removed. Ultrasonic troughing was carried out to further refine the occlusal access cavity. Initially, four canals were noted (MB, ML, DB and DL). Working lengths were determined using an electronic apex locator and confirmed radiographically. Further ultrasonic troughing was carried out between the isthmus joining the MB and ML canal to reveal an additional middle mesial canals (MM). All canals were confluent in the apical 1/3rd of the mesial and distal roots. Chemomechanical preparation was completed using 1 % sodium hypochlorite solution and rotary endodontic files (ProTaper Next). An intracanal medicament of calcium hydroxide was placed for a 4-week period (Fig. 7.34).

At the obturation appointment, the patient was asymptomatic. A final rinse of 1 % sodium hypochlorite, saline and 17 % EDTA was used. The canals were dried prior to commencement of obturation. A cone-fit radiograph was taken to verify master apical gutta-percha points in the mesial canals. Obturation was completed using a warm vertical compaction technique using AH plus cement. In the mesial root, all cones were cemented in place prior to individual down packing. Following down pack, a mid-fill radiograph was taken to confirm homogeneity of apical gutta-percha. Backfill was completed using Obtura and System B. A further radiograph was taken to confirm final obturation. A void was noted in the apical 1/3rd of the distal canal (Fig. 7.34). Further use of energised spreading was carried out using an ultrasonically activated K-file to working lengths. A coronal temporary restoration of IRM and glass ionomer cement was placed and the patient advised to see his general dental practitioner for definitive coronal restoration. Final radiograph demonstrated homogenous dense fills in five canals with patency confirmed by sealer puffs in both mesial and distal roots (Fig. 7.35). The patient was warned of the possibility of post-operative sensitivity and followed up a week later. He remained asymptomatic at which time he was discharged back to the care of his general dental practitioner.

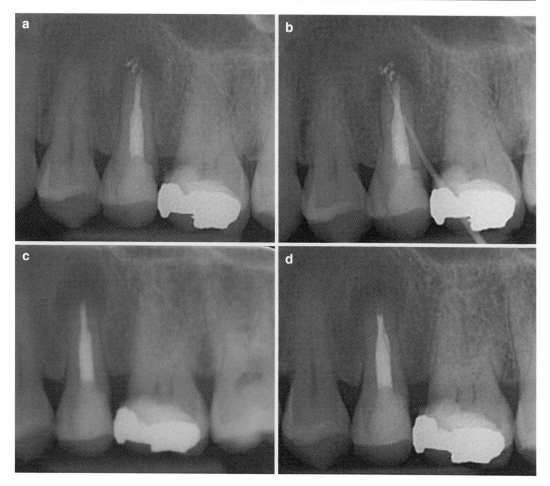

Fig. 7.33 Clinical radiographs demonstrating (**a**) preoperative view of tooth 25. Note overprepared root canal with surplus root filling material beyond the confines of the canal system. A periradicular lesion can be seen. (**b**) Gutta-percha sinus tracing radiograph tracked to the periapex and surplus endodontic material associated with tooth 25. (**c**) Granulation tissue and excess endodontic material removal and root resection carried out. (**d**) Retrograde preparation completed using ultrasonics and placement of retrograde Biodentine (similar opacity to adjacent dentine)

Case 5 Non-surgical root canal treatment of tooth 47 with internal root resorption and complex distal root anatomy treated with a combination of warm vertical and warm lateral compaction

A 49-year-old male patient who suffered from well-controlled hypertension was referred for endodontic management of tooth 47. The patient had been experiencing increasing pain and sensitivity with the tooth eventually culminating in acute pulpitis. Following emergency pulp extirpation by his general dental practitioner, all his symptoms subsided. The patient was referred for completion of endodontic treatment. At time of consultation, clinical examination revealed an intact occlusal dressing. Tooth 47 was asymptomatic with no pain on palpation or percussion. Radiographic examination confirmed prior endodontic access. An unusual radiolucency was noted in the coronal 1/3rd of the distal root canal system. The distal root appeared bulbous with possible bifurcation in the apical 1/3rd (see Fig. 7.36).

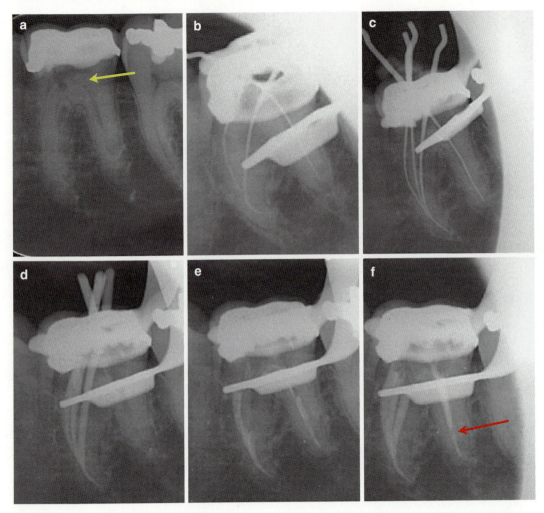

Fig. 7.34 Clinical radiographs demonstrating nonsurgical root canal treatment of tooth 36. Note (**a**) preoperative view showing calcified coronal pulp chamber, previous access with intact dentine overlying the distal roots (*yellow arrow*). (**b**) IAF radiograph showing MB, ML, and D canals (note DB and DL canals confluent in apical 1/3). (**c**) Following the use of ultrasonic troughing in the mesial root, an additional middle mesial canal was located. All three canals were confluent in the apical 1/3. (**d**) Master apical gutta-percha cones checked for fit in the mesial root. (**e**) Mid-fill radiograph demonstrating downpack and apical gutta-percha fill. A warm vertical compaction technique using AH Plus, System B, and Obtura was used. (**f**) Following completion of backfill, a void was noted in the apical 1/3 of the distal canal (*red arrow*). A warm lateral compaction technique was used with an energized ultrasonic K-file to working length, fine finger spreader, and corresponding accessory cones

Access cavity refinement revealed four canals. Chemomechanical canal preparation was completed using rotary files following glide path preparation. The distal root bifurcated in the apical 1/3rd with two separate apical foramina (Vertucci 1–2 canal configuration). Patency was maintained in all canals and supplemental sonic irrigation was carried out using the EndoActivator.

An intra-canal dressing of calcium hydroxide was placed for a period of 4 weeks.

At time of obturation, the tooth remained asymptomatic. A final irrigation regime of 1 % sodium hypochlorite and 17 % EDTA was used as a rinse. The canals were dried and master cones seated to length coated with AH plus cement. A warm vertical compaction technique

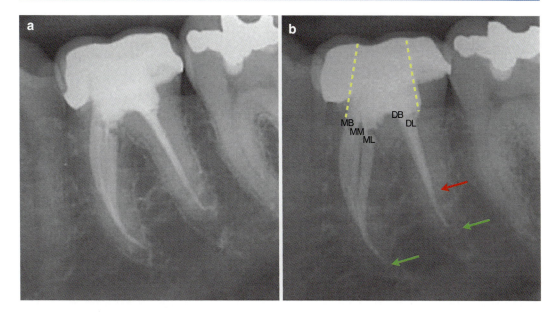

Fig. 7.35 (**a, b**) Radiographic examination showing completed nonsurgical root canal treatment of tooth 36. Note access cavity through existing crown (*dotted yellow line*), five canals cleaned and shaped, apical 1/3 void removed (*red arrow*) and sealer puffs in mesial and distal apices confirming maintenance of apical patency (*green arrows*)

was used using System B and Obtura with gutta-percha.

Additional warm lateral compaction (energised spreading technique) was used in the distal root canal system to ensure a homogenous root filling was obtained both in the apical 1/3rd (level of bifurcation) and the coronal 1/3rd (internal root resorption defect).

A temporary double seal coronal restoration of IRM and glass ionomer cement was placed prior to discharge. The patient was advised to see his general dental practitioner for placement of a permanent cast cuspal coverage restoration.

Case 6 Non-surgical root canal treatment of tooth 38 which had been transplanted into the 35 positions. Mesial canals obturated with warm vertical compaction using AH plus cement and gutta-percha. Distal canal obturated with MTA/gutta-percha

A fit and healthy 24-year-old and healthy patient was referred for endodontic management of tooth 38. The patient recently had his infraoccluded ankylosed second deciduous mandibular molars removed. The permanent successors (teeth 35 and 45) were congenitally missing. The patient was then seen by an oral-maxillofacial surgeon for removal of impacted mandibular wisdom teeth. A decision was made to extract both lower 38 and 48 and transplant the teeth to the 35 and 45 spaces (see Fig. 7.37). Following transplantation, the patient was reviewed and tooth 38 (transplanted to tooth 35 position) was diagnosed as non-vital. An endodontic referral was made for further management.

At time of endodontic consultation, a draining sinus was noted in the overlying buccal mucosa of tooth 38. A gutta-percha sinus-tracing radiograph confirmed the sinus originated from the mesial root of tooth 38. A provisional diagnosis of chronic apical periodontitis with suppuration of tooth 38 was made. After a lengthy discussion with the patient, a decision was made to proceed with non-surgical endodontic therapy.

Access cavity preparation confirmed three canals (as seen by previous cone-beam CT scan) (see Figs. 7.37 and 7.38).

Chemomechanical canal preparation was completed with a combination of stainless-steel hand files and rotary files using 1 % sodium

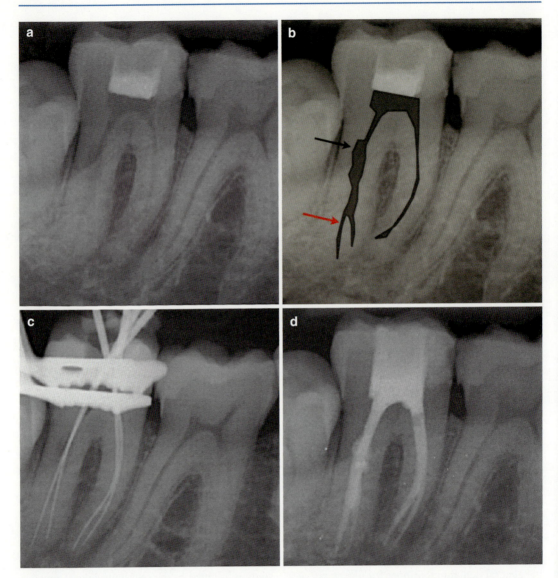

Fig. 7.36 Clinical radiographs demonstrating nonsurgical root canal treatment of tooth 47 using a warm vertical compaction/warm lateral compaction technique with AH Plus cement and gutta-percha. Note (**a**) preoperative view of tooth 47. (**b**) Unusual canal configuration demonstrating internal root resorption in the middle 1/3 of the distal canal (*black arrow*) and Vertucci 1–2 canal configuration in apical 1/3 (*red arrow*). (**c**) Master apical file radiograph following chemomechanical preparation using 1 % sodium hypochlorite solution. (**d**) Final completed obturation. Note the internal resorption defect has been obturated as well as the complex apical anatomy in the distal root

hypochlorite solution. The mesial canals were prepared using rotary files. Ultrasonic troughing was carried out between the isthmus joining the MB and ML canal revealing a large communication. The distal canal was a large ovoid-shaped canal system (size #100). Working length determination was carried out using a combination of electronic, radiographic and

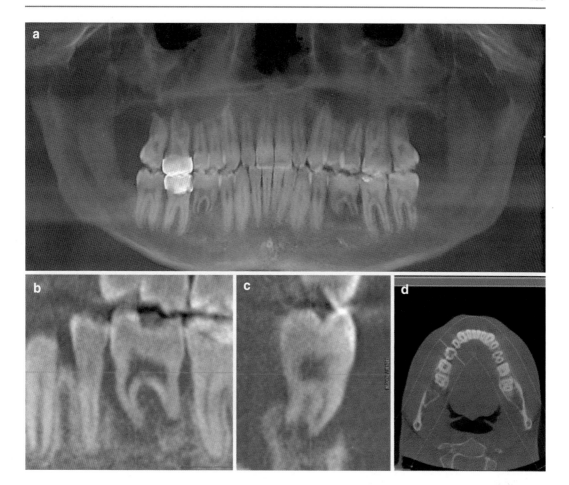

Fig. 7.37 Cone beam CT scan showing (**a**) transplanted teeth 38 and 48 into 35 and 45 positions. Teeth 35 and 45 were congenitally missing. (**b**) Coronal view of tooth 38 demonstrating periapical pathology. (**c**) Sagittal cross-sectional (buccolingual) view. (**d**) Axial view showing internal anatomy

paper points. An intra-canal calcium hydroxide dressing was placed 4 weeks. The patient was reviewed at the 4-week period and the draining sinus in relation to tooth 38 had resolved. A further appointment was scheduled for completion of endodontic treatment.

Obturation of the mesial canals was completed using a warm vertical compaction technique using AH plus cement, gutta-percha, system B and Obtura. The distal canal was obturated using MTA in the apical 5 mm followed by gutta-percha backfill (see Fig. 7.39). A temporary coronal restoration of Biodentine and glass ionomer cement was placed prior to discharge back to his general dental practitioner. The patient was reviewed at 3 months and he remained asymptomatic. Tooth 48 remained asymptomatic but non-responsive to pulp sensibility testing. Further review appointments were scheduled to monitor periapical healing of tooth 38 and monitoring of the pulp status of tooth 48 (Fig. 7.40).

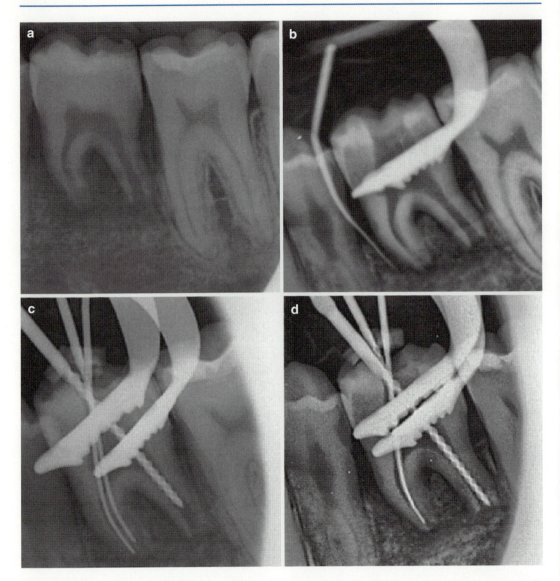

Fig. 7.38 Clinical radiographs demonstrating nonsurgical root canal treatment of transplanted tooth 38. Note (**a**) preoperative parallel long-cone conventional digital radiograph demonstrating periradicular infection associated with the periapex of tooth 38. (**b**) A gutta-percha sinus tracing radiograph confirming intraoral draining sinus in overlying attached buccal mucosa is related to the mesial root of tooth 38. (**c**) Initial apical file radiograph. Working length established for mesial canals #50 K-files. Distal canal had a wide open apex with bleeding making electronic working length determination difficult. (**d**) Master apical file radiograph. The distal canal length was determined using a combination of electronic apex and paper point technique. MAF file size in distal canal was #100

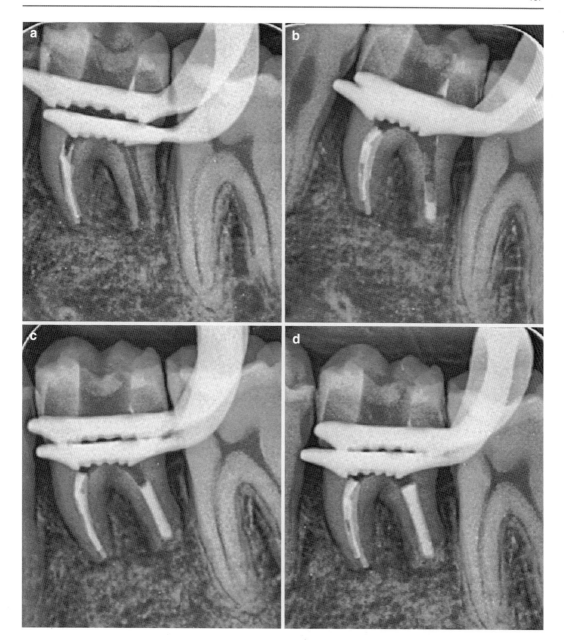

Fig. 7.39 Clinical radiographs demonstrating obturation of tooth 38. The mesial canals were obturated using AH Plus cement and a warm vertical compaction technique using AH Plus cement. The distal canal was obturated using MTA in the apical/middle portion of the canal and backfill using gutta-percha in the remaining coronal portion of the canal. Note (**a**) completed warm vertical compaction using gutta-percha in the mesial root system. (**b–c**) MTA fill. (**d**) Completed obturation

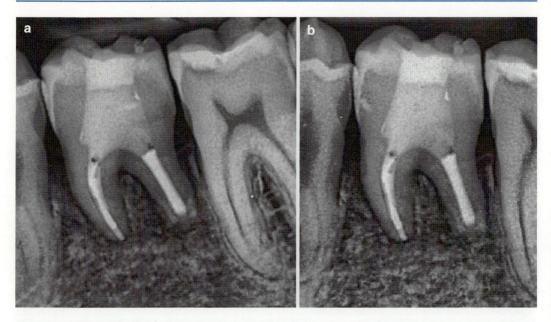

Fig. 7.40 Clinical radiographs of completed nonsurgical root canal treatment of transplanted tooth 38. Note (**a**) immediate postoperative completed filling. (**b**) A 3-month review radiograph

Clinical Hints and Tips to Avoid Obturation Mishaps

- **Preoperative assessment**
  It is important to identify preoperatively any neural structures or proximal risk to anatomical structures such as the maxillary sinus in relation to the tooth undergoing endodontic therapy. Consider referral when warranted.
- **Working length determination**
  Working length is essential and maintaining an apical foramen as small as possible is important during the cleaning and shaping procedures.
- **Resistance form**
  Tapered preparations should be created to ensure that an apical stop has been created to limit extrusion of material beyond the confines of the canal.
- **Technique used**
  The final obturation technique selected should bear in mind any anatomical constraints such as resorptive defects that may increase the likelihood of overfilling. In general, cold lateral techniques will lead to the least risk of extrusion compared to warm vertical compaction.

- **Material selection**
  Do not use toxic materials such as N2 or Endomethasone which are no longer recommended.
- **Apical barriers**
  May be considered to further prevent extrusion of material, particularly in cases where teeth are in close proximity to neurovascular bundles
- **Sealer volume**
  Should be kept to minimal not only to prevent long-term risk of dissolution and shrinkage but also the immediate risk of extrusion and complications

References

1. Kakehashi S, Stanley HR, Fitzgerald RJ. The effects of surgical exposures of pulps in germ-free and conventional rats. Oral Surg Oral Med Oral Pathol. 1965;20:340–9.
2. Peters OA, Laib A, Gohring TN, Barbakow F. Changes in root canal geometry after preparation assessed by high-resolution computed tomography. J Endod. 2001;27:1–6.
3. Nair PNR. Light and electron microscopic studies of root canal flora and periapical lesions. J Endod. 1987;13:29–39.

4. Sjogren U, Hagglund B, Sundqvist G, Wing K. Factors affecting the long-term results of endodontic treatment. J Endod. 1990;16:498–504.

5. Gorni F, Gagliani M. The outcome of endodontic retreatment: a 2-yr follow-up. J Endod. 2004;30:1–4.

6. Seltzer S, Soltanoff W, Smith J. Biologic aspects of endodontics: V – periapical tissue reactions to root canal instrumentation beyond the apex and root canal fillings short of and beyond the apex. Oral Surg Oral Med Oral Pathol. 1973;36:725–37.

7. Chugal NM, Clive JM, Spångberg LS. Endodontic infection: some biologic and treatment factors associated with outcome. Oral Surg Oral Med Oral Pathol Oral Radiol Endod. 2003;96:81–90.

8. Grossman L. Endodontic practice. 10th ed. Philadelphia: Lea & Febiger; 1981. p. 279.

9. Jasper E. Adaption and tolerance of silver point canal filling. J Dent Res. 1941;4:355.

10. Goldberg F. Relation between corroded silver points and endodontic failures. J Endod. 1981;7(5):224–7.

11. González-Martín M, Torres-Lagares D, Gutiérrez-Pérez JL, Segura-Egea JJ. Inferior alveolar nerve paraesthesia after overfilling of endodontic sealer into the mandibular canal. J Endod. 2010;36(8):1419–21.

12. Sargenti A, Richter SL. Rationalized root canal treatment. New York: AGSA Scientific Publications; 1959.

13. Kaufman AY, Rosenberg L. Paraesthesia caused by Endomethasone. J Endod. 1980;6(4):529–31.

14. Kleier DJ, Averbach RE. Painful dysesthesia of the inferior alveolar nerve following use of a paraformaldehyde-containing root canal sealer. Dent Traumatol. 1988;4(1):46–8.

15. Schwandt NW, Gound TG. Resorcinol-formaldehyde resin "Russian Red" endodontic therapy. J Endod. 2003;29(7):435–7.

16. Friedman CE, Sandrik JL, Heuer MA, Rapp GW. Composition and physical properties of gutta-percha endodontic filling materials. J Endod. 1977;3(8):304–8.

17. Goodman A, Schilder H, Aldrich W. The thermomechanical properties of gutta-percha. II. The history and molecular chemistry of gutta-percha. Oral Surg Oral Med Oral Pathol. 1974;37:954–61.

18. Schilder H, Goodman A, Aldrich W. The thermomechanical properties of gutta-percha. V. Volume changes in bulk gutta-percha as a function of temperature and its relationship to molecular phase transformation. Oral Surg Oral Med Oral Pathol. 1985;59:285–96.

19. Cunningham KP, Walker MP, Kulild JC, Lask JT. Variability of the diameter and taper of size# 30, 0.04 gutta-percha cones. J Endod. 2006;32(11):1081–4.

20. Cardoso CL, Kotaka CR, Redmerski R, Guilhermetti M, Queiroz AF. Rapid decontamination of gutta-percha cones with sodium hypochlorite. J Endod. 1999;25(7):498–501.

21. Gordon MP, Love RM, Chandler NP. An evaluation of .06 tapered gutta-percha cones for filling of .06 taper prepared curved root canals. Int Endod J. 2005;38:87–96.

22. Schafer E, Koster M, Burklein S. Percentage of gutta-percha-filled areas in canals instrumented with nickel-titanium systems and obturated with matched single cones. J Endod. 2013;39(7):924–8.

23. Tomson RM, Polycarpou N, Tomson PL. Contemporary obturation of the root canal system. Br Dent J. 2014;216(6):315–22.

24. Bailey GC, Ng YL, Cunnington SA, Barber P, Gulabivala K, Setchell DJ. Root canal obturation by ultrasonic condensation of gutta-percha. Part II: an in-vitro investigation of the quality of obturation. Int Endod J. 2004;37:694–8.

25. Van Zyl SP, Gulabivala K, Ng YL. Effect of customization of master gutta-percha cone on apical control of root filling using different techniques: an ex vivo study. Int Endod J. 2005;38(9):658–66.

26. McSpadden JT. Presentation to the meeting of American Association of Endodontists. Atlanta, Georgia; 1979.

27. Tagger M, Tamse A, Katz A, Korzen BH. Evaluation of the apical seal produced by hybrid root canal filling method, combining lateral condensation and thermatic compaction. J Endod. 1984;10:299–303.

28. Schilder H. Filling root canals in three dimensions 1967. J Endod. 2006;32:281–90.

29. Buchanan LS. The continuous wave of obturation technique: 'centred' condensation of warm gutta-percha in 12 seconds. Dent Today. 1996;15:60–2. 64–7.

30. Yee FS, Marlin J, Krakow AA. Gron Three-dimensional obturation of the root canal using injection-moulded, thermo plasticized dental gutta-percha. J Endod. 1977;3:168–74.

31. Johnson WB. A new-gutta-percha technique. J Endod. 1978;4:184–8.

32. Cantatore G. Thermafil versus System B. Endod Prac. 2001;5:30–9.

33. Whitworth J. Methods of filling root canals: principles and practices. Endod Top. 2005;12:2–24.

34. Grossman LI. Improved root canal cement. J Am Dent Assoc. 1958;56:381–5.

35. Markowitz K, Moynihan M, Liu M, Kim S. Biologic properties of eugenol and zinc oxide-eugenol: a clinically oriented review. Oral Surg Oral Med Oral Pathol. 1992;73(6):729–37.

36. Spångberg L. Biologic effect of root canal filling materials: the effect on bone tissue of two formaldehyde-containing root canal filling pastes, N2 and Riebler's paste. Oral Surg Oral Med Oral Pathol. 1974;38:934–44.

37. Desai S, Chandler N. Calcium hydroxide-based root canal sealers: a review. J Endod. 2009;35(4):475–80.

38. Zmener O, Spielberg C, Lamberghini F, Rucci M. Sealing properties of a new epoxy resin-based root-canal sealer. Int Endod J. 1997;30(5):332–4.

39. Kim YK, Grandini S, Ames JM, Gu LS, Kim SK, Pashley DH, Gutmann JL, Tay FR. Critical review of

methacrylate resin-based root canal sealers. J Endod. 2010;36(3):383–99.

40. Gencoglu N, Turkmen C, Ahiskali R. A new silicon-based root canal sealer (Roekoseal Automix). J Oral Rehabil. 2003;30:753–7.

41. Özok AR, van der Sluis LW, Wu MK, Wesselink PR. Sealing ability of a new polydimethylsiloxane-based root canal filling material. J Endod. 2008;34(2):204–7.

42. Camilleri J. Evaluation of selected properties of mineral trioxide aggregate sealer cement. J Endod. 2009;35:1412–7.

43. Shanahan DJ, Duncan HF. Root canal filling using Resilon: a review. Br Dent J. 2011;211(2):81–8.

44. Li GH, Niu LN, Zhang W, Olsen M, De-Deus G, Eid AA, Chen JH, Pashley DH, Tay FR. Ability of new obturation materials to improve the seal of the root canal system: a review. Acta Biomater. 2014;10(3): 1050–63.

45. Rafter M. Apexification: a review. Dent Traumatol. 2005;21(1):1–8.

46. Simon S, Rilliard F, Berdal A, Machtou P. The use of mineral trioxide aggregate in one-visit apexification treatment: a prospective study. Int Endod J. 2007; 40(3):186–97.

47. Ricucci D, Langeland K. Apical limit of root-canal instrumentation and obturation, part 2. A histological study. Int Endod J. 1998;31:394–409.

48. Sjögren U, Sundqvist G, Nair PNR. Tissue reaction to gutta-percha particles of various sizes when implanted subcutaneously in guinea pigs. Eur J Oral Sci. 1995;103(5):313–21.

49. López-López J, Estrugo-Devesa A, Jané-Salas E, Segura-Egea JJ. Inferior alveolar nerve injury resulting from overextension of an endodontic sealer: non-surgical management using the GABA analogue pregabalin. Int Endod J. 2012;45(1):98–104.

50. Seddon HJ. Three types of nerves injuries. Brain. 1943;66:237–88.

51. Grotz K, Al-Nawas B, de Aguiar EG, Schulz A, Wagner W. Treatment of injuries to the inferior alveolar nerve after endodontic procedures. Clin Oral Investig. 1998;2:73–6.

52. Hauman CH, Chandler NP, Tong DC. Endodontic implications of the maxillary sinus: a review. Int Endod J. 2002;35(2):127–41.

53. Legent F, Billet J, Beauvillain C, Bonnet J, Miegeville M. The role of dental canal fillings in the development of Aspergillus sinusitis. A report of 85 cases. Arch Otorhinolaryngol. 1989;246:318–20.

54. Giardion L, Pontieri F, Savoldi E, Tallarigo F. Aspergillus myetoma of the maxillary sinus secondary to overfilling of a root canal. J Endod. 2006;32(7):692–4.

55. Nair PN, Sjogren U, Krey G, Kahnberg KE, Sundqvist G. Intraradicular bacteria and fungi in root-filled, asymptomatic human teeth with therapy-resistant periapical lesions: a long-term light and electron microscopic follow-up study. J Endod. 1990;16: 580–8.

56. Lin LM, Pascon EA, Skribner J, Gangler P, Langeland K. Clinical, radiographic, and histologic study of endodontic treatment failures. Oral Surg Oral Med Oral Pathol. 1991;71:603–11.

57. Baumgartner JC, Falkler Jr WA. Bacteria in the apical 5 mm of infected root canals. J Endod. 1991;17: 380–3.

58. Ng YL, Mann V, Gulabivala K. A prospective study of the factors affecting outcomes of nonsurgical root canal treatment: part 1: periapical health. Int Endod J. 2011;44(7):583–609.

59. Ng YL, Mann V, Gulabivala K. A prospective study of the factors affecting outcomes of non-surgical root canal treatment: part 2: tooth survival. Int Endod J. 2011;44(7):610–25.

60. Estrela C, Holland R, Estrela A, Alencar AH, Sousa-Neto MD, Pécora JD. Characterization of successful root canal treatment. Braz Dent J. 2014;25(1):3–11.

Endodontics in the Deciduous/ Mixed Dentition

8

8

Bobby Patel

Summary

Formocresol pulpotomy was the standard of care when used for vital primary pulp therapy. Concern has been expressed as to the safety of formocresol use in paediatric dentistry. From the published data, available ferric sulphate, mineral trioxide aggregate (MTA) and indirect pulp treatment (IPT) appear to be promising alternatives to the single-visit formocresol pulpotomy for cariously exposed vital primary molar teeth. Ferric sulphate use is technique-sensitive and MTA has cost implications. The modified stepwise excavation technique is discussed as an alternative to IPT to prevent pulpal exposure in teeth with deep caries. Desensitising pulp therapies and pulpectomy procedures are also discussed as alternative options when trying to maintain a deciduous tooth.

Clinical Relevance

Various treatment concepts have been recommended for the management of deep carious lesions and pulpal exposures. Indirect and direct pulp-capping procedures, stepwise excavation and pulpotomy techniques are discussed in relation to primary teeth and permanent teeth with open apices (immature root development) including indications and rationale.

B. Patel, BDS MFDS MClinDent MRD MRACDS
Specialist Endodontist, Brindabella Specialist Centre,
Canberra, ACT, Australia
e-mail: bobbypatel@me.com

8.1 Overview of the Literature

Recent times have shown a paradigm shift whereby treatment procedures involving the pulp are led by biologically based strategies, which attempt to allow healing of a diseased pulp or prevent the progression of disease in a vital pulp. In cases where apical periodontitis is present, the rationale for endodontic treatment, by providing the best root filling, has been proven as an effective treatment modality for most cases.

The management of an unexposed pulp due to caries or trauma remains straightforward. Provided the pulp is protected by a biologically compatible restoration, then the potential for repair is good. The management of an exposed pulp remains controversial. Therapies aimed at preserving the vitality of the pulp, including pulp capping or partial or full pulpotomies, have very good success rates where trauma has been the cause. Treatment options for the management of deep caries in an attempt to prevent carious pulp exposures include indirect pulp-capping procedures and stepwise excavation techniques. Direct pulp-capping procedures and pulpotomies are indicated where a carious pulp exposure has occurred and the aim is to preserve the vitality of the pulp. The rationale for any selected treatment is ultimately based on whether the underlying pulp is deemed vital or nonvital [1–3].

There is poor correlation between clinical symptoms and the histopathological conditions of the pulp, which further complicates the accurate diagnosis of the pulp [4]. Without histological examination to determine the extent of inflammation, we can only make assumptions regarding the probable pulpal status of any given tooth. A thorough clinical history and examination is essential in determining the likely pulpal status of the tooth concerned and will therefore help determine the most appropriate treatment.

A detailed history of the complaint will reveal the characteristics of the pain, which is often helpful in determining the likely pulp status. A distinction between provoked pain that ceases following removal of the causative factor (chemical, thermal or mechanical irritants) and spontaneous pain should be made. The former is usually indicative of a probable diagnosis of reversible pulpitis that will be more amenable to pulp preservation treatments (indirect pulp-capping, direct pulp-capping and pulpotomy procedures). Spontaneous pain, such as constant unprovoked throbbing pain, or pain that continues long after the stimulus has been removed is usually associated with extensive degeneration in the root canals that will require more extensive pulp therapies aimed at treating the diseased radicular pulp tissue (pulpectomy procedures) [5, 6]. One should bear in mind, as is often the case, that the pulp can suffer a complete breakdown without having any previous history of pain [7].

Clinical signs and symptoms such as redness, swelling, severe dental decay, ditched or fractured restorations and draining sinuses or parulis may indicate further evidence of underlying pulpal pathology. Mechanical allodynia (percussion sensitivity) may be unreliable in a child due to psychological aspects in determining a normal response compared to a lowered pain threshold due to pulpal inflammation. Tooth mobility in the primary dentition is also an unreliable sign due to teeth that may be near to exfoliation as a result of normal physiological resorption [2].

Clinical examination will include sensitivity testing, such as electric pulp testing and thermal testing which is unreliable in primary teeth [8]. In teeth with incomplete root formation, the aforementioned tests are also of limited value due to varied responses from immature teeth, unreliable responses due to apprehension and fear from the child and difficulties in understanding or communicating accurately the tests themselves [9, 10].

Interpretation of radiographic findings in the primary dentition is often complicated by the underlying permanent successor and surrounding tooth follicle. Misdiagnosis of pulpal pathology mistaken for the underlying follicle may occur leading to errors in diagnosis and subsequent management.

Research has shown that when the marginal ridge has spontaneously broken away over dental caries, the pulp tissues are already compromised [11]. Pulpotomies, pulpectomies and conventional preformed metal crowns (stainless steel) have an excellent record of success and play a major role in providing quality dental care for children [12].

Retention of the pulpally involved deciduous tooth is usually advisable to prevent or minimise mesial drift of permanent successors. This may be of benefit in reducing subsequent crowding and resultant malocclusions [13].

In the developing dentition, a more conservative pulp preservation procedure (such as indirect and direct pulp capping or pulpotomy or apexogenesis) may be indicated to allow completion of root formation provided the tooth is deemed vital. Further dentine deposition along the root will strengthen the immature tooth, which has thin dentinal roots helping to diminish future root fracture [14, 15] (Fig. 8.1).

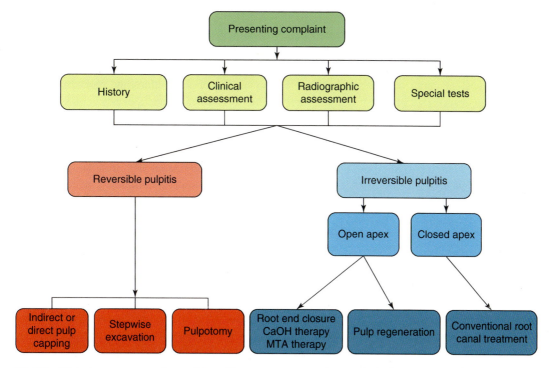

Fig. 8.1 Clinical management of reversible and irreversible pulpitis in the mixed/permanent dentition. Note if the apex is open, then root-end closure procedures or pulpal regeneration may be indicated to allow for continued root development

Indirect pulp capping is a treatment modality that has gained increased popularity recently that can be undertaken in a single-visit appointment (indirect pulp capping) or a two-stage procedure (stepwise excavation) [3, 16, 17]. The premise of either treatment is to prevent exposure of the pulp during deep carious excavation by leaving the deepest carious dentine overlying the pulp in place to preserve vitality. Residual dentine thickness is an important prognostic factor for reactionary dentinogenesis and the ability of surviving odontoblasts to secrete tertiary dentine allowing continued pulp survival.

A suitable lining material is placed to allow for reparative dentine stimulation [18]. There is no general agreement as to what type of lining material is ideal although calcium hydroxide, mineral trioxide aggregate (MTA), composite resins and glass ionomer cements have all appeared to be satisfactory in their ability to induce a calcific barrier formation [19]. The placement of a high-quality temporary and final restoration is essential for success.

In the stepwise approach for caries excavation, various amounts of carious dentine are sealed off by a temporary restoration for a period of time. Re-entry is carried out in anticipation of the possibility of remineralisation of softened noninfected dentine over the pulp and hard tissue repair. The intent is to carry out further excavation of remaining caries without ensuing pulpal exposure [20, 21].

A potential disadvantage of carrying out these types of procedures is delaying the inevitable pulpectomy and possible difficulties thereof due to ensuing pulpal reactions and calcifications that can lead to negotiation difficulties. Unfortunately, treatments are guided to either invasive pulp therapy or procedures aimed at maintaining pulpal integrity based on the probable pulpal status, which can only be verified following careful follow-up. The advantage in an immature tooth with continued root development is obvious, but in a mature tooth, the obvious benefits must be weighed up against the possibility of developing a peri-radicular apical lesion, which reduces the success rate of root canal treatment [22].

Direct pulp-capping procedures are required when an inadvertent pulp exposure has occurred. The decision to avoid a pulpectomy is based on the assumption that the radicular pulp remains vital and only superficial inflammation is present confined to a few millimetres at the site of exposure. Controversy has plagued this treatment modality, and its success depends on various issues including the size of pulpal exposure, presence of infected dentinal chips, control of haemorrhage, type of pulp-capping material used and the quality of the 'dentinal bridge' formed [23]. The technique is not normally advocated for carious primary molars [24].

A pulpotomy procedure should be performed on a tooth that is judged vital. The coronal pulp is amputated, and then the radicular pulp is either fixed using formocresol, preserved using a haemostatic agent such as ferric sulphate or sodium hypochlorite solution to form a clot barrier or bridged by using calcium hydroxide or mineral trioxide aggregate [30–32]. The success of the technique is highly dependent on achieving a good coronal seal, which will effectively cut off the nutritional supply for any remaining dentinal bacteria and will prevent further bacterial microleakage. It has been strongly recommended that adhesive restorations or preformed crowns be employed following any primary molar pulp therapy procedure [25–28].

There has been a suggestion that the use of formocresol in paediatric dentistry is unwarranted due to safety concerns. Studies have linked formocresol with nasopharyngeal cancer in both human and animal studies based on exposure to formaldehyde at very high doses. The evidence in the literature suggests that formocresol is probably not a potent human carcinogen under low-exposure conditions. Nevertheless, the fixation of radicular pulp stumps using formocresol is no longer recommended, and alternatives using either ferric sulphate or mineral trioxide aggregate have been advocated using clinical studies to demonstrate equal if not better results [27–30].

Ferric sulphate (5–15 %) promotes pulpal haemostasis by forming a protective metal-protein clot at the surface of the vital radicular pulp stumps. A zinc oxide eugenol base is then usually applied over the radicular pulpal tissue.

MTA has been used successfully in adult endodontic procedures since 1993 and has been recommended for pulp capping, pulpotomy, apical barrier formation in teeth with open apexes, repair of root perforations and root canal filling. The constituents include tricalcium silicate, dicalcium silicate, tricalcium aluminate, tetracalcium aluminoferrite, calcium sulphate and bismuth oxide. The material has excellent bioactive properties and essentially stimulates cytokine release from pulpal fibroblasts, which in turn stimulates hard tissue formation. In pulp-capping or pulpotomy procedures, it is mixed with sterile water to a sandy consistency, which is gently packed against the radicular pulp stumps. The material is hydrophilic and takes up to 4 h to set completely [32].

Desensitising pulp therapies have been recommended primarily for deciduous teeth and also used by some clinicians for the permanent dentition [33]. This two-stage technique uses paraformaldehyde paste to fix and devitalise hypersensitive coronal pulp tissue. In view of increasing concerns about the use of formaldehyde (as previously mentioned), an alternative approach, using Ledermix paste, has been recommended [34]. Ledermix is a readily available paste containing triamcinolone acetonide (steroid) and demeclocycline (antimicrobial). It is used widely in adult endodontic procedures and has been shown to reduce pulpal inflammation and pain.

Pulpectomy is indicated where the radicular pulp is nonvital or irreversibly inflamed. It is contraindicated when there is evidence of extensive internal or external root resorption or if more than one-third of the root length has been lost. The most commonly used medicaments for primary molar root canal therapy are zinc oxide eugenol (ZnOE) paste, iodoform paste and calcium hydroxide [35, 36]. Slow-setting pure zinc oxide eugenol paste has traditionally been the material of choice as a primary molar root filling material. However, concerns have been expressed regarding the slow removal of zinc oxide eugenol by the body (if extruded through the root apex) and the differential rate of resorption between this material and the tooth itself. The use of Vitapex (a mixture of calcium hydroxide and iodoform paste) has a superior success rate to that of zinc oxide eugenol and is removed more readily if extruded through an apex [37].

A recent systematic review of the literature summarised that because of the lack of good studies, it is not possible to determine whether an injured pulp as a result of deep caries can be maintained or whether it should be removed and replaced with a root canal filling. Both randomised studies and prospective observational studies are needed to investigate whether a pulp exposed to deep caries is best treated by measures intended to preserve it or by pulpectomy and root filling [38]. Current practice is dictated by best clinical judgement as to the pulpal diagnosis and appropriate treatment thereafter. Indirect pulp-capping, pulpotomy and pulpectomy procedures are indicated in deciduous teeth in order to remain as space maintainers avoiding crowding if the tooth was lost early. Immature teeth with incomplete root formation would be teeth that gain most benefit from pulp preservation procedures rather than less conservative pulpectomy treatments. Root canal procedures are reserved for those cases where apical periodontitis has been confirmed and extraction is to be avoided.

8.2 Indirect Pulp Capping

The procedure is acceptable for the management of a deep carious lesion where the patient has no signs or symptoms indicative of pulpal pathosis. The aim is to remove the entire carious lesion except for the last remaining stained dentine overlying the pulp. The rationale is to arrest the carious process and to provide conditions conducive to the formation of reactionary dentine. The remaining carious dentine (stained) is allowed to remineralise, promoting pulpal healing and preserving the vitality of the pulp without inadvertent frank carious exposure.

The procedure consists of the following steps:

1. Preoperative radiograph such as a parallel bitewing and parallel periapical confirming carious lesion and proximity to pulp.

2. Standard local anaesthetic protocol to provide adequate anaesthesia.
3. The use of rubber dam to isolate the tooth being treated.
4. All caries is removed at the enamel-dentine junction (periphery of the cavity).
5. Careful removal of soft deep carious dentine (using slow-speed hand-piece with a round stainless-steel bur and excavators) overlying the pulp region with care avoiding a pulpal exposure.
6. Placement of appropriate lining material such as hard-setting calcium hydroxide cement, reinforced glass ionomer cement or zinc oxide eugenol.
7. Placement of a definitive restoration. An excellent coronal seal needs to be provided to prevent further micro-leakage (Fig. 8.2).

8.3 Modified Stepwise Excavation

The stepwise excavation technique has been used for the management of deep carious lesions to avoid inadvertent pulpal exposure. A less invasive approach, whereby the deepest caries is left in situ at the first appointment, has been modified at an attempt to change an active carious lesion into an arrested lesion. The aim of the first excavation is to change the carious environment without removing the softened carious dentine, which is in close proximity to the pulp. If one were to try and remove all the caries close to the dentine-pulpal border, then a pulpal exposure may be created. The active soft yellowish dentine will eventually become darker, harder and drier demineralised dentine resembling a slowly progressing lesion. The tooth is re-entered at a later stage to complete the caries removal process.

The stepwise excavation technique consists of the following steps:

1. Preoperative radiograph such as a parallel bitewing and parallel periapical confirming carious lesion and proximity to pulp.
2. Standard local anaesthetic protocol to provide adequate anaesthesia.

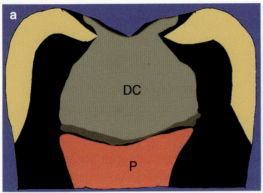

Fig. 8.2 Diagrammatic representation of the indirect pulp capping procedure. (**a**) Preoperative view demonstrating deep caries (*DC*) overlying pulp (*P*) and (**b**) post-operative following caries removal. Note stained dentine overlying pulp (S) is left in situ. A suitable lining material [L] and an excellent coronal seal (*CS*) are placed

3. The use of rubber dam to isolate the tooth being treated.
4. All caries is removed at the enamel-dentine junction (periphery of the cavity).
5. Careful removal of the central outermost softened carious dentine using an excavator only to ensure that a provisional restoration can be placed.
6. No attempt is made to excavate as close to the pulp as possible in order to remove all infected dentine, thereby reducing the risk of pulpal exposure.
7. A provisional restoration is selected on the basis of the interim dressing period from 6 to 8 months.
8. A second final excavation is carried out whereby careful removal of deep carious dentine (using slow-speed hand-piece with a round stainless-steel bur and excavators) overlying the pulp region with care avoiding a pulpal exposure. As per the indirect pulp-capping treatment, any hard stained dentine overlying the pulp can be left in situ to avoid exposure.
9. Placement of appropriate lining material such as hard-setting calcium hydroxide cement, reinforced glass ionomer cement or zinc oxide eugenol.
10. Placement of a definitive restoration. An excellent coronal seal needs to be provided to prevent further micro-leakage (Figs. 8.3 and 8.4).

8.4 Direct Pulp Capping

This treatment option is limited to the permanent dentition and not recommended for the management of pulpal exposures in the primary dentition. The aim of the treatment is to encourage the formation of a dentine bridge at the site of pulpal exposure by encouraging the formation of reparative dentine. This allows the preservation of the underlying pulp and its continuing vitality based on the assumption that the tooth is asymptomatic and the tooth is considered vital.

The procedural steps include:

1. Preoperative radiograph such as a parallel bitewing and parallel periapical confirming carious lesion and proximity to pulp.
2. Standard local anaesthetic protocol to provide adequate anaesthesia.
3. The use of rubber dam to isolate the tooth being treated.
4. Gross caries is removed using either a sharp spoon excavator or a large, round slow-speed tungsten carbide bur. Caries detector dye can be used with appropriate magnification (operating dental microscope).
5. As the pulp is approached, the cavity can be flushed with sodium hypochlorite solution to reduce the bacterial load.
6. The remaining affected carious tissue is removed.

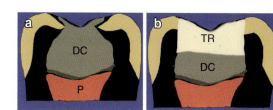
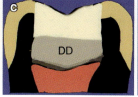
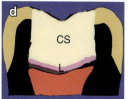
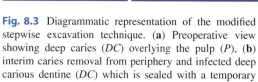

Fig. 8.3 Diagrammatic representation of the modified stepwise excavation technique. (**a**) Preoperative view showing deep caries (*DC*) overlying the pulp (*P*), (**b**) interim caries removal from periphery and infected deep carious dentine (*DC*) which is sealed with a temporary restoration (*TR*) for 6–8 months (**c**) note deep carious dentine has changed to a harder demineralised dentine (*DD*) which is easier to remove without causing a pulpal exposure at the 6–8-month second appointment and (**d**) final coronal seal (*CS*) with appropriate lining (*L*) overlying the pulp

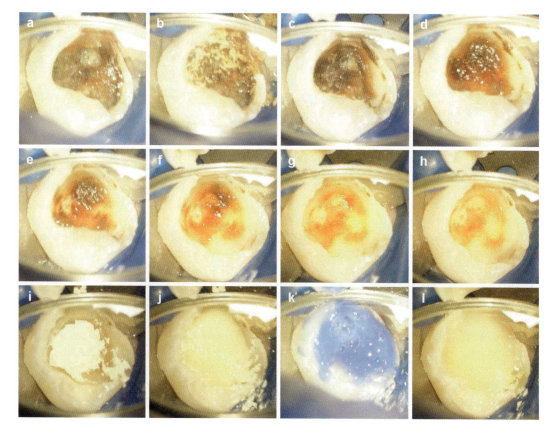

Fig. 8.4 Clinical photographs demonstrating indirect pulp capping procedure using MTA. Note (**a–h**) caries removal leaving in situ stained dentine overlying pulp, (**i**) MTA placement, (**j**) GIC base, (**k**) acid etching and (**l**) placement of composite resin restoration

7. Pulpal bleeding can be controlled by either gentle application of cotton wool pledget soaked in water/saline or sodium hypochlorite for up to 10 min. Care should be taken to avoid the application of too much pressure on the pulp.

8. Once haemostasis has been achieved, application of hard-setting calcium hydroxide or MTA (thickness of at least 2 mm).

9. A definitive restoration ensuring good coronal seal is placed. If MTA is used, then a moistened cotton wool pledget is placed over this to

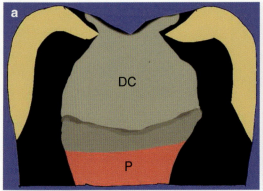 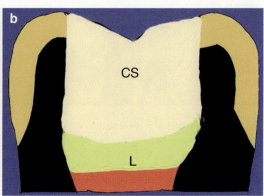

Fig. 8.5 Diagrammatic representation showing (**a**) pre-operative view showing extensive deep caries (*DC*) involving the pulp (*P*) and (**b**) post-operative view following caries removal. Note suitable lining material such as MTA placed over pulp exposure (*L*) and overlying definitive coronal seal restoration (*CS*) which is necessary to prevent further pulpal insult. This treatment is not recommended for primary deciduous teeth

allow for complete setting and a temporary restoration is placed. The tooth is re-entered 5–10 days later for placement of a definitive restoration (Fig. 8.5).

8.5   Pulpotomy

A pulpotomy procedure involves the removal of the irreversibly inflamed coronal pulp and protection of the underlying non-inflamed healthy radicular pulp. The tooth should be generally asymptomatic and the treatment considered in those cases where a carious or mechanical exposure due to trauma has occurred resulting in exposure of the vital coronal pulp tissue.

The procedural steps include:

1. Parallel preoperative radiograph showing all roots and apices.
2. Standard local anaesthetic protocol to provide adequate anaesthesia.
3. The use of rubber dam to isolate the tooth being treated.
4. All caries is removed.
5. Complete removal of the roof of the pulp chamber. Recommended to use a nonend-cutting bur.
6. Coronal pulp tissue is removed using either a sharp spoon excavator or a large, round slow-speed stainless-steel bur (Fig. 8.6).
7. Pulpal bleeding should be controlled within 5 min using gentle application of cotton wool pledget soaked in water/saline.
8. Appropriate medicament is selected for direct application to the radicular pulp stumps which can include:
   (a) 15.5 % ferric sulphate solution (Astringedent) can be burnished on the pulp stumps with a micro-brush for 15 s or used with a cotton wool pledget and gently applied with pressure. Thorough rinsing and drying is carried out.
   (b) 20 % (1:5 dilution) Buckley's formocresol solution is applied to the radicular pulp stumps using a cotton wool pledget for 5 min to achieve superficial tissue fixation.
   (c) MTA paste is applied over the radicular pulp stumps with appropriate carrier.
   (d) Well-condensed layer of calcium hydroxide applied directly over the radicular pulp stump (Fig. 8.7).
9. A suitable lining material is placed such as resin-modified glass ionomer cement or zinc oxide eugenol cement.
10. A definitive restoration is placed to ensure an excellent coronal seal. Note in the case of primary teeth, a preformed metal crown should be placed or an adhesive restoration.

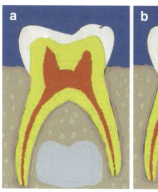
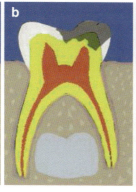
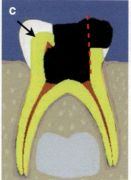
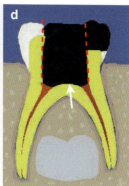

Fig. 8.6 Diagrammatic representation of primary pulp amputation (vital pulpotomy). The procedure is carried out using local anaesthetic and rubber dam isolation (salivary ejector and cotton wool rolls can be used as an alternative). (**a**) The pulp chamber of deciduous molar teeth are very large relative to the external dimensions of the crown. The enamel and dentine walls of these teeth are fairly thin and the distance between the pulp horns and the enamel surface is sometimes as little as 2 mm. (**b**) Carious primary tooth with an infected, irreversibly inflamed coronal pulp. (**c**) Caries is excavated, the pulp chamber is opened widely and the coronal pulp is removed with a sterile round bur running at low speed. Care must be taken to ensure the entire roof of the pulp chamber is removed (*dotted red line*) and no remnants of pulp tissue have been left (*black arrow*). (**d**) Care must also be taken in avoiding weakening of the fragile walls of the tooth and also perforation of the pulpal floor (*white arrow*)

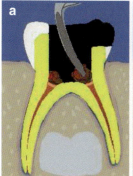
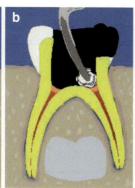
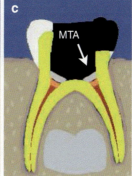
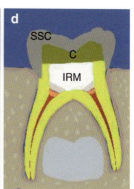

Fig. 8.7 Diagrammatic representation of vital pulpotomy procedure (continued from Fig. 8.6). (**a**) Irrigation of the pulp chamber with either saline or local anaesthetic solution will help to dislodge coronal pulp remnants and dentine debris. The cavity is dried with cotton wool pledgets and the pulp stumps identified. The natural cessation of bleeding from the radicular pulp contraindicates the need for pulpectomy. (**b**) A cotton wool pledget moistened in ferric sulphate or saline is applied to the pulp stumps to facilitate haemorrhage control. After a 5 minute application the tissue at the entrance to the canals should be cauterized and no longer be bleeding. (**c**) Mineral Trioxide Aggregate (*MTA*) is placed over the radicular pulp stumps. (**d**) Intermediate restorative material (*IRM*) and core material (*C*) is placed over the MTA and a stainless steel crown (*SSC*) is cemented using glass ionomer cement to maintain the coronal seal and prevent catastrophic tooth fracture in the long term

8.6   Pulpectomy

Pulpectomy can be carried out in the primary dentition with appropriate patient selection in order to maintain the tooth until expected exfoliation. The clinician must be aware of complicating factors such as molar radicular morphology, close proximity to the permanent successor tooth and inherent physiological resorption that will occur. The aim of this procedure is to remove irreversibly inflamed or necrotic radicular pulp tissue, clean and shape the canal spaces and obturate the root canals with a filling material. The selection of root filling material is critical and must be selected on the basis that it will resorb at the same rate as the primary tooth and not cause any detrimental damage and be eliminated rapidly if extruded beyond the confines of the fine canals.

The clinical procedural steps include:

1. Preoperative radiograph demonstrating all roots, apices and position/presence of permanent successor.
2. Standard local anaesthetic protocol to provide adequate anaesthesia.
3. The use of rubber dam to isolate the tooth being treated.
4. Removal of all caries.
5. Removal of entire roof of pulp chamber preferably with a nonend-cutting bur (Endo Z).
6. Coronal pulp tissue is removed using either a sharp spoon excavator or a large, round slow-speed stainless-steel bur.
7. Root canals identified and working lengths established keeping 2 mm short of root apices.
8. Irrigation regime using 1 % sodium hypochlorite solution or 0.2 % chlorhexidine solution.
9. Canal shaping carried out either with hand files or rotary files; Note: do not overprepare/enlarge the canals due to thin walls; ideally less than size #30.
10. Non-setting calcium hydroxide paste used to dress canals and tooth temporised for 7–10 days.
11. Appropriate root canal filling material selected depending on whether physiological resorption expected or not, i.e. if the permanent successor is not present, (a) then the primary tooth may be a long-term solution as a space maintainer. On the other hand, if a permanent successor is present, (b) then normal physiological resorption will be expected.
    (a) The canals are dried with paper points and obturated with gutta-percha root filling and conventional root canal sealer of choice.
    (b) The canals are dried with paper points and obturated with a resorbable paste such as slow-setting pure zinc oxide eugenol, non-setting calcium hydroxide paste or a mixture of iodoform/calcium hydroxide paste.

8.7 Clinical Cases

Case 1: MTA Pulpotomy in a Permanent Tooth A fit and healthy 32-year-old lady was referred for endodontic management of tooth 27. The patient had had an extensive temporary restoration placed with suspected caries involving the pulp (Fig. 8.8). Clinical examination revealed the tooth had remained asymptomatic with no tenderness to percussion or palpation. Special tests revealed the tooth responded to both electric pulp testing and thermal stimulus (CO_2 snow). The patient was highly anxious in the dental setting and could not tolerate rubber dam treatment for prolonged periods of time. Radiographic examination confirmed an extensive restoration overlying the pulp chamber. A decision was made to carry out a pulpotomy.

The tooth was isolated under rubber dam and temporary restoration was dismantled. Caries was removed confirming pulp exposure. Coronal pulp tissue was removed and bleeding of the coronal pulp stumps achieved. An MTA pulpotomy dressing was placed and the tooth re-temporised. A week later following no pain or discomfort, the tooth was permanently restored with a bonded composite restoration. In normal circumstances, a complete pulpectomy and root canal treatment would have been performed. Due to the patient's anxieties and intolerance of rubber dam, a decision was made to carry out a simple procedure with the possibility of extraction if pulpal symptoms ensue in the future. The patient was made aware of the long-term prognosis and warned of the possibility of failure.

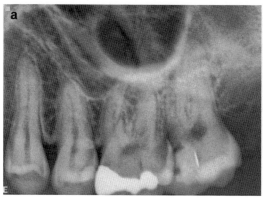 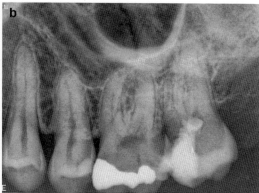

Fig. 8.8 Clinical case 1 demonstrating radiographs showing (**a**) preoperative view showing tooth 27 with failing temporary restoration and caries in close proximity to the pulp in an adult patient with complete root development. The patient was very apprehensive and could not tolerate rubber dam for long sessions. Caries removal was carried out under local anaesthetic and rubber dam isolation. A carious pulpal exposure was noted and a decision made to carry out a coronal pulpotomy. Haemorrhage was controlled using light pressure and irrigation with 1 %sodium hypochlorite solution. 4 mm of MTA was placed in the coronal pulp chamber and a wet cotton wool pledget and temporary restoration seal. (**b**) The patient was reviewed a week later and a permanent bonded composite restoration placed and post-operative radiograph taken. The patient remained asymptomatic

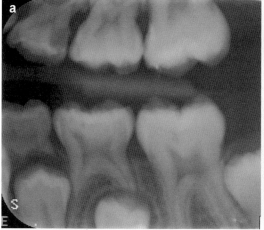 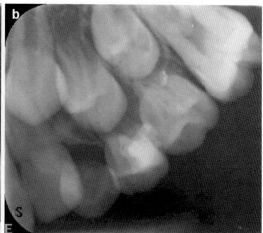

Fig. 8.9 Clinical case 2 showing clinical radiographs demonstrating (**a**) gross DO caries in tooth 64. The 9-year-old patient was asymptomatic at time of presentation. (**b**) Pulpotomy carried out with ferric sulphate and MTA filling followed by bonded adhesive restoration

Case 2: MTA Pulpotomy in a Deciduous Tooth A 9-year-old fit and healthy child (my daughter) was seen for gross caries affecting tooth 64 (Fig. 8.9). Pulpal symptoms had become noticeable with pain on eating occasionally. The tooth was isolated with rubber dam and all caries removed. A pulpotomy procedure was carried out (Fig. 8.10) using ferric sulphate to control the bleeding. Once haemorrhage was controlled, an MTA filling was placed in the tooth. The tooth was then restored using the 'sandwich technique' using glass ionomer cement and composite resin restoration. The tooth remained asymptomatic until exfoliation.

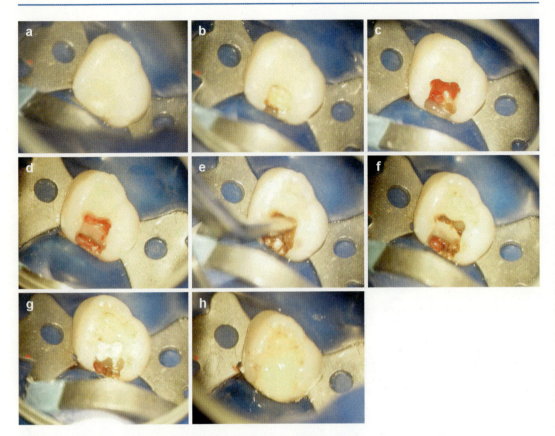

Fig. 8.10 Clinical case 2 demonstrating clinical photographs showing step-by-step procedure of a vital pulpotomy carried out in a deciduous tooth using 15.5 % ferric sulphate and MTA cement overlying radicular pulp stumps. Note (**a**) preoperative view demonstrating intact enamel, (**b**) gross caries, (**c**) pulpal exposure following caries removal with bleeding from the pulp, (**d**) following irrigation with 1 % sodium hypochlorite solution to reduce bacterial load further, (**e**) application of ferric sulphate to radicular pulp stumps, (**f**) clot barrier formation following application of haemostatic agent, (**g**) application of MTA over radicular pulp stumps and (**h**) final bonded restoration

---

Clinical Hints and Tips
(i) **Indirect pulp capping**
- This procedure purposely avoids a pulpal exposure by leaving the deepest decay in place.
- A thin layer of demineralised stained dentine can be left in place.
- Caries dye indicators are useful with appropriate illumination and magnification.
- Re-entry is not attempted.

(ii) **Stepwise excavation**
- Caries excavation is a two-appointment procedure.
- Initially the lesion's periphery is made caries-free.

- The central caries is partially removed to leave soft carious dentine overlying the pulp.
- Calcium hydroxide is placed and a suitable long-term temporary restoration placed.
- At 6–12 months, the tooth is re-entered and all carries are removed.

(iii) **Direct pulp capping**
- Use 1 % sodium hypochlorite irrigation solution and cotton wool pledgets with gentle pressure if bleeding does not stop following simple irrigation.
- Continuous profuse bleeding after 5 min may indicate severe pulp inflammation requiring a more radical approach.

- Consider either calcium hydroxide/resin-modified glass ionomer cement or MTA as a suitable seal over the exposure.

(iv) **Pulpotomy**

- Consider using either 15.5 % ferric sulphate or MTA instead of formocresol.

(v) **Pulpectomy**

- Take care and avoid overpreparation due to thin roots associated with primary teeth; recommended preparation size should not be greater than #30 hand files in a molar tooth.
- Consider using resorbable material that is relatively inert such as non-setting calcium hydroxide paste or calcium hydroxide and iodoform paste if the tooth is prone to normal physiological resorption due to exfoliation.
- Consider using gutta-percha and sealer if no permanent successor is present and exfoliation due to normal physiological resorption unlikely.

References

1. Fuks AB, Chosack A, Klein H, Eidelman E. Partial pulpotomy as a treatment alternative for exposed pulps in crown-fractured permanent incisors. Dent Traumatol. 1987;3:100–2.
2. Chailertvanitkul P, Papungkornkit J, Sooksantisakoonchai N, Pumas N, Pairojamornyoot W, Leela-apiradee N, & Abbott PV. Randomised control trial comparing calcium hydroxide and mineral trioxide aggregate for partial pulpotomies in cariously-exposed pulps of permanent molars. Int Endod J. 2014;47(9);835–42.
3. Bjørndal L, Reit C, Bruun G, Markvart M, Kjældgaard M, Näsman P, Thordrup M, Dige I, Nyvad B, Fransson H, Lager A, Ericson D, Petersson K, Olsson J, Santimano EM, Wennström A, Winkel P, Gluud C. Treatment of deep caries lesions in adults: randomized clinical trials comparing stepwise vs. direct complete excavation, and direct pulp capping vs. partial pulpotomy. Eur J Oral Sci. 2010;118:290–7.
4. Dummer PMH, Hicks R, Huws D. Clinical signs and symptoms in pulp disease. Int Endod J. 1980;13(1): 27–35.
5. Patel B. Examination and diagnosis. In: Patel B. Endodontic Diagnosis, Pathology and Treatment planning. Mastering clinical practice. Switzerland: Springer; 2015.
6. Baume LJ, Holz J. Long term clinical assessment of direct pulp capping. Int Dent J. 1981;31: 251–60.
7. Michaelson PL, Holland GR. Is pulpitis painful? Int Endod J. 2002;35:829–32.
8. Andreasen JO, Bakland LK, Flores MT, Andreasen FM, and Andersson L. Traumatic dental injuries: a manual. Oxford, UK: Wiley-Blackwell; 2013.
9. Klein H. Pulpal responses to electric pulp stimulator in the developing permanent anterior dentition. J Dent Child. 1978;45:199–202.
10. Fuss Z, Trowbridge H, Bender IB, Rickoff B. Assessment of reliability of electric and thermal pulp testing agents. J Endod. 1986;12:301–5.
11. Duggal MS, Nooh A, High A. Response of the primary pulp to inflammation: a review of the Leeds studies and structural challenges for the future. Eur J Paediatr Dent. 2002;3:111–4.
12. Duggal MS, Gautam SK, Nichol R, Robertson AS. Paediatric dentistry in the new millennium: 1. Quality care for children. Dent Update. 2003;30:230–4.
13. Fanning E. Effect of extraction of deciduous molars on the formation and eruption of their successors. Angle Orthod. 1962;32:44.
14. Cvek M, Cleaton-Jones PE, Austin JC, Andreasen JO. Pulp reactions to exposure after experimental crown fractures or grinding in adult monkeys. J Endod. 1982;8:391–7.
15. Shabahang S. Treatment options: Apexogenesis and Apexification. J Endod. 2013;39(3):S26–9.
16. Coll JA. Indirect pulp capping and primary teeth: is the primary tooth pulpotomy out of date? J Endod. 2008;34:S34–9.
17. Bjorndal L. Indirect pulp therapy and stepwise excavation. J Endod. 2008;34:S29–33.
18. Goldberg M, Smith AJ. Cells and extracellular matrices of dentin and pulp: a biological basis for repair and tissue engineering. Crit Rev Oral Biol Med. 2004;15(1):13–27.
19. Whitworth JM, Myers PM, Smith J, Walls AWG, McCabe JF. Endodontic complications after plastic restorations in general practice. Int Endod J. 2005;38:409–16.
20. Leskell E, Ridell K, Cvek M, Majare I. Pulp exposure after stepwise vs direct complete excavation of deep carious lesions in young posterior teeth. Endod Dent Traumatol. 1996;12:192–6.
21. Bjorndal L, Larsen T, Thylstrup A. A clinical and microbiological study of deep carious lesions during stepwise excavation using long term treatment intervals. Caries Res. 1997;31:411–7.
22. Ng YL, Mann V, Gulabivala K. A prospective study of the factors affecting outcomes of nonsurgical root canal treatment: part 1: periapical health. Int Endo J. 2010;44(7):583–609.
23. Cho SY, Seo DG, Lee SJ, Lee J, Lee SJ, Jung IY. Prognostic factors for clinical outcomes according to time after direct pulp capping. J Endod. 2013;39(3):327–31.

24. Al-Zayer MA, Straffon LH, Feigal RJ, Welch KB. Indirect pulp treatment of primary posterior teeth: a retrospective study. Paediatr Dent. 2003;25:29–36.
25. Guelmann M, Bookmyer KL, Villalta P, Garcia-Godoy F. Microleakage of restorative techniques for pulpotomised primary molars. J Dent Child. 2004;71:209–11.
26. Kindelan SA, Day P, Nichol R, Willmott N, Fayle SA. UK National Clinical Guidelines in Paediatric Dentistry: stainless steel preformed crowns for primary molars. Int J Paediatr Dent. 2008;18:20–8.
27. Simon S, Perard M, Zanini M, Smith AJ, Charpentier E, Djole SX, Lumley PJ. Should pulp chamber pulpotomy be seen as a permanent treatment? Some preliminary thoughts. Int Endod J. 2013;46: 79–87.
28. Rodd HD, Waterhouse PJ, Fuks AB, Fayle SA, Moffat MA. Pulp therapy for primary molars. Int J Paed Dent. 2006;16(s1):15–23.
29. Milnes A. Is Formocresol Obsolete? A fresh look at the evidence concerning safety issues. J Endod. 2008;34:S40–6.
30. Erdem AP, Guven Y, Balli B, Ilhan B, Sepet E, Ulukapi I, Aktoren O. Success rates of mineral trioxide aggregate, ferric sulfate, and formocresol pulpotomies: a 24-month study. Pediatr Dent. 2011;33(2):165–70.
31. Parirokh M, Torabinejad M. Mineral trioxide aggregate: a comprehensive literature review—part I: chemical, physical, and antibacterial properties. J Endod. 2010;36(1):16–27.
32. Fernández CC, Martínez SS, Jimeno FG, Lorente Rodríguez AI, Mercadé M. Clinical and radiographic outcomes of the use of four dressing materials in pulpotomized primary molars: a randomized clinical trial with 2-year follow-up. Int J Paediatr Dent. 2013;23: 400–7.
33. Garcia-Godoy F. A 42-month evaluation of glutaraldehyde pulpotomies in primary teeth. J Pedod. 1986;10:148–55.
34. Hansen HP, Ravn JJ, Ulrich D. Vital pulpotomy in primary molars. a clinical and histological investigation of the effect of zinc-oxide eugenol cement and Ledermix. Scand J Dent Res. 1971;79:13–23.
35. Llewelyn DR. UK National Guidelines in Paediatric Dentistry: the pulp treatment of the primary dentition. Int J Paediatr Dent. 2000;10:248–52.
36. Kubota K, Golden BE, Penugonda B. Root canal filling materials for primary teeth: a review of the literature. ASDC J Dent Child. 1992;58:225–7.
37. Mortazavi M, Mesbahi M. Comparison of zinc oxide and eugenol, and Vitapex for root canal treatment of necrotic primary teeth. Int J Paediatr Dent. 2004;14:417–24.
38. Bergenholtz G, Axelsson S, Davidson T, Frisk F, Hakeberg M, Kvist T, Norland A, Petersson A, Portenier I, Sandberg H, Tranaeus S, Mejare I. Treatment of pulps in teeth affected by deep caries – a systematic review of the literature. Singapore Dent J. 2013;34(1):1–12.

Apexogenesis, Apexification, Revascularization and Endodontic Regeneration

9

Bobby Patel

Summary

Apexogenesis is a vital pulp therapy procedure to encourage continued root development and maturation with normal root thickness. Apexification is an endodontic procedure that aims to either induce a hard tissue barrier in a tooth with an open apex or the continued apical development of an incomplete root in teeth with apical periodontitis. Revascularization and regeneration procedures are newer methods that allows for new living tissue to form in the cleaned canal space allowing for continued root development in terms of both length and thickness.

Clinical Relevance

Apexification is a method for treating and preserving immature permanent teeth that have lost their pulp vitality. Traditionally calcium hydroxide was the material of choice for creating a calcific barrier at the root apex inducing closure over several months. One-visit apexification using MTA has also been recommended as a predictable method for creating an artificial barrier at the apex. Recently, a number of case reports have emerged whereby immature necrotic permanent teeth have been treated with a triple antibiotic paste protocol allowing continued root development and normal thickness. These procedures, as a result of revascularization as opposed to regeneration, show promise for future treatment strategies aimed at continued root development and possibly pulp vitality maintenance. The concept of regenerating the pulp-dentine complex by tissue engineering is in its infancy, but continued research may one day result in the ability to 'regrow' a pulp and completely change the management of apical periodontitis both in the immature and mature tooth.

9.1 Overview of Endodontic Apexogenesis, Apexification, Revascularization and Regeneration

The completion of root development and closure of the apex occur up to 3 years after eruption in the permanent dentition [1]. Treatment of teeth that have sustained injuries, resulting in either necrotic pulps or apical periodontitis, during

B. Patel, BDS MFDS MClinDent MRD MRACDS
Specialist Endodontist, Brindabella Specialist Centre, Canberra, ACT, Australia
e-mail: bobbypatel@me.com

© Springer International Publishing Switzerland 2016
B. Patel (ed.), *Endodontic Treatment, Retreatment, and Surgery*,
DOI 10.1007/978-3-319-19476-9_9

this transitional period provides a significant challenge for the clinician [2]. Two common approaches for managing such cases include apexogenesis or apexification [3, 4]. Apexogenesis is a 'vital pulp therapy procedure performed to encourage continued physiological development and formation of the root end' (Fig. 9.1).

Apexification is defined as a 'method to induce calcified barrier in a root with an open apex or the continued apical development of an incomplete root in teeth with necrotic pulps' [5].

Traditionally the clinical protocol for 'apexification' involved the placement of calcium hydroxide as an intra-canal medicament to eliminate intra-radicular infection and induce an apical barrier requiring multiple visits and a protracted treatment, which could take several months [3, 6]. Recently, an alternative one-visit apexification protocol involving the use of mineral trioxide aggregate has gained popularity as a means of creating an artificial barrier at the open apex to which a hard tissue barrier can readily form with similar outcomes to using cal-

cium hydroxide. In the apical barrier technique, a biocompatible barrier material is placed at the apex to facilitate obturation. Mineral trioxide aggregate is the material of choice due to its optimal sealing ability, biocompatibility and ability to induce hard tissue and set in a moist environment. The advantage of using this technique is that the treatment time is reduced to one or two appointments with significant expedition of treatment with similar outcomes and prognosis [7–12]. The disadvantage of using either calcium hydroxide or mineral trioxide aggregate has been the inconsistency of achieving continued root maturation. Teeth treated with either techniques are at greater risk to root fracture as a consequence of thin dentinal walls resulting in the premature loss of the tooth [13–16].

Revascularization of avulsed and replanted immature teeth with open apices is well established and achievable provided optimal replantation techniques are used. Prompt replantation with minimal extra-oral dry periods and ideal root development stage (open apices of

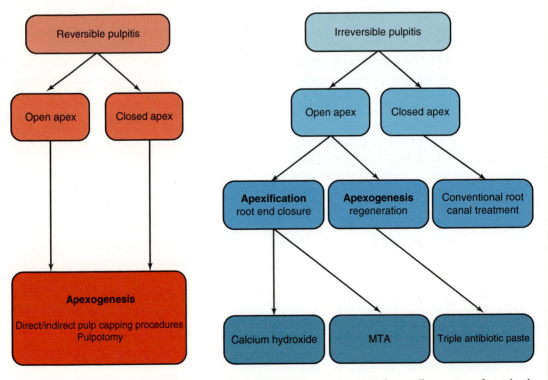

Fig. 9.1 Showing treatment options for the management of immature permanent teeth according to stage of root development (i.e., complete or incomplete)

greater than 1.1 mm) are the prerequisites for revascularization [17]. Regeneration (revitalization) of infected necrotic pulp tissue has been an important issue in endodontics for more than a decade. Regenerative endodontics has been defined as 'biologically-based procedures designed to physiologically replace damaged tooth structures, including dentine and root structures, as well as cells of the pulp-dentine complex' [5]. Based on a series of case reports, there appears to be evidence that new soft tissue can enter the root canal with the potential for subsequent hard tissue deposition resulting in continued root maturation [18]. Current approaches for treating the traumatized immature tooth with pulpal necrosis do not reliably achieve the desired clinical outcomes, consisting of healing of apical periodontitis, promotion of continued root development and restoration of the functional competence of pulpal tissue. An optimal approach for treating the immature permanent tooth with a necrotic pulp would be to regenerate functional pulpal tissue [19, 20].

Over the last decade, a number of case reports have been reported in the literature demonstrating this new revitalization approach in achieving tissue generation and regeneration. Continued root development has been demonstrated in cases that presented as infected and necrotic with occasional draining sinuses. As a result, it may be predicted that traditional apexification methods employed may become of historical interest only [21, 22]. These case reports advocate the use of a triple antibiotic paste to eliminate the intraradicular infection, a prerequisite for setting the conditions to allow for subsequent revascularization [23–29]. The triple antibiotic paste in these cases consists of a combination of ciprofloxacin, metronidazole and minocycline, which has been shown to reliably disinfect the root canal system. The disinfection of the root canal is carried out without any mechanical debridement. Irrigation using sodium hypochlorite is used and then the antibiotic paste placed for a period of time. At the second appointment, a blood clot is produced to the level of the cemento-enamel junction to provide a scaffold for the ingrowth of new tissue. The cervical portion of the tooth is sealed with MTA and a bonded resin composite restoration [30]. The formation of a blood clot is the key to success, and this crucial step, which is essential for the stimulation of revascularization, is unpredictable. Currently research strategies are underway in order to understand fully the true nature of this 'regenerated tissue' and provide future potential synthetic matrices, which will act as more predictable scaffolds [31].

Although regenerative endodontic treatment causes root development, there are several drawbacks and unfavourable outcomes that can occur [32]. Tooth discolouration has been cited and is related to the use of either minocycline in the triple antibiotic paste or MTA coronally [33, 34]. Ideal root development is not achieved in all cases, suboptimal barrier placement has been an issue, and there has been failure to induce bleeding in some reports [34, 35].

In summary, the question is no longer 'can regenerative endodontic procedures be successful?' Instead, the important question facing us is 'what are the issues that must be addressed to develop a safe, effective, and consistent method for regenerating a functional pulp-dentine complex in our patients?' [36]. Additional translational studies and clinical trials evaluating the different aspects of this procedure are required in order to understand the many interrelated aspects that could result in better and more predictable outcomes [37]. The idea of replacing severely compromised teeth or missing teeth in the future using stem cells as a precursor may well be on the horizon making dentures and dental implants obsolete [38].

9.2   Apexification with Calcium Hydroxide

The formation of a hard tissue barrier at the open apex of an immature permanent tooth has traditionally been performed using long-term calcium hydroxide dressings and has been an accepted endodontic procedure with a high degree of success. The calcium hydroxide is placed in the root canal to stimulate a hard tissue (cementoid or osteoid) barrier across the wide-open apex prior to placement of a permanent root filling. The barrier formation prevents over-extension of root filling material into the surrounding peri-apical tissues. Studies have demonstrated that repeated dressing changes initially at 1 month, and then 3-month intervals thereafter can result in barrier formation anywhere from 4 to 9 months. The calcium hydroxide acts as a mild inflammatory stimulant that initially causes necrosis of the tissue surface with calcification over time. Calcium hydroxide is antibacterial due to its inherent high pH (12.2), which creates an environment that is not conducive for the survival of bacteria. Calcium hydroxide pastes release hydroxyl (OH-) ions readily, which is essential for barrier formation. Several commercial calcium hydroxide pastes are available including those made with saline (EndoCal and Calasept) or methylcellulose (Pulpdent and TempCanal). The latter are less soluble with a creamier consistency ideal for placement within the canal with less extrusion and dissolution over time. The wider the opening at the apex, the greater the chance of dissolution making the saline-based products more susceptible to being washed out. The clinical steps when using calcium hydroxide include:

1. Treatment is carried out under local anaesthesia and rubber dam isolation utilizing a dental operating microscope.
2. Straight-line access is established. Direct visualization of the apical foramen should be attempted using the dental operating microscope.
3. The root canal is chemomechanically debrided with copious irrigation using sodium hypochlorite solution (this can be delivered ultrasonically or using sonic activation such as the EndoActivator).
4. Minimal shaping is required due to thin dentinal walls. Working length is determined using electronic apex locators, paper points and radiographs.
5. An interim dressing of Ledermix paste or 50:50 mix of Ledermix and Pulpdent paste is placed to control any infection and prevent any inflammatory resorption that may be present. A double seal temporary restoration of Cavit and glass ionomer cement is then placed.
6. At the second appointment, the canal is re-irrigated, dried and dressed with a suitable calcium hydroxide paste. The calcium hydroxide can be packed at the apex using either pluggers or thick paper points. The canal is then backfilled with calcium hydroxide to ensure that reinfection does not occur during the interim period. Radiographs are taken to check that the apical level of calcium hydroxide is satisfactory and to ensure that an overfill has not occurred. The canal should appear radiopaque indicating that the entire canal has been filled with calcium hydroxide. A well-sealing temporary restoration is then replaced to the level of the root orifice (Fig. 9.2).
7. The patient is reviewed at 3-month intervals, and a further radiograph can be taken to assess whether an apical barrier has formed and whether the calcium hydroxide dressing has been washed out. If no washout is evident, then the dressing need not be replaced. Where evidence of washout is clear, indicated by the absence of radiopaque material within the canal, then the dressings can be replaced. The progress of barrier formation can be assessed using paper points. A large paper point is selected to check for the presence of an apical barrier by gently pressing at the apex and checking whether any evidence of blood/exudate is present and whether the paper point can be introduced beyond the apex easily. If no barrier is confirmed, then a further dressing is introduced to the level of the apex where barrier formation is desired.
8. Once a barrier has been confirmed, a final root filling is placed using either a cold lateral chloroform dip technique or warm vertical compaction technique after a further 3-month period. On completion the access cavity is permanently restored accordingly (Fig. 9.3).

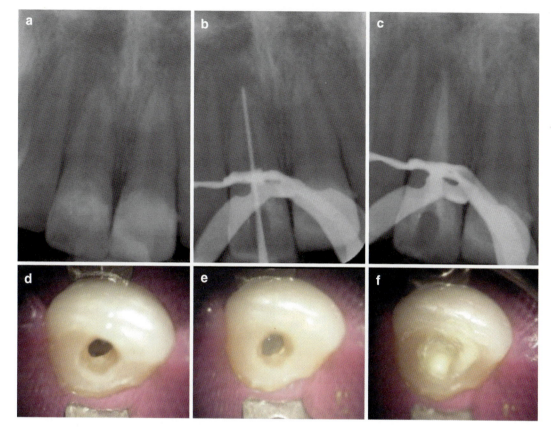

Fig. 9.2 Clinical radiographs and photographs showing (**a**) pre-operative radiograph, (**b**) MAF radiograph confirmed using #100K file, (**c**) calcium hydroxide dressing, (**d**) access preparation, (**e**) chemo-mechanical preparation using 1 % sodium hypochlorite solution, and (**f**) calcium hydroxide dressing placed using a lentilo spiral filler to ensure a homogenous dressing was placed

9.3 One-Step Apexification with MTA

Despite the demonstrated clinical success associated with calcium hydroxide apexification, there are a number of drawbacks. The unpredictability of an apical hard tissue barrier formation, lengthy procedures often requiring several visits and the associated increased risks of cervical root fracture have led clinicians to adopt a one-step apexification procedure. Studies have demonstrated that using mineral trioxide aggregate as an apical matrix, single-appointment obturation of the canal can be achieved with high success rates. MTA has been shown to induce apical hard tissue formation without an inflammatory response owing to its excellent biocompatibility. Furthermore, newly formed bone, cementum and periodontal ligament have been shown to attach to the MTA layer pro-

viding an excellent seal. The wet environment, as a consequence of wide-open apices, means that a suitable hydrophilic material such as MTA is ideal in terms of setting ability without the risk of being washed away. The only disadvantage when using MTA is related to its handling and manipulation, which, like any technique, requires careful practice, skills and knowledge developed before appropriate use. As a result, MTA should be considered the material of choice when considering one-step apexification procedures in cases of immature developing teeth with wide-open apices:

1. Appropriate anaesthesia, rubber dam application and adequate straight-line access are achieved utilizing a dental operating microscope to visualize the peri-apex and apical tissues beyond.
2. The root canal system is chemomechanically debrided using appropriate disinfectants

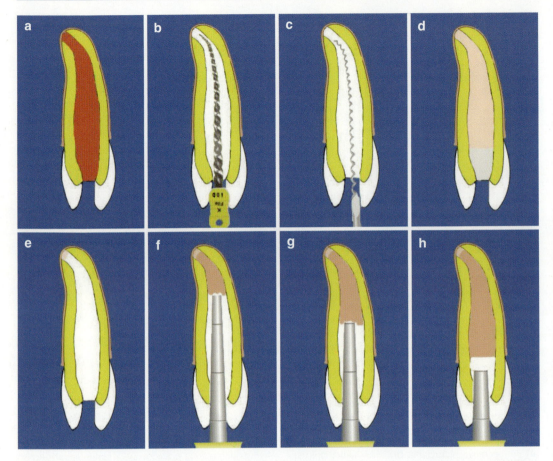

Fig. 9.3 Diagrams showing clinical steps for achieving apexification using calcium hydroxide. Note (**a**) preoperative view of immature permanent tooth with large apical foramen, (**b**) MAF greater than #100 K-file, (**c**) placement of calcium hydroxide using Lentulo spiral filler, (**d**) interim calcium hydroxide changed every 3 months until (**e**) apical hard tissue barrier formation complete, and (**f–h**) obturation completed with gutta-percha root filling material. Note apical closure complete but root development remains incomplete

(sodium hypochlorite) with minimal shaping. Ultrasonic or sonic activation is desirable to ensure a bacteria-free environment is created.

3. The canal is dried with paper points ensuring that any remnants of calcium hydroxide have been thoroughly removed.

4. The MTA powder is mixed with sterile saline to create a thick creamy paste according to manufacturer's recommendations (Fig. 9.4).

5. The MTA is then deposited 1 mm short of the working length using an appropriate carrier and further condensed with minimal pressure using appropriate-sized paper points. The paper points will reduce the chances of apical extrusion of material as well as controlling the moisture present in the MTA mix, readily absorbing or imparting moisture as necessary. A resorbable matrix can be introduced to the apex prior to placement of MTA to further prevent extrusion of material. Preselected Schilder pluggers as well as paper points can be used to introduce the apical barrier (Fig. 9.4 and 9.5).

6. The MTA plug placement is verified with a radiograph ensuring a thickness of at least 4–5 mm is achieved. Further adaptation, to avoid voids, is achieved using ultrasonics. This can be carried out, by touching the plugger used to place the MTA, with an ultrasonic tip, creating enough vibration to further compact the material. If the radiograph demonstrates that the apical plug is not satisfactory, then the MTA can be removed using saline

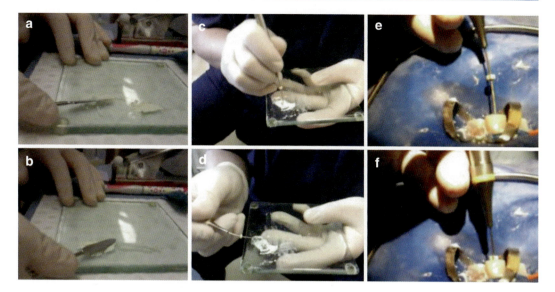

Fig. 9.4 Clinical photographs showing (**a, b**) mixing of MTA with sterile water (**c, d**) the use of MAP system to carry MTA and (**e, f**) placement of MTA inside root canal using suitable carrier

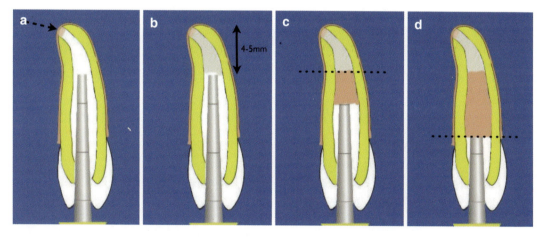

Fig. 9.5 Clinical diagrams showing (**a**) placement of apical barrier (*dotted arrow*), (**b**) MTA plug 4–5 mm, (**c**) introduction of heated gutta-percha using Obtura, and (**d**) backfill to level of cementoenamel junction. Note the coronal access cavity is restored with a resin composite restoration to reinforce the root

irrigation allowing the filling procedure to be repeated (Fig. 9.5).

7. A wet cotton wool pledget can be placed against the MTA and left for at least 24 h to allow complete setting of the cement. At the second appointment, following removal of the cotton wool pledget, the entire canal can be filled with gutta-percha filling material. A softened thermoplasticized technique using Obtura is preferred to cold/warm lat-

eral compaction and the use of finger spreaders. The latter can create wedging forces within the root canal increasing risk of root fractures (Fig. 9.5).

8. The cervical canal space is then reinforced with composite resin to below the to cemento-enamel junction in order to further strengthen the tooth and increase the resistance to fracture.

9. Routine recall (1 month, 6 months and 12 months) should be carried out to determine

the success of treatment and ensure that apical periodontitis does not persist.

9.4 Apexogenesis Procedures

Vital pulp therapies aimed to treat reversible pulpal injuries include indirect pulp-capping procedures following deep caries removal or direct pulp-capping and pulpotomy procedures following pulpal exposure. Apexogenesis is a therapeutic procedure aimed at amputating the coronal necrotic and possibly infected pulp. This creates an environment that is conducive to continued radicular pulp preservation. The premise is to avoid the inherent clinical problems that are associated with nonvital immature developing teeth with wide-open apices, reversed tapered canals (blunderbuss) and thin dentinal walls.

A traditional pulpotomy involves the removal of the coronal pulp to the floor of the chamber. This procedure usually results in pulp canal obliteration and is usually followed by a complete pulpectomy and endodontic treatment. In comparison, a Cvek pulpotomy or partial pulpotomy involves removal of 2 mm of the pulp adjacent to the exposure. Its goal is to maintain pulp vitality indefinitely and allow root development to continue. The procedure consists of the following steps:

1. Pulp tissue is removed 2 mm apical to the exposure with a high-speed diamond bur with copious water coolant.
2. Haemorrhage is controlled with saline or diluted sodium hypochlorite solution (2.5 %) soaked on a cotton wool pledget.
3. The pulp is covered with either a layer of MTA or calcium hydroxide (Fig. 9.6).

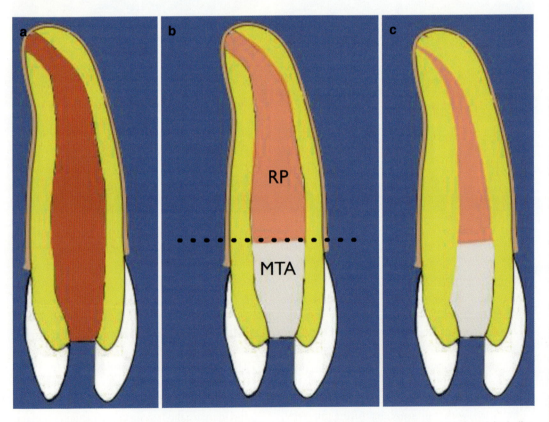

Fig. 9.6 Diagrams showing (**a**) immature developing tooth with large open apex and (**b**) Cvek pulpotomy with removal of coronal 2–3 mm pulp leaving intact the radicular pulp (*RP*) and placement of coronal seal including MTA at the level of CEJ to allow for (**c**) continued root development and apical closure

4. The coronal aspect of the tooth is sealed with a double seal consisting of IRM and glass ionomer cement to ensure that no coronal leakage is possible.

5. The patient is re-evaluated 1 month postoperatively and then every 3 months for the first year and yearly thereafter until root development is completed. The pulpal status is reviewed including sensitivity tests to assess vitality.

9.5   Revitalization, Revascularization and Regeneration

Revascularization of a necrotic pulp was once thought of as only possible after an avulsion injury of an immature permanent tooth. The advantage of this outcome is the possibility of continued root development resulting in thin dentinal walls being further strengthened to reduce the risk of root fracture long term. Outcome is dependent on a minimal extra-oral alveolar time, large open apices (usually >1.1 mm) and short roots that allow new tissue to grow into the tooth. The pulp is presumed to be necrotic but not infected such that it can act as a scaffold for the newly developing tissue.

Recently, a number of case reports have been reported in the literature whereby revascularization of infected necrotic immature teeth, once thought impossible, has been carried out successfully. The procedure relies on effective disinfection within the canal followed by the creation of a scaffold into which new tissue can grow. Chemomechanical disinfection with sodium hypochlorite alone is not sufficient to reliably create an environment conducive for revascularization of the infected necrotic pulp. This has led to the additional use of a triple antibiotic paste, developed by Hoshino and colleagues, consisting of ciprofloxacin, metronidazole and minocycline. The necrotic immature tooth is disinfected without mechanical instrumentation using sodium hypochlorite solution. The canal is then dressed with the triple antibiotic paste (prepared by a compounding pharmacist) for up to 1 month.

At the second appointment, following resolution of clinical signs and symptoms, a suitable scaffold using a blood clot is created. This step requires over instrumentation beyond the apex to create bleeding within the canal. A blood clot is produced at the level of the cemento-enamel junction. MTA is placed coronal to the blood clot to ensure that a good seal is achieved and the tooth restored with a bonded composite restoration. The tooth is then monitored over time to verify continuing thickening of dentinal walls, further root development and absence of apical periodontitis (see Fig. 9.7).

Presently this type of procedure is still in its infancy and can be described as experimental in nature. Questions have been raised as to issues with the use of local antibiotics including sensitivity and staining, inherent problems with reliable scaffold creation and the predictability of the procedure. The true nature of the tissue that is recreated is also questionable and whether this is in fact regenerated pulp tissue or simply the ingrowth of periodontal tissues allowing revascularization. Future treatment directions may one day lead to the ability to routinely place synthetic scaffolds that predictably allow the regrowth of pulp tissues eliminating the need for placement of endodontic obturating materials. Our understanding of the biology associated with routine clinical treatments continues to evolve through future research and highlights the merits of clinical decision making underpinned with robust evidence-based practice.

9.6   Clinical Cases

Case 1: Apexification Procedure of Tooth 21 Using Interim Calcium Hydroxide Dressing, MTA and Gutta-Percha Without an Apical Barrier A fit and healthy 10-year-old girl was referred for endodontic management of tooth 21. The patient recalled sustaining traumatic blow to this tooth about a year ago at a water slide park. The patient reported the tooth flared up recently with localized pain and swelling in the region of tooth 21. Her general dental practitioner placed an emergency pulp dressing and

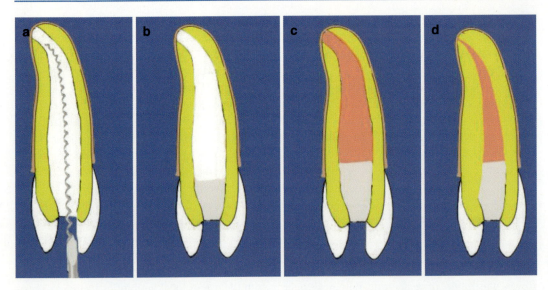

Fig. 9.7 Diagrammatic representation showing the key steps during revascularization procedure. Note (**a**, **b**) placement of triple antibiotic paste within canal space following minimal instrumentation and irrigation using sodium hypochlorite solution. After an interim period of 1 month, the tooth is reentered and (**c**) a scaffold is created by overinstrumentation beyond the apex creating bleeding within the canal. A blood clot to the level of the cementoenamel junction followed by a coronal seal using MTA. Continued monitoring should show (**d**) continuation of root development and apical closure over time

arranged for further management with a specialist. At time of consultation, the patient was asymptomatic. Clinical examination revealed tooth 21 was non-tender to percussion and palpation. An intact palatal dressing was confirmed. Tooth 11 responded positively to both electric pulp testing and thermal stimulus (CO2 snow). Radiographic examination revealed an immature open apex associated with tooth 21. A periradicular radiolucency was noted with the periapex of tooth 21 (Fig. 9.8).

Treatment options were discussed with the patient including extraction and replacement. The parents were informed that a dental implant option could not be considered until growth had stopped (estimated age 25). After a lengthy discussion, the parents were in agreement to try and retain the tooth for as long as possible. They understood that long term there was a higher chance of root fracture due to arrested root development and the large open apex.

At the first treatment appointment, the access cavity was refined to ensure straight-line access was achieved and all pulp horns were incorporated. An open apex was confirmed with apical file size #120. Working length was confirmed using both the electronic apex locator and radiographic examination. Minimal canal preparation was carried out and irrigation to working length was supplemented with ultrasonics. An intra-canal dressing of calcium hydroxide was placed for an interim period of 1 month. Post-operative films confirmed a well-obturated canal space and overfill at the peri-apex of tooth 21. The patient was warned of the possibility of post-operative discomfort and to contact if any problems occurred. A further review appointment was scheduled 4 weeks later.

At the 1-month review appointment, the patient remained asymptomatic. A decision was made to leave the dressing in for a further 2 months. At the 3-month review appointment following initial canal dressing placement, a radiograph confirmed some intra-canal medicament resorption. The peri-radicular overfill had diminished in size but was still evident. A decision was made to complete the endodontic treatment using MTA and gutta-percha backfill.

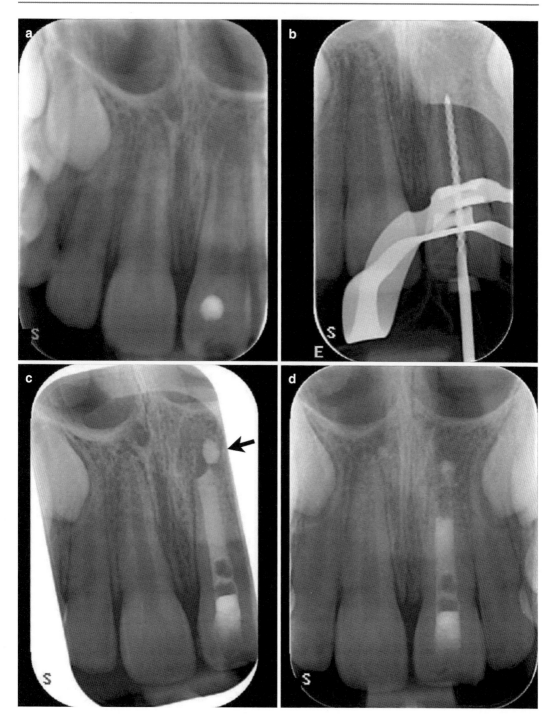

Fig. 9.8 Clinical radiographs demonstrating nonsurgical root canal treatment of tooth 21. An immature wide open apex was noted at time of examination. The patient had previously sustained trauma to the tooth which had flared up with localized pain and discomfort. Her general dental practitioner had placed an endodontic dressing and referral was sought for further management. Note (**a**) preoperative view of tooth 21 demonstrating prior endodontic access (incomplete). An extensive periradicular radiolucency was evident. Note normal root end closure of tooth 11 compared to the wide open apex of tooth 21. (**b**) Estimated electronic working length film. (**c**) Following minimal canal preparation and irrigation, an intra-canal dressing of calcium hydroxide was placed. Note overfill of medication (*black arrow*). (**d**) Three-month follow-up showing resorption of intra-canal medicament and overfill

MTA was introduced into the canal using the MAP system and carefully packed to working length estimate using paper points (size #100). The apical 5 mm of the canal was obturated with MTA (see Fig. 9.9) and allowed to set prior to gutta-percha backfill placement. An IRM and glass ionomer cement restoration was placed to ensure coronal seal prior to visiting her general dentist for placement of a permanent tooth-coloured restoration (see Fig. 9.9). The patient was placed on yearly reviews to ensure that continued healing occurred.

Case 2: One-Step Apexification Procedure of Tooth 11 Using MTA and Gutta-Percha with an Apical Barrier A fit and healthy 11-year-old boy (the son of our practice receptionist) was seen for endodontic management of tooth 11 (Fig. 9.10). Three years ago, he had sustained a complicated crown fracture of the tooth following a skateboarding accident. The patient had previously been undergoing apexification using calcium hydroxide therapy for the past 18 months. Clinical examination revealed the tooth was within normal limits with no pain or tenderness of note. Radiographic examination revealed a large open apex associated with tooth 11.

The tooth was accessed under rubber dam and checked for any calcific hard tissue barrier at the apex (none was confirmed). The working length was established using an electronic apex locator and confirmed radiographically (see Fig. 9.10). Irrigation was carried out using 1 % sodium hypochlorite solution. Minimal canal preparation was carried out with stainless-steel instruments. The master apical size was #110.

The canal was dried and a decision made to complete treatment using a single-visit MTA apexification procedure. A Bio-Oss barrier was placed at the terminal end point of preparation. MTA was placed in the apical 5 mm using the MAP system. Gutta-percha was placed in the remaining middle/coronal 1/3 of the canal using AH Plus cement. A double seal temporary restoration was placed using IRM and glass ionomer cement. The patient subsequently attended for fixed orthodontic appliance therapy for a

2-year period. Following debonding of all the maxillary dentition, the patient saw a prosthodontist for intermediate restoration of the tooth. A long-term provisional Luxatemp resin crown restoration and titanium temporary post was placed. The patient has been advised that this should 'buy him some time' until the age of 18–25 years when dentoalveolar growth slows down and a permanent cast post and core restoration with a ceramo-metal or all-ceramic crown can be considered. The patient has also been advised of the long-term possibility of root fracture and need for replacement with a dental implant if indicated in the future (see Fig. 9.10).

Case 3: Single-Visit Apexification Procedure of Tooth 21 Using MTA and Gutta-Percha Without an Apical Barrier A 23-year-old patient who suffered from coeliac disease was referred for endodontic management of tooth 21. Endodontic treatment was started by the general dental practitioner, and referral sought for further management due to difficulty establishing the working length. At time of consultation, the patient was asymptomatic. Past medical history revealed the patient had been treated for cleft lip and palate repair with a bone graft in the anterior maxilla. Clinical examination revealed tooth 21 was non-tender to percussion and palpation. An intact palatal access dressing was seen. Radiographic examination confirmed prior endodontic access. Incomplete root development was noted with a wide-open apex (Fig. 9.11).

Access cavity design was refined prior to establishing working length. Working length was determined using a #100 K-file and electronic apex locator. Further determination of the apical limit of preparation/obturation was determined using premeasured paper points (#90). An irrigation regime of 1 % NaOCl was used and minimal preparation was carried out. No exudate was noted in the canal.

An MTA carrier was pre-fitted short of working length and verified radiographically (Fig. 9.11). MTA was mixed to the desired consistency and placed at working length

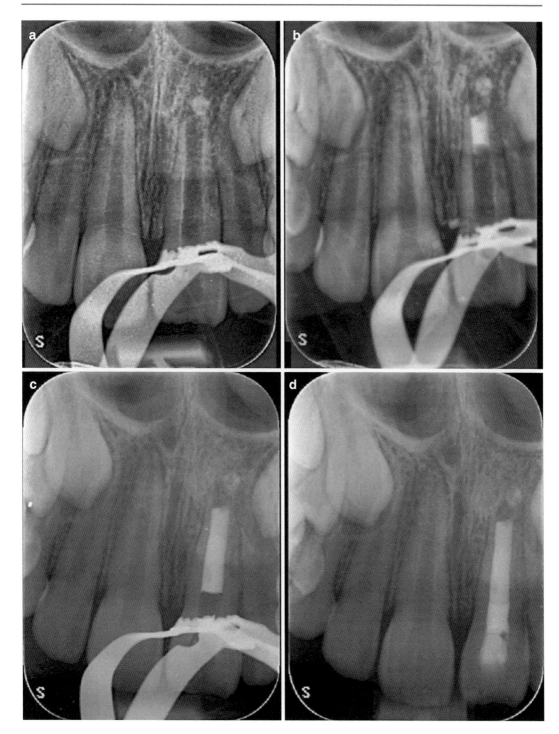

Fig. 9.9 Clinical radiographs demonstrating nonsurgical root canal treatment of tooth 21. Note (**a**) radiographic examination confirming removal of intra-canal medicament. (**b**) Apical 5 mm obturated with MTA. (**c**) Remaining coronal canal space obturated with AH Plus cement and gutta-percha root filling. (**d**) Temporary IRM and glass ionomer cement restoration

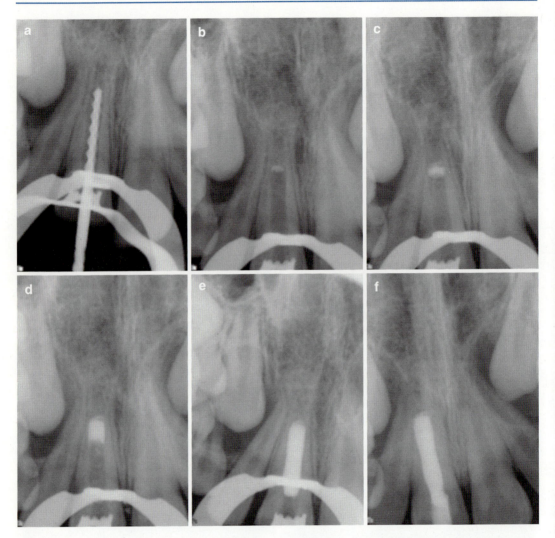

Fig. 9.10 Clinical case showing single-visit apexification using MTA in a 9-year-old boy. Tooth 11 sustained trauma resulting in necrosis of the root canal. The patient had been seen previously for a period of 18 months during which time calcium hydroxide apexification had been attempted. Due to the protracted treatment and increasing number of appointments, the patient's mother had sought a referral to the practice. Radiographic series showing (**a**) master apical file. Note blunderbuss roots with large apical foramen >1.1 mm, (**b**) barrier placement to prevent extrusion of MTA, (**c, d**) MTA apical 5 mm, (**e**) gutta-percha backfill, and (**f**) final radiograph with coronal seal

using the pre-fitted MTA carrier. Premeasured paper points were then used to further compact the MTA apically prior to further MTA placement.

Radiographs were taken periodically to assess the apical MTA fill to ensure adequate compaction and no overfilling was occurring (Fig. 9.12). Once an adequate apical fill was confirmed, the MTA was allowed to set prior to obturation of the remaining canal system.

Obturation of the remaining canal was completed using AH Plus cement and gutta-percha using system B and Obtura. After the initial backfill and compaction, a radiograph was taken to confirm whether a homogenous root filling was present. Radiograph confirmed a void at the MTA/gutta-percha interface (Fig. 9.13). Further downpacking was carried out with an 8 % system B tapered plugger 2 mm short of the MTA interface. Following heating of the existing

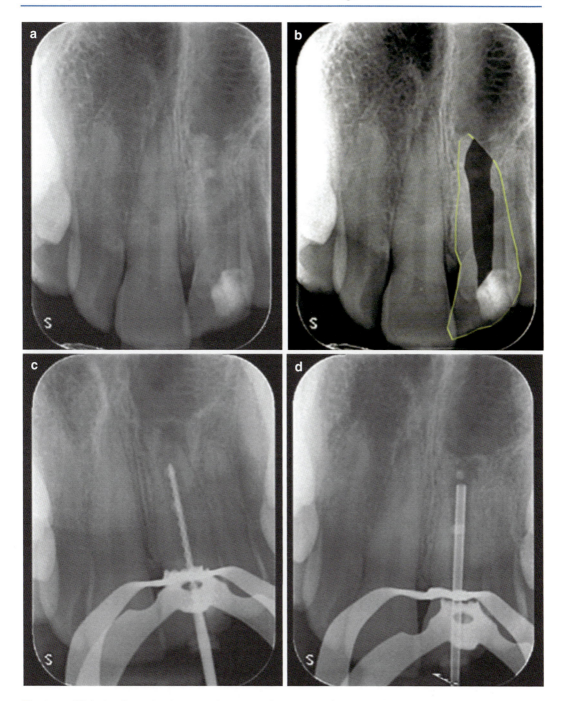

Fig. 9.11 Clinical radiographs demonstrating nonsurgical root canal treatment of tooth 21 using single-visit apexification using MTA and gutta-percha without an apical barrier. Note (**a**, **b**) preoperative view confirming prior endodontic access with an incompletely developed root. (**c**) Initial apical file placement size #70 K-file to show the size of apical foramen in comparison. (**d**) Pre-fitting of MTA plugger prior to MTA obturation of apical 3–5 mm

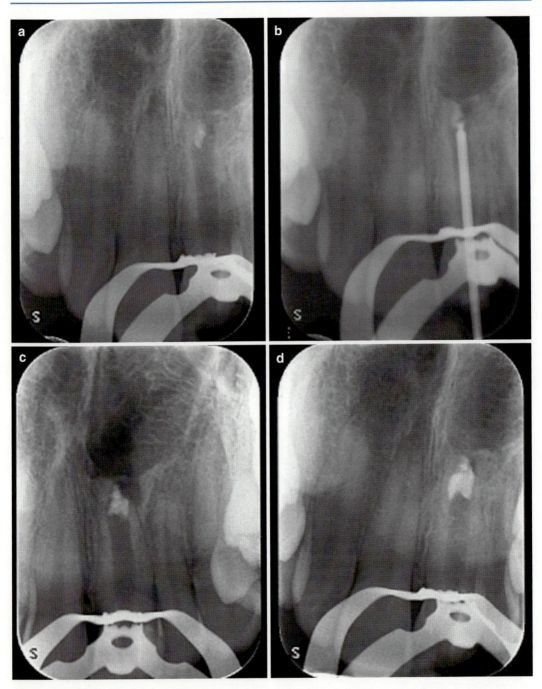

Fig. 9.12 Clinical radiographs demonstrating nonsurgical root canal treatment of tooth 21 using single-visit apexification using MTA and gutta-percha without an apical barrier. Note (**a–d**) MTA obturation of apical 3–5 mm. After placement of the MTA, it is further condensed using pre-fitted paper points. Radiographs are taken to ensure that adequate obturation is achieved with minimal overfilling

gutta-percha, further compaction was carried out using a pre-fitted plugger. Further radiographic examination confirmed the void had been addressed (Fig. 9.13).

Further backfilling of the remaining portion of the coronal root canal system was completed to the cervical aspect of the tooth. A temporary double seal was achieved using IRM and glass

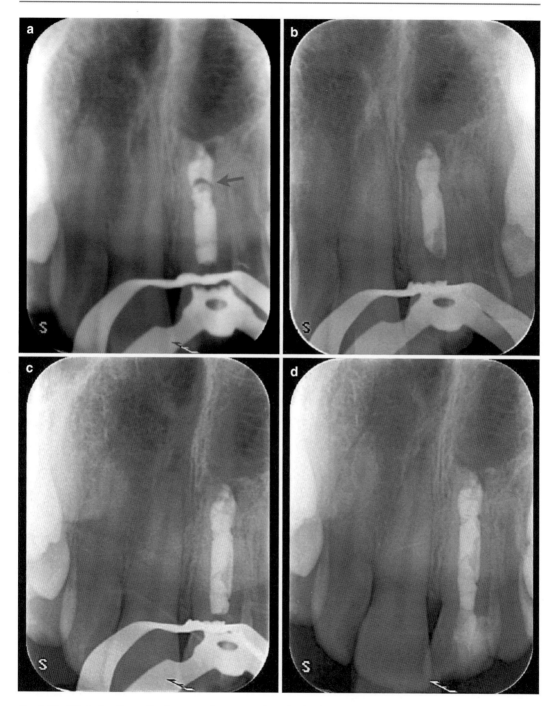

Fig. 9.13 Clinical radiographs demonstrating nonsurgical root canal treatment of tooth 21 using single-visit apexification using MTA and gutta-percha without an apical barrier. Note (**a–c**) backfill of remaining canal with gutta-percha using Obtura and System B following setting of the MTA. A void (*green arrow*) was noted requiring further downpacking and condensation to ensure adequate compaction. Care must be taken to ensure that the apical plug of MTA does not get further condensed resulting in overfilling. (**d**) Final postoperative radiograph with temporary double coronal seal

ionomer cement. The patient was referred back to her general dental practitioner for permanent coronal restoration.

Clinical Hints and Tips for Apexification Procedures Using MTA

- Prior to MTA plug placement, the tooth should be minimally prepared with hand files and chemomechanically debrided using sodium hypochlorite solution. An interim antibacterial dressing is recommended.
- A resorbable barrier can be used at the apex to prevent extrusion of MTA.
- The MTA is mixed to thick creamy consistency and an appropriate carrier is selected. Premeasurements using the carrier or paper points are carried out to ensure that it can be taken to full working length with ease.
- MTA should be placed 1 mm short of the intended working length and can then be gently compacted to length using paper points.
- If the MTA plug is not in the correct position, then saline can be used to wash out the filling material prior to re-plugging.
- The MTA plug should be 4–5 mm and a wet cotton wool pledget left in situ for at least 6 h prior to backfilling with gutta-percha.
- A resin composite restoration should be placed in the coronal aspect of the tooth to reinforce the root further.
- Routine follow-up radiographs and recall appointments are recommended to ensure that healing is taking place.

References

1. Logan WHG, Kronfeld R. Development of the human jaws and surrounding structures from birth to the age of fifteen years. J Am Dent Assoc. 1933;20(3):379–427.
2. Trope M. Treatment of immature teeth with non-vital pulps and apical periodontitis. Endod Top. 2006;14:51–9.
3. Rafter M. Apexification: a review. Dent Traumatol. 2005;21(1):1–8.
4. Tenca JI, Tsamtsouris A. Continued root development: apexogenesis and apexification. J Pedodon. 1978;2:144–57.
5. American Association of Endodontics. Glossary of endodontic terms. 8th ed. Chicago: American Association of Endodontist; 2012.
6. Cvek M. Treatment of non-vital permanent incisors with calcium hydroxide. I. Follow-up of periapical repair and apical closure of immature roots. Odontol Revy. 1972;23(1):27.
7. Shabahang S, Torabinejad M. Treatment of teeth with open apices using mineral trioxide aggregate. Pract Periodont Aesthet Dent. 2000;12:315–20.
8. Witherspoon DE, Ham K. One visit apexification: technique for inducing root end-barrier formation in apical closures. Pract Proced Aesthet Dent. 2001;13:455–60.
9. Steinig TH, Regan JD, Gutmann JL. The use and predictable placement of Mineral Trioxide Aggregate in one-visit apexification cases. Aust Endo J. 2003;29:34–42.
10. Aminoshariae A, Hartwell GR, Moon PC. Placement of Mineral Trioxide Aggregate using two different methods. J Endod. 2003;29:679–82.
11. Felippe WT, Felippe MC, Rocha MJ. The effect of mineral trioxide aggregate on the apexification and periapical healing of teeth with incomplete root formation. Int Endod J. 2006;39:2–9.
12. Simon S, Rilliard F, Berdal A, Machtou P. The use of mineral trioxide aggregate in one-visit apexification treatment: a prospective study. Int Endod J. 2007;40(3):186–97.
13. Cvek M. Prognosis of luxated non-vital maxillary incisors treated with calcium hydroxide and filled with gutta-percha. A retrospective clinical study. Dent Traumatol. 1992;8:45–55.
14. Sheehy EC, Roberts GJ. Use of calcium hydroxide for apical barrier formation and healing in non-vital immature permanent teeth: a review. Br Dent J. 1997;183:241–6.
15. Katebzadeh N, Dalton RC, Trope M. Strengthening immature teeth during and after apexification. J Endod. 1998;24:256–9.
16. Andreasen JO, Farik B, Munksgaard EC. Long-term calcium hydroxide as root canal dressing may increase risk of root fracture. Dent Traumatol. 2002;18:134–7.
17. Garcia-Godoy F, Murray PE. Recommendations for using regenerative endodontic procedures in permanent immature traumatized teeth. Dent Traumatol. 2012;28(1):33–41.
18. Andreasen JO, Bakland LK. Pulp regeneration after non-infected and infected necrosis, what type of tissue do we want? A review. Dent Traumatol. 2012;28(1):13–8.

19. Wigler R, Kaufman AY, Lin S, Steinbock N, Hazan-Molina H, Torneck CD. Revascularization: a treatment for permanent teeth with necrotic pulp and incomplete root development. J Endod. 2013;39(3): 319–26.
20. Hargreaves KM, Diogenes A, Teixeira FB. Treatment options: biological basis of regenerative endodontic procedures. J Endod. 2013;39(3):S30–43.
21. Chueh LH, Huang GTJ. Immature teeth with periradicular periodontitis or abscess undergoing apexogenesis: a paradigm shift. J Endod. 2006;32(12): 1205–13.
22. Huang GTJ. Apexification: the beginning of its end. Int Endod J. 2009;42:855–66.
23. Sato I, Ando-Kurihara N, Kota K, Iwaku M, Hoshino E. Sterilization of infected root-canal dentine by topical application of a mixture of ciprofloxacin, metronidazole and minocycline *in situ*. Int Endod J. 1996;29:118–24.
24. Hoshino E, Kurihara-Ando N, Sato I, et al. In-vitro antibacterial susceptibility of bacteria taken from infected root dentine to a mixture of ciprofloxacin, metronidazole and minocycline. Int Endod J. 1996;29:125–30.
25. Yanpiset K, Trope M. Pulp revascularization of replanted immature dog teeth after different treatment methods. Dent Traumatol. 2000;16:211–7.
26. Iwaya S, Ikawa M, Kubota M. Revascularization of an immature permanent tooth with apical periodontitis and sinus tract. Dent Traumatol. 2001;17:185–7.
27. Ritter AL, Ritter AV, Murrah V, Sigurdsson A, Trope M. Pulp revascularization in replanted immature dog teeth after treatment with minocycline and doxycycline assessed by laser Doppler flowmetry, radiography, and histology. Dent Traumatol. 2004;20:75–84.
28. Banchs F, Trope M. Revascularization of immature permanent teeth with apical periodontitis: new treatment protocol? J Endod. 2004;30:196–200.
29. Winley W, Teixeira F, Levin L, Sigurdsson A, Trope M. Disinfection of immature teeth with a triple antibiotic paste. J Endod. 2005;31:439–43.
30. Paryani K, Kim SG. Regenerative endodontic treatment of permanent teeth after completion of root development: a report of 2 cases. J Endod. 2013; 39(7):929–34.
31. Torabinejad M, Faras H, Corr R, Wright KR, Shabahang S. Histologic examinations of teeth treated with 2 scaffolds: a pilot animal investigation. J Endod. 2014.
32. Nosrat A, Homayoufar N, Oloomi K. Drawbacks and unfavourable outcomes of regenerative endodontic treatments of necrotic immature teeth: a literature review and report of a case. J Endod. 2012; 38(10):1428–34.
33. Kim J, Kim Y, Shin S, Park J, Jung I. Tooth discolouration of immature permanent incisor associated with triple antibiotic therapy: a case report. J Endod. 2010;36:1086–91.
34. Petrino J, Boda K, Shambarger S, Bowles W, McClanahan S. Challenges in regenerative endodontics: a case series. J Endod. 2010;36:536–61.
35. Chen MH, Chen KL, Chen CA, Tayebaty F, Rosenberg PA, Lin LM. Responses of immature permanent teeth with infected necrotic pulp tissue and apical periodontitis/abscess to revascularization procedures. Int Endo J. 2012;45(3):294–305.
36. Hargreaves KM, Geisler T, Henry M, Wang Y. Regeneration potential of the young permanent tooth: what does the future hold? J Endod. 2008; 34(7):S51–6.
37. Diogenes A, Henry MA, Teixeira FB, Hargreaves KM. An update on clinical regenerative endodontics. Endod Top. 2013;28(1):2–23.
38. Nair PNR. What is on the horizon? J Conserv Dent. 2014;17:1.

Non-surgical Root Canal Retreatment

10

Bobby Patel

Summary

Non-surgical endodontic retreatment is one option for the management of persistent apical periodontitis associated with a root-filled tooth or where new disease has emerged after root filling. Consideration should always be given as to whether or not the tooth in question is of strategic importance. A cost-benefit analysis must take into account alternative treatment options including surgical apicectomy or extraction. Retreatment typically consists of regaining access to the canal, followed by complete removal of foreign material from within the canal system. Adequate re-instrumentation and disinfection protocols used for primary cases are recommended.

Clinical Relevance

Gaining access to pulp chambers previously root treated may require dismantling of crowns, bridges and post and core restorations. Previous root-filling materials including gutta-percha, carrier-based obturation material, silver points and paste-/cement-type fillings may be encountered requiring appropriate techniques for removal. Goals to achieve success in retreatment cases will be similar to untreated primary cases although previous errors such as canal obstructions, transportations, perforations or apical blockages may prevent adequate disinfection. The clinician must be aware of the technical difficulties encountered and strategies employed to overcome such errors aimed at ensuring success over the long term.

10.1 Overview of Non-surgical Root Canal Retreatment

Indications for root canal re-treatment include either teeth with inadequate root canal fillings with radiological findings of developing or persisting apical periodontitis and/or symptoms or teeth with inadequate root canal fillings when the coronal restoration requires replacement or the coronal dental tissue is to be bleached [1]. Root canal treatment usually fails when treatment falls short of acceptable standards leading to persistent microbial infection in the root canal system [2]. The primary cause of endodontic treatment

B. Patel, BDS MFDS MClinDent MRD MRACDS
Specialist Endodontist, Brindabella Specialist Centre,
Canberra, ACT, Australia
e-mail: bobbypatel@me.com

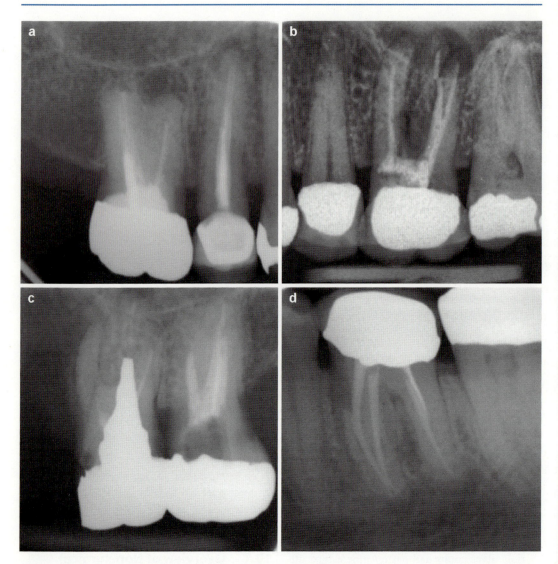

Fig. 10.1 Clinical radiographs demonstrating inadequate root canal fillings with or without poor coronal restorations. Note (**a**) well-fitting post and core restoration with untreated MB2 and poorly treated MB1, DB, and P canals. (**b**) Well-fitting cast restoration with poorly treated root canals. Suspect furcal perforation to be also present. (**c**) Poor-fitting cast post restoration with poorly condensed and inadequately treated canals. (**d**) Well-fitting cast restoration with periradicular pathology associated with both mesial and distal roots. Ineffective treatment protocols likely to have resulted in failure

failure can be attributed to inadequacies in three-dimensional cleaning, shaping and obturation resulting in persistent intra-radicular biofilm infections [3]. Missed canals, iatrogenic events (canal transportation, zipping and perforation), radicular fractures or reinfection of the root canal system where the coronal seal is lost after completion of root canal treatment can all lead to failure [4] (see Fig. 10.1). Less common reasons for failure include extra-radicular infections, foreign body reactions and nonmicrobial causes such as radicular cysts [5–9].

Healing after endodontic therapy is monitored by strict criteria based on clinical examination and interpretation of periodic radiographs (see Table 10.1). Clinical follow-up studies show that a large proportion of treated cases with chronic apical periodontitis show signs of healing within 1 year of treatment and in some instances as early as 2–6 months [10, 11] (Fig. 10.2). Some studies

Table 10.1 Endodontic treatment outcomes based on strict criteria assessed by clinical and radiographic signs and symptoms to determine whether the treated case has healed or failed

Healed	Both clinical and radiographic presentations are normal (Fig. 10.2). No further follow-up is required
Healing	A reduced radiolucency combined with normal clinical presentation can be interpreted as healing in progress (Fig. 10.2). Further follow-up is required
Failing (uncertain)	Radiolucency has persisted without change. Clinical presentation is normal. Further follow-up reviews are necessary to ascertain whether the case has failed
Failed	Radiolucency has emerged, persisted without change or increased in size. Clinically signs and symptoms may be present (Fig. 10.1)

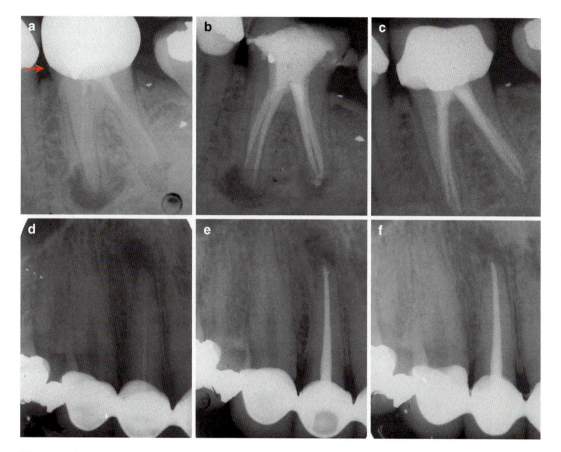

Fig. 10.2 Clinical radiographs demonstrating healing dynamics in re-treatment cases. Both cases have been grossly underfilled with the likelihood of ineffective disinfection of residual infection. Note (**a**) preoperative radiograph demonstrating extensive periradicular radiolucency associated with mesial and distal apices of tooth 46. Crown margin was defective mesially warranting removal and restorability assessment prior to proceeding (*red arrow*). (**b**) Re-treatment completed with chemomechanical debridement of all canals using intra-canal calcium hydroxide medicament in between visits. (**c**) 6-month recall radiograph demonstrating healed case. (**d**) Preoperative radiograph demonstrating single-cone obturation in tooth 14. Note extensive periradicular pathology. (**e**) Root canal re-treatment procedure completed through existing cast restoration (periapical changes already demonstrated). (**f**) 6-month recall radiograph demonstrating further healing at periapex. Both cases were treated with 2 % stainless steel instruments and cold lateral compaction techniques

have demonstrated that follow-up periods of 4 years or longer may be required when determining success of treatment in some cases. Late periapical changes have been observed radiographically more than 10 years after treatment, whereby healing appeared to have been disturbed and delayed by extension of root canal filling material into the periapical tissues. Small radiolucencies around surplus material should not be misinterpreted as failure [12, 13]. Root-filled teeth should be followed up at least a year after completion to determine whether a favourable outcome has been achieved. Absence of pain, swelling and other symptoms including sinus tract, no loss of function and radiological evidence of a normal periodontal ligament space around the root all indicate success [1].

If radiographic examination reveals the lesion has remained the same size or has diminished but not resolved, then the outcome is considered (uncertain). In this situation the lesion should be assessed until it has either resolved or for a minimum period of 4 years. If a lesion persists after 4 years, then it may be considered to be associated with post-treatment disease and probable failure [1].

During the follow-up period, if the tooth that has been treated exhibits clinical signs and symptoms of infection or a radiologically visible lesion that has either appeared subsequent to treatment or increased in size or if the lesion has remained the same size or diminished but not resolved during the 4-year assessment period, then the treatment can be considered a failure requiring either retreatment or extraction [1].

Scar tissue poses a significant diagnostic dilemma with difficulties to differentiate such a lesion from a radiolucency of pathological origin (apical periodontitis). Clinicians should be aware that although the incidence of this phenomenon is very low, this clinical entity must be taken into account when assessing failure of a treated case. These uncertain cases of healing are demonstrated radiologically by lesions that may have reduced in size but not completely resolved. Provided there are no clinical signs and symptoms, then these types of cases can be monitored for further periods to ensure that no increased lesion size has occurred (which would indicate failure) [1, 14–16].

If root canal treatment has failed, there are usually four possible treatment options, namely, review, retreatment, apical surgery and extraction. Root canal retreatment is often the pre-ferred means of treating a failed root canal treatment, especially when the failure is due to a technical deficiency. The existing root canal filling is removed and the infected root canal system disinfected using irrigants and medicaments. Root canal retreatment is often much more complicated compared to initial treatment, since restorations need to be dismantled and root canal filling materials (including both conventional gutta-percha fillings and unconventional paste fills) have to be removed in order to gain access to the canal system. Iatrogenic errors such as fractured instruments, perforations and canal transportations can further complicate matters. It is imperative to assess that the tooth is restorable prior to embarking on prolonged and often expensive treatment. Longitudinal tooth cracks and fractures that principally occur in the vertical plane or long axis of the crown and/or root can lead to particular uncertainty in terms of diagnostic and treatment decisions. Such cracks and fractures can lead to ongoing symptoms that can often be mistaken for lesions of endodontic origin. Once confirmation of an unfavourable crack or fracture has been made, then extraction will be indicated (Fig. 10.3). If the tooth is deemed unrestorable or unfavourable, then extraction should be considered with suitable replacement if indicated [17].

The decision to gain direct access through an existing restoration or dismantle first must be based on the vulnerability of recontamination during root canal retreatment. It is crucial that the coronal seal be maintained both during and after endodontic treatment to prevent reinfection of the canal space. It is well documented that if coronal leakage occurs (especially when a poor coronal restoration is combined with a poor root filling), then failure is likely to occur [18–20]. If the crown is judged to be of good quality (both clinically and radiographically) with no obvious marginal discrepancies macroscopically, then retreatment can be carried out with a conservative access preparation which can be sealed using either adhesive or amalgam Nayyar core restorations upon completion [21]. In a laboratory study using incisor teeth, cutting an access cavity resulted in a 15 % reduction in relative strength,

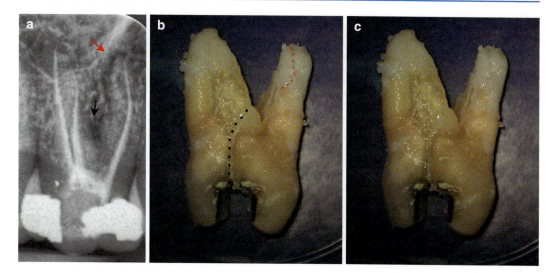

Fig. 10.3 Clinical radiograph and photographs demonstrating longitudinal fracture in tooth 26. Note (**a**) preoperative radiograph showing previously root-treated tooth. A periradicular radiolucency can be seen with the MB root (*red arrow*) and in the furcation (*black arrow*). Probing profile at time of presentation was within normal limits. Root canal re-treatment or extraction with prosthodontic replacement was discussed and the patient decided on the latter. (**b**) and (**c**) Longitudinal root fractures associated with the MB root (*dotted red line*) and furcation region (*dotted black line*). Root canal re-treatment would have been a pointless exercise in this case

and subsequent amalgam restoration resulted in a 5 % reduction in relative strength [22]. Restoration of a crowned tooth with a plastic restoration following completion of endodontic treatment ensures that coronal seal is maintained not requiring replacement of the crown.

Dismantling of the coronal restoration is necessary if crown margins are defective or undermined by caries. Retaining such a restoration risks jeopardising further success in the future due to reinfection. For temporary crown and bridge, the restorations can be removed easily using either a scaler or large spoon excavator. Various methods used for permanent crown removal include sectioning, using lifting devices and ultrasonics and can be classified according to whether the method is deemed conservative (prosthesis remains intact), semi-conservative (minor damage to the prosthesis but can potentially be reused) and destructive (prosthesis is damaged and not reusable) [23, 24] (see Table 10.2).

Post removal has been shown to be a predictable procedure using appropriate techniques. Methods for removal of cast, preformed and ceramic posts include ultrasonics and use of post

Table 10.2 Classification for crown and bridge disassembly

Conservative	Richwill Crown and Bridge Remover Ultrasonic Sliding hammer Matrix bands
Semi-conservative	WAMkey Metalift Crown and Bridge Remover System
Destructive	Crown and bridge sectioning using tungsten carbide burs

Adapted from Bartley and Hayes [23]

pulling devices (Ruddle post removal kit, Masserann Kit, Eggler post remover, Thomas post remover) [23–31]. Fibre posts may need to be drilled out [32, 33]. Risks of post removal include root fracture [34] and generation of excessive heat causing necrosis of the surrounding bone [35].

Historically numerous materials have been advocated for filling root canals including gutta-percha, gutta-percha carrier devices, synthetic polymer-based polycaprolactone thermoplastic material (Resilon), silver points and endodontic pastes/cements [36] (see also Chap. 7).

Gutta-percha can be removed mechanically using hand or rotary instruments aided by heat or solvents or with the use of ultrasound. Methods employed are dependent on the quality (poorly condensed or well condensed), method of gutta-percha root filling (cold lateral, warm lateral, warm vertical or single cone technique), type of sealer used and personal preference [37–40].

Solvents have been advocated to soften gutta-percha and sealer pastes and assist in its removal. Several solvents have been proposed including chloroform, eucalyptol, rectified turpentine and orange solvent. In general, all solvents are toxic to some degree, and their use should be limited and handled with care [41–45] (see Table 10.3).

Gutta-percha carrier devices such as Thermafil were traditionally comprised of gutta-percha moulded around a plastic or metal carrier. A variety of techniques have been proposed to remove Thermafil obturations including mechanical instrumentation with solvents, heated pluggers and rotary instrumentation. Success of retreatment depended more on the ability to remove the carrier than the technique of gutta-percha removal [46–49]. Recently the manufacturer of Thermafil (Dentsply, Tulsa Dental Specialties, Tulsa, OK) has developed a carrier-based system using a proprietary cross-linked gutta-percha core instead of

plastic carriers. GuttaCore can be removed with greater ease than other carrier-based systems. Unlike normal gutta-percha, this core material does not readily dissolve with solvents and is not amenable to plasticising with heat. The manufacturer recommends the use of NiTi instrumentation such as ProTaper retreatment files for the removal of this obturating material [50–52].

Resilon a synthetic polymer-based alternative to gutta-percha can be thermoplastically condensed and combined with a resin-based sealer to create a "monobloc" root filling. Its removal in retreatment is similar to the removal of condensed gutta-percha [53].

The "dirty fills" of endodontic pastes and cements have a poor track record and should be considered obsolete primarily due to their inherent properties of shrinkage, provision of an inadequate seal and serious risk of adverse reactions if inadvertently extruded beyond the confines of the canal system. Non-setting pastes/cements can be easily removed using a combination of solvents, hand and rotary instrumentation and ultrasonics. Hard-setting pastes such as resorcinol-formalin root filling (SPAD, Traitement SPAD, Quetigny, Les Dijon, France) also known as "Russian Red", due to the colour, sets extremely hard. Tags are formed within the dentinal tubules making retreatment very difficult if not impossible. The use of ultrasound is necessary to remove the hard-setting cement without overzealous preparation or perforation risk compared to the use of burs or drills. The use of Endosolv R (Spécialités Septodont, Saint-Maur, France) is available to aid in the removal of such pastes although clinically its effectiveness is limited with very little effect, if any [54–59].

Silver point fillings although once popular are now considered obsolete. Although ductile enabling easy placement and radiographically appealing, these fillings resulted in voids due to cross-sectional round silver points attempting to obturate a three-dimensional root canal system relying on a sea of sealer to plug the gaps. Over time sealer dissolution and silver point corrosion products as a result of tissue-fluid contact resulted in failure and their ultimate demise. Retreatment cases occasionally require the removal of silver

Table 10.3 Properties of commonly used gutta-percha solvents

Chloroform	High efficacy in dissolving gutta-percha and root canal sealers Antimicrobial High toxicity if inhaled or extruded beyond confines of the canal
Eucalyptol	Low efficacy in dissolving gutta-percha and root canal sealers Antimicrobial activity unknown Low toxicity if inhaled or extruded beyond confines of the canal
Rectified oil of turpentine	Low efficacy in dissolving gutta-percha High antimicrobial activity High toxicity if inhaled or extruded beyond confines of the canal
Orange oil	High efficacy in dissolving gutta-percha and root canal sealers Antimicrobial activity unknown Nil toxicity if inhaled or extruded beyond confines of the canal

point fillings. Successful removal of silver points is dependent on the ability to expose the silver point during disassembly without avoiding further fracture, loosening the silver point from the surrounding cement casing and gaining an adequate purchase in order to extract it from the root canal. If the head of the silver point has been exposed correctly and not fractured at the level of the root canal, then a surgical haemostat, artery forceps or Steiglitz forceps can be used to grasp the silver point and aiding removal. If the silver point is flushed with the root canal orifice, then the use of ultrasonics, Masserann Kit (Micro-Mega, Besancon, France) or Cancellier Kit (SybronEndo, Orange, CA, USA) may be advantageous in trephining and engaging the silver point for removal purposes [60–63].

Chemomechanical preparation and disinfection protocols used for the management of primary untreated cases can be applied to previously root-treated teeth. Multi-visit appointments with the use of intra-canal inter-appointment medicaments are mandatory since the time to properly disinfect the root canal system in a single visit is often impossible. Dismantling of existing restorations and previous root-filling materials and renegotiating canals to length are time-consuming procedures requiring proper disinfection procedures to be postponed until the second appointment [64].

The outcome of endodontic treatment is generally better than root canal retreatment, and this difference may be attributed to both the nature and location of the infection and treatment difficulties encountered when trying to rectify previous treatment errors. A systematic review of 17 studies published between 1961 and 2005 reported that the pooled success rates of root canal retreatment ranged between 70 and 80 % [65]. A systematic review of 63 studies published between1922 to 2002 reported the pooled success rate of root canal treatment ranged between 68 and 85 % when strict criteria were used [66]. The major difference between the outcomes of primary and secondary root canal retreatment resides only in the ability to predictably access and negotiate the root canal system to the (residual) apical infection. Outcome data offers a very

favourable prognosis for non-surgical root canal retreatment provided it is performed to acceptable guideline standards [67].

A few studies have compared non-surgical retreatment and endodontic surgery. A Cochrane review concluded that the short-term healing rates might be higher in the surgically treated cases [68]. The two randomised controlled trials comparing outcome of non-surgical retreatment vs. surgery hypothesised that the surgical treatment resulted in a more rapid bone fill but was associated with higher risk of "late failures" [69, 70]. The most recent meta-analysis comparing the outcomes of non-surgical root canal retreatment and endodontic microsurgery concluded that the latter was a reliable treatment option with favourable initial healing and a predictable outcome [71]. Bearing in mind that the cause of failure is usually residual infection within the root canal system, then non-surgical root canal retreatment should be the treatment of first choice. In cases where apical anatomy has been altered (canal transportation or blockage), whereby rendering re-treatment procedures ineffective or impossible, then surgery may be the only alternative treatment option. An informed decision by the patient should be reached based on careful case assessment and known prognostic factors that may influence treatment outcomes. One must also take into consideration the estimated cost-benefit analysis for all options including extraction and replacement when considering any treatment. A typical example is an anterior tooth with a well-fitting cast post and core restoration where dismantling is not only a costly exercise but also carries the risk of potential root fracture. Such cases may be more amenable to a surgical approach rather than non-surgical retreatment.

10.2   Disassembly Techniques for Crown Removal

Gaining access to root canals for non-surgical root canal retreatment procedures may involve the removal of existing restorations, cores, crowns, posts and materials from the orifice of root canals. Successful treatment depends on achieving this goal, which can be complex and challenging with additional risks of failure if incorrect dismantling techniques are employed. Longevity of the tooth will be dependent on preserving the remaining sound tooth structure and minimising further losses when attempting to re-enter the canal system. Financial implications are also of primary concern for the patient particularly if they have already made a costly investment by way of a cast restoration following completion of primary root canal treatment previously.

If the existing cast restoration is deemed to be good in quality, i.e. clinically and radiographically there does not appear to be any marginal discrepancies, then the crown may be retained.

Root canal retreatment can be carried out by way of a conservative access through the existing cast restoration and subsequently sealed following completion of treatment (Fig. 10.4). The patient must be warned, nevertheless, the inherent risks when working through crowns including the risk of fracture (porcelain), debonding and the possibility of removal and replacement if microscopic evidence of microleakage is evident during treatment.

If the crown has an obvious defective margin or has been undermined by caries, then removal is indicated. Retaining a compromised restoration will only serve to reinforce failure in the future by way of microleakage and reinfection. Removal of the restoration will allow

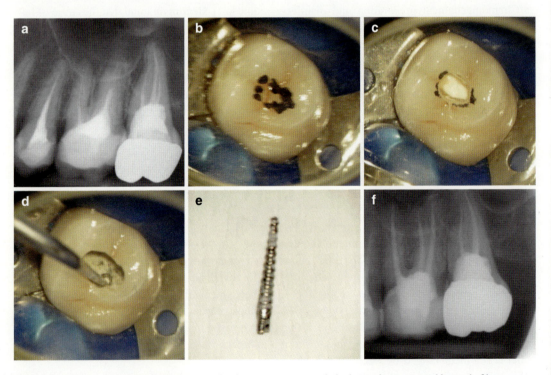

Fig. 10.4 Clinical radiograph and photographs demonstrating root canal re-treatment procedure through a well-fitting cast restoration. Note (**a**) preoperative radiograph demonstrating poorly treated tooth 26 with peri-radicular pathology in relation to the mesial root. A serrated post was noted in the palatal canal. (**b**) and (**c**) Access preparation through the existing cast restoration. Once the core was revealed, ultrasonics were used instead of burs to prevent post fracture and retrieval difficulties. (**d**) Post located and (**e**) removed using ultrasonics. (**f**) Final obturation completed. Note minimal access cavity has been restored with an adhesive restoration to ensure coronal seal is maintained

for a careful assessment of remaining tooth structure and restorability prior to endodontic retreatment. Additionally removal allows improved vision and accessibility, particularly in cases where there is obvious crown-root misalignment.

Methods employed to remove cast restorations include conservative (where the prosthesis remains intact), semi-conservative (where minor damage to prosthesis occurs but it can potentially be reused) and destructive (a new cast restoration will need to be fabricated).

Conservative methods

1. The Richwill Crown and Bridge Remover (Richwill laboratories, Orange, CA, USA)

A water-soluble thermoplastic resin is available that can be softened in hot water and then placed on the tooth undergoing treatment. The patient is asked to bite down and compress the resin block to about two-thirds of the original thickness. When the resin has cooled, it will set hard and the patient is instructed to open their mouth quickly, resulting in lifting or loosening of the existing restoration. The patient must be warned of the risk of loosening or removing the opposing restoration (see Fig. 10.5).

2. Siqveland matrix band placement

This involves the application of a Siqveland matrix band over the crown, which is burnished into the undercuts and then pulled vertically. This can be a relatively simple successful method for the removal of some crowns, particularly if they have been temporarily cemented in place.

3. Sliding hammer crown and bridge remover

A suitable tip is selected to engage the crown margin, and then a weight is slid along the shaft of the instrument in a series of short successive taps aimed at loosening the restoration. This method can be uncomfortable for the patient and

if forces are incorrectly directed pose risk of considerable damage to the underlying tooth and core. The use of this technique should be reserved for metal cast restorations where these are not risk of porcelain fracture.

Semi-conservative methods

1. Wamkeys (Dentsply, Weybridge, UK)

These are key-like instruments available in 3 sizes. A hole must be cut through the crown bucally or lingually parallel to the occlusal surface and at an imaginary level of the underlying core. A key is then inserted and rotated 90° resulting in a force in the path of insertion of the crown resulting in loosening or dislodgment. Care must be taken during initial hole preparation and rotation with porcelain crowns due to the risk of porcelain fracture.

Destructive methods

1. Sectioning

Sectioning the crown with a suitable tungsten carbide bur is an effective way of removal. A groove needs to be cut extending from the mid-buccal gingival aspect to the occlusal aspect of the crown. A similar groove is made on the mid-lingual aspect. The two sides are then connected by a further groove on the occlusal surface of the crown. Care must be taken to ensure that the groove does not extend beyond the margins of the crown to the underlying core with inadvertent risk of unnecessary tooth damage. Following groove preparation a suitable instrument such as a flat plastic can be inserted into the groove and rotated in order to separate the crown into two fragments. Occasionally a further groove may need to be created in a mesial-distal direction if the restoration proves to be very difficult to remove. It is important to ensure that the restoration is severed at the gingival margins otherwise prising the crown apart will be very difficult (Fig. 10.6).

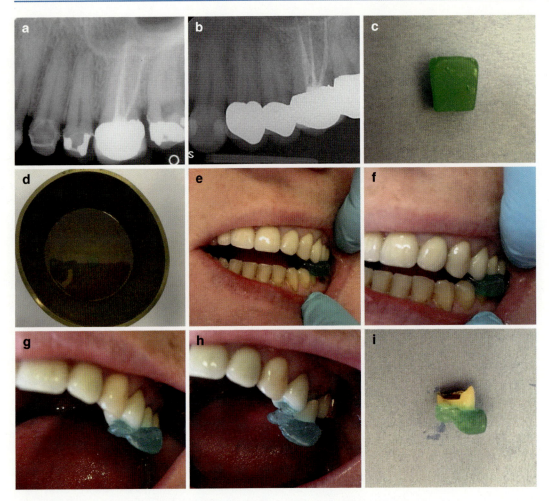

Fig. 10.5 Clinical photographs demonstrating the use of the Richwill crown and bridge remover. Note (**a**) preoperative view of teeth 24, 25, 26, and 27 which were treatment planned for replacement crowns. (**b**) Following crown preparation and cementation procedures, the patient complained of pain and tenderness associated with tooth 25. Acute apical periodontitis was suspected and the patient referred for endodontic treatment. The prosthodontist had cemented tooth 25 with temporary cement to ease crown removal prior to endodontic therapy. (**c**) The water-soluble pliable resin crown remover. (**d**) The remover is placed in warm tap water (145° F) for 1–2 min. The remover is ready when it compresses slightly when a firm force is applied between the thumb and index finger. (**e**) The remover is placed directly under the occlusal surface of tooth 25 and (**f**) the patient is asked to bite down. (**g**, **h**) Once the resin is cooled down, the patient is asked to forcefully open their mouth quickly resulting in (**i**) successful removal of the restoration

10.3   Disassembly Techniques for Core Removal

Underlying cores are generally constructed from amalgam or composite. The Nayyar amalgam core has been advocated as a means of restoring posterior teeth without the placement of posts. Amalgam is normally packed 2–4 mm into the coronal portion of the root canals. Removal of amalgam cores in the coronal 1/3 of the root canal should be carried out under direct visualisation using a dental operating microscope. Core material should be removed with the use of ultrasonic tips, and burs should not be used due to risk of iatrogenic damage and perforation. Composite core material can be effectively removed using

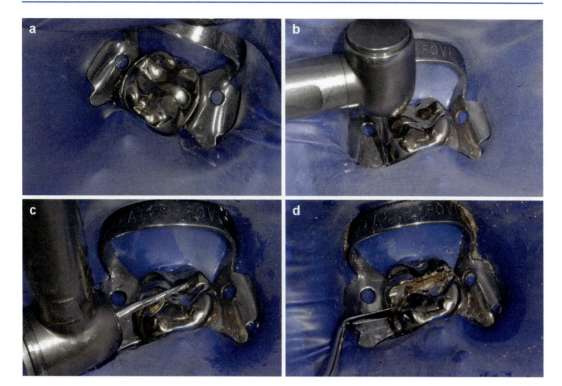

Fig. 10.6 Clinical photographs demonstrating destructive method of removing a cast restoration. (**a**) Preoperative view of the tooth, (**b**) gingival-occlusal reduction of cast restoration, (**c**) occlusal reduction, and (**d**) the use of a flat plastic instrument to separate two halves of sectioned crown

ultrasonic vibration, although visualisation can be hampered if the colour of the core is similar to the surrounding dentine. Intermittent use of water spray within the access cavity may help distinguish between core material and adjacent dentine with differing translucencies when observed under the microscope. The CPR2, BUC1 and ProUltra2 tips are diamond coated and effective at removing amalgam and composite.

10.4 Disassembly Techniques for Post Removal

Post removal has been shown to be a fairly predictable procedure provided appropriate techniques have been employed. The two main risks when removing posts are the potential for root fracture and periodontal ligament damage. The former may result if inappropriate techniques are employed, and the latter may occur as direct damage from overheating when using ultrason-

ics. All patients should be informed of the relative low risk of root fracture following post removal. Periodontal ligament damage is preventable by ensuring the ultrasonic unit is set at a low power setting and the assistant is able to provide a constant spray of water coolant to the ultrasonic tip/post to dissipate and counteract the heat generated.

Post removal devices

1. Ultrasonics

The use of ultrasonics has been shown to be highly effective when attempting to remove posts. The post must be separated from the core ensuring that the margins are undermined and any obvious cement lute is removed (Figs. 10.7 and 10.8).

The ultrasonic tip can be applied to the post head and vibrated out requiring an average time of 10 min. Well-cemented posts may be difficult to remove, and if there does not seem to be any

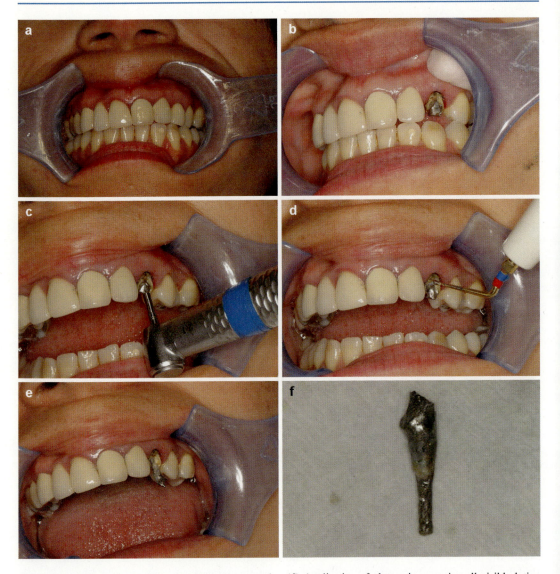

Fig. 10.7 Clinical photographs showing cast tapered post and core restoration removal using ultrasonics. Note (**a**) preoperative view of tooth 23 ceramic post and core restoration. (**b**) Removal of ceramic crown reveals underlying post and core restoration. (**c**) Core reduced in size.

(**d**) Application of ultrasonics ensuring all visible luting cement has been disrupted. Constant water cooling with 3 in 1 used throughout the procedure to ensure no damage to the periodontal ligament occurs. (**e**) Post vibrated out and (**f**) post and core restoration dismantled

evidence of movement after sufficient time (5–15 min approximately), then alternative methods of removal may need to be used.

The clinician should always endeavour to work at the lowest power setting that will efficiently and safely accomplish the task at hand. The selected ultrasonic instrument is initially moved circumferentially around the post to ensure that no remnants of cement lute are

present. Specific ultrasonic instruments designed to transfer energy directly to the post are available ensuring optimal energy transfer required to promote cement/bond failure and post dislodgement. The instrument is energised and moved around the post. As stated earlier the by-product of ultrasonic energy is the production of heat and countermeasures should be taken.

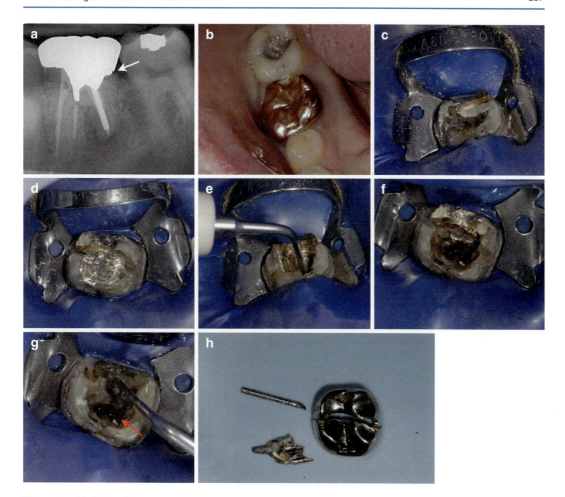

Fig. 10.8 Clinical radiograph and photographs showing dismantling of failed endodontically treated tooth 36. Note (**a**) pre-operative view demonstrating marginal discrepancy (*white arrow*). Parallel prefabricated post present in distal canal with peri-radicular radiolucency noted. (**b**) Pre-operative clinical view of full gold crown restoration. (**c**) Following sectioning of crown and placement of rubber dam. (**d**) Underlying cast post and core restoration sectioned into mesial and distal halves. (**e**) Removal of mesial cast post using ultrasonics. (**f**) Distal cast restoration and post. Care needs to be taken to avoid post fracture to the level of orifice which will increase difficulty when attempting removal. (**g**) Following dismantling of core, cemental lute is removed and post vibrated using ultrasonics. Cotton wool is placed in the mesial canals (*red arrow*) to prevent potential canal blockages from occurring during the post removal procedure. (**h**) Final crown, post and core restoration removed

If a screw or metallic post is present, the ultrasonic tip can be worked around the post in an anticlockwise direction to help loosen and unscrew it (Figs. 10.8 and 10.9).

Removal of the fibre post is generally specific to the post system, with different manufacturers supplying different removal kits. Often a pilot hole needs to be created followed by drilling through the entire post using increasing diameter drills. When hollowing through the post, the removal drills must be orientated centrally to reduce the risk of possible perforation or initiation of vertical fractures.

2. The Ruddle post removal device

This system was devised to mechanically engage and remove different kinds of posts and intra-canal obstructions whose cross-sectional diameters are 0.60 mm or greater. The kit consists

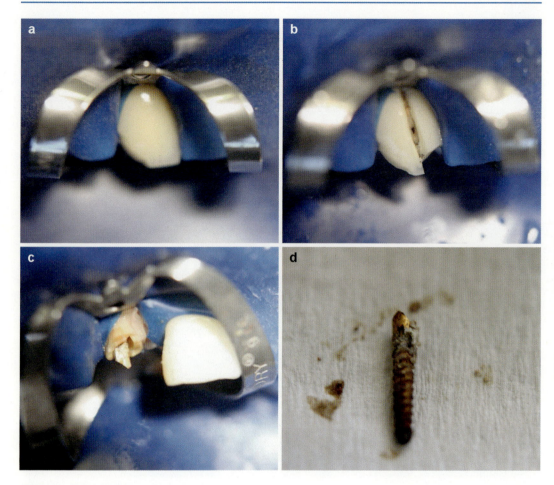

Fig. 10.9 Clinical photographs demonstrating (**a**) preoperative image of fractured screw post-retained ceramic restoration, (**b**) crown sectioned, (**c**) cement lute removed from around the screw post prior to (**d**) removal

of extracting pliers, a trans-metal bur, five trephines of varying diameters, five corresponding tubular taps whose internal diameters range from 0.6 to 1.60 mm, a torque bar, tube spacers and a selection of rubber bumpers. Prior to using this system, complete circumferential visualisation of the post within the pulp chamber is essential.

Core material is first reduced in size to ensure that a trephine drill from the kit can be used to mill the post core into a cylinder. The trephines are rotated in a latch-type slow handpiece at 15,000 rpm in a clockwise direction. The trephine is used to machine down a 2–3 mm length of the most coronal aspect of the exposed post. A rubber

bung is fitted onto the shaft of the remover and used to rest on the root surface thereby protecting it. The tubular tap is then screwed onto the remains of the post that has been previously milled by the trephine bur in a counterclockwise direction. The jaws of the extracting pliers are placed between the head of the remover and rubber bungs and opened by rotating a screw. As the jaws open a force is exerted along the long axis of the post enabling its removal (Figs. 10.10 and 10.11).

If turning the screw knob becomes increasingly difficult, the clinician should consider using the indirect ultrasonic technique to further attempt vibration of the post-engaged tubular tap.

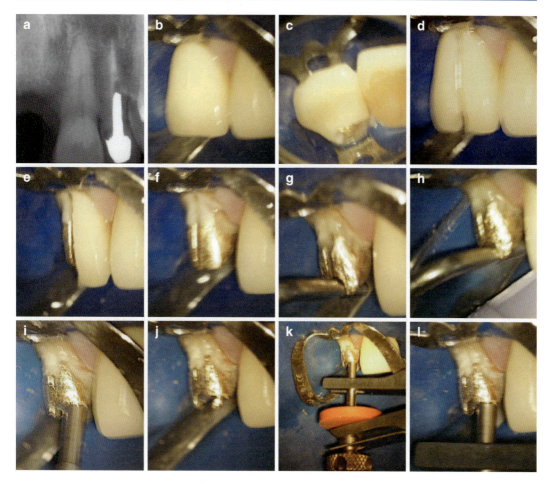

Fig. 10.10 Clinical photographs demonstrating post and core restoration removal in tooth 12. Note (**a**) preoperative radiograph with periapical radiolucency associated with the periapex. (**b**) and (**c**) Buccal and palatal views of existing cast restoration. Note marginal discrepancy on the palatal aspect warranting dismantling. (**d**, **e**) Crown sectioned and removed (**f**) underlying cast post and core revealed (**g**) application of ultrasonics used to vibrate post and core restoration and (**h**) water coolant constantly used. (**i**) After 15 min of ultrasonics decision to use Ruddle post remover kit. The post head is prepared with a trephine bur. (**j**) A number 3 trephine has machined down the coronal 3 mm of the post. (**k**) The assembled Ruddle post system mounted in place and (**l**) close-up view of the tubular tap which has been turned counterclockwise to form threads on the trephined post head

10.5   Retreatment of Gutta-Percha-Treated Canals

There are a number of methods to remove gutta-percha during root canal retreatment. These include mechanical (stainless steel or nickel-titanium rotary files), thermal (System B), chemical (solvents such as chloroform) or a combination of any of the aforementioned.

Mechanical methods

1. Stainless steel hand instruments

Mechanical methods alone are only useful if the root filling consists of a standardised single cone that has been cemented in place or the existing filling is poorly condensed (Fig. 10.12). In both scenarios space will be present between the

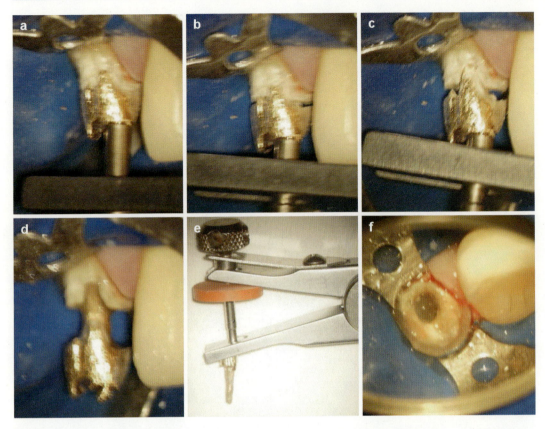

Fig. 10.11 Clinical photographs demonstrating use of Ruddle post remover system to retrieve post and core restoration. Note (**a**) the tubular tap has been secured. The rubber surface has been seated against the occlusal surface to protect the tooth (**b–e**) the jaws of the extracting pliers are opened by turning the screw clockwise. As the jaws slowly open the post can be seen safely withdrawn from the long axis of the tooth. (**f**) Post removal completed

root filling and root canal wall allowing the insertion of a Hedström file and engagement of the filling material. The file is rotated a quarter turn clockwise to ensure further engagement before withdrawing the file from the canal. The loose filling should be withdrawn easily. Occasionally the use of a Hedström braiding technique whereby two to three files are inserted, engaged and twisted prior to withdrawal (Fig. 10.13). This technique can be particularly useful for removing overextended root fillings.

Removal of gutta-percha will vary according to the obturation technique previously employed. On occasion single cones or poorly condensed root fillings may be mechanically removed in one single motion using only hand instrumentation. Well condensed root fillings, canal length, curvature, internal anatomy and cross sectional diameter may all influence the ease of removal and often require a combination of additional gutta-percha removal techniques to be used.

2. Nickel-titanium rotary instruments

Rotary nickel-titanium files can be used to remove gutta-percha root fillings. ProTaper retreatment files have been specifically designed for this purpose. These rotary files are used at a set speed of between 500 and 700 rpm allowing effective engagement and removal of the obturating material. The ProTaper D1 file (30/09) is rotated into the coronal mass of gutta-percha to create friction, heat and allowing penetration of the instrument deeper into the canal. The file should be removed frequently for removal of gutta-percha debris from the flutes. Once the

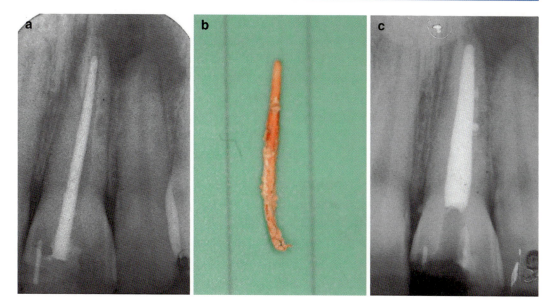

Fig. 10.12 Clinical radiograph and photograph of endodontic re-treatment of tooth 21. Note (**a**) preoperative radiograph demonstrating single-cone gutta-percha treatment. A periradicular radiolucency was associated with this tooth. Adjacent tooth 22 responded positively to thermal and electric pulp testing, (**b**) gutta-percha cone removed using combination of mechanical and thermal methods. (**c**) Completed case using warm vertical compaction technique

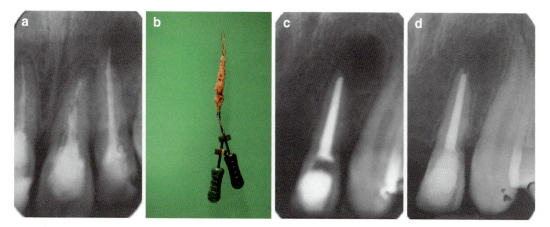

Fig. 10.13 Clinical radiographs and photograph of endodontic re-treatment of tooth 22. Note (**a**) preoperative radiograph demonstrating overfilled tooth 22 with a distinct periradicular lesion, (**b**) gutta-percha cones removed using combination of mechanical (Hedstrom braiding technique) and thermal methods. (**c**) Completed case using warm vertical compaction technique. (**d**) 6-month review radiograph demonstrating reduction in lesion size and ongoing healing

instrument has safely instrumented the coronal 1/3, the next instrument ProTaper D2 file (25/08) can be selected. This instrument allows removal of gutta-percha from the middle 1/3 of the canal. When appropriate, the ProTaper D3 file (20/07) can be used to instrument and enable gutta-percha removal from the apical 1/3 of the canal. Small-sized hand files should be used for the last 1–2 mm apically to allow negotiation of the canal. Care must be taken particularly in curved canals where heavy pressing may result in canal transportation and possible perforation.

3. Ultrasonic instruments

The use of ultrasonics with an appropriate tip can be particularly useful for removing gutta-percha in the coronal 1/3 of the canal. Often any gutta-percha remaining on the canal wall can be visible under the operating microscope, and precise application of an ultrasonic instrument can allow safe removal without risk of iatrogenic damage.

Thermal methods

Heat directly applied to condensed gutta-percha root fillings can allow softening, facilitating direct removal or indirectly creating further space for hand or rotary instruments in combination with chemical means to engage and remove root-filling remnants. When using any heated device in the root canal, care must be taken not to apply excessive heat to avoid periodontal ligament damage. Heated instrument should only be activated in short intermittent bursts as opposed to continuous application.

1. Use of open flame

Hand instruments are passed through an open flame until red-hot and then the instrument is transferred to the tooth resulting in superficial softening of the gutta-percha. Disadvantages of this technique include poor heat transfer, since the instrument will begin to cool down as soon as it is removed from the flame and also there is a risk of inadvertent injury to the patient.

2. Touch 'n Heat (SybronEndo, Orange, CA, USA)
3. System B Heat Source (SybronEndo, Orange, CA, USA)

These devices eliminate the need for open flame in the operatory resulting in added safety and controlled heat delivery to the working site. Various electrically heated spreaders or pluggers are available with touch activation and adjustable heat intensity that can be introduced into the mass of gutta-percha. Upon activation the gutta-percha is heated and softened. The spreader or plugger is allowed to cool down again before a quick burst of heat activation to allow removal of spreader/plugger along with any softened gutta-percha clinging to the cooled spreader/plugger. These instruments can be used effectively to within 5–7 mm of the apical constriction (depending on curvature) allowing further mechanical and chemical removal as necessary.

10.5.1 Chemical Solvents

Mechanical removal of gutta-percha with or without the use of heat will help clear the bulk of gutta-percha root filling. However, there will be remnants of gutta-percha attached to canal walls and in the critical apical portion of the tooth that will require the use of solvents. Solvent use to soften gutta-percha is a quick and reliable method (Figs. 10.14 and 10.15). Inadvertent extrusion of solvent can be harmful to the patient resulting in acute pain and possible allergic reactions; therefore, solvents should be confined to within the canal system only.

1. Chloroform

The solvent should be drawn up in a small syringe and marked to avoid confusion with other irrigants that may be used during the procedure. Once the bulk of gutta-percha has been removed from the coronal and middle 1/3 of the canal, the solvent can be introduced into the canal. A reservoir of the solvent can be introduced with care not to overfill, since excessive solvent will result in rubber dam dissolution and puncture requiring replacement. Once the solvent has been introduced, hand stainless steel or nickel-titanium rotary instruments can be used to further soften the remaining gutta-percha root filling. The softened gutta-percha can be engaged with Hedström files as discussed previously. On removal the file should be cleaned and further solvent may be required to aid removal.

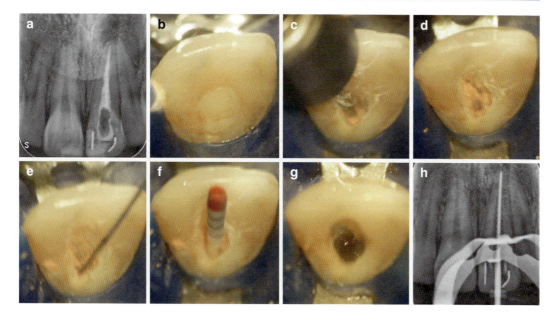

Fig. 10.14 Clinical radiographs and photographs demonstrating re-treatment of tooth 21 using a combination of mechanical re-treatment rotary files and chemical solvent (chloroform). Note (**a**) preoperative radiographs of tooth 21, (**b**) palatal access cavity prior to treatment, (**c**) the use of D1 ProTaper re-treatment file, (**d**) space created, (**e**) introduction of chloroform solvent, (**f**) paper point wicking of gutta-percha, (**g**) the use of sodium hypochlorite irrigation following removal of all remnants of gutta-percha, and (**h**) MAF confirming all gutta-percha has been effectively removed

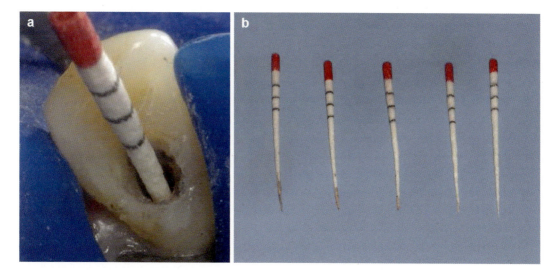

Fig. 10.15 Clinical photographs demonstrating the chloroform wicking technique. Once the majority of gutta-percha has been removed using mechanical, thermal, and chemical means, any final remnants of material are removed by the "wicking technique." (**a**) The root canal is flushed with the solvent (chloroform) followed by drying with paper points. This helps to remove any final remnants of gutta-percha particularly in the apical 1/3 of the canal. (**b**) As we move from left to right, paper points introduced into the canal system remove remaining remnants of gutta-percha until none is left

Once all the gutta-percha has been removed, the canal can be flooded with solvent, and a "wicking technique" using paper points can be applied to remove any remaining remnants of gutta-percha. Once there are no signs of gutta-percha on the paper point, you can be confident that the gutta-percha has been removed (Fig. 10.15). Radiographic assessment may be required to confirm removal has been completed.

10.6 Retreatment of Gutta-Percha Carrier-Based Fillings

A gutta-percha carrier device or obturator is composed of gutta-percha moulded around a plastic or metal carrier (Thermafil). The metal carrier devices have become obsolete due to difficulties of retrieval. The plastic carrier devices have recently been replaced by a proprietary cross-linked gutta-percha core, which is claimed to facilitate retreatment if required (GuttaCore). Removal of the plastic carriers can be carried out either mechanically using Hedström files with or without the solvent. Heat application to the head of the carrier has also been proposed whereby the plastic carrier is softened and adheres to the cooled spreader/plugger, which can then be withdrawn. Techniques utilising rotary files at high speeds have also been advocated whereby insertion of the file alongside the carrier until resistance is met creates friction and heat softening the gutta-percha and carrier for ease of removal. Care must be taken, particularly in curved canals where canal transportation is possible. Removal of carriers can be problematic particularly if the carrier fractures leaving an apical segment beyond the curvature. Ideally a space should be created beside the carrier to allow for surrounding gutta-percha and sealer to be removed using small files and solvents before trying to remove the carrier whole. If the gutta-percha has not been effectively removed, then the carrier will remain adherent to the remaining gutta-percha, and there is greater risk of carrier fracture.

10.7 Retreatment of Paste Fills

Although no longer advocated in modern endodontics, cases for retreatment may still be encountered, particularly patients from Eastern Europe where this method of filling root canals remain popular. Effective removal of paste/cement depends on whether the material is non-setting (soft) or hard setting. Non-setting materials can easily be removed using a combination of solvent action and mechanical instrumentation. Hard-setting pastes, such as resorcinol-formalin root fillings (SPAD, Traitement SPAD, Quetigny, Les Dijon, France), set by forming resin tags attached to the dentinal tubules, making retreatment very difficult. Removal will be dependent on the extent of the filling and whether it is accessible to ultrasonic files that can break up the residual material in a controlled fashion. Difficulties arise in curved canals where instruments can no longer be visualised with the aid of a microscope greatly increasing iatrogenic perforation risk. Additional solvent use has been recommended (Endosolv R, Spécialités Septodont, Saint-Maur, France) but only in conjunction with mechanical means of removal.

10.8 Retreatment of Silver Point Fillings

Once a popular technique for root canal obturation, these types of fillings have fallen out of fashion and considered obsolete. Nevertheless there will still be cases requiring retreatment where a silver point filling requires retrieval. The first step to ensure successful retrieval will be to separate the core from the silver point, which often protrudes into the coronal pulp chamber. The core material can be carefully dismantled using ultrasonics ensuring the head of the silver point is left intact without weakening or fracturing it. Separation of the silver point to the level of the canal orifice will make retrieval very difficult requiring principles used to manage separated instruments (see Chap. 11). Prior to attempting removal the silver point must be loose. Silver points are round in cross-section, so their ability to seal the root canal system was reliant on a

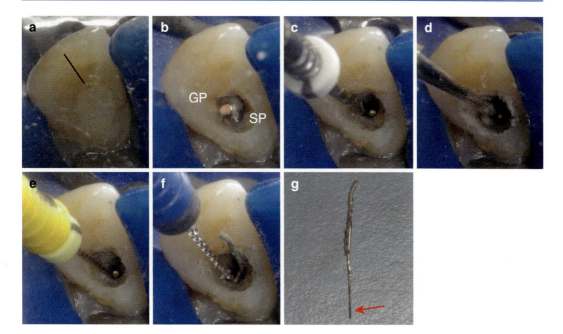

Fig. 10.16 Clinical photographs demonstrating step-by-step procedure for removing a silver point. (**a**) Preoperative palatal aspect of tooth 22. (**b**) Note following careful dismantling of the coronal restoration the underlying gutta-percha and silver point is exposed, (**c**) gutta-percha removed using mechanical re-treatment files, (**d**) use of ultrasonics to remove any remnants of cement lute/sealer surrounding the silver point, (**e**) checking for space beside silver point instrument and canal wall, (**f**) insertion of Hedstrom file to attempt retrieval once space verified and silver point judged to be loose. (**g**) Extracted silver point (note corrosion as evident by black staining (*red arrow*)

large volume of sealer to fill the remaining space. This sealer component has to be loosened to ensure that the silver point is free ensuring withdrawal without fracture (Fig. 10.16).

A mechanical file should be inserted beside the silver point and circumferentially worked to loosen the silver point within the canal. Use of solvents may be helpful for dissolution of sealer remnants and breakage of cement lute. Once the point is deemed to be loose, extraction of the silver point will require a point of purchase at the exposed coronal portion. The use of surgical haemostat, artery forceps and specialised forceps (Steiglitz forceps) can be helpful. The Cancellier kit (SybronEndo, Orange, CA, USA) is a microtube removal method that can be used to engage an intracanal obstruction such as a silver point. It contains four different sized microtubes (diameters of approximately 0.50, 0.60, 0.70 and 0.80 mm) selected to pre-fit the exposed head of the coronally exposed obstruction. The use of adhesive allows the hollow tube and silver point to set, enabling extraction. Caution should be exercised in terms of the amount of adhesive used, which could inadvertently block the canal.

If the silver point has fractured in the middle 1/3 or apical 1/3 of the canal or a sectional silver point was used, then retrieval will be very difficult. Removal will be dependent on the position of the instrument, whether it is beyond the curvature of the canal and whether it can be bypassed or not. Occasionally a surgical approach may need to be adopted to facilitate removal.

10.9   Removal of Root Canal Sealers

Traditional endodontic root canal sealers based on zinc oxide eugenol or calcium hydroxide can be readily removed using a combination of mechanical instrumentation supplemented with the aid of solvents. However, removal of glass ionomer cements, epoxy or other resin-based sealers can prove to be more difficult to remove due to their adherence to the canal walls and insolubility in the presence of solvents. Effective removal of these sealers will require the use of ultrasonics which is more time consuming and risky.

10.10 Clinical Cases

Endodontic failures are the result of a multitude of aetiological factors including coronal leakages, missed canals, underfillings (indicating underprepared canals), ledges, perforations and transportations. Irrespective of aetiology the predominant factor underlying the failure is bacterial, either reinfection by way of coronal leakage or inadequate management of the residual bacterial load in the first instance. Success of retreatment will not only be dependent on regaining apical access but often involving complex disassembly techniques that if not correctly carried out may further compromise the tooth in question. Costly retreatment procedures may be better suited for clinicians with the skills and expertise and understanding beforehand as to what is required to achieve success. Referral to a specialist may be prudent to ensure a favourable outcome.

Case 1: Retreatment Due to Missed Canal Anatomy A fit and healthy 36-year-old patient was referred for endodontic retreatment of tooth 25. The general dental practitioner had been unable to locate the additional palatal canal, and the patient was experiencing intermittent pain from the tooth. Access cavity preparation was carried out followed by refinement with the use of ultrasonic instrumentation to locate the additional palatal canal. Gutta-percha was removed from the buccal canal using rotary ProTaper retreatment files and solvent action in the apical 1/3. Patency was confirmed in both canals and chemomechanical preparation completed using 1 % sodium hypochlorite solution. Additional sonic irrigation was carried out before placement of an interim calcium hydroxide dressing for 4 weeks. A double seal temporary restoration was placed using Cavit and glass ionomer cement. Root canal obturation was completed using a warm vertical compaction technique (System B and Obtura) using AH plus cement. The patient

was referred back to the general dental practitioner for placement of a permanent cast cuspal coverage restoration (Fig. 10.17).

Case 2: Retreatment Due to the Enlargement of Peri-radicular Radiolucent Lesion Associated with a Root-Treated Tooth A 41-year-old patient with well-controlled hypertension was referred for endodontic retreatment of tooth 46. The patient had been experiencing discomfort with this tooth, which had been previously endodontically treated 12 months ago by an endodontic specialist. The general dental practitioner was concerned about the possibility of root fracture and uncertain as to the possible cause of failure. Clinical examination revealed a ditched temporary occlusal access dressing. Tooth 46 was tender to percussion and radiographic examination confirmed the presence of a peri-radicular radiolucency (Fig. 10.18).

Previous gutta-percha was removed using a combination of rotary retreatment files and chloroform wicking. Patency was re-established, working lengths determined and chemomechanical preparation completed using 1 % sodium hypochlorite solution. An interim calcium hydroxide dressing was placed for 4 weeks. The canals were obturated using a warm vertical compaction technique using AH plus cement. The patient was referred back to the general dental practitioner for placement of a permanent core restoration. An orthodontic band was left in situ to prevent coronal fracture, and a decision was made to delay placement of a cast restoration until definitive signs of periapical healing. The patient was reviewed at 6 months at which time there were clear signs of apical healing.

Case 3: Retreatment Due to Technical Deficiency A fit and healthy 31-year-old patient was referred for endodontic assessment of tooth 36. The patient previously had tooth 37 root treated, but this tooth had been extracted due to vertical root fracture and subsequently replaced with a dental implant. The general dental practitioner was considering placement of a crown restoration on tooth 36 to prevent future demise but was concerned with the suboptimal root canal treatment (Fig. 10.19).

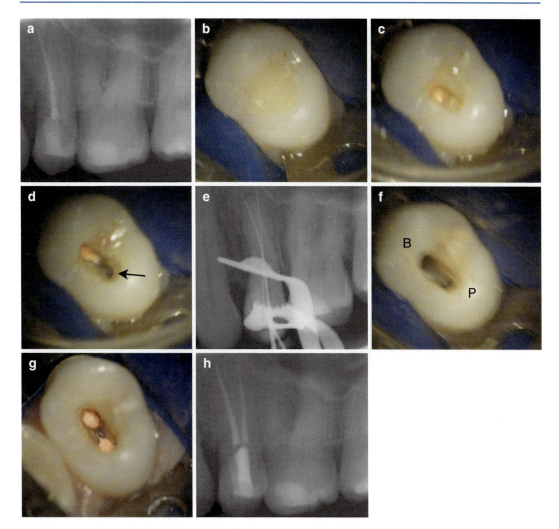

Fig. 10.17 Clinical radiographs and photographs demonstrating root canal re-treatment of tooth 25. Note (**a**) preoperative film demonstrating two root canals and only the buccal canal has been treated. (**b**) Intraoral view demonstrating coronal restoration, (**c**) access cavity preparation revealing obturated buccal canal, (**d**) refinement of access to locate untreated palatal canal (*black arrow*), (**e**) master apical file radiograph showing working lengths of buccal and palatal canals (buccal canal was retreated using mechanical/chemical measures), (**f**) intraoral view of buccal and palatal canals following completion of chemomechanical debridement, (**g**) obturated canals, and (**h**) final postoperative radiograph demonstrating well-obturated canals and coronal double seal temporary restoration

Clinical examination revealed the tooth was asymptomatic. Radiographic examination confirmed previous endodontic fillings short of respective apices. A widened periodontal ligament was noted with the mesial roots. A decision was made to embark on root canal retreatment.

A coronal access cavity preparation was carried out through the existing core restoration. The composite core material required careful ultrasonic troughing with the aid of the operating microscope. Gutta-percha root-filling material was removed using rotary retreatment files and solvent action. Patency was achieved in the confluent mesial canals. The distal canals were blocked and patency could not be regained. Chemomechanical preparation was completed using 1 % sodium hypochlorite solution. An interim dressing of calcium hydroxide was placed

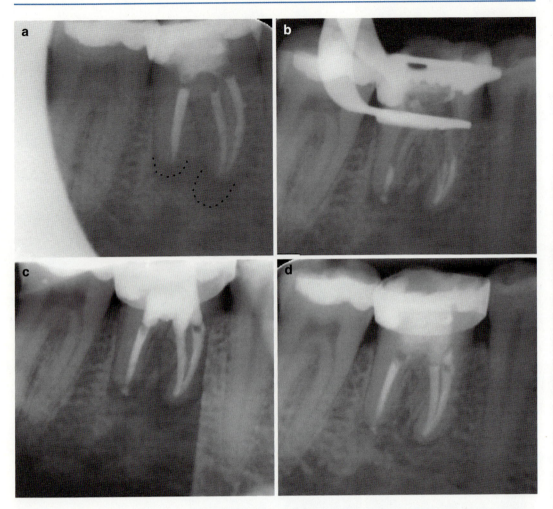

Fig. 10.18 Clinical radiographs demonstrating endodontic re-treatment of tooth 46. Note (**a**) pre-operative radiograph showing primary treatment completed by a specialist endodontist. The coronal temporary restoration was still in place despite treatment completed twelve months ago. Obturation appears well condensed. A periradicular radiolucency was noted and the tooth was symptomatic. A decision was made to proceed with root canal re-treatment. (**b**) Mid-fill radiograph. (**c**) Post-treatment obturation using a warm vertical compaction technique. The patient was advised to have a permanent resin core placed but to delay placement of a cast restoration until healing was evident. An orthodontic band was left in place as a precaution during this interim period. (**d**) The patient was reviewed at 6 months. Note complete peri-apical healing. The patient was advised to return to his general dental practitioner for a cast cuspal coverage restoration to prevent potential for both tooth fracture and coronal leakage

for a 4-week period. Obturation was completed using a warm vertical compaction technique using AH plus cement. The patient was referred back to the general dental practitioner for placement of a permanent cast cuspal coverage restoration. At 6 months review the patient remained asymptomatic.

Case 4: Retreatment Through a Cast Post Restoration Without the Need for Dismantling A fit and healthy 68-year-old gentleman was referred for endodontic retreatment of tooth 46. Clinical examination revealed a ceramic crown restoration with good marginal integrity. Radiographic examination revealed a

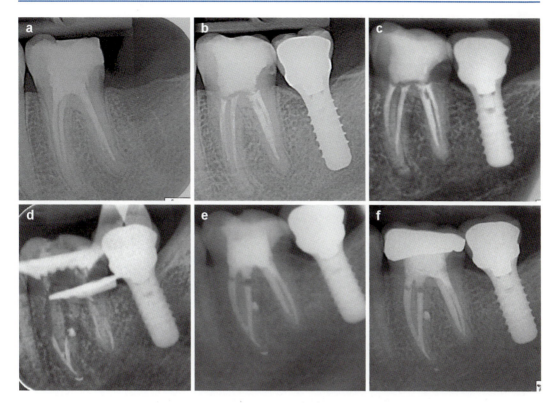

Fig. 10.19 Clinical radiographs demonstrating root canal re-treatment of tooth 36 due to technical deficiencies. The general dental practitioner was keen to place a cast restoration on this tooth to avoid root fracture. Note (**a**) preoperative view showing acquired loss of tooth 37 due to vertical root fracture. (**b**) A dental implant was placed in the 37 socket. (**c**) Preoperative view showing four root-filled canals short of respective apices (>3 mm). (**d**) Mid-fill radiograph demonstrating lateral canal. (**e**) Postoperative view demonstrating retreated 36. (**f**) 6-month review radiograph following placement of a cast restoration

post-retained restoration with poorly condensed root fillings. A peri-radicular radiolucency was associated with the peri-apex of tooth 46. A decision was made to access the crown and post removal without crown disassembly. The patient was warned of the possibility of ceramic fracture and debonding following post removal. Access was carried out initially using a tungsten carbide bur until core material was encountered. Ultrasonic files were used to dismantle the core to prevent post fracture. The post was removed using ultrasonic vibration. Gutta-percha was removed using rotary retreatment files and solvent action. Patency was achieved in all canals and chemomechanical preparation completed using 1 % sodium hypochlorite solution.

An interim calcium hydroxide dressing was placed for 4 weeks. Obturation was completed using a warm vertical compaction technique using AH plus cement. No post preparation space was left in the distal canal, since the post was not contributing to retention of the pre-existing crown or core. A reinforced zinc oxide eugenol and glass ionomer restoration was placed as a temporary measure. The patient returned to his general dental practitioner who placed a composite core restoration in the access cavity. The patient was reviewed at 6 months, and radiographic examination revealed continued periapical healing. The patient was advised a further follow-up review in 12 months to determine healing of the preoperative periapical lesion (Fig. 10.20).

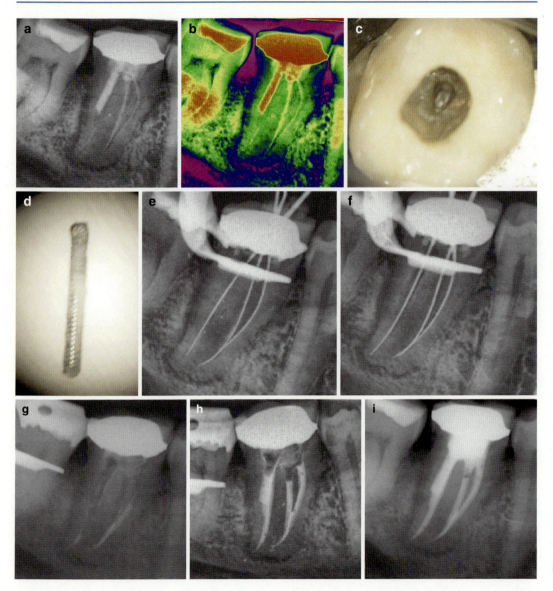

Fig. 10.20 Clinical radiographs and photographs demonstrating endodontic re-treatment of tooth 46. Note (**a**) and (**b**) preoperative digital films showing previous suboptimal root canal treatment. A parallel post was evident in the distal canal. A periradicular radiolucency was present. The case had been treated more than 4 years ago and a provisional diagnosis of failed RCT was made. (**c**) Intraoral view following access preparation and core dismantling to reveal the post. (**d**) Post removal following application of ultrasonics. (**e**) Initial apical file and (**f**) master apical file radiographs. Note confluent mesial canal anatomy. (**g**) Mid-fill radiograph following downpack. (**h**) Backfill using a warm vertical compaction technique with AH Plus cement, System B, and Obtura. (**i**) 6-month review radiograph showing completed case

Case 5: Endodontic Retreatment of a Tooth with Unusual Apical Anatomy A 43-year-old gentleman was referred for endodontic retreatment of tooth 21. The patient had undergone root canal treatment over 15 years ago in South Africa. During a routine examination his general dental practitioner had noted an incidental lateral periradicular radiolucent lesion associated with this

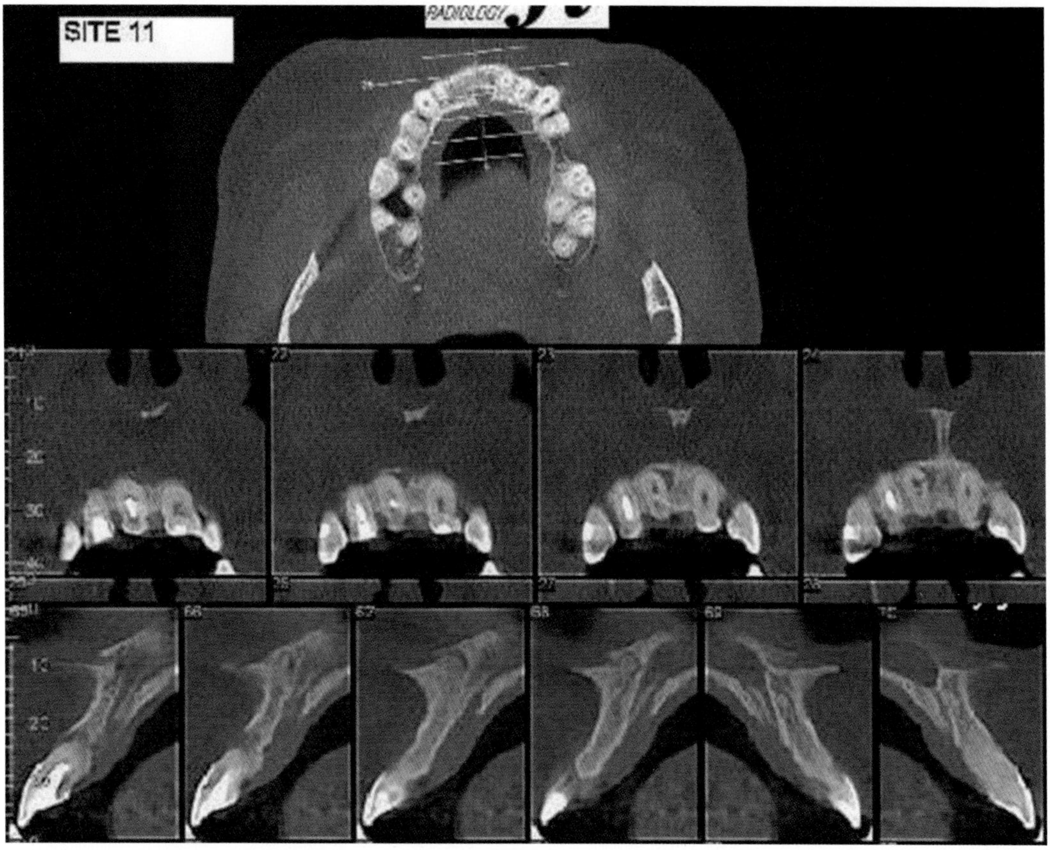

Fig. 10.21 Cone beam CT multiplanar images showing axial, coronal and sagittal images of tooth 11. The impression of a prominent accessory canal in tooth 11 was noted. Localised bone loss on the mesial aspect of tooth 11 is best appreciated in coronal slices 22–24. The lateral (accessory) canal is best seen on coronal slice 24

tooth. Clinically the tooth was asymptomatic. Radiographic examination confirmed previous endodontic treatment. A lateral peri-radicular radiolucency was confirmed. Treatment options were discussed, and the patient was keen to attempt retreatment in the first instance. The patient was sent for a cone beam CT scan of the maxilla only to rule out the possibility of an apical root fracture. The cone beam CT report stated the probability of a lateral canal in the apical 1/3 of tooth 11 with an associated peri-radicular radiolucency (Fig. 10.21).

Non-surgical root canal retreatment was carried out under a rubber dam. Previous root fillings were removed using mechanical and chemical means (rotary retreatment files and chloroform wicking). Apical patency was confirmed. A lateral canal was instrumented and confirmed radiographically. A gutta-percha sinus-tracing radiograph was traced to the lateral radiolucent lesion associated with tooth 11. Chemomechanical instrumentation was carried out and master apical file size confirmed #90. An intra-canal medicament of calcium hydroxide was placed for 4 weeks and the patient reviewed accordingly (Fig. 10.22). At the review appointment the sinus had healed. A periapical radiograph confirmed that the intra-canal dressing had dissolved (Fig. 10.22). A further dressing of calcium hydroxide was placed, and radiographic examination confirmed extrusion of dressing material (Fig. 10.23). The patient was warned of the possibility of post-operative sensitivity. The patient was reviewed a further 8 weeks later. At the review appointment the tooth

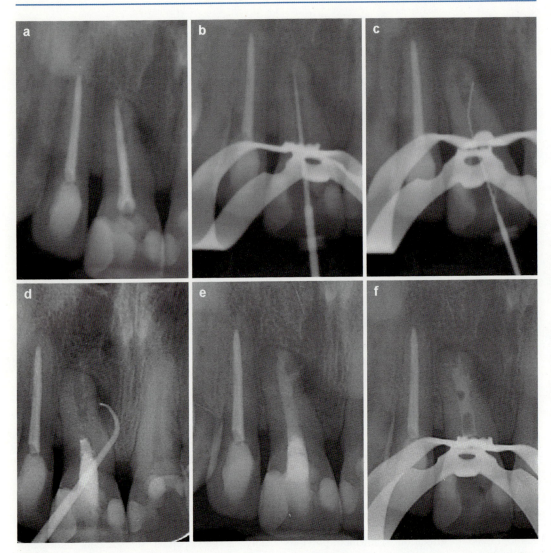

Fig. 10.22 Clinical radiographs demonstrating root canal re-treatment of tooth 11. Note (**a**) preoperative view demonstrating lateral periradicular lesion and initial root canal treatment. (**b**) IAF radiograph following removal of previous root filling material. (**c**) Lateral canal working length radiograph. (**d**) Gutta-percha sinus tracing radiograph demonstrating sinus in relation to lateral lesion. (**e**) Calcium hydroxide dressing placement. (**f**) 1-month review showing dissolution of dressing material

remained asymptomatic. A decision was made to obturate the canal. A pretreatment radiograph was taken to confirm presence of calcium hydroxide in the lateral lesion. The canal was reaccessed, and a final irrigation was carried out using 1 % sodium hypochlorite solution and 17 % EDTA. A master gutta-percha cone was cone fitted using a chloroform customisation technique.

The canal was dried and AH plus sealer introduced using paper points. The master gutta-percha cone was cemented to length and a warm vertical compaction technique was carried out. Downpack was carried out to the lateral canal position. A mid-fill radiograph was taken to confirm the apical 1/3 gutta-percha fill (Fig. 10.23). The remaining middle 1/3 and coronal aspects of the canal

Fig. 10.23 Clinical
radiographs demonstrating
(**a**) further dressing
material placement for a 3
month period. (**b**)
Pre-obturation radiograph
demonstrating dissolution
of dressing and extrusion
of calcium hydroxide
dressing into the lateral
lesion. (**c**) Mid-fill
radiograph following
chloroform cold lateral
customization and warm
vertical compaction using
AH plus cement. Note the
extrusion noted laterally is
the previous calcium
hydroxide dressing that
has not yet dissolved. (**d**)
Final post operative view
demonstrating well
obturated case

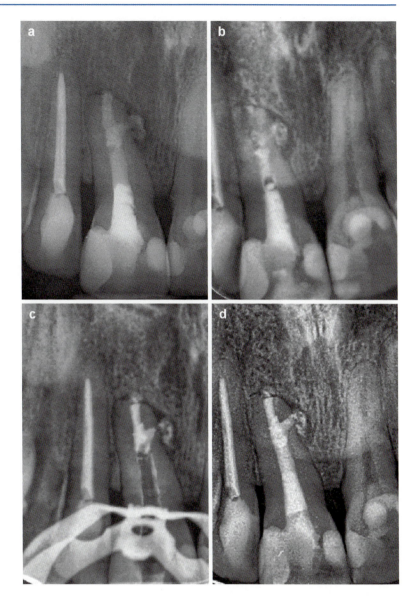

was obturated using Obtura backfill. A temporary double seal coronal restoration was placed using IRM and glass ionomer cement. The patient was referred back to his general dental practitioner for permanent restoration of the tooth.

Case 6: Endodontic Retreatment of Tooth 36 Previously Treated with Silver Point Fillings A fit and healthy 85-year-old gentleman was referred for endodontic retreatment of tooth 36. The patient had previously undergone root canal treatment in 1960 during his time in the naval forces. The tooth had remained asymptomatic until 2 months ago when he became aware of intermittent pain and discomfort. The pain was exacerbated by biting and chewing and localised to tooth 36. Clinical examination revealed a full gold crown restoration with an intact overlying buccal class V restoration on the mesial aspect. The tooth was tender to percussion. Radiographic examination revealed the presence of silver point root fillings in the mesial and distal roots. An untreated

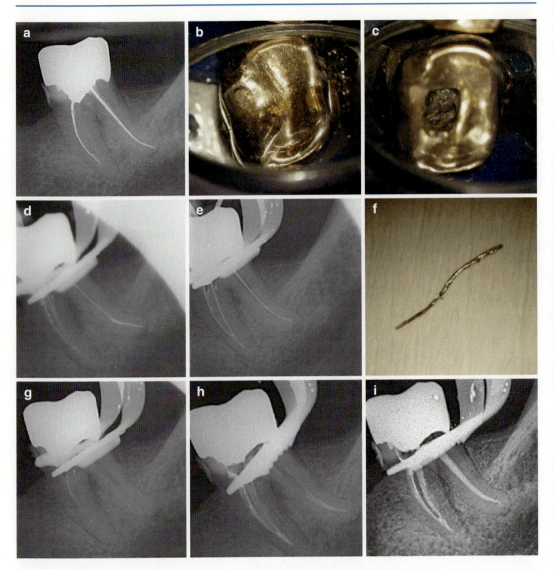

Fig. 10.24 Clinical radiographs and photographs demonstrating endodontic re-treatment of tooth 36. Note (**a**) preoperative radiograph demonstrating silver point root fillings placed 30 years previously. (**b**) Full gold crown restoration. (**c**) Access cavity demonstrating underlying amalgam core. Ultrasonics were used to carefully break up the core material without disrupting the silver points. (**d**) MB silver point filling was removed and additional untreated ML canal located which was confluent with the MB canal. No further length could be achieved mesially. The distal silver point had sectioned at the curvature. The silver point was initially bypassed and could be visualized under the dental operating microscope. The point was carefully vibrated with ultrasonics and retrieved. (**e**) MAF radiograph. (**f**) Retrieved distal silver point which had fractured in the apical 1/3. (**g**) Radiograph confirming removal of all silver points. (**h**) Mid-fill radiograph following warm vertical compaction using gutta-percha and AH Plus cement. (**i**) Radiograph following backfill using Obtura

mesial canal was noted and the mesial root filling was short of the radiographic apex. A peri-radicular radiolucency was noted with the distal root. A provisional diagnosis of acute exacerbation of chronic apical periodontitis was made and treatment options discussed. The patient was keen to try and retain the tooth avoiding a free end saddle situation in his lower left posterior region. Access cavity was prepared through the existing cast restoration. The underlying amalgam core

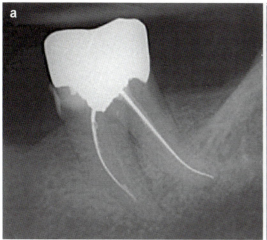
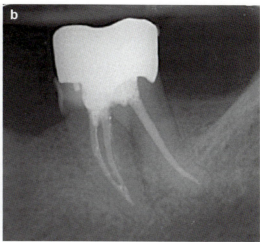

Fig. 10.25 Clinical radiographs demonstrating (**a**) pre-operative view of tooth 36 with untreated ML canal and silver point fillings in MB and D canals. (**b**) Post-operative view of completed re-treatment. The patient was asked to return to his general dental practitioner for placement of a permanent coronal restoration. The mesial canals were confluent in the apical 1/3 but blocked beyond this point. Despite attempts of negotiating further no canal patency could be achieved. Following completion of chemo-mechanical preparation to this level and intra-canal medicament the tenderness associated with the tooth settled down completely. The patient was warned of possible surgery in the future if any further symptoms were to occur and the patient was still keen to retain the tooth

was dismantled carefully ensuring that the silver points were left undisturbed. Troughing of core material was carried out at a low-power setting until both silver points could be visualised. The mesial point in the mesiobuccal canal was progressively bypassed using K files up to size #20. Chloroform was used to dissolve any remnants of sealer. A Hedström file was then placed in the space created and used to engage the silver point and remove it. Further ultrasonic troughing was carried out more lingually to locate the untreated mesiolingual canal. The silver point in the distal canal was also initially bypassed to working length, and progressively larger file sizes up to #25 were introduced. Initial irrigation was carried out with chloroform to help dissolve any sealer within the canal. A Hedström braiding technique was used to retrieve the silver point. On retrieval the apical portion beyond the curvature had separated. The point could be bypassed and visualised using the dental operating microscope. The silver point was gently vibrated using an ultrasonic narrow tip at a very low power setting. The separated silver point was ultrasonically vibrated, loosened and retrieved using a Hedström file size #50. Chemomechanical preparation was carried out using 1 % sodium hypochlorite solution. The mesial canals were blocked at the level of previous instrumentation. No further length could be achieved (Fig. 10.24).

A standard rotary preparation was completed using ProTaper Next files. An intra-canal medicament of calcium hydroxide was placed for 4 weeks. At the obturation appointment, the patient's symptoms had resolved and the patient remained asymptomatic. Obturation was completed using a warm vertical compaction technique using gutta-percha and AH plus cement. Following completion of obturation, a temporary double seal was placed in the access cavity (IRM/glass ionomer cement) prior to discharge back to the patient's general dental practitioner (Fig. 10.25).

> **Clinical Hints and Tips for Root Canal Treatment and Retreatment Procedures to Ensure Optimal Management of Root Canal Infection**
> - The use of rubber dam is essential to facilitate an aseptic technique.
> - Canal preparation should be to the canal terminus ensuring no space has been left untreated.

- Sufficient taper should be given to the canal preparation to optimise disinfection procedures and facilitate obturation.
- Optimal irrigation of the canal system should be carried out using a suitable disinfectant with tissue-dissolving properties.
- The use of an antiseptic intra-canal dressing of the canal system in between visits.
- The use of a biologically acceptable "double" temporary coronal seal of the root canal system after disinfection procedures is essential to ensure reinfection does not occur between visits.
- Correct extension of a homogenous root canal filling to the canal terminus without extrusion is ideal.
- Optimal final cast cuspal coverage restoration should be advised to prevent bacterial recontamination of the canal system and fracture of the tooth.

References

1. European Society of Endodontology. Consensus report of the European society of Endodontology on quality guidelines for endodontic treatment. Int Endod J. 2006;39:921–30.
2. Nair PNR, Sjögren U, Kahnberg KE, Krey G, Sundqvist G. Intraradicular bacteria and fungi in root-filled, asymptomatic human teeth with therapy resistant periapical lesions: a long-term light and electron microscopic follow-up study. J Endod. 1990;16:580–8.
3. Ricucci D, Siqueira Jr JF, Bate AL, Pitt-Ford TR. Histologic investigations of root canal-treated teeth with apical periodontitis: a retrospective study from 24 patients. J Endod. 2009;3:493–502.
4. Lin LM, Rosenberg PA, Lin J. Do procedural errors cause endodontic treatment failure? J Am Dent Assoc. 2005;136:187–93.
5. Nair PNR, Schroeder HE. Periapical actinomycosis. J Endod. 1984;10:567–70.
6. Sjögren U, Happonen RP, Kahnberg KE, Sundqvist G. Survival of Arachnia propionica in periapical tissues. Int Endod J. 1988;21:277–82.
7. Figdor D, Sjögren U, Sorlin S, Sundqvist G, Nair PNR. Pathogenicity of Actinomyces Israelii and Arachnia propionica; experimental studies in guinea pigs and phagocytosis and intra-radicular killing by human polymorphonuclear leukocytes in vitro. Oral Microbiol Immunol. 1992;7:129–36.
8. Nair PNR. Non-microbial etiology: foreign body reaction maintaining post-treatment apical periodontitis. Endod Top. 2003;6:96–113.
9. Nair PNR. Non-microbial etiology: periapical cysts sustain post-treatment apical periodontitis. Endod Top. 2003;6:114–34.
10. Ørstavik D. Time-course and risk analyses of the development and healing of chronic apical periodontitis in man. Int Endod J. 1996;29:150–5.
11. Kerosuo E, Ørstavik D. Application of computerized image analysis to monitoring endodontic therapy: reproducibility and comparison with visual assessment. Dentomaxillofac Radiol. 1997;26:79–84.
12. Strindberg L. The dependence of the results of pulp therapy on certain factors. An analytic study based on radiographic and clinical follow-up examination. Acta Odontol Scand. 1956;14:99–101.
13. Molven O, Halse A, Fristad I, MacDonald-Jankowski D. Periapical changes following root canal treatment observed 20–27 years postoperatively. Int Endod J. 2002;35:784–90.
14. Molven O, Halse A, Grung B. Incomplete healing (scar tissue) after periapical surgery – radiographic findings 8–12 years after treatment. J Endod. 1996;22:264–8.
15. Nair PNR, Sjögren U, Figdor D, Sundqvist G. Persistent periapical radiolucencies of root-filled human teeth, failed endodontic treatments, and periapical scars. Oral Surg Oral Med Oral Pathol Oral Radiol Endod. 1999;87:617–27.
16. Sathorn C, Parashos P. Monitoring the outcomes of root canal re-treatments. Endod Top. 2011;19:153–62.
17. Pitt-Ford TR, Rhodes JS. Root canal re-treatment: 1. Case assessment and treatment planning. Dent Update. 2004;31:34–9.
18. Saunders WP, Saunders EM. Coronal leakage as a cause of failure in root canal therapy: a review. Endod Dent Traumatol. 1994;10:105–8.
19. Ray HA, Trope M. Periapical status of endodontically treated teeth in relation to the technical quality of the root filling and coronal restoration. Int Endod J. 1995;28:12–8.
20. Tronstad L, Asbjornsen K, Doving L, Pedersen I, Eriksen HM. Influence of coronal restorations on the periapical health of endodontically treated teeth. Int Endod J. 2003;30:361–8.
21. Nayyar A, Walton RE, Leonard LA. An amalgam coronal-radicular dowel and core technique for endodontically treated posterior teeth. J Prosthet Dent. 1980;43:511–5.
22. Yu YC, Abbott PV. The effect of endodontic access cavity preparation and subsequent restorative procedures on incisor crown retentions. Aust Dent J. 1994;39:247–51.
23. Bartley A, Hayes SJ. Crown and bridge disassembly – when, why and how. Dent Update. 2007;34:140–50.
24. Olivia RA. Review of methods for removing cast gold restorations. J Am Dent Assoc. 1979;99:840–7.

25. Krell KV, Jordan RD, Madison S, Aquilino S. Using ultrasonic scalers to remove fractured posts. Int Endod J. 1986;36:687–90.
26. Crane DL. Posts, points and instruments: how to retrieve them II. Compendium. 1990;11:626–8.
27. Hülsmann M. Methods for removing metal obstructions from the root canal. Endod Dent Traumatol. 1993;9:223–37.
28. Ruddle CJ. Non-surgical endodontic re-treatment: post removal simplified. J Endod. 1993;19:366–9.
29. Machtou P, Sarfati P, Cohen AG. Post removal prior to re-treatment. J Endod. 1998;15:552–4.
30. Hauman CH, Chandler NP, Purton DG. Factors influencing the removal of posts. Int Endod J. 2003;36:387–90.
31. Williams VD, Bjorndal AM. The Masserann technique for the removal of fractured posts in endodontically treated teeth. J Prosthodont Res. 1983;49:46–8.
32. Linderman M, Yaman P, Dennison J, Herrero A. Comparison of effectiveness of various techniques for removal of fibre posts. J Endod. 2005;31:520–2.
33. de Rijk WG. Removal of fibre posts from endodontically treated teeth. Am J Dent. 2000;13(Spec no):19B–21.
34. Abbott PV. Incidence of root fractures and methods for post removal. Int Endod J. 2002;35:63–7.
35. Dominici JT, Clark S, Scheetz J, Eleazer PD. Analysis of heat generation using ultrasonic vibration for post removal. J Endod. 2005;31:301–3.
36. Whitworth JM. Methods of filling root canals: principles and practices. Endod Top. 2005;12:2–24.
37. Good LM, McCammon A. Removal of gutta-percha and root canal sealer: a literature review and an audit comparing current practice in dental schools. Dent Update. 2012;39:703–8.
38. Stabholz A, Friedman S. Endodontic retreatment – case selection and technique. Part 2 – treatment planning for retreatment. J Endod. 1988;14:607–14.
39. Friedman S, Stabholz A, Tamse A. Endodontic retreatment – case selection and technique. Part 3: retreatment techniques. J Endod. 1990;18:543–9.
40. Mandel E, Friedman S. Endodontic retreatment: a rational approach to root canal reinstrumentation. J Endod. 1992;11:565–9.
41. McDonald MN, Vire DE. Chloroform in the endodontic operatory. J Endod. 1992;18:301–3.
42. Hansen MG. Relative efficacy of solvent used in endodontics. J Endod. 1998;24:38–40.
43. Whitworth JM, Boursin EM. Dissolution of root canal sealer cements in volatile solvents. Int Endod J. 2000;33:19–24.
44. Friedman S, Moshonov J, Trope M. Efficacy of removing glass ionomer cement, zinc-oxide eugenol and epoxy resin sealers from re-treated root canals. Oral Surg Oral Med Oral Pathol. 1992;73:609–12.
45. Wilcox LR. Endodontic re-treatment: ultrasonics and chloroform as the final step in reinstrumentation. J Endod. 1989;15:125–8.
46. Johnson WB. A new gutta-percha technique. J Endod. 1978;4:184–8.
47. Bertrand MF, Pellegrino JC, Rocca JP, Klinghofer A, Bolla M. Removal of Thermafil root canal filling material. J Endod. 1997;23:54–7.
48. Guess GM. Predictable Thermafil removal technique using the system-B heat source. J Endod. 2004;30:61.
49. Wilcox LR, Juhlin JJ. Endodontic retreatment of Thermafil verses laterally condensed gutta-percha. J Endod. 1994;29:115–7.
50. Gutmann JL. The future of root canal obturation. Dent Today. 2011;39:130–1.
51. Gu LS, Ling JQ, Wei X, Huang XY. Efficacy of ProTaper Universal rotary retreatment system for gutta-percha removal from root canals. Int Endod J. 2008;41:288–95.
52. Beasley RT, Williamson AE, Justman BC, Qian F. Time required to remove Guttacore, Thermafil Plus and thermoplasticized gutta-percha from moderately curved root canals with Protaper files. J Endod. 2013;39:125–8.
53. Ezzie E, Fleury A, Soloman E, Spears R, He J. Efficacy of retreatment techniques for a resin-based root canal obturation material. J Endod. 2006;32:341–4.
54. Matthews Jr JD. Pink teeth resulting from Russian endodontic therapy. J Am Dent Assoc. 2000;131:1598–9.
55. Schwandt NW, Gound TG. Resorcinol-formaldehyde resin "Russian Red" endodontic therapy. J Endod. 2003;29:435–7.
56. Negm MM. Biological evaluation of SPAD. II: a clinical comparison of Traitment SPAD with the conventional root canal filling technique. Oral Surg Oral Med Oral Pathol. 1987;63:487–93.
57. Krell KV, Neo J. The use of ultrasonic endodontic instrumentation in the re-treatment of a paste-filled endodontic tooth. Oral Surg Oral Med Oral Pathol. 1985;60:100–2.
58. Jeng HW, ElDeeb ME. Removal of hard paste fillings from root canals by ultrasonic instrumentation. J Endod. 1987;13:295–8.
59. Vranas RN, Hartwell GR, Moon PC. The effect of endodontic solutions on Resorcinol-formalin paste. J Endod. 2003;29:69–72.
60. Krell KV, Fuller MW, Scott GL. The conservative retrieval of silver cones in difficult cases. J Endod. 1984;10:269–73.
61. Hülsmann M. Retrieval of silver cones using different techniques. Int Endod J. 1990;23:298–303.
62. Nagai O, Yani N, Kayaba Y, Kodama S, Osada T. Ultrasonic removal of broken instruments in root canals. Int Endod J. 1986;19:298–304.
63. Spriggs K, Gettleman B, Messer HH. Evaluation of a new method of silver point removal. J Endod. 1990;16:335–8.
64. Zehnder M, Paque F. Disinfection of the root canal system during root canal re-treatment. Endod Top. 2011;19:58–73.

65. Ny YL, Mann V, Gulabivala K. Outcome of secondary root canal treatment: a systematic review of the literature. Int Endod J. 2008;41:1026–46.
66. Ng YL, Mann V, Rahbaran S, Lewsey J, Gulabivala K. Outcome of primary root canal treatment: systematic review of the literature – part 1. Effects of study characteristics on probability of success. Int Endod J. 2007;40:921–39.
67. Ng YL, Gulabivala K. Outcome of non-surgical retreatment. Endod Top. 2011;18:3–30.
68. Del Fabbro M, Taschieri S, Testori T, Francetti L, Weinstein L. Surgical versus non-surgical endodontic re-treatment for periradicular lesions. Cochrane Database Syst Rev. 2007;3, CD005511.
69. Danin J, Strömberg T, Forsgren H, Linder LE, Ramsköld LO. Clinical management of nonhealing periradicular pathosis. Surgery versus endodontic retreatment. Oral Surg Oral Med Oral Pathol Oral Radiol Endod. 1996;82:213–7.
70. Kvist T, Reit C. Results of endodontic retreatment: a randomized controlled trial study comparing surgical and non-surgical procedures. J Endod. 1999;25:814–7.
71. Kang M, Jung HI, Song M, Kim SY, Kim HC, Kim E. Outcome of nonsurgical retreatment and endodontic microsurgery: a meta analysis. Clin Oral Investig. 2015;1–14.

Separated Endodontic Instruments

11

Bobby Patel

Summary

The mishap of an instrument fracture is an inherent risk with endodontic treatment, which can be detrimental to the long-term success. A combination of torsional and cyclic fatigue is responsible for file fracture following excessive rotational bending or repeated torsion beyond the limits of recovery. Mechanisms of fracture, contributing factors, prognosis and management are discussed.

Clinical Relevance

A combination of factors including operator proficiency; access cavity design; instrumentation technique employed; use of torque-controlled motors and rotational speeds employed; anatomy of the root canal including canal curvature position, length, radius and angle of curvature; number of instrument uses; and manufacturing process may all contribute to failure. Clinical methods employed to reduce this occasionally unforeseen circumstance are discussed. Where breakage occurs, the patient should be informed from the outset and due consideration given to whether the instrument should be removed or left in situ. Clinical methods of removal or bypassing are discussed including methods currently used in specialist practice. Managed correctly, the presence of a separated instrument should not adversely affect the outcome.

11.1 Overview of Instrument Fracture

Endodontic file fracture has traditionally been considered an uncommon event; however, a recent perception of increased fracture incidence with rotary nickel-titanium (NiTi) instruments has emerged. It is mandatory that the patient be informed if instrument fracture occurs during treatment or if a fractured file is discovered during a routine radiographic examination. When a file fractures during root canal treatment, there are several treatment options available to the clinician. Fractured instruments are a definite hindrance to the goals of cleaning, shaping and filling of root canals, and therefore their presence can adversely affect endodontic treatment outcome. The definitive management and decision

B. Patel, BDS MFDS MClinDent MRD MRACDS
Specialist Endodontist, Brindabella Specialist Centre, Canberra, ACT, Australia
e-mail: bobbypatel@me.com

© Springer International Publishing Switzerland 2016
B. Patel (ed.), *Endodontic Treatment, Retreatment, and Surgery*,
DOI 10.1007/978-3-319-19476-9_11

259

to remove a fractured file should be carefully weighed against the possible benefits of bypassing or risks of file retention. Although modern techniques employed in endodontic practice have improved the clinician's ability to remove fractured files, removal may not always be possible or even desirable given the risks of further damage. A plethora of different methods have been employed to remove fractured instruments, and although successful, these techniques usually require the use of the dental operating microscope and specialist care. Removal of a fractured file is not without considerable risk, particularly in the narrow apical regions of the root canal, beyond the curvature of the canal. Attempts at removal may result in excessive enlargement of the canal and risk the possibility of perforation of the root. Therefore, leaving the fragment in situ should be considered if referral is not possible (Fig. 11.1).

Within the endodontic literature, it appears that retained fractured instruments do not reduce the prognosis of endodontically treated teeth if apical periodontitis is absent. However, in cases where peri-radicular disease is present, healing is likely to be significantly compromised. The hindrance posed by the presence of an endodontic instrument is particularly evident in those cases where separation has occurred early before adequate canal disinfection has been achieved. Considering the risks associated with file removal, perhaps this should only be attempted if apical disease is present [1–3].

The majority of endodontic instruments are made of stainless steel, nickel-titanium (NiTi) alloy or carbon-steel under ISO/ANSI specifications [4, 5]. Fractured root canal instruments may include endodontic files, finger spreaders, spiral fillers and Gates Glidden burs.

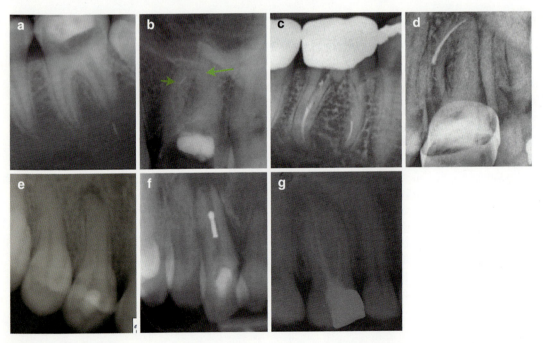

Fig. 11.1 Clinical radiograph demonstrating various instrument fractures referred to specialist endodontic practice. Note (**a**) instrument inadvertently pushed beyond the confines of the canal after the general dental practitioner attempted retrieval. (**b**) Two separated instruments were noted in the MB and DB canals (*green arrows*). The patient was a lawyer and had not been informed of the mishaps. (**c**) and (**d**) Instrument fractures present in the apical 1/3 of the canal system at and beyond the canal curvatures. (**e**) Separated Lentulo spiral filler likely due to minimal canal preparation prior to dressing the tooth. (**f**) A fractured rosehead bur. (**g**) Endodontically treated tooth with a separated stainless steel hand file in the MB canal

Nickel-titanium was developed 40 years ago by Buehler and colleagues in the Naval Ordnance Laboratory [6]. Walia and associates first proposed the use and development of NiTi alloy for the fabrication of endodontic instruments due to their special characteristics of super elasticity and shape memory [7]. Super elasticity is associated with the occurrence of a phase transformation of the alloy upon the application of stress or temperature above a critical level. The low temperature phase is called martensitic and the high temperature phase is known as austenitic. The stress-induced martensitic transformation reverses spontaneously upon release of the stress returning to its original shape and size. This special property manifests as an enhanced elasticity of the NiTi alloy, allowing the material to recover after large strains. NiTi instruments appear highly flexible and elastic, hence the possibility of use in a continuous rotary fashion even in a curved canal. Despite these advantages, unexpected instrument fracture is not uncommon and represents a major concern in clinical use.

Two distinct fracture mechanisms responsible for file separation, acting alone or in combination, have been described in the literature – namely, torsional stress and cyclic fatigue [8–10]. The twisting of a file about its longitudinal axis at one end whilst the other end is fixed generates torsional stress. This can happen in straight or curved canals if the tip binds resulting in friction against the canal wall. When the elastic limit of the metal is exceeded, the rotary instrument undergoes plastic deformation (unwinding). The file will ultimately fracture if the load is sufficiently high. Cyclic fatigue results in failure of the file when repeated cycles of tension and compression occurring during bending are sufficient to cause structural breakdown and eventual fracture. Clinically, rotation of a file in a curved canal contributes to the tension/compression cycling as a file is rotating. In reality, both factors work together to weaken a rotary file and ultimately cause file fracture with little to no warning.

Many manufacturing design characteristics of rotary NiTi files can influence their resistance to fatigue and fracture. As a general rule, fine and flexible files are vulnerable to torsional stress but more resistant to cyclic fatigue. Conversely rigid, larger files can have a greater torque applied without torsional failure and a greater propensity towards failure by cyclic fatigue. Conventional stainless steel K-files have a total cutting length of 16 mm and a standardized increase in diameter by 0.02 mm per millimetre. This increase in diameter is termed a taper of 2 %. For example, an instrument designated as size 25 is 25/100 thick at the tip (0.25 mm). At the end of the cutting edge, it is 16×0.02 mm $= 0.32$ mm thicker (i.e. $0.25 + 0.32$ mm $= 0.57$ mm). 6 % tapered NiTi instruments have less resistance to fracture compared to 4 and 2 % [11]. Moreover, an acute canal curvature coronally is more likely to lead to instrument fracture compared to a gradual apical curve.

It is well known that the nature of the alloy and the manufacturing process greatly affect the instruments' mechanical behaviour. To improve fracture resistance of NiTi files, manufacturers have either introduced new alloys to manufacture NiTi files or developed new manufacturing processes. M wire (used in Vortex Blue and WaveOne) has been developed by a series of proprietary thermo-cycling processing procedures creating instruments that are more flexible and more resistant to failure compared to traditional NiTi alloy [12–14]. Another novel approach has been the development of the Twisted File using a combination of heat treatment and twisting of a ground blank nickel-titanium wire. A raw nickel-titanium wire is selected in its austenite crystalline structure, and then by means of heating and cooling procedures, a completely new crystalline phase (R phase) is created. The Twisted File is created by twisting the R phase wire into the desired shape, heating and cooling it to maintain the shape and then converting it back to its austenite crystalline structure. The instrument is deemed more resistant to cyclic fatigue, and the manufacturing process deems it less susceptible to microfracture points along the length of the file since it is not ground like conventional NiTi files [15, 16]. Recently, NiTi rotary instruments made from a NiTi-controlled memory wire (CM Wire; DS Dental, Johnson City, TN) have been introduced. The major advantage of the Typhoon CM

File is that its shape memory has been removed or controlled by a special thermo-mechanical process. This unique file can be prebent or curved retaining its shape without any attempt at straightening. In curved root canals, the instrument will follow the natural root canal anatomy without undue disproportionate lateral forces resulting in transportation and straightening. The Typhoon CM File has increased torsional strength and increased resistance to cyclic fatigue resulting in a file that is more likely to unwind as opposed to unexpected fracture [17, 18].

Instrument fracture can be a serious iatrogenic mishap that can complicate or compromise the outcome of endodontic treatment. Several factors have been identified in the literature, which may be responsible for the ultimate demise of an instrument and methods that can help prevent nickel-titanium rotary fracture (Table 11.1).

Studies have demonstrated that higher rates of NiTi rotary instrument fracture occur with less experienced operators whose tactile sensation may not be adept at recognizing when a file may undergo excessive torsional resistance, taper lock and ultimately fracture. Preclinical training in extracted teeth or blocks and hands-on courses allows the clinician time to acquire the necessary competence, proficiency and tactile skills required to avoid procedural mishaps. Examination of instruments prior to and after use is recommended whereby flutes are inspected for deformities and signs of unwinding due to

Table 11.1 Factors identified that can either contribute towards or prevent instrument fracture

File flexibility and taper
Manufacturing process
Operator proficiency
Inappropriate access design
Reproducible glide path
Anatomical constraints
Angle of curvature and radius of curvature
Repeated use of instruments
Instrumentation technique and manipulation
Rotational speed
Use of torque-controlled motors
Use of irrigation and/or lubrication
Reciprocation vs. continuous rotation

excessive torsional stresses. Instruments should be used according to manufacturer's instructions with appropriate torque settings and speed of rotations always avoiding the use of excessive forces, especially apical pressures [19, 20].

Inappropriate and inadequate access cavity design features during preparation procedures will result in complications during the cleaning and shaping process. Ideal access preparations should ensure straight-line, unimpeded access to the root canal orifices with all obstructions such as dentine or calcifications having been removed. Ideally direct access to the apical portion of the canal or to the point of the first curvature should be achieved avoiding overzealous preparation for fear of stripping or perforations. Endodontic instruments that are then passively introduced into the canal will follow the natural canal anatomy with less torsional and cyclic fatigue stresses on the instrument. Deviation from the original canal curvature, which can lead to procedural errors such as zipping, stripping and perforations, is also minimized. Correct access preparation and design is a crucial first step before the introduction of instruments necessary to avoid catastrophic mishaps and fractures [21, 22].

A smooth reproducible glide path extending from the canal orifice to the apex of the root in theory should be created before introducing NiTi rotary instruments into the canal. This can be achieved using either traditional stainless steel instruments or using the recently developed PathFile system (see Chap. 3). The premise is that unwanted anatomical interferences and canal obstructions are eliminated reducing the unexpected file separations during rotary preparation. The use of stainless steel instruments has the advantages of excellent tactile sensation especially with respect to torsional stresses and the enhanced ability to negotiate blockages and calcifications often encountered in root canal systems. The use of rotary NiTi files for creating such a path has been found to cause less canal aberration and less modification of the original canal anatomy in stimulated root canals [23–26]. The PathFile system consists of three instruments, with 21–25–31 mm length and 0.02 taper; they have a square cross section. The PathFile #1 (purple) has an ISO 13 tip size; the PathFile #2 (white) has an ISO 16 tip size; the PathFile #3 (yellow) has an ISO 19 tip size. The manufacturer suggests using the first PathFile immediately after a #10 hand K-file has been used to scout the root canal to full working length.

Anatomical constraints and variation in root canal anatomy within a tooth increase the likelihood of instrument fracture in certain cases. Hidden challenges such as merging canals, curvatures (S shaped, abrupt angles of curvature, double curvature, abrupt radius of curvatures), dilacerating or dividing canals, isthmuses, fins and aberrations may all result in unexpected instrument fracture. The clinician must be aware that both the angle of curvature and radius of curvature in combination with instrument size selected will influence the possibility of failure. As the angle of curvature increases, there is an increased possibility of instrument fracture using larger less flexible instruments. With regard to the radius of curvature as the radius decreases, the instrument stress and strain increases with the likelihood of instrument fracture [9, 27–29].

The repeated use of endodontic NiTi or stainless steel instruments results in a higher risk of failure and fracture compared to single-use instruments. The more cycles of rotation an endodontic instrument endures, the greater the working stress that is created within the file resulting in deformation and failure [9, 30, 31]. Recently, the emergence of variant Creutzfeldt–Jakob disease (vCJD) has highlighted issues regarding the decontamination protocols commonly used for reuse of surgical and dental instruments. The resistance of prion agents to inactivation and the notorious difficulty associated with cleaning endodontic instruments has led to the emergence of single-use endodontic NiTi rotary instruments in recent times [32–35].

Endodontic instruments have been designed with tips that are described as passive or active. An active instrument has non-landed active cutting blades, which are effective at removing dentine. Passive instruments on the other hand have a radial land between cutting edge and flute, which reduces the cutting ability. In general, active instruments cut more efficiently and aggressively compared to passive instruments, which have less tendency to straighten the canal that can result in transportation and ledges [36]. During instrumentation, the rotary file should always passively follow the canal pathway, and no attempt should be made to apply any apical pressure. The more apical pressure applied, the greater the risk that the NiTi instrument will encounter 'taper lock' undergoing structural fatigue and failure [10, 37, 38]. The term 'taper lock' describes the situation when an instrument dimension closely approaches the canal's size and taper.

The manufacturing process of NiTi instruments during the machining and milling of the alloy during the production phase can lead to lattice structure distortion, microhardness inconsistency and surface microcracks. These could be the prelude to an imminent, further deterioration of the instrument and could explain the reported increased breakage of these instruments under normal operative conditions [39, 40].

Rotational speed of the instrument has been cited as a cause of fatigue fracture of NiTi instruments and that this is less likely to occur with lower rates of speed [41, 42]. Manufacturers advocate predetermined rotational speeds according to the instrument selected for use, and clinicians are recommended to adhere to these guidelines to minimize the risk of instrument fracture accordingly.

Torque-controlled motors were introduced with a built in feedback mechanism that limits the maximum torque delivered to a handpiece to reduce the risk of torsional fatigue of an endodontic NiTi instrument. Instruments will show differing torsional strengths according to file geometry (cross-sectional shape and area). Once the preset torque (preprogrammed into the circuitry of the machine according to manufacturer's recommendations) is reached, the motor either stops or automatically reverses. This is to prevent excessive build up of stress in the instrument whereby limiting the applied torque to below the ultimate strength of the material reducing the risk of torsional failure. Note frequent engagement of the autoreverse function also carries a risk of torsional fatigue of the instrument.

The use of such motors has been demonstrated to be beneficial in canals with limited accessibility [19, 38, 43, 44].

The use of irrigation and lubrication during the cleaning and shaping procedures has been shown to reduce root canal clogging of dentinal mud, bacteria and inorganic debris that can accumulate as a result. Irrigant and lubricant use has been shown to act synergistically to reduce frictional resistance and undue torsional stresses placed on the instrument reducing the likelihood of torsional failure. Canals should be copiously irrigated using sodium hypochlorite solution, and lubricants such as ethylenediaminetetraacetic acid (EDTA) can be used as adjuncts during the preparation phase [45, 46].

Rotary instrument manipulation has been shown to be one of the most important factors contributing to instrument fatigue and failure. Instruments should be used in a smooth, light apical motion and continuous pecking motion without allowing the instrument to rotate in any one particular area for an extending period of time. It has also been shown that as the length of this pecking motion increased, the number of rotations to fracture also increased [11, 37, 47].

NiTi root canal instruments have been traditionally used in a continuous clockwise rotation within the tooth overlaying a preparatory shape on the original anatomy of the root canal. Two single file systems – RECIPROC (VDW, Munich, Germany) and WaveOne (Dentsply Maillefer, Ballaigues, Switzerland) – have been recently introduced following a new reciprocating concept. The reciprocating sequence consists of a counterclockwise movement and a clockwise movement to prepare the root canal system achieving adequate shapes with efficient cleaning ability [48]. The reciprocating motion of the file theoretically reduces the cyclic fatigue placed on the instrument, thereby reducing the propensity to separate and increasing the lifespan of the instrument. Theoretically, this 'balanced force' type of technique also allows for more centred canal preparations which are helpful when managing curved canal systems where repeated compression and flexion can lead to instrument fracture [49–53].

11.2   Outcome and Prognosis

The impact of a retained fractured instrument on endodontic treatment prognosis has been assessed by two retrospective case control studies. The conclusion drawn from both studies was that a retained fractured instrument per se generally did not adversely affect endodontic case prognosis. In addition, the presence of a preoperative radiolucency was significantly associated with a reduced chance of healing [54, 55]. On the basis of the current best available evidence, the prognosis for endodontic treatment when a fractured instrument fragment is left within the root canal is not significantly reduced [56]. The success of removing a fractured instrument is closely related to whether the fragment can be visible using a dental operating microscope. In those cases where the fragment is not visible, the probability of successful removal is reduced significantly [57].

Several methods have been proposed for the removal of fractured instruments within the root canal system with varying limitations and success. Techniques include the use of the Masserann Kit [58], Endo Extractor [59], Canal Finder System [60], ultrasonic devices [61–63], staging platforms [64] and the Instrument Removal System (IRS) [65]. The inherent problems associated with all these devices include the risk of excessive removal of root canal dentine, ledging, perforation, limited application in narrow and curved canals and the possibility of extrusion of the separated instrument through the apex [60, 62, 66] (see fig. 11.1).

Successful removal of any retained fragment is dependant on factors such as the position of the instrument in relation to canal curvature, depth within the canal (apical, middle or coronal) (Fig. 11.2), whether the instrument is visible using the dental operating microscope and type of instrument that has separated (NiTi or stainless steel files). The more apically positioned the instrument, the greater the risk of iatrogenic damage, including root perforation or fracture. Conservation of root dentine is paramount to long-term longevity of the tooth, and this must be balanced against the proviso of straight-line

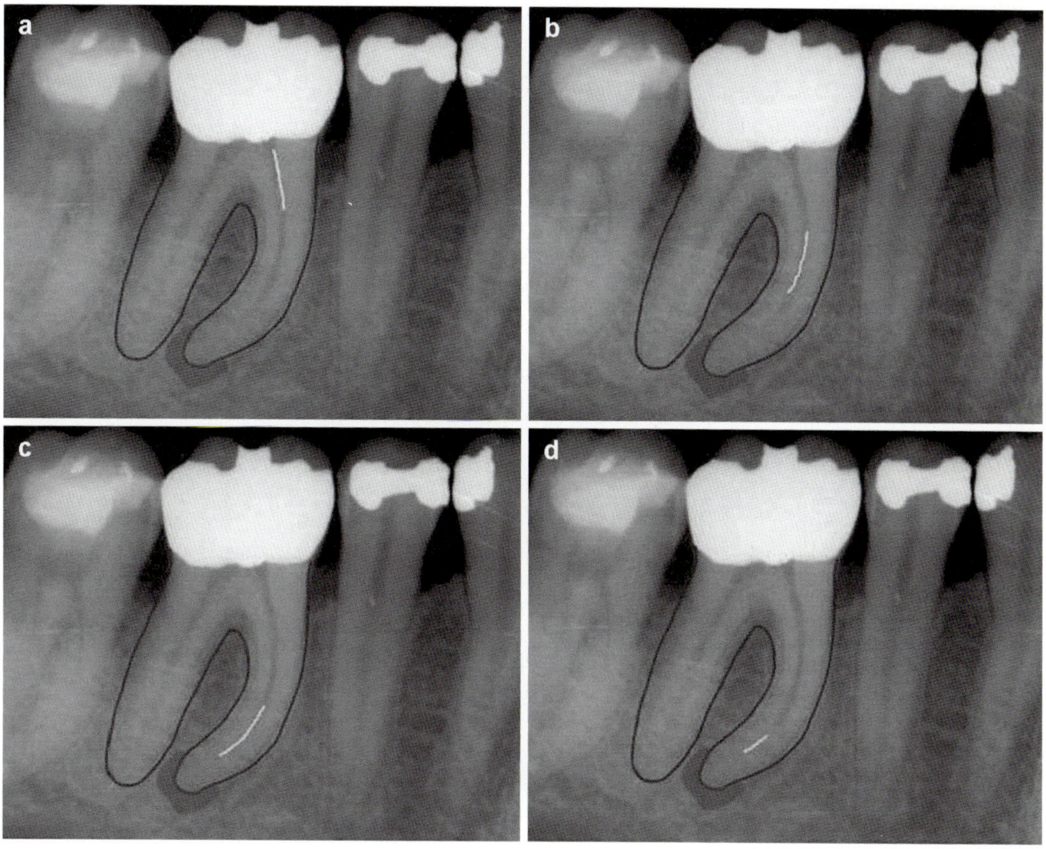

Fig. 11.2 Diagrammatic representation of location of instrument and ease of removal. Note (**a**) coronal fragment, (**b**) middle 1/3 and (**c**) apical at level of curvature. (**d**) Presence of an instrument beyond the curvature where retrieval attempt is the most difficult and adverse risk is greatest

access necessary to visualize the instrument. In some cases, it would be advisable to consider leaving the instrument in situ especially if the instrument can be bypassed or the instrument is at or beyond the curvature where visibility is less than ideal or not possible [67].

Another consideration when determining whether to bypass/leave a separated instrument as opposed to removal is when instrument breakage has occurred. Early instrument breakage increases the likelihood of inadequate chemomechanical canal enlargement, debridement and ineffective microbial load reduction. If the instrument cannot be bypassed and then provided, it is not at the apex or beyond the curvature instrument removal could be recommended, particularly if a peri-radicular preoperative radiolucent lesion is present.

Careful adherence to recommended principles when using rotary NiTi instrumentation would minimize the unfortunate occurrence of instrument fracture. Where instrument fracture has occurred, the patient should be informed, and appropriate referral sought to an endodontist for case assessment. The decision to bypass or leave the instrument in situ must be weighed up with the benefits of removal. Intraoperative factors such as timing of separation, type of instrument fractured, length of instrument fracture, position of fractured instrument (apical, middle and coronal), level of apical curvature in relation to fractured instrument, presence or absence of apical periodontitis, possibility of merged canals, residual dentine thickness and visibility must all be considered before making a decision.

11.3   Retrieval Methods

Manual Retrieval Techniques

The use of hand files (usually Hedstrom files), excavators and various gripping devices such as a fine haemostat or Stieglitz forceps has been advocated for the removal of separated instruments. Hedstrom files can be inserted to varying depths within the root canal system, whereas the other instruments are only useful when the metal object requiring removal extends into the pulp chamber. The use of these instruments is only beneficial when attempting removal of silver points or metal objects that are not bound within the root canal and easily accessible from within the pulp chamber itself (see chapter).

The Masserann Kit

The Masserann Kit (Micro-Mega, Besancon, France) has been used for removal of broken metal objects in the root canal including separated endodontic files. The technique requires removal of excessive amounts of dentine in order to accommodate the various trephines used to expose the metal fragment. This method is not suitable in narrow and curved canals where there is an increased risk of perforation. The kit is ideal for fragments located in the coronal aspect of the root canal where the trephine drill is least likely to result in perforation of the root. The trephine drill is used to expose and accommodate the metal object in its centre whilst cutting a circumferential trough around the object. The smallest tubular extractors have diameters of about 1.20 and 1.50 mm, which limit their safe use to generally larger canals in the anterior teeth.

The Canal Finder System

This system connects to an air motor providing a simultaneous watch winding and reciprocation movement. The amplitude of reciprocal movement is up to 1 mm and increasing the speed decreases the amplitude of motion. The system has been used to bypass and remove fractured instruments within the root canal with varying degrees of success.

Cancellier Kit

The Cancellier Extractor Kit (SybronEndo; Orange, California) contains four different-sized microtubes with diameters of approximately 0.50, 0.60, 0.70 and 0.80 mm. An ultrasonic instrument is typically used to trephine around and expose the coronal 3 mm of an obstruction allowing the internal diameter of the microtube to fit over the coronally exposed obstruction. The pre-fit microtube may now be bonded onto the obstruction with an adhesive, such as cyanoacrylic glue. This removal method is effective for retrieving a non-fluted broken instrument or when there is difficulty retrieving a separated file that is already loose within the root canal. Caution should be exercised to not use too much adhesive, which could inadvertently block a canal.

Instrument Retrieval System (IRS)

The Instrument Removal System (IRS) is a mechanical method for the removal of intracanal obstructions such as silver points, carrier-based obturators or broken endodontic files. The IRS is indicated for the removal of broken instruments that are lodged in the straight portions of the root or partially around the canal curvature. Three instruments with diameters ranging from 0.60 (yellow), 0.80 (red) and 1.00 mm (black) are available comprising of a microtube and screw wedge. Each microtube has a small-sized plastic handle to enhance vision during placement, a side window to improve mechanics and a 45° bevelled end to "scoop up" the coronal end of a broken instrument. The clinician must utilize ultrasonic instrumentation to circumferentially expose 2–3 mm of the separated file. An IRS microtube is then selected that can passively slide through the pre-enlarged canal and drop over the exposed broken instrument. Once the microtube has been positioned, the same colour-coded screw wedge is inserted and slid internally through the microtube's length until it contacts the obstruction. The obstruction is engaged by gently turning the screw wedge handle counterclockwise (CCW). A few degrees of rotation will serve to tighten, wedge and, oftentimes, displace the head of the obstruction through the microtube window. If any given colour-coded screw wedge is unable to achieve a strong hold on the obstruction, then another colour-coded screw wedge may be chosen to improve engagement and successful removal.

Ultrasonics

The most widely used device to remove a broken instrument is to utilize piezoelectric ultrasonic technology and specific ultrasonic instruments. An ultrasonic unit should be set within the lower power settings, and ultrasonic instruments should have a contra-angled design to provide good access and visualization when using the dental operating microscope. Various working tips and dimensions are available and selected whereby the length of the ultrasonic instrument will reach the broken obstruction and its diameter will passively fit affording a favourable line of sight within the canal. Troughing tips such as diamond-coated CPR 3D (15 mm), 4D (20 mm) and 5D (25 mm) (Spartan CPR instruments, Fenton, Missouri), BUC3 (Spartan instruments) and titanium CPR 6 (red 20 mm), CPR 7 (blue 24 mm) and CPR 8 (green 27 mm) are recommended. CPR 3D–5D are active along the sides of the instrument, whereas CPR 6–8 are end cutting and only active at the tips.

To facilitate this straight-line access to the head of the broken instrument, preparation of a 'staging platform' may be necessary. The tip of this ultrasonic instrument is placed in close contact against the obstruction and typically activated within the lower power settings. The clinician should always work at the lowest power setting that will allow for efficiency and safety without the risk of further mishap. The main risks when using ultrasonic instruments deep in the canal are excessive heat generation leading to damage to the attachment apparatus, guttering of root dentine resulting in an increased perforation risk and further separation of the fragment reducing the possibility of retrieval or ultimately fracture of the ultrasonic instrument itself. Ultrasonic preparation below the orifice is conducted dry so the clinician has constant visualization of the energized tip against the broken instrument. Ultrasonic tips have been manufactured with a coating of zirconium nitride (ProUltra ultrasonic instruments; Dentsply, Tulsa, Oklahoma) specifically to function dry. To maintain vision, the dental assistant can direct a continuous stream of air to blow out dentinal dust and use irrigation from time to time. Irrigation not only allows removal of dentine dust that is created thereby improving visibility but also ensures that any potential heat that is generated is dissipated preventing any harmful effects to the surrounding attachment apparatus.

The selected ultrasonic instrument is moved lightly, in a CCW direction, around the obstruction creating a trough and space. This ultrasonic action aims to precisely peel away dentine, exposing the coronal few millimetres of the obstruction safely.

During ultrasonic use, the obstruction should begin to loosen, unwind and then eventually spin within the root canal. Gently wedging the energized tip between the tapered file and canal wall will often cause the broken instrument to abruptly "jump out" of the canal. In other instances, the exposed broken instrument can be 'grabbed' and pulled out using one of the currently available extraction devices discussed earlier.

11.4 Guidelines for Removing a Separated Instrument

Removal of a separated instrument from the root canal is a demanding task that requires time, manual skills and suitable equipment irrespective of which third of the canal the separation has occurred. The knowledge of root canal anatomy and the use of a dental operating microscope to ensure visualization are a prerequisite before considering such a task. Some general recommendations are given:

1. Establish and confirm the location of the instrument fragment radiographically and clinically by tactile sensation. If the fragment is at or beyond the level of the curvature, then retrieval is less predictable.
2. Consider the timing of instrument fracture. The earlier the instrument fractured, the less likely adequate debridement has taken place and the more likely it will be a problem.
3. Consider the presence of a preoperative radiolucency, which may compromise long-term prognosis particularly if a separated instrument is present.

4. Initially an attempt should be made to try and bypass the instrument using small manual K-file instruments. The majority of root canals are elliptical so when an instrument is lodged it may be feasible to bypass. In some cases where apical confluence exists, it may be possible to bypass the instrument utilizing the other canal. No attempt should be made to try and prepare a bypassed instrument using rotary instrumentation. Occasionally when the bypassed instrument is prepared with larger file sizes, the instrument can be loosened or dislodged with further ultrasonics.

5. If bypass is not possible and there is likelihood that the presence of the instrument will jeopardize the prognosis of the case (due consideration to points 1–3 taken into account), then it may be worthwhile considering appropriate referral.

6. Straight-line access to the coronal end of the fragment is important to ensure safe troughing of dentine as possible avoiding the creation of any zipping, transportation and perforation. A 'staging platform' to create straight-line access is created with either modified Gates Glidden (GG) drills or LightSpeed instruments. Careful attention to the anatomy of the root must be made since there is high risk of root perforation and a microscope is a prerequisite before any pre-enlargement. Selecting an appropriate-sized GG drill whose maximum cross-sectional diameter is slightly larger than the visualized instrument creates the staging platform. The GG sizes 1–4 are most typically employed in furcated teeth and have maximum diameters of 0.50, 0.70, 0.90 and 1.10 mm. Cutting it perpendicular to its long axis at its maximum cross-sectional diameter alters the tip of the GG drill. This modified GG is carried into the pre-enlarged canal, rotated at a reduced speed of approximately 300 RPM and directed apically until it lightly contacts the most coronal aspect of the obstruction. This clinical step creates a small staging platform, which facilitates the introduction of an ultrasonic instrument. If properly performed, straight-line coronal and radicular access, in conjunction with magnification and lighting, should enable the clinician to fully visualize the most coronal aspect of a broken instrument. To facilitate excellent vision to the intra-radicular obstruction, the canal should be vigorously flushed and thoroughly dried prior to beginning ultrasonic procedures. Note the GG drill should only be used in the straight portion of the canal and no attempts made to attempt any negotiation of canal curvatures (Fig. 11.3).

7. Prior to performing any radicular instrument removal techniques, it is wise to place cotton pellets over other exposed orifices, if present, to prevent the nuisance re-entry of the fragment into another canal system during the removal process.

8. Appropriate ultrasonic instrumentation is carried out to create a trough of 2–3 mm deep around the coronal fragment circumferentially. Troughing tips are selected according to location of the fragment, and the process is carried out in a controlled and predictable manner with the aid of illumination and appropriate magnification. Care must be taken when using titanium alloy ultrasonic instruments such as CPR 6–8, which are slender, long and parallel sided enabling cutting at the tip. Although extremely flexible, the tip of the instrument can be prone to breakage if too much force is applied or the power setting is too high. Extreme caution should be exercised when using these instruments and a light touch (similar to using a lead pencil) is advocated. The tips are moved counterclockwise around the fractured instrument to disengage it from the surrounding dentine. The process of dentine removal is carried out slowly and carefully ensuring intermittent water and air coolant use. Occasionally the application of a second diamond-coated CPR 5D tip can be activated once in contact the metal fragment only. Care must be taken when this tip is used near dentine since it is very aggressive. The application of two different types of metal tips at two different frequencies can produce an effect whereby the metal fragment can bounce

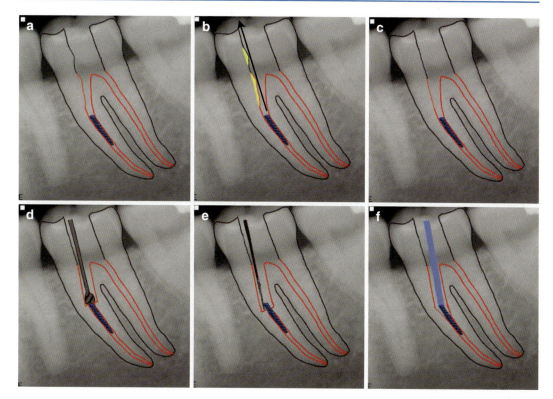

Fig. 11.3 Clinical diagrams representing removal of a separated instrument. Note (**a**) preoperative view demonstrating presence of separated file in the middle 1/3 of the mesial root. (**b**) and (**c**) First step is to remove all coronal interferences and ensure straight-line access is present.

(**d**) A modified gates glidden drill is used to create a staging platform. (**e**) Ultrasonics are used to carefully trephine around the file. (**f**) Removal of the loosened file can be carried out using appropriate retrieval technique of choice

within the canal more coronally. A stainless steel metal fragment will absorb the ultrasonic energy bodily showing movement earlier on. A nickel-titanium file on the other hand will absorb the energy at the tip at point of contact, which can result in the fragment getting smaller as the flutes are worn away. It is therefore important to not touch the fragment as much as possible, and any ultrasonic energy that is applied is relayed through the surrounding dentine ensuring the whole file fragment can be removed (Fig. 11.3).

9. When the fragment shows movement, a small 06 or 08 K-file can be used to try and bypass the loose piece. Once bypassed, you have regained the lost canal space on initial separation. Larger file diameters should be gradually bypassed further opening canal space around the instrument. Further ultrasonic instrumentation will help to jar the instrument causing further bouncing more coronally. It is important to remember that once bypassed this apical patency beyond the separated fragment should be maintained. It is very easy to push the loosened fragment further apically particularly if larger K-files are advanced in succession too quickly.

10. It is ill advised to pass another rotary instrument alongside the separated fragment if it has not been removed. Introduction of a Hedstrom file may be possible to try and further engage the loose fragment to allow removal. If the fragment lies in the coronal or middle 1/3, it may be possible to use one of the retrieval methods discussed earlier.

11. Attempts at removal of an instrument beyond the apical curvature are high risk and probably futile. The amount of dentine that can be safely removed is minimal and the risk of

perforation is high. Remember not all cases result in retrieval. Occasionally if the instrument has been successfully bypassed, then canal shaping and sealing the fragment in place may be successful.

12. Should retrieval attempts prove unsuccessful without any further compromise to the tooth and symptomology continues, then alternative treatment options such as apical surgery, intentional reimplantation or extraction should be considered.

13. The patient must always be informed of the presence of any instrument fracture and the potential risks outlined prior to considering retrieval. Treatment objectives should be aimed at conserving as much tooth as possible. The ability to access and remove a broken instrument will be influenced by the cross sectional diameter, length and curvature of the canal. As a rule of thumb if the separated instrument cannot be visualized it will be highly unlikely to be retrieved. Furthermore retrieval attempts of any such obstruction will increase the chances of iatrogenic complications such as root perforation further compromising the outcome.

11.5 Clinical Cases

Case 1: Bypassing a Separated Instrument A fit and healthy 29-year-old patient was referred for endodontic retreatment of tooth 16. The general dental practitioner noted a separated stainless steel K-file was present in the mesiobuccal root. Clinical examination revealed the tooth was asymptomatic. Radiographic findings confirmed previous endodontic treatment with scantily condensed root fillings short of respective apices. A separated instrument was confirmed in the apical 1/3 of the MB root beyond the curvature. An extensive peri-radicular radiolucency was seen. The tooth was dismantled, restorability assessed and deemed suitable for cast restoration post treatment. Previous root fillings were removed using mechanical and chemical means (Hedstrom files and chloroform wicking). Patency was gained in the DB and P canals. The MB1 canal was blocked and the instrument could not be bypassed. Ultrasonic troughing was carried out mesially to reveal additional untreated MB2 and MB3 canals. MB1, MB2 and MB3 canals all merged at the peri-apex. Chemomechanical preparation was completed using stainless steel hand files with a 0.5 mm step-back increment using sodium hypochlorite 2.5 % solution. An intra-canal dressing of calcium hydroxide was placed for 4 weeks. The five canals were obturated using cold lateral compaction apically and warm lateral compaction using ZnOE sealer (Roth cement). The tooth was restored with an amalgam Nayyar core. This case demonstrates the complexity of assessing each case individually, and the decision to remove, leave and bypass an instrument not only depends on the location of the instrument but also additional factors. In this case, the presence of extra canals allowed chemical disinfection to be carried out in the apical 1/3 of the mesial root increasing the probability of success. Removal of the instrument would have risked perforation, and apicectomy would have been the only option if healing was not evident (Fig. 11.4).

Case 2: Leaving a Separated Instrument in Situ A 46-year-old gentleman was referred to specialist practice for the management of a separated instrument in the apical 1/3 of the mesio-buccal root of the tooth 46 (Fig. 11.5). The general dental practitioner had attempted root canal treatment through the existing cast restoration and had fractured a 25/06 nickel-titanium rotary instrument during chemomechanical preparation. The patient was asymptomatic at clinical examination. Radiographic examination confirmed the presence of a separated instrument in the apical 1/3 beyond the curvature in the mesio-buccal root. Access preparation confirmed the presence of the instrument, which could not be bypassed. The instrument could not be visualized under the dental operating microscope, and so there was no indication to carry out any staging platform procedures. The risk of perforation was deemed high. Since the patient was asymptomatic, a decision was made to leave the instrument in situ knowing that many further problems would require either surgical apicectomy or extraction. Chemomechanical preparation was completed, and an intra-canal dressing of

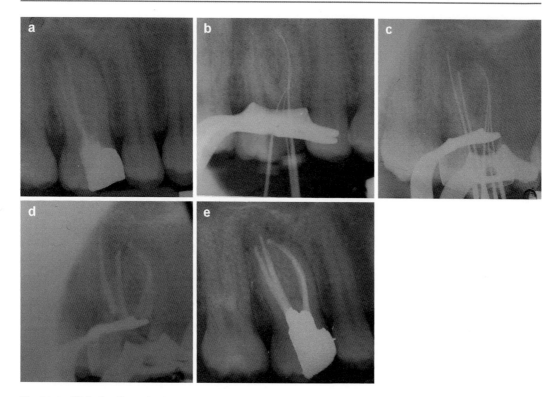

Fig. 11.4 Clinical radiographs demonstrating endodontic re-treatment and bypassing of a separated instrument in tooth 16. Note (**a**) preoperative view of tooth 16 showing an extensive periradicular radiolucency associated with the periapex of tooth 16. A separated stainless steel K-file was noted in MB1 in the apical 1/3 beyond the curvature. (**b**) Removal of previous gutta-percha root filling material, apical patency in P and DB canals and ultrasonic trough- ing mesially to confirm additional MB2 and MB3. Note MB1, MB2 and MB3 were confluent in the apical 1/3. The MB1 instrument could not be removed or bypassed. A decision was made to leave the instrument in situ. (**c**) Master apical file radiograph of P, DB, MB1, MB2 and MB3 canals. (**d**) Mid-fill radiograph and (**e**) post-opera- tive view following obturation and amalgam coronal restoration

calcium hydroxide was placed for 3 months. The patient remained asymptomatic and was keen to retain the tooth at the review appointment. Obturation of the case was completed using a warm vertical compaction technique using AH plus cement. The tooth was temporized accord- ingly and returned to the general dental practitio- ner for permanent coronal core restoration.

Case 3: Removal of a Separated Instrument in the Coronal 1/3rd A 56-year-old patient was referred to specialist practice for the management of tooth 26. A separated instrument (endodontic explorer) was present in the palatal canal and so prevented canal preparation (Fig. 11.6). Clinical radiographs confirmed a radiopaque tapered object in the palatal canal. A peri-radicular

radiolucency was associated with the palatal root. Access was refined and the instrument verified clinically. Using the operating dental microscope, the instrument could be fully visualized. Careful ultrasonic troughing was performed circumferen- tially around the instrument resulting in its removal.

Case 4: Removal of Separated Lentulo Spiral Filler A 30-year-old female patient was referred for endodontic management of tooth 14. The patient had recently experienced severe pain and discomfort with the tooth prompting her to seek dental treatment. Her general dental practitioner had carried out an emergency pulp extirpation with minimal mechanical preparation. During placement of an inter-appointment dressing, a

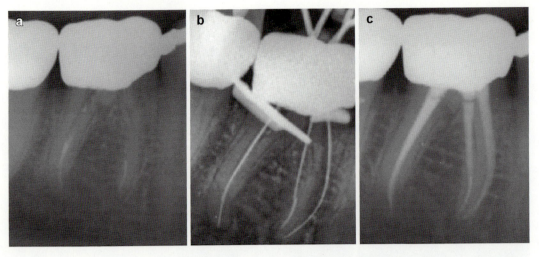

Fig. 11.5 Clinical radiographs demonstrating endodontic treatment of tooth 46 with a separated 25/06 NiTi instrument in the mesiobuccal root. Note (**a**) preoperative treatment confirming radio-opaque dressing in the distal canal and separated instrument in the MB root. The instrument was in the apical 1/3 beyond the curvature. (**b**) Working length radiograph. Note the instrument in the MB root could not be visualized with the dental operating microscope. Staging platform creation would have resulted in unnecessary coronal/middle 1/3 over-preparation with risk of perforation that could lead to early demise of the tooth. The patient remained asymptomatic despite instrument fracture. (**c**) Completed obturation using warm vertical compaction and AH Plus cement. The instrument that fractured was a finishing file and so much of the chemomechanical disinfection has been completed prior to separation. The patient understands that any future problems including persistence or enlargement of the periapical lesion will require a further surgical procedure or extraction

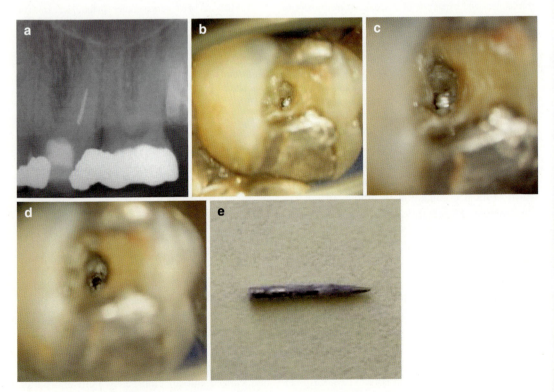

Fig. 11.6 Clinical photographs and radiographs showing (**a**) preoperative view with separated endodontic explorer in the palatal canal (**b**) and (**c**) microscopic views showing instrument at both low and high power (note space between the instrument and canal wall). (**d**) and (**e**) Removal of instrument following the use of ultrasonic instrumentation

#25 Lentulo spiral filler had fractured in the buccal canal. Clinical examination revealed the tooth was slightly tender to percussion although most of her symptoms had improved. Radiographic examination confirmed a Lentulo spiral filler that had separated. A peri-radicular radiolucency was noted at the peri-apex. Access cavity preparation was refined with care to avoid further fracture of the coronal segment of the instrument. The Lentulo spiral filler could be visualized in the coronal access chamber. Initially the palatal canal was instrumented and patency achieved. Small 08 and 10 K-files were used to bypass the Lentulo spiral filler fragment in the buccal canal, and patency was achieved. Further instrument sizes #15 and greater could not negotiate to length.

Ultrasonics was applied at a low power setting and the instrument was loosened. Stieglitz forceps were used to grasp the end of the spiral filler fragment, and using an anticlockwise motion, the fragment was removed from the canal. Chemomechanical preparation was completed with no further complications (Fig. 11.7).

Case 5: Removal of a Separated Instrument in the Apical 1/3ʳᵈ During root canal treatment, a 25/06 nickel-titanium rotary file separated in the mesial root of tooth 46. The instrument had separated at the apex of the mesiobuccal root. Following access cavity preparation, the instrument could be visualized using

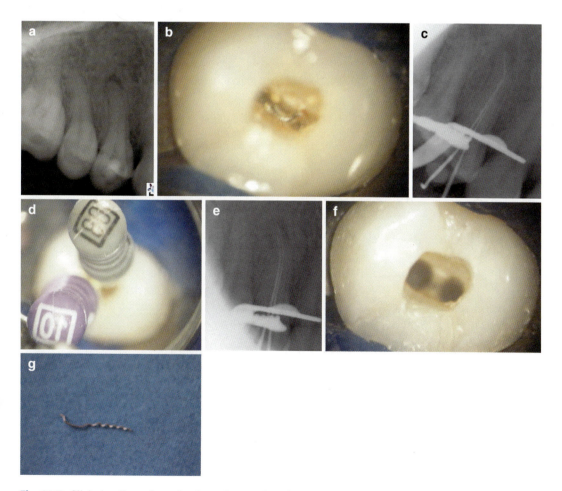

Fig. 11.7 Clinical radiographs and colour photographs demonstrating removal of a fractured Lentulo spiral filler in tooth 14. Note (**a**) preoperative view demonstrating separated instrument fragment. (**b**) View of instrument under the microscope. (**c**) and (**d**) Initial bypassing of instrument. (**e**) Working length radiograph confirming removal of instrument. (**f**) Access cavity and B and P canals following canal preparation completion. (**g**) Separated instrument following removal

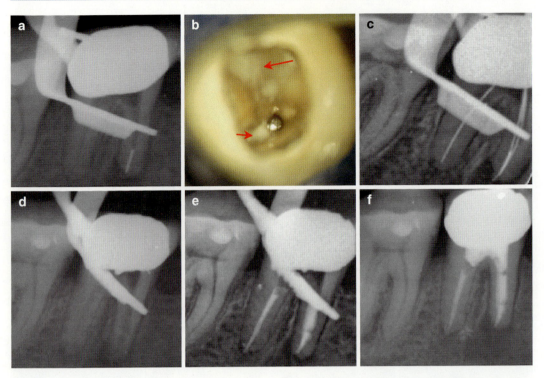

Fig. 11.8 Clinical radiographs and photograph demonstrating instrument removal in the apical 1/3rd of the mesio-buccal root of tooth 46. Note (**a**) pre-operative radiograph demonstrating instrument located in the apical 1/3rd of the mesio-buccal root at the apex. Minimal curvature was noted. (**b**) Intra-operative microscopic view. The distal and mesio-lingual canals were temporarily sealed with cotton wool (*red arrows*) to prevent the instrument accidentally falling into and causing further blockage. The instrument could be visualized. (**c**) Master apical file radiograph showing the instrument could be bypassed. (**d**) Following staging platform creation with a modified gates glidden drill and careful ultrasonic application the instrument was removed safely. (**e**) and (**f**) Completed obturation. Note over-preparation in the mesial root as a result of instrument removal techniques. Care must always be observed since overzealous preparation can result in root perforation and increased risk of root fracture in the long term. Instruments separated at the apex may also be inadvertently pushed beyond the confines of the canal requiring a further surgical procedure

a dental operating microscope. A staging platform was created using a modified Gates Glidden drill with care to avoid overpreparation in the danger zones. K-files were used and the instrument could be bypassed. The distal canal and mesiolingual canal were temporarily sealed with cotton wool to avoid further instrument blockage should the instrument be removed. Ultrasonic troughing was carefully applied with minimal apical pressure circumferentially around the instrument. After 10 min of application, the instrument could be seen to loosen eventually resulting in its removal. Chemomechanical preparation was completed and an intra-canal dressing of calcium hydroxide placed for 7 days. The patient was seen for

obturation of the canals prior to being sent back to his general dental practitioner for permanent coronal restoration placement (Fig. 11.8).

Clinical Hints and Tips for Strategies Aimed to Reduce File Breakage
- Always create a glide path and ensure patency with small hand files (#10).
- Ensure straight-line access.
- Use a crown-down technique depending on the instrument system ensuring a torque-controlled electric motor at the recommended manufacturer's settings for that particular instrument is used.

- Avoid triggering the autoreverse mode by advancing the instrument slowly or switching to a high torque setting.
- Use a light touch only, never pushing hard on any instrument until resistance is met.
- Use a pecking motion with increments as large as possible depending on canal anatomy.
- Do not prepare root canals in a dry operating field.
- Practice is key and attending workshops/courses and utilizing extracted teeth and blocks will allow the operator to gain valuable tactile skills needed to prevent instrument failure.
- Do not leave any rotary file in one place, particularly in curved canals.
- Examine the files and flutes regularly during use, preferably with magnification. Evidence of unwinding of any instrument should alert the clinician to difficult anatomy and the file discarded immediately.
- Instrumentation of root canals should be a timely procedure with due care.
- Difficult canal anatomy should be recognized early. Radius of curvatures and angles of curvatures should be predetermined to alert the clinician to the possibility of an adverse outcome.
- Care should be excised in cases where confluent canals exist. Typically mesial roots of lower molars where an abrupt curvature due to confluence will increase the risk of file separation.

References

1. McGuigan MB, Louca C, Duncan HF. Endodontic instrument fracture: causes and prevention. Br Dent J. 2013;214(7):341–8.
2. McGuigan MB, Louca C, Duncan HF. Clinical decision-making after endodontic instrument fracture. Br Dent J. 2013;214(8):395–400.
3. McGuigan MB, Louca C, Duncan HF. The impact of fractured endodontic instruments on treatment outcome. Br Dent J. 2013;214(6):285–9.
4. Rzhanov EA, Belyaeva TS. Design features of rotary root canal instruments. ENDO (Lond Engl). 2012; 6(1):29–39.
5. ISO 3630–1. Dentistry – root canal instruments – part 1: general requirements and test methods. 2nd ed. Switzerland: International Organization for Standardization; 2008.
6. Buehler WH, Cross WB. 55-Nitinol unique wire alloy with memory. Wire J. 1969;2:41–9.
7. Walia HM, Brantley WA, Gerstein H. An initial investigation of the bending and torsional properties of Nitinol root canal files. J Endod. 1988;14:346–51.
8. Cho OI, Versluis A, Cheung GS, Ha JH, Hur B, Kim HC. Cyclic fatigue resistance tests of Nickel-Titanium rotary files using simulated canal and weight loading conditions. Restor Dent Endod. 2013;38(1):31–5.
9. Pruett JP, Clement DJ, Carnes Jr DJ. Cyclic fatigue testing of nickel-titanium endodontic instruments. J Endod. 1997;23(2):77–85.
10. Sattapan B, Palamara JE, Messer HH. Torque during canal instrumentation using rotary nickel-titanium files. J Endod. 2000;26(3):156–60.
11. Yao JH, Schwartz SA, Beeson TJ. Cyclic fatigue of three types of rotary nickel-titanium files in a dynamic model. J Endod. 2006;32(1):55–7.
12. Alapati SB, Brantley WA, Lijima M. Metallurgical characterization of a new nickel-titanium wire for rotary endodontic instruments. J Endod. 2009;35: 1589–93.
13. Al-Hadlaq SMS, Aljarbou FA, Althumairy RI. Evaluation of cyclic flexural fatigue of M-Wire nickel-titanium rotary instruments. J Endod. 2010; 36:305–7.
14. Ye J, Gao Y. Metallurgical characterization of M-Wire nickel-titanium shape memory alloy used for endodontic rotary instruments during low cyclic-fatigue. J Endod. 2012;38:105–7.
15. Gambarini G, Grande NM, Plotino G, Somma F, Garala M, De Luca M, Testarelli L. Fatigue resistance of engine-driven rotary nickel-titanium instruments produced by new manufacturing methods. J Endod. 2008;34:1003–5.
16. The twisted file brochure. Orange: Sybron Endo; 2008. Instructions for the use of the Twisted file system. Available at http://www.devosendo.nl/uploads/pdf/56_Twisted%20File.pdf (Accessed on 1st Dec 2015).
17. Shen Y, Qian W, Abtin H, Gao Y, Haapasalo M. Fatigue testing of controlled memory wire nickel-titanium rotary instruments. J Endod. 2011;37: 997–1001.
18. Shen Y, Zhou HM, Zheng YF, Campbell L, Peng B. and Haapasalo M. Metallurgical characterization of controlled memory wire nickel-titanium rotary instruments. J Endod 2011; 37(11);1566–1571.
19. Yared GM, Bou Dagher FE, Machtou P. Failure of profile instruments used with high and low torque motors. Int Endod J. 2001;34(1):471–5.
20. Yared GM, Bou Dagher FE, Machtou P, Kulkarni GK. Influence of rotational speed, torque and operator proficiency on failure of Greater Taper Files. Int Endod J. 2002;35(1):7–12.
21. Patel S. Rhode J. A Practical guide to endodontic access cavity preparation in molar teeth. Brit Dent J 2007;203;133–140
22. Yared GM, Kulkarni GK. Failure of profile Ni-Ti instruments used by inexperienced operator under

access limitations. Int Endod J. 2002;35(6): 536–41.

23. Mounce R. Endodontic K-files: invaluable endangered species or ready for the Smithsonian? Dent Today. 2005;24:102–4.

24. Varela-Patino P, Martin-Biedman B, Rodriguez LC, Cantatore G, Bahillo JG. The influence of a manual glide path on the separation rate of Ni-Ti Rotary instruments. J Endod. 2005;31:114–6.

25. Van der Vyver PJ. Creating a glide path for rotary instruments: part one. Endod Prac. 2011:40–3.

26. Van der Vyver PJ. Creating a glide path for rotary instruments: part two. Endod Prac. 2011:46–53.

27. Sontag D, Stachniss-Carp S, Stachniss V. Determination of root canal curvatures before and after canal preparation (part 1): a literature review. Aust Endod J. 2005;31(3):89–93.

28. Gunday M, Sasak H, Garip Y. A comparative study of three different root canal curvature measurement techniques and measuring the canal access angle in curved canals. J Endod. 2005;31:796–8.

29. Schneider SW. A comparison of canal preparations in straight and curved root canals. Oral Surg Oral Med Oral Pathol. 1971;32:271–5.

30. Zuolo ML, Walton RE. Instrument deterioration with usage: nickel-titanium vs stainless steel. Quintessence Int. 1997;28:397–402.

31. Gambarini G. Cyclic fatigue of profile rotary instruments after prolonged clinical use. Int Endod J. 2001;34:386–9.

32. Arens FC, Hoen MM, Steiman HR, Dietz Jr GC. Evaluation of single use rotary nickel-titanium instruments. J Endod. 2003;29:664–6.

33. Yared G. Canal preparation using only one Ni-Ti rotary instrument; preliminary observations. Int Endod J. 2008;41:339–44.

34. Azarpazhooh A, Fillery ED. Prion disease: the implications for dentistry. J Endod. 2008;34(10):1158–66.

35. Walker T, Budge C, Vassey M, Sutton JM, Raven ND, Marsh PD, Bennett P. vCJD and the cleanability of endodontic files: a case for single use. Quintessence Int. 2009;3(2):115–20.

36. Walsh H. The hybrid concept of nickel-titanium rotary instrumentation. Dent Clin N Am. 2004;48: 183–202.

37. Li UM, Lee BS, Shih CT, Lan WH, Lin CP. Cyclic fatigue on endodontic nickel-titanium rotary instruments: static and dynamic tests. J Endod. 2002; 28(6):448–51.

38. Yared GM, Bou Dagher FE, Machtou P. Influence of rotational speed, torque and operator's proficiency on ProFile failure. Int Endod J. 2001;34:47–53.

39. Rapisarda E, Bonaccorso A, Tripi TR, Condorelli GG, Torrisi L. Wear of nickel-titanium endodontic instruments evaluated by scanning electron microscopy: effect of ion implantation. J Endod. 2001; 27:588–92.

40. Kuhn G, Tavernier B, Jordan L. Influence of structure on nickel-titanium endodontic instruments failure. J Endod. 2001;27:516–20.

41. Gabel WP, Hoen M, Steiman HR, Pink FE, Dietz R. Effect of rotational speed on nickel-titanium file distortion. J Endod. 1999;25:752–4.

42. Martin B, Zelada G, Varela P, Bahillo JG, Magan F, Ahn S, Rodriguez C. Factors influencing the fracture of nickel-titanium rotary instruments. Int Endod J. 2003;36:262–6.

43. Gambarini G. Rationale for the use of low-torque endodontic motors in root canal instrumentation. Endod Dent Traumatol. 2000;16:95–100.

44. Berutti E, Negro AR, Lendini M, Pasqualini D. Influence of manual pre-flaring and torque on the failure rate of ProTaper rotary instruments. J Endod. 2004;30:228–30.

45. Baumgartner JC, Mader CL. A scanning electron microscopic evaluation of four root canal irrigation regimes. J Endod. 1987;13:147–57.

46. McSpadden JT. Mastering endodontic instrumentation. Ramsey: Arbor Books; 2007. p. 49.

47. Dederich DN, Zakariasen KL. The effect of cyclic axial motion on rotary endodontic instrument fatigue. Oral Surg Oral Med Oral Pathol. 1986;61:192–6.

48. Gernhardt CR. One shape- a single file NiTi system for root canal instrumentation used in continuous rotation. Quintessence Int. 2013;7(3):211–6.

49. Roane JB, Sabala C, Duncanson Jr MG. The 'balanced forced' concept for instrumentation of curved canals. J Endod. 1985;11:203–11.

50. Roane JB, Sabala C. Clockwise or counter clockwise? J Endod. 1984;10:349–53.

51. Southward DW, Oswald RJ, Natkin E. Instrumentation of curved molar root canals with the Roane technique. J Endod. 1987;13:479–89.

52. Varelo-Patino P, Ibanez-Parraga A, Rivas-Mundina B, Cantatore G, Otero XL, Martin-Biedma B. Alternating versus continuous rotation: a comparative study on the effect of instrument life. J Endod. 2010;36: 157–9.

53. De-Deus G, Moreira EJ, Lopes HP, Elias CN. Extended cyclic fatigue life of F2 ProTaper instruments used in reciprocating movement. Int Endod J. 2010;43:1063–8.

54. Crump MC, Natkin E. Relationship of broken root canal instruments to endodontic case prognosis: a clinical investigation. J Am Dent Assoc. 1970; 80:1341–7.

55. Spili P, Parashos P, Messer HH. The impact of instrument fracture on outcome of endodontic treatment. J Endod. 2005;31:845–50.

56. Panitvisai P, Parunnit P, Sathorn C, Messer HH. Impact of a retained instrument on treatment outcome: a systematic review and meta-analysis. J Endod. 2010; 36(5):775–80.

57. Nevares G, Cunha RS, Zuolo ML, Da Silveira Bueno CE. Success rates for removing or bypassing fractured instruments: a prospective clinical study. J Endod. 2012;38(4):442–4.

58. Masserann J. New method for extracting metallic fragments from canals. Inf Dent. 1972;54: 3987–4005.

59. Gettleman BH, Spriggs KA, ElDeeb ME, Messer HH. Removal of canal obstructions with the Endo Extractor. J Endod. 1991;17:608–11.
60. Hulsmann M. Methods for removing metal obstructions from the root canal. Endod Dent Traumatol. 1993;9:223–37.
61. Souyave LC, Inglis AT, Alcalay M. Removal of fractured endodontic instruments using ultrasonics. Br Dent J. 1985;159:251–3.
62. Nagai O, Tani N, Kayabe Y, Kodama S, Osada T. Ultrasonic removal of broken instruments in root canals. Int Endod J. 1986;19:298–304.
63. Plotino G, Pameijer CH, Grande NM, Somma F. Ultrasonics in endodontics: a review of the literature. J Endod. 2007;33(2):81–95.
64. Ruddle CJ. Micro-endodontic non-surgical retreatment. Dent Clin North Am. 1997;41:429–54.
65. Ruddle CJ. Broken instrument removal. The endodontic challenge. Dent Today. 2002;21:70–2. 4, 6.
66. Souter NJ, Messer HH. Complications associated with fractured file removal using an ultrasonic technique. J Endod. 2005;31:450–2.
67. Al-Fouzan KS. Incidence of rotary profile instrument fracture and the potential for bypassing in vivo. Int Endod J. 2003;36:864–7.

Iatrogenic Perforations

12

Bobby Patel

Summary

Root perforation may occur during endodontic procedures compromising both the tooth and periodontium and affecting the long-term prognosis. Crestal level perforations are difficult to manage due to proximity to the epithelial attachment resulting in inflammation, bone resorption and necrosis. Management of root perforations is dependant on time of perforation to repair, location and size. Methods to treat perforations are outlined including the internal matrix concept and use of materials capable of inducing osteogenesis and cementogenesis where applicable.

Clinical Relevance

Accidental root perforations can occur due to a number of iatrogenic errors involving access preparation, canal identification and location, during root canal instrumentation and post space preparation. Methods employed to avoid such errors and diagnosis and management where present are discussed. Once a perforation has been confirmed, appropriate management for immediate sealing including referral where necessary is a prerequisite to ensure success in the long term. In particular, crestal perforations and their intimate relationship with surrounding epithelial attachment risk long-term unfavourable outcome if not managed in a timely and correct fashion.

B. Patel, BDS MFDS MClinDent MRD MRACDS
Specialist Endodontist, Brindabella Specialist Centre, Canberra, ACT, Australia
e-mail: bobbypatel@me.com

12.1 Overview of Root Perforations and Their Management

A root perforation is a mechanical or pathologic communication formed between the supporting periodontal apparatus of the tooth and the root canal system [1–3]. Perforations are caused by either iatrogenic (endodontic and restorative treatments) or pathological (root resorption) errors or caries [4].

A study evaluating the aetiology and location of 55 root perforations seen in a dental school found that almost 50 % of the perforations were due to endodontic treatment and slightly more than 50 % were due to prosthodontic treatment. The maxillary canine tooth was the most frequently perforated tooth, followed by the lateral incisor, premolars and first molars. The anterior teeth resulted in buccal perforations due to access problems. In 53 % of cases reported, the perforation was a direct result of post space preparation [5].

The prognostic factors that determine success of a perforation repair are the time interval between occurrence of perforation and its repair, the location of the perforation and the size. Time of occurrence is significant in terms of risk of apical migration of the epithelium attachment resulting in a periodontal pocket and associated defect. The best time to repair a perforation to minimize emergence of an infection is immediately after occurrence [6]. The location of the perforation in terms of its position in relation to the level of epithelium attachment and crestal bone is critical to long-term success. The prognosis for cases where the perforation defect is near to this anatomical area is poor due to microbiological contamination [6]. Furcal perforations, which are not treated immediately, can lead to persistent inflammation, rapid periodontal breakdown and a permanent communication with the oral cavity [6]. Larger size perforations may not respond to repair as well compared to a smaller defects [7] (Fig. 12.1).

The diagnosis of an iatrogenic root perforation is made by good vision and lightning (use of the dental operating microscope), radiographic assessment and use of electronic apex locators. Crown-root alignment should be evaluated particularly where a cast restoration has been placed. Radiographs to evaluate the size, shape and depth of the pulp chamber, relative to the furcal floor, are an essential preoperative prerequisite. The author recommends taking a parallel bitewing radiograph as well as a parallel periapical and a 15° horizontal tube shift x-ray as part of the routine endodontic assessment of a case [8–11]. Cone beam CT radiography has been shown to have a higher sensitivity to detect strip perforations and root perforations after root canal treatment in mandibular molar teeth [12].

A narrow isolated periodontal defect may be a possible sign of periodontal breakdown as a result of a perforation and must be differentiated from the differential diagnosis of localized periodontal disease and vertical root fracture [13].

The first step in managing non-surgical orthograde root perforations is to control the haemorrhage at the site of the perforation using either pressure or irrigation. Care must be taken not to irrigate sodium hypochlorite solution through the perforation site into the surrounding tissues for risk of a hypochlorite accident [14]. An internal matrix technique using a resorbable matrix such as decalcified freeze-dried bone, hydroxyapatite and calcium sulfate and restorable collagen with MTA may be placed in which a sealing material can be condensed [7, 15–18]. Numerous sealing materials have been used over the years with varying degrees of success. Glass ionomer cement, resin-ionomers and mineral trioxide aggregate depending on type of perforation (size and location) have been recommended and used with success [19–23].

Indications for a surgical approach include large perforations, perforations as a result of resorption and failure of healing following a non-surgical orthograde approach [24]. Guided tissue

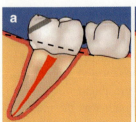 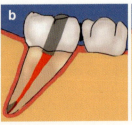 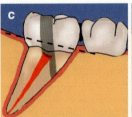 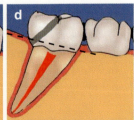

Fig. 12.1 Representing different levels of perforation and their associated prognosis. (**a**) A lateral perforation coronal to the attachment level can be included in the restoration, and provided a seal is achievable should have no bearing on outcome. (**b**) and (**c**) Lateral perforations in the middle or apical portion of the root canal are treated like accessory anatomy, and provided a good endodontic seal is achievable, then this should have no bearing on prognosis in the long term. (**d**) A lateral perforation at or just apical to the attachment level and furcal perforations have the least favourable prognosis

regeneration has been attempted in the management of endodontic perforations with some success in case reports by acting as barrier for apical epithelial migration [25].

Perforation repairs can be performed with a high level of success, but long-term studies, ideally prospective, are still lacking to evaluate their success [26].

12.2 Classification of Root Perforations

The following table is a classification of root perforations which is based on the key prognostic factors that affects long-term outcome, namely, size and location of perforation and timeline from diagnosis to repair (Table 12.1).

12.3 Diagnosis of Root Perforations

Early recognition of a root perforation is crucial to the long-term prognosis. Sudden bleeding or pain during instrumentation of the root canals or post space preparation in the teeth is an important sign that should alert the clinician to the possibility of an iatrogenic error resulting in a perforation. The presence of blood on paper points, particularly on the coronal or middle 1/3, may also be indicative of such a mishap. One must be aware that over-instrumentation beyond the apical foramina or remaining pulp tissue remnants within the canal system can also result in evidence of blood on a paper points.

A more reliable method is to use an electronic apex locator (EAL). The working length should always be verified with an EAL, and a premature reading significantly shorter than the estimated length in combination with profuse bleeding is often a good indicator of the presence of a perforation.

The diagnostic value of a radiograph can be useful when a file is placed to this level often demonstrating that the file is misplaced beyond the confines of the canal into the periodontal tissues. If the perforation is either buccal or lin-

Table 12.1 Root perforation classification and prognosis according to type

(i) *Fresh perforation*
Perforation that has occurred and treated at the same time under aseptic conditions. The prognosis should be favourable
(ii) *Old perforation*
Previously not treated with likely bacterial infection. The prognosis is questionable depending on apical migration of epithelium as a result of chronic inflammation/presence of narrow probing profile
(iii) *Small perforation*
A perforation whose diameter is smaller than a #20 endodontic instrument. Mechanical damage to adjacent tissue is minimal and the opportunity to seal is easy. The prognosis is good
(iv) *Large perforation*
This type of perforation may occur during post preparation, during access preparation or as a result of over-instrumentation/strip perforation resulting in significant tissue damage and difficulty in providing an adequate seal. The prognosis is deemed questionable
(v) *Coronal perforation*
A perforation that is coronal to the level of the crestal bone and epithelial attachment with minimal damage to the adjacent supporting tissues. The ability to seal in terms of access to the perforation site is good. The prognosis is good
(vi) *Crestal perforation*
The perforation is at the level of the epithelial attachment into the crestal bone. The prognosis is questionable
(vii) *Apical perforation*
The perforation site is apical to the crestal bone and epithelial attachment. The prognosis should be good provided the perforation site remains aseptic with no microbial contamination. The prognosis should be good provided no orthograde root filling material is extruded through this artificial anatomy

Adapted from Fuss and Trope 1996 [3]

gual, then the diagnostic yield of the radiograph is limited.

The use of a dental operating microscope is another effective tool in the detection of perforations and management thereafter. High magnification combined with illumination will often allow direct unimpeded visualization of the perforation within the straight portion of the root canal.

If a perforation has been present for some time and there has been communication with the perforation site and attachment level at crestal bone level, then a narrow probing profile may be detected in this area. The ingress of bacteria within this communication will result in further apical migration of epithelial attachment resulting in a narrow pocket depth.

12.4 Iatrogenic Causes of Root Perforation

Access preparation

A well-designed and executed access cavity is an essential objective whereby straight-line access is gained to the root canal system without overzealous tooth removal thereby preserving the overall integrity of the tooth (Fig. 12.2).

Due consideration should be given to the orientation of the tooth in question and in particular any deviation of the crown and root along the long axis of the tooth. This can typically occur in cases where a crown has been placed or where the tooth is dilacerated, rotated or imbricated (Fig. 12.3).

Furcation perforations occurring typically in the floor of the posterior molar teeth usually occur during access preparation when due care has not been given to the level of the furcation relative to the crown. A preoperative bitewing radiograph will give the clinician an excellent idea as to the approximate depth to the pulp chamber. Digital radiographic systems allow for manipulation of the image taken and

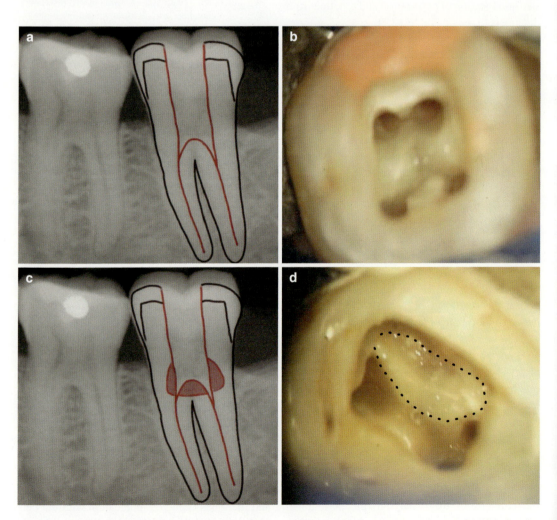

Fig. 12.2 Clinical photograph demonstrating (**a**) and (**b**) straight-line access and retention of as much tooth structure as possible and (**c**) and (**d**) inappropriate access preparation resulting in over-preparation and risk of perforation (*dotted area*)

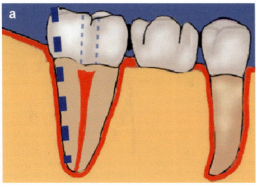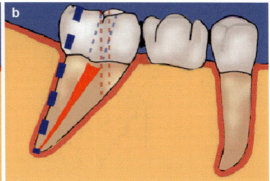

Fig. 12.3 Diagrams showing crown-root mismatch which can account for iatrogenic perforation during access cavity preparation. High risk when the crown of the tooth is a crown or bridge abutment. Careful preoperative clinical and radiographic assessment is imperative. Note the pulp chamber is often in the centre of the tooth at the level of the cementoenamel junction (CEJ). Note (**a**) thick *dotted blue line* indicating long axis of root/tooth and *thin dotted blue line* showing correct access. (**b**) Note *red dotted line* indicating perforation possibility if crown-root axis is not correctly aligned with the bur during access preparation

measurements to be made. Provided the bitewing is a parallel image with minimal distortion, then the measurement should be fairly accurate.

Canal identification

Canal identification can be problematic in those cases where obvious calcification has occurred in the coronal pulp chamber resulting in iatrogenic perforations.

Chronic insults whereby reparative dentine is laid down will result in sclerosed canals and diminished pulp chambers. Anatomical features pertinent to the tooth in question as well as preoperative radiographs will alert the clinician to the expected number of root canals and their likely position. Once an initial access preparation has been made, the individual canals can be located usually following the 'road map' of root canal anatomy which is darker compared to the whiter axial walls. Pulp chamber calcifications can often be observed using a dental operating microscope and illumination highlighting the colour difference between surrounding anatomies. Ultrasonic tips are often useful when removing small amount of dentine in search of canal orifices. No burs should be used to gouge the floor of the pulp chamber and risk perforation.

Canal preparation

The advent of nickel titanium rotary instrumentation techniques means the ideal canal shape should be a continuously tapered preparation, maintaining canal anatomy and keeping the apical foramen as small as possible. The clinician should bear in mind the danger zones in relation to root canal anatomy and care during preparation procedures to ensure no strip perforation occurs due to overzealous instrumentation (Fig. 12.4).

Incautious preparations without taking into account the original anatomy and overzealous use of either rotary instruments or large tapered Gates Glidden burs can result in apical or crestal strip perforations. Large inflexible instruments used in curvatures can also result in zipping of the canal anatomy leading to perforations. A glide path should always be used prior to negotiating any canal curvature whether straight or curved (Fig. 12.5).

Post space preparation

Post space preparation should be carried out ideally at time of obturation. Clinically 4–5 mm of gutta-percha should remain apical to the post space to maintain an apical seal. A safe preparation should be taken under the guidance of the dental operating microscope to avoid risk of perforation due to deviation of post bur from the long axis of the root. The canal anatomy should be assessed for any changes in curvature along the root length, which would risk perforation.

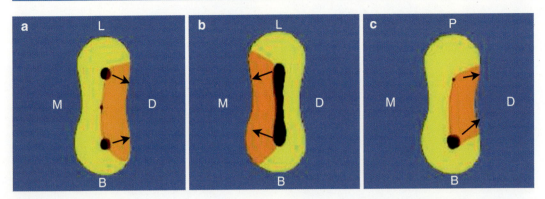

Fig. 12.4 Diagrams representing danger areas typically encountered in posterior molar teeth. (**a**) Mesial roots of mandibular molars, (**b**) distal roots of mandibular molars and (**c**) mesiobuccal roots of maxillary molars. Instrumentation towards the danger areas (*orange*) such as the furcations or root concavities can increase the likeli-

hood of a strip perforation. Overzealous coronal canal preparation using gates glidden burs, for example, can easily result in this unfavourable outcome. Care must be taken to identify correctly the danger zone in the root area and avoid unnecessary preparation of this area

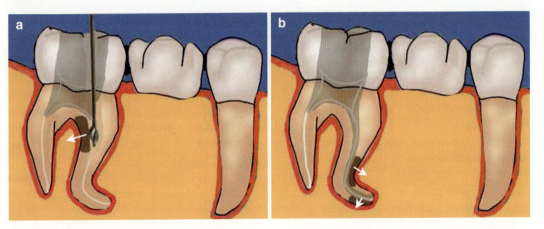

Fig. 12.5 Diagrams showing how a strip perforation can occur when (**a**) preparing the coronal 1/3 of the canal with rotary instrumentation such as gates glidden drills. These drills are used only in the straight portion of the canal remembering never to prepare the root canal more than 1/3 of the root diameter. Overzealous preparation must be avoided. Overaggressive preparation (**b**) in a severely

curved root canal can result in preferential removal of root dentine from the inside of the curve in the middle 1/3 of the canal and similar removal of dentine on the outside of the curve in the apical 1/3 of the canal due to the tendency for the file to straighten out. This can lead to both a strip perforation and tear-shaped apical preparation, both of which are difficult to obturate

12.5　Non-surgical Perforation Repair

A prerequisite for non-surgical management is that the perforation site can be visualized using the dental operating microscope. In those instances where a strip perforation has been created, then the canal space beyond the perforation must be obturated prior to repair of the perforation. The first step in order to visualize the

perforation site is to stem any bleeding which may be present. Local anaesthetic, sodium hypochlorite or triamcinolone acid soaked on a cotton wool pledget and pressed against the site of perforation should be sufficient to control haemorrhage (Fig. 12.6).

To avoid extrusion of filling material into the periodontal tissues and risk of further inflammation, delayed healing or need for a surgical procedure for debridement, an internal modified matrix

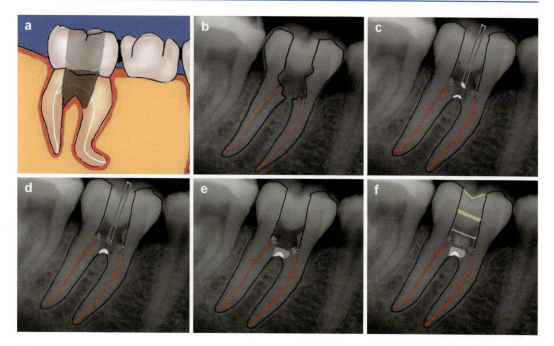

Fig. 12.6 Diagrams showing steps in repair of a furcal perforation. (**a**, **b**) Furcal perforation, (**c**) placement of cotton wool over canal orifices to prevent any reparative material dislodging into canals, (**d**) placement of barrier material, (**e**) placement of artificial floor repair material which is packed against the barrier such as MTA and (**f**) cotton wool and interim dressing to allow setting of MTA. Note the canals have been prepared at this stage ready to obturate at the second appointment. The artificial barrier is assessed at the second appointment for integrity ensuring a permanent seal is present

technique can be used. Sterile inorganic bovine bone (ABB; Bio-Oss, Geistlich AG, Wolhusen, Switzerland) is packed into the perforation defect. Once the matrix is in place, the artificial floor barrier can be placed using either glass ionomer cement, MTA or Biodentine without the risk of pushing the material into the surrounding bone and supporting tissues.

If MTA has been used, then the access cavity is sealed with a temporary moist cotton wool pledget to ensure that the site has sealed and the MTA has set (Fig. 12.7).

12.6 Surgical Perforation Repair

A surgical approach may be indicated in cases with large perforations that are not amenable to an orthograde approach, failure of healing following a non-surgical approach, surgical repair of an overfill following perforation repair and inaccessible perforations where a surgical approach is feasible. Before surgery is undertaken, non-surgical root canal treatment must be completed. Where a surgical approach is used to manage an apical perforation, then resection is carried out to this level provided the crown-root ratio remains favourable. A surgical approach and its success in attempting repair are dependant upon adequate accessibility. A general presurgical assessment is necessary prior to considering this type of approach (see Chap. 13).

12.7 Clinical Cases

Case 1: Furcal Perforation Repair with Internal Matrix and MTA A fit and healthy 46-year-old gentleman was referred regarding tooth 36 which failed to settle despite repeated intra-canal dressings (Figs. 12.8 and 12.9). Clinical examination revealed tooth 36 had an intact occlusal dressing which was tender to percussion. Mobility was within normal limits and

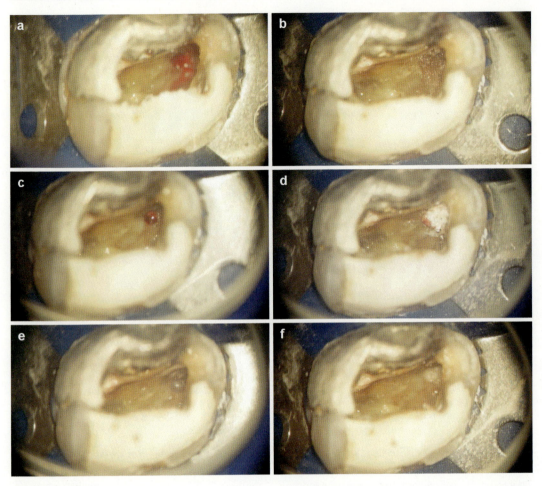

Fig. 12.7 Clinical photographs demonstrating an iatrogenic perforation after the dentist had been searching for a calcified canal. He reported using a bur to remove further dentine in the MB region. (**a**) Following removal of temporary dressing, obvious bleeding was noted in the MB region. (**b**) Placement of cotton wool soaked in local anaesthetic to control the bleeding. (**c**) Perforation diameter greater than a size 20 endodontic instrument. (**d**) and (**e**) Placement of freeze-dried bone at the site of the perforation (internal matrix concept) and (**f**) placement of MTA over the site of perforation to maintain seal

periodontal probing profile was within normal limits. Radiographic examination confirmed previous endodontic access in tooth 36. A furcal radiolucency was evident suggestive of possible iatrogenic perforation. Following dismantling of the temporary restoration, bleeding was evident in the floor of the pulp chamber. The access cavity was gently irrigated with sodium hypochlorite and the furcal perforation identified mesial to the distal canal. The perforation site was sealed with an internal matrix of Bio-Oss followed by MTA repair of the furcal defect. The MB, ML and D canals were chemomechanically prepared and working lengths established. An intra-canal dressing of calcium hydroxide was placed. A wet cotton wool pledget was placed over the MTA perforation repair and the tooth re-temporized. The patient was reviewed a week later. All his symptoms had resolved. The tooth was re-accessed, and the three canals were obturated using a warm vertical compaction technique and AH Plus cement. An IRM and glass ionomer double seal temporary restoration was placed. The patient was referred back to his general dental practitioner for permanent restoration of the tooth.

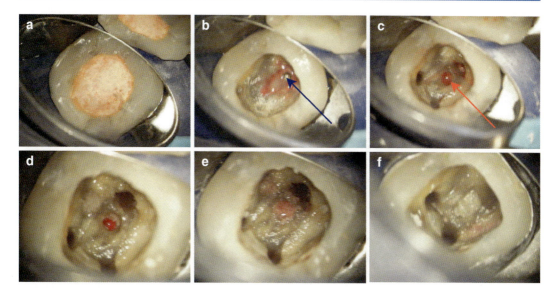

Fig. 12.8 Clinical photographs showing (**a**) preoperative temporary restoration, (**b**) bleeding and pus on the floor of the pulp chamber. (**c**) Following irrigation with sodium hypochlorite, it is clear that bleeding from an iatrogenic perforation exists in the furcation region (*blue arrow*); (**d**) the bleeding is controlled (*red arrow*) and (**e**) an internal matrix utilized prior to (**f**) placement of MTA as the repair material for the artificial floor of the pulp

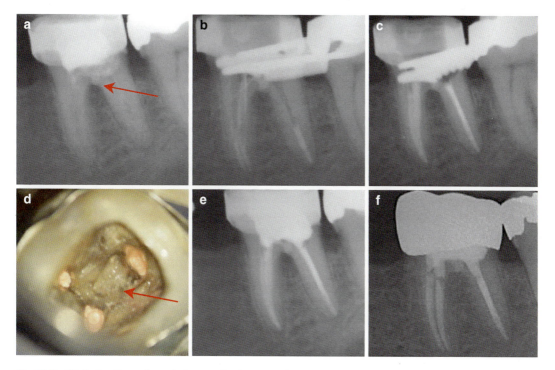

Fig. 12.9 Clinical radiographs and photographs demonstrating (**a**) post perforation repair at first visit; (**b**) mid-fill radiograph demonstrating apical 1/3 obturation; (**c**) radiograph demonstrating backfill; (**d**) MB, DB and D canals obturated and MTA repair site covered with glass ionomer cement; (**e**) post-operative radiograph demonstrating completed case. No periodontal defect was noted in the furcation region and the patient remained completely pain-free. The patient was advised to have the orthodontic band removed and replaced with a cast cuspal coverage restoration. (**f**) 3-year follow-up radiograph showing normal appearance in furcation region. *Red arrow* shows perforation repair using MTA/Glass ionomer cement

The perforation was recognized early by the referring practitioner and prompt referral organized. Time taken from perforation to repair was minimal with no periodontal destruction prior to repair noted. The long-term prognosis for this tooth was good with minimal risk of periodontal breakdown. The patient was reviewed 3 years later following an endodontic referral for another tooth. Radiographic examination confirmed excellent healing in the furcation region adjacent to the perforation repair site (Fig. 12.9).

Case 2: Mesial Cervical Perforation Repair with Glass/Ionomer Cement and Biodentine A fit and healthy 68-year-old lady was referred for endodontic management of tooth 37 (Figs. 12.10, 12.11 and 12.12). The patient had had a crown constructed on the tooth 12 months previously.

Recently the tooth had become very painful, and the dentist had attempted root canal treatment but had noted difficulties accessing the canals due to possible calcification. The patient reported intermittent sensitivity with the tooth. Clinical examination revealed tooth 37 had been restored with a ceramic crown with an occlusal access cavity, which was temporarily sealed. Radiographic examination confirmed tooth 36 was missing. Tooth 37 had a crown-root misalignment with mesial tilting of tooth 37. A radiolucency was noted on the mesial aspect of the crown at crestal bone level. The temporary restoration was dismantled and access orientation was noted to be misaligned mesially. A perforation was confirmed on the mesial aspect. Access cavity was refined and three necrotic canals located. Chemomechanical preparation was completed using 1 % sodium hypochlorite solution and NiTi

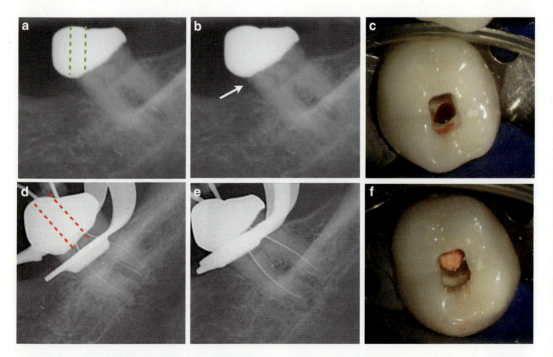

Fig. 12.10 Clinical radiographs and photographs demonstrating cervical perforation repair in tooth 37. Note (**a**) and (**b**) pre-operative radiograph demonstrating crown-root misalignment resulting in incorrect access preparation (*dotted green line*) and mesial cervical perforation (*white arrow*). (**c**) Intra-oral view following coronal temporary restoration removal. Excessive bleeding with direction of access cavity suggests mesial perforation which was confirmed when a probe was placed through the defect. (**d**) Correct straight line access (*dotted red line*). (**e**) Master apical file radiograph confirming identification of all canal anatomy. (**f**) Following chemo-mechanical preparation the root canals were temporarily sealed with gutta-percha

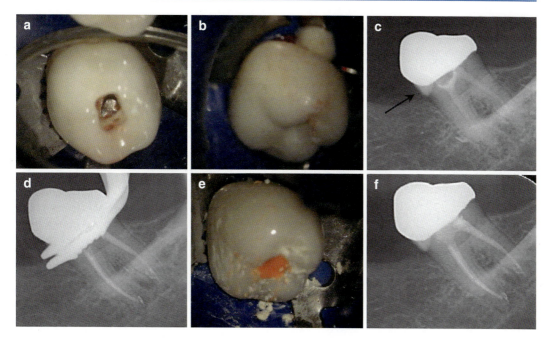

Fig. 12.11 Clinical radiographs and photographs demonstrating cervical perforation repair in tooth 37. Note (**a**) flat plastic instrument can be passed mesially in the area of the suspected perforation and confirmed intra-orally through the crown access. The instrument was used to prevent excessive spillage of glass ionomer cement repair material into the cervical aspect of the tooth. (**b**) Placement of glass ionomer cement into mesial defect to repair perforation site. (**c**) Post-treatment radiograph demonstrating intra-canal medicament and satisfactory repair of the perforation site (*black arrow*). (**d**) The patient was seen four weeks later for completion of endodontic treatment. A warm vertical compaction technique was used. (**e**) Temporary coloured glass ionomer cement restoration used to seal the access cavity. (**f**) A Biodentine filling was placed over the coronal pulp orifices to minimize future coronal leakage

rotary files. A gutta-percha temporary seal was placed overlying the mesial and distal canals to prevent any repair material inadvertently blocking the canals. The mesial perforation site was explored confirming an extensive mesial perforation. Cotton wool soaked in hypochlorite solution was placed through the perforation site to stop the bleeding. Glass ionomer cement was placed on the mesial aspect to seal the perforation site. The canals were dressed with calcium hydroxide and the tooth was re-temporized and a follow-up review arranged 4 weeks later. The patient remained asymptomatic and a decision to proceed to obturation was made.

At the obturation appointment, the mesial perforation site was examined under the dental operating microscope to ensure that an adequate seal was present. Mesially no probing defect was noted. The three canals were obturated using a warm vertical compaction technique using AH Plus cement. Biodentine was placed directly overlying the coronal root canal orifices to ensure that if the mesial perforation repair deteriorated in the future, then the coronal seal could be maintained. The Biodentine was mixed according to manufacturer instructions and the coronal pulp chamber was sealed. A temporary coloured coronal restoration was placed to prevent any further risk to the mesial repair site and underlying Biodentine seal.

This case highlights the difficulties encountered with access preparation, particularly in tilted molar teeth where there is crown-root misalignment due to the coronal cast restoration. Access cavity design should have been carried out in a distal orientation in alignment with root morphology as opposed to the mesial tilted crown.

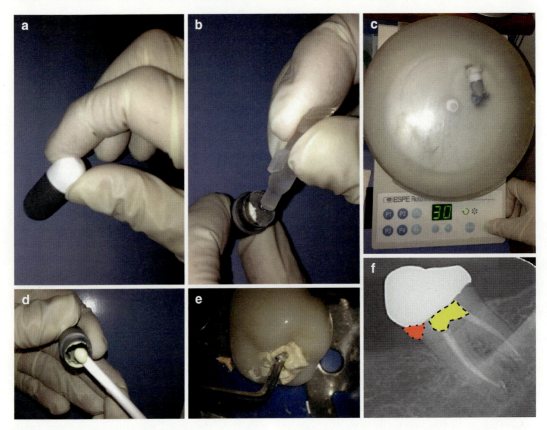

Fig. 12.12 Clinical photographs and radiograph demonstrating the use of Biodentine as a permanent seal overlying the canal orifices to prevent any coronal leakage that may result from the mesial defect. (**a**) The capsule containing Biodentine is gently tapped on a hard surface to loosen the powder. (**b**) Five drops of sterile water are placed in the capsule containing the Biodentine powder. (**c**) The capsule is placed in a mixing device at a speed of 4000 rpm for 30 s. (**d**) The capsule is opened and the Biodentine is checked for material consistency. If a thicker consistency is desired, then wait for 30 s to 1 min before checking again. (**e**) The Biodentine is transferred to tooth 37 and packed into the coronal pulp chamber using a hand plugger. (**f**) Note final post-operative radiograph demonstrating glass ionomer perforation repair (*red*) and Biodentine orifice seal (*yellow*)

Case 3: Labial Perforation Repair at Cervical Margin Using Internal Matrix and MTA A fit and healthy 59-year-old lady was referred to specialist practice for non-surgical endodontic treatment of tooth 21 (Figs. 12.13 and 12.14). The patient had been experiencing a dull pain in the region intermittently which resulted in a lip swelling. She attended her general dental practitioner who prescribed antibiotics and attempted root canal treatment. The dentist was unable to locate the canal due to calcification and a referral was sought. The patient was still symptomatic at time of consultation. Past dental history revealed the patient had sustained trauma to the tooth as a teenager. No endodontic treatment had been indicated, but the patient had noticed that the tooth

had gradually discoloured over time. A few years ago, the patient had had a ceramic crown placed for aesthetic reasons. Radiographic examination confirmed previous endodontic access, which was misaligned. The root canal system appeared completely sclerosed. A peri-radicular radiolucency was associated with the peri-apex of the tooth. Access cavity preparation revealed bleeding and suspected labial perforation. Straight-line access was created with orientation towards the palatal aspect of the tooth. Ultrasonic troughing was carried out using the dental operating microscope until a sticky point was noted. Initial canal preparation was carried out using small K-files 08 and 010 until patency was achieved. Working length was established and chemomechanical

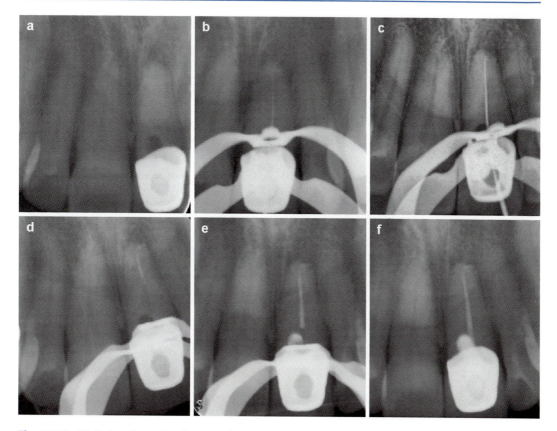

Fig. 12.13 Clinical radiographs demonstrating non-surgical root canal treatment and perforation repair of tooth 21. Note (**a**) preoperative radiograph demonstrating well-fitting ceramic crown restoration, pulp canal obliteration and misaligned access preparation. (**b**) Correct straight-line access gained and following ultrasonic troughing the canal orifice located and initial apical file with patency. (**c**) Master apical file confirming working length. (**d**) Obturation of canal using warm vertical compaction and AH Plus cement. (**e**) Perforation repair using MTA. (**f**) Final post-operative film demonstrating root canal obturation and perforation repair

preparation was completed using 1 % sodium hypochlorite solution. An intra-canal dressing of calcium hydroxide was placed within the root canal and at the labial perforation site. The patient was seen 4 weeks later for obturation of the tooth and perforation repair. Obturation was completed using a warm vertical compaction technique using AH Plus cement. Gutta-percha was placed below the level of the labial perforation. Bleeding at the perforation site was controlled using cotton wool soaked in hypochlorite solution. An internal Bio-Oss matrix was placed and the perforation site sealed with MTA. The crown was temporarily sealed with IRM and glass ionomer cement.

Case 4: Lingual-Cervical Perforation Repair with Internal Matrix and Glass Ionomer Cement An apprehensive well-controlled hypertensive 56-year-old female patient was referred for endodontic management of tooth 46. The patient had had a cast restoration placed on the tooth 12 months earlier. She developed pain and tenderness in relation to this tooth exacerbated when biting or chewing. The general dental practitioner attempted access preparation through the cast restoration and was unable to locate the distal canal system. The tooth was dressed with Ledermix and referral sought. Clinical examination revealed tooth 46 was asymptomatic.

Radiographic examination confirmed previous endodontic access. Dentine removal was noted overlying the distal root canal system with overextension. A peri-radicular radiolucency was noted with the distal root apex. Root canal treatment was initiated, and following

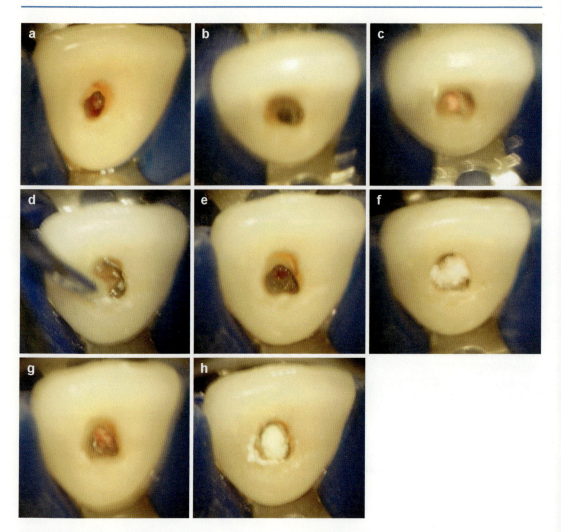

Fig. 12.14 Clinical photographs demonstrating non-surgical root canal treatment and labial cervical perforation repair of tooth 21. Note (**a**) perforation confirmed by bleeding following initial access to the tooth. The access cavity was misaligned and labially placed resulting in a labial perforation. (**b**) Correct access cavity preparation more centred and towards palatal (straight line access) allowed eventual canal location and preparation following extensive ultrasonic troughing. (**c**) Gutta-percha root filling completed using a warm vertical compaction technique. (**d**) Bleeding arrested using cotton wool soaked in sodium hypochlorite solution. (**e**) Labial perforation site with adequate bleeding control. (**f**) Placement of internal matrix of Bio-Oss. (**g**) Labial perforation site following matrix placement. (**h**) Placement of MTA to seal perforation site

removal of temporary access cavity material, excessive bleeding was noted in the distal aspect of the tooth. Gentle irrigation with sodium hypochlorite solution was carried out and file placed into the suspected distal canal orifice. Electronic apex locator and subsequent radiograph confirmed an iatrogenic perforation in the disto-lingual aspect of the tooth (Figs. 12.15 and 12.16).

Further ultrasonic troughing was carried out to reveal the true distal canal orifice. Chemomechanical preparation was completed using 1 % NaOCl solution and rotary files. The perforation site was visualized under the dental operating microscope, and a decision was made to use an internal matrix technique to prevent any extrusion of restorative material into the surrounding alveolar bone. A master gutta-percha

Fig. 12.15 Clinical radiographs demonstrating non-surgical root canal treatment of tooth 46. Note (**a**) preoperative radiograph showing prior endodontic access. The general dentist had placed a cast cuspal coverage restoration and the tooth had become symptomatic soon after. Access opening was carried out but the distal canal could not be located. Note extensive distal exploration. (**b**) IAF radiograph demonstrating perforation in the distolingual aspect verified by file. (**c**) Ultrasonic troughing was carried out to locate the untreated distal canal. (**d**) MAF preparation completed

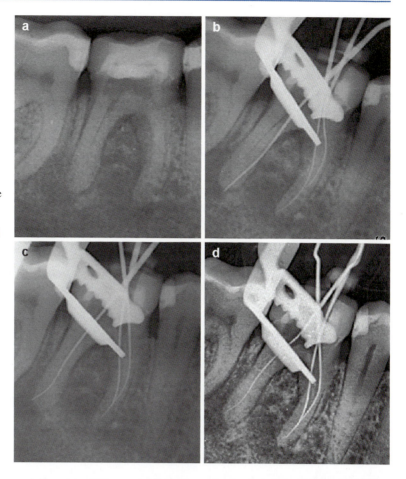

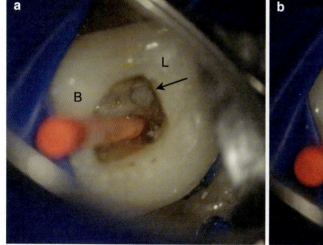
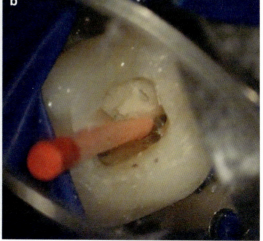

Fig. 12.16 Clinical radiographs demonstrating perforation repair in tooth 46 using an internal matrix technique. Note (**a**) gutta-percha has been placed in the prepared distal canal to prevent perforation repair material blocking the canal. An internal matrix using Bio-Oss was placed (*black arrow*) to prevent extrusion of perforation repair material into the distolingual furcation area. (**b**) Glass ionomer cement restorative material was used to seal the perforation. Once the material had set, the gutta-percha cone was removed and a calcium hydroxide dressing placed for a further four weeks

cone was placed in the distal canal to prevent accidental blockage of the canal with perforation repair material. A cotton wool pledget soaked in NaOCl solution was placed over the bleeding perforation site to arrest haemorrhage. Bio-Oss was used as an internal matrix and packed into the perforation site. Glass ionomer cement restorative material was then placed over the perforation site/matrix to seal the perforation. Once the glass ionomer restorative material had set, the gutta-percha cone was removed, canal was re-irrigated and canals were dressed with an inter-appointment calcium hydroxide dressing. The patient was reviewed at 4 weeks and remained asymptomatic. No periodontal probing defect was detected disto-lingually. A decision was made to proceed with obturation.

At the obturation appointment, the tooth was re-accessed and the perforation repair site was examined to ensure that the repair was satisfactory. Obturation of the root canal system was completed using a warm vertical compaction technique using AH Plus cement, gutta-percha, system B and Obtura (Fig. 12.17).

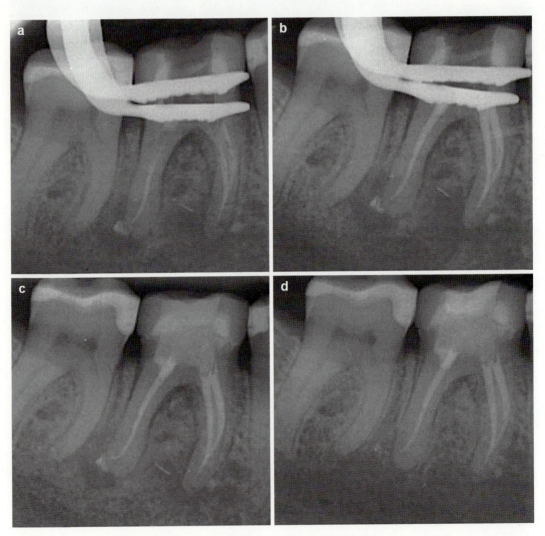

Fig. 12.17 Clinical radiographs demonstrating completed root canal treatment of tooth 46. (**a**) Mid-fill radiograph using warm vertical compaction technique with AH Plus cement and gutta-percha. Note extruded sealer at the distal apex. (**b**) Backfill completed using System B and Obtura. (**c**) Post-operative view demonstrating completed treatment. (**d**) 12-month review radiograph showing periapical healing. The patient remained asymptomatic with no abnormal periodontal defect in the area of the perforation

A Biodentine restoration was placed over the root canal orifices and perforation repair to prevent any coronal micro-leakage. A temporary glass ionomer cement (pink) was placed in the occlusal access cavity overlying the Biodentine restoration to ease visualization for the general dental practitioner when placing his permanent core. The patient was reviewed at a 12-month follow-up at which time she remained asymptomatic. Clinical examination revealed no abnormal probing profile. Radiographic examination confirmed periapical healing with significant reduction in the distal periapical lesion. Sealer extrusion material had also been resorbed. The patient was reassured as to the long-term prognosis for the tooth and discharged back to her general dental practitioner.

Clinical Hints and Tips for the Prevention and Management of Endodontic Perforations

(i)   **Preoperative assessment**
      Assess crown-root alignment.
      Good quality parallel periapical radiographs at different angles (horizontal tube shift) and use of a parallel bitewing radiograph to determine coronal pulp chamber depth, size and shape relative to furcal floor.

(ii) **During access preparation**
      Care should be taken when accessing the teeth with narrow and calcified pulp chambers.
      Root orientation must be determined prior to rubber dam placement and access preparation in the teeth with cast restorations.

(iii) **During root canal preparation**
      Strip perforations should be avoided by overzealous preparation techniques. Coronal pre-flaring with Gates Glidden drills should be avoided and pre-enlargement of the danger zones avoided (e.g. furcation areas).

(viii) **During post preparation**
      Ideal post diameter, length and type (custom-made or prefabricated) should be determined according to tooth types, confluence of canals, root

thickness and length. Overzealous post preparation should be avoided with conservation of radicular dentine in mind.

(v)   Once a perforation has been identified, care must be taken with irrigation techniques to avoid a hypochlorite accident. Alternative use of chlorhexidine may be considered until anatomical site, position and size of perforation are verified and visualized as possible.

(vi) Haemorrhage at the perforation site must be controlled prior to repair. If the perforation is present in the coronal pulp chamber and is easily visualized under the dental microscope, then pressure application using a cotton wool pledget previously immersed in hypochlorite will achieve the desired result.

(vii) The use of a sealing material that is biologically compatible and supports both osteogenesis and cementogenesis is preferable. Materials of choice include MTA and Biodentine. A resorbable internal matrix may be useful prior to condensation of sealing material.

(viii) Apical perforations can either be sealed with an osteogenic-/cementogenic-inducing material or using conventional endodontic principles provided haemorrhage control is achievable. Infected or bleeding apical perforations may require use of antibacterial intra-canal dressing placement for at least 1 week prior to obturation.

(ix) Crestal perforations must be sealed as soon as possible to improve prognosis due to proximity to the epithelial attachment. Large furcal perforations may require the use of an internal matrix technique to avoid extrusion of repair material into the surrounding periodontal tissues. Temporary sealing of the remaining root canals must be ensured to avoid accidental spillage and blockage.

References

1. American Association of Endodontists. Glossary of endodontic terms. 7th ed. Chicago: American Association of Endodontists; 2003. p. 1–51.
2. Alhadainy HA. Root perforation. A review of the literature. Oral Surg Oral Med Oral Pathol. 1994;78:368–74.
3. Fuss Z, Trope M. Root perforations: classification and treatment choices based on prognostic factors. Endod Dent Traumatol. 1996;12:255–64.
4. Torabinejad M, Lemon RR. Procedural accidents. In: Walton RE, Torabinejad M, eds. Principles and Practice of Endodontics, 3rd edn. Philadelphia: WB Saunders, 2002: 312–331.
5. Kvinnsland I, Oswald RI, Halse A, Gronningdeter AG. A clinical and roetgenotological study of 55 cases or root perforation. Int Endod J. 1989;22: 75–84.
6. Seltzer S, Sinai I, August D. Periodontal effects of root perforations before and during endodontic procedures. J Dent Res. 1970;49(2):332–9.
7. Lemon RR. Nonsurgical repair of perforation defects. Internal matrix concept. Dent Clin North Am. 1992;36:439–57.
8. McCabe PS. Avoiding perforations in endodontics. J Ir Dent Assoc. 2006;52:139–48.
9. Moreinis SA. Avoiding perforation during endodontic access. J Am Dent Assoc. 1979;98:707–12.
10. Wong R, Cho F. Microscopic management of procedural errors. Dent Clin North Am. 1997;41:455–79.
11. Fuss Z, Assooline LS, Kaufman AY. Determination of location of root perforations by electronic apex locators. Oral Surg Oral Med Oral Pathol Oral Radiol Endod. 1996;82:432–9.
12. Shemesh H, Cristescu RC, Wesselink PR, Wu MK. The use of cone-beam computed tomography and digital periapical radiographs to diagnose root perforations. J Endod. 2011;37:513–6.
13. Tamse A. Vertical root fractures in endodontically treated teeth: diagnostic signs and clinical management. Endod Top. 2006;13:84–94.
14. Zhu WC, Gyamfi J, Niu LN, Schoeffel GJ, Liu SY, Santarcangelo F, Khan S, Tay KC, Pashley DH, Tay FR. Anatomy of sodium hypochlorite accidents involving facial ecchymosis – a review. J Dent. 2013;41(11):935–48.
15. Hartwell GR, England MC. Healing of furcation perforations in primate teeth after repair with decalcified freeze-dried bone: a longitudinal study. J Endod. 1993;19:357–61.
16. Rafter M, Baker M, Alves M, Daniel J, Remeikis N. Evaluation of healing with the use of an internal matrix to repair furcation perforations. Int Endod J. 2002;35:775–83.
17. Alhadainy HA, Himel VT, Lee WB, Elbaghdady YM. Use of hydroxyapatite based material and calcium sulfate as artificial floors to repair furcal perforations. Oral Surg Oral Med Oral Pathol Oral Radiol Endod. 1998;86:723–9.
18. Bargholtz C. Perforation repair with mineral trioxide aggregate: a modified matrix concept. Int Endod J. 2005;38:59–69.
19. Dragoo MR. Resin-ionomer and hybrid-ionomer cements: part II – clinical and histological wound healing responses in specific periodontal lesions. Int J Periodontics Restorative Dent. 1997;17:75–87.
20. Ford TR, Torabinejad M, McKendry DJ, Hong CU, Kariyawasam SP. Use of mineral trioxide aggregate for repair of furcal perforations. Oral Surg Oral Med Oral Pathol Oral Radiol Endod. 1995;79:756–63.
21. Holland R, Filho JA, de Souza V, Nery MJ, Bernabe PF, Junior ED. Mineral trioxide aggregate repair of lateral root perforations. J Endod. 2001;27:281–4.
22. Main C, Mirzayan N, Shabahang S, Torabinejad M. Repair of root perforation using mineral trioxide aggregate: a long term study. J Endod. 2004;30:80–3.
23. Krupp C, Bargholz C, Brüsehaber M, Hülsmann M. Treatment outcome after repair of root perforations with mineral trioxide aggregate: a retrospective evaluation of 90 teeth. J Endod. 2013;39:1364–8.
24. Regan JD, Witherspoon DE, Foyle DM. Surgical repair of root and tooth perforations. Endod Top. 2005;11:151–78.
25. Barkhordar RA, Javid B. Treatment of endodontic perforations by guided tissue regeneration. Gen Dent. 2000;48:422–6.
26. Pontius V, Pontius O, Braun A, Frankenberger R, Roggendorf MJ. Retrospective evaluation of perforation repairs in 6 private practices. J Endod. 2013;39:1346–58.

Endodontic Microsurgery

13

Roberto Sacco, Anthony Greenstein,
and Bobby Patel

Summary

Traditional endodontic surgery involves the surgical management of a tooth with a periapical lesion that cannot be resolved by conventional non-surgical endodontic treatment/retreatment. The main objective of periradicular surgery is to promote tissue regeneration. Indications for surgery include complex root canal anatomy, irretrievable materials in the root canal, procedural accidents requiring surgery, persistent symptomatic cases, refractory lesions and where biopsy may be needed. This can be achieved by the surgical removal of periapical pathological tissue (surgical curettage) and by removing/occluding irritants within the confines of the apical portion of the root canal system and isthmuses (retrograde root resection, root end preparation and retrograde obturation). Endodontic microsurgery combines unsurpassed magnification and illumination using a dental operating microscope and specific micro-instruments that significantly affects case selection, predictability and post-operative healing sequelae. These major advances in surgical technique, instrumentation and materials have occurred over the last twenty years. Supported by research they have not only led to the overall improvement in treatment success but the ability to save what were once considered hopeless teeth

R. Sacco, CDT, DDS, MSc, PG Cert Sed
Oral Surgery Specialist, Senior Clinical
Teaching Fellow, UCL-Eastman Dental Institute,
123 Gray's Inn Road, London WC1X 8WD, UK

Oral Surgery Specialist Dentist, King's College
Hospital NHS Trust, Denmark Hill,
London SE5 9RS, UK

A. Greenstein, BM BS, MRCS, BDS, MFDS RCS (ED)
Oral and Maxillofacial Surgery, Pan Scotland
Rotation, Honorary Lecturer at University
of Aberdeen School of Medicine and Dentistry,
Aberdeen, UK

B. Patel, BDS MFDS MClinDent MRD MRACDS (✉)
Specialist Endodontist, Brindabella Specialist Centre,
Canberra, ACT, Australia
e-mail: bobbypatel@me.com

© Springer International Publishing Switzerland 2016
B. Patel (ed.), *Endodontic Treatment, Retreatment, and Surgery*,
DOI 10.1007/978-3-319-19476-9_13

The use of the dental operating microscope, surgical micro-instruments, ultrasonic instrumentation and biocompatible root-end filling materials has resulted in a more favourable outcome with greater predictability. The art of microsurgical techniques is based on both an understanding of a biological approach and utilizing surgical expertise to contribute to a positive healing response. The endodontist can easily incorporate these techniques and concepts into their everyday practice enhancing available treatment strategies for the management of peri-radicular disease.

13.1 Overview of Surgical Endodontics

Root canal treatment is carried out when the pulp is nonvital or has been removed to prevent or treat apical periodontitis [1]. It has been well established that apical periodontitis is an inflammatory process in the peri-radicular tissues sustained by microorganisms in the necrotic root canal system [2–4]. The success of primary root canal treatment is dependent on effective removal of this bacterial load below a critical threshold to allow for healing.

Success rates up to 97 % have been demonstrated for primary root canal treatment [5]. Nevertheless failure may occur after treatment. Endodontic failures are primarily due to the persistence of bacteria within the anatomically complexities of the root canal [6], persistent extra-radicular infection [7, 8], foreign body reactions to gutta-percha root filling materials [8] and radicular cysts [9].

Previously treated teeth with persistent periapical lesions can be treated either with non-surgical retreatment or endodontic surgery. Non-surgical retreatment is generally most beneficial because it seeks to eliminate the bacteria from within the root canal system. Surgery for intra-canal infections can isolate, but not eliminate, the bacteria from the root canal and would be limited to those cases where non-surgical retreatment is not judged to be possible [10]. When the aetiology is independent of the root canal system [6–9], surgery is the most beneficial treatment (Fig. 13.1). Non-surgical retreatment may still be indicated in these cases, especially when intra-canal infection cannot be ruled out [10].

Systematic reviews comparing the outcome of non-surgical root canal retreatment and surgical endodontics suggest that the latter offers more favourable initial success. However, non-surgical retreatment offers a more favourable long-term outcome [11, 12]. If the root canals

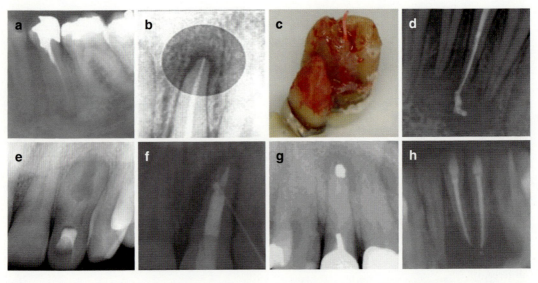

Fig 13.1 Clinical radiographs and photographs showing endodontic cases which have failed despite attempts at treatment. (**a**) Missed anatomy, (**b**) persistent disease despite well-obturated canal system, (**c**) overextension resulting in extraction, (**d**) overfill causing possible foreign body reaction, (**e**) complex anatomy, (**f**) suspected root fracture, (**g**) previous surgical failure, and (**h**) persistent apical pathosis despite re-treatment attempts

are accessible, then non-surgical retreatment is the treatment of choice [13].

Pre-surgical rinsing with chlorhexidine mouth rinse helps to reduce bacterial load and plaque formation, which in turn promotes healing of the surgical site [14]. There is no indication to provide preoperative prophylactic antibiotics prior to periapical surgery to prevent post-operative infections in a healthy patient with no medical indications [15]. Preemptive use of oral non-steroidal drug therapy should be considered prior to surgery as an effective method of reducing post-operative pain [16].

The use of the dental operating microscope in terms of enhanced magnification and illumination to facilitate and enhance each phase of endodontic surgery has been well documented [17–20].

The generation of successful intraoperative anaesthesia and haemostasis are critical pillars supporting the foundation of effective endodontic surgical procedures. Local anaesthesia with a vasoconstrictor is useful in terms of minimizing pain and providing effective haemorrhage control [21]. Tissue blanching is a characteristic sign of effective vasoconstriction.

Management of soft tissues is important from an aesthetically successful treatment point of view [22]. When designing a tissue flap, various methods of incision can be selected depending on the flap selected. It is important that incision, elevation and reflection of soft tissue are performed in a way that is conducive for healing by primary intention. This goal is facilitated by ensuring all incisions are complete, sharp and placed on sound bone. Great care must be taken throughout the surgical procedure ensuring tissue damage is kept to a minimum. Tearing or severing of tissue should be avoided during elevation and flap reflection [22]. The tissues should be kept moist and prevented from drying out throughout the procedure by applying a damp gauze using saline. This will help minimize tissue shrinkage, which would result in further difficulty with tissue re-approximation and higher tension when suturing [23]. The use of a papillary preservation flap can be considered where feasible to further minimize recession post-operatively, particularly where gingival biotype is thick and flat and aesthetics is of primary concern [24, 25].

Flap retraction is dependent on correct retractor selection and placement on sound bone not soft tissues, which would result in further trauma.

It has been demonstrated that leaving bleeding tissue tags intact on the exposed bone or periodontal ligament fibres that were severed on flap reflection will facilitate healing [26] (Fig. 13.2).

The uncertainty in knowing the true extent of the periapical lesion combined with the increased

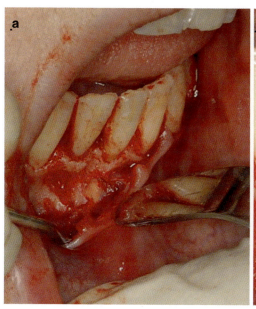
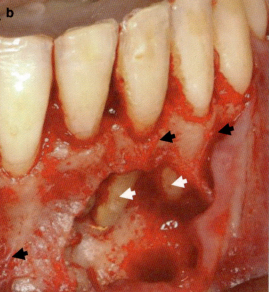

Fig 13.2 Clinical photographs showing (**a**) flap reflection and (**b**) bleeding tags of tissue attached to overlying cortical bone (*black arrows*) and exposed root surfaces (*white arrows*). These tags should never be intentionally removed

risk of scarring means submarginal flaps such as Ochsenbein-Luebke semilunar flaps are no longer recommended [27].

Osteotomy is a critical step, where cortical bone is still intact, allowing adequate access and facilitating subsequent removal of soft tissue lesion surrounding the apical and/or lateral aspects of the root apex. This unimpeded access is critical to ensure root-end resection, and preparation is carried out correctly without compromising adjacent structures. If the cortical plate has already been breached or thinned by underlying pathology, then curettes may be used to expose the apex of the root. Bone removal is recommended with an appropriate bur (surgical round bur) using a reverse-air handpiece (Impact Air 45) to reduce the risk of surgical emphysema [28]. Copious amounts of sterile water or saline should be used throughout the procedure to prevent overheating of the surrounding bone [29]. Steel and tungsten carbide burs have been shown to produce less heat than diamond burs resulting in the possibility of compromised healing [30]. The osteotomy should be carried out with a light shaving motion to further reduce any heat generated. A bony lid technique has been advocated in the past for accessing the apical region of mandibular teeth. With the advent of modern microsurgical techniques, which are more conservative, these techniques are likely obsolete [34].

After the cortical bone is removed to expose the lesion, the soft tissue is curetted from the crypt (peri-radicular curettage). The majority of soft tissue should be removed if possible and sent for histopathological diagnosis. Numerous case reports have been presented in the literature where suspected periapical pathosis was in fact something more sinister [35–37]. In some instances it may not be possible to remove the lesion in its entirety due to risk of damaging adjacent structures. In this case further excision may be possible following root resection.

Usually removal of the granulation tissue, which is chronically inflamed, will reduce the amount of bleeding within the surgical crypt [38]. Haemostasis in the surgical crypt can also be managed by several pharmacological techniques including resorbable sponges containing epinephrine and calcium sulphate paste [39] or direct application of ferric sulphate [40]. Potential

delayed wound healing may occur if the entire ferric sulphate is not removed [41].

Root-end resection should be carried near perpendicular to the long axis of the root where possible. This makes it much easier for the operator to resect the root end completely, to detect multiple or aberrant canals and subsequent ease of retrograde preparation [31–33]. Dentinal tubules are also more perpendicular in orientation to the long axis of the tooth so this type of resection will expose fewer tubules [42]. It has been shown that 98 % of apical canal anomalies and 93 % of lateral canals system ramifications occur in the apical 3 mm [43]. Where possible it is recommended to remove at least 3 mm of root end with an appropriate bur (Lindemann H151) with appropriate water cooling.

The resected root end should be inspected under magnification and illumination using a micro-mirror to ensure resection is complete and there are no cracks in the root and to check for any anatomical canal irregularities, missed canals or isthmuses. The bevelled root surface can also be inspected after staining with a neutral, buffered, sterile dye such as methylene blue [31–33]. A radiograph can be taken at this stage to ensure resection has been carried out to the appropriate level.

The aim of root-end preparation using ultrasonic instrumentation is to clean and shape the apical 3 mm of the root canal system. The instrumentation is parallel and confined to within the root canal. Aberrant anatomies such as fins and isthmuses are cleaned without damaging the remaining dentinal walls [31–33].

Root-end preparation may create a smear layer, consisting of organic and inorganic substances, which may prevent complete adaptation of root-end filling material. Removal of this smear layer using EDTA or citric acid may be beneficial [44].

Prior to root-end filling, the surgical crypt should be isolated from fluids, bleeding controlled and root-end preparation dried. There are several methods of root-end filling each having been used with various degrees of success. Amalgam is no longer recommended based on its increased micro leakage compared to other materials, risk of tissue argyria and no evidence of its ability to support tissue regeneration and unfavourable biocompatibility [45–48]. Current evidence suggests the use of MTA, ZOE cements,

Diaket and Retroplast is acceptable dependent on prevailing clinical conditions [49–53].

A final debridement of the crypt is carried out using sterile saline to ensure that no foreign material is left in situ. Radiographic evidence of the quality of the root-end filling is recommended prior to wound closure.

Good tissue re-approximation with minimal tension using an appropriate suturing technique will allow for optimal healing by primary intention. Non-absorbable sutures in sizes 5-0 to 8-0 are preferred using gentle manipulation with microsurgical instruments. The smallest number of sutures should be used, thereby minimizing tension, foreign body reaction and irritation [23–25, 54]. Compression of the repositioned tissues with a saline moistened piece of gauze will reduce the coagulum to a thin fibrin layer between the repositioned tissue and cortical bone. This will further reduce post-operative bleeding and swelling [54]. Sutures can be removed 48–96 h postoperatively provided the wound is stable [54].

In summary, the expected outcome of apical surgery is good, and therefore, before considering tooth extraction and replacement, apical surgery should be attempted when it is feasible [55].

13.2 Indications and Contraindications

When endodontic treatment fails, the clinician and patient are faced with the dilemma of either considering endodontic retreatment or surgery to maintain the tooth. There is an agreement that non-surgical retreatment prior to a surgical approach will offer the tooth the best chance of success because all possible sites of infection are treated (clinical case 3, 4, 5 and 6). The decision-making process for retreatment and/or surgery is usually driven by periodontal assessment, restorative considerations and endodontic status of the tooth (see Fig. 13.3). A cost-benefit analysis is carried out including extraction and replacement options. A well-fitting coronal cast restoration does not preclude retreatment since minimal access cavities can be prepared through the crown and restored without complication upon completion. Conversely a poor coronal restoration needs to be sacrificed and dismantled to assess restorability prior to considering retreatment. In those cases, which have been restored with posts, sacrificing the crown is not always necessary. Endodontic access and post removal are still possible through the crown in

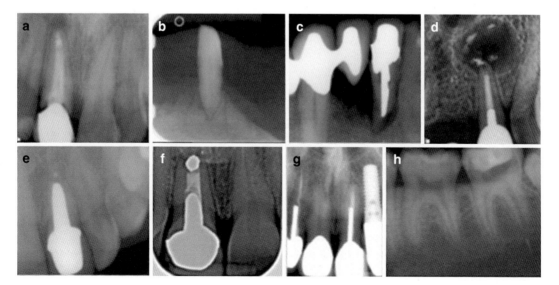

Fig 13.3 Clinical radiographs showing indications and contraindications to endodontic surgery or re-surgery. Note (**a–c**) poor restorability or periodontal support contraindicating a surgical approach, (**d, e**) well-fitting post crown restorations which would support a surgical approach, (**f**) failing post crown restoration which would not be suited to re-surgery, and (**g, h**) separated instruments which would only be amenable to a surgical approach for removal

some cases although if the post was placed for retention of the crown, then debonding is highly likely. The benefit of post removal must be weighed up against the risk of further weakening of the tooth and possible root fracture.

Well-fitting post crown restorations may be more amenable to microsurgical techniques with favourable outcomes (clinical Case 2) (Fig. 13.33).

The other situations where surgery is more beneficial compared to endodontic retreatment are those cases where the aetiology of the endodontic lesion is independent of the root canal system such as foreign body reactions to gutta-percha (clinical case 1) (Fig. 13.32), extra-radicular infections and true cysts (radicular).

Intra-canal obstructions and aberrant anatomy preventing access to the apical tissues will all require surgery to rectify the problem (clinical Case 4) (Fig. 13.35, Table 13.1).

13.3   Microsurgical Versus Traditional Approaches

Endodontic microsurgery encompasses the magnification and illumination provided by the dental operating microscope with the use of specifically designed micro-instruments. The use of the operating microscope during surgery offers the clinician a number of advantages including higher magnification enabling precise anatomical detail to be observed including root apex identification and anatomical details including microfractures, isthmuses and lateral canals; precise and complete removal of diseased tissue; conservative ultrasonic root-end preparations; and precise root-end filling placement. Traditional endodontic surgery had a number of disadvantages including difficulties with root apices identification, large osteotomies and long resection angles that would invariably lead to destruction of surrounding cortical bone and root length. Soft tissue management has also changed with the use of micro-instruments enabling precise incisions to be made preserving papilla, thereby reducing post- operative complications

Table 13.1 Indications and contraindications for surgical endodontics

A. Indications
(i) Peri-radicular disease associated with a well-treated previous root treatment where retreatment would be deemed detrimental to the tooth or where no improvement may be gained
(ii) Peri-radicular disease associated with anatomical deviations such as tortuous roots, sharp angle bifurcations, pulp stones and calcifications preventing non-surgical retreatment to be undertaken
(iii) Peri-radicular disease associated with procedural errors such as instrument fractures, ledges, blockages or perforated canals, which cannot be corrected non-surgically
(iv) Where a biopsy of the peri-radicular tissues is indicated
(v) Exploratory surgery to visualize the peri-radicular tissues and tooth/root is required when perforation or fracture is suspected

B. Contraindications
(i) *Anatomical factors* Proximity to neurovascular bundles, unusual bone or root configurations, proximity to maxillary sinus, lower second molars with thick cortical plate and lingual inclination of roots. Limited mouth opening resulting in reduced surgical access
(ii) *Periodontal and restorative factors* Poor supporting structures, active moderate-severe periodontal disease and failing or failed coronal restorations
(iii) *Medical factors* Severe systemic disease (ASA III–IV), patients with diseases such as leukaemia or severe neutropenia in the active stage and uncontrolled diabetes or patients who have recently undergone cardiac or cancer therapy
(iv) *Surgeons skill and ability* The clinician's surgical skills and knowledge. Where in doubt a referral should be made to an appropriate endodontist

including gingival recession and scar formation. The use of smaller suture materials such as 5-0 or 6-0 monofilaments result in not only less trauma but also more rapid healing. Atraumatic tissue retraction using a groove technique (i.e. placement and prevention of retractor slippage is facilitated by making a resting groove in bone) aims to further reduce the risk of post-operative pain and swelling (see Table 13.2 and 13.7).

Endodontic microsurgery uses state-of-the-art equipment, instruments and materials aimed at

Table 13.2 Differences between traditional and microsurgical approaches in surgical endodontics

	Traditional	Microsurgery
Osteotomy size	Large 8–10 mm	Small 3–4 mm
Bevel angle	Long 45–65°	Shallow 0–10°
Resected root surface inspection	Not possible with standard instruments	Always possible
Isthmus identification	Impossible	Possible
Root-end preparation	Difficult to ensure only within the canal	Always within the canal
Root-end filling material	Amalgam often used	MTA or Super EBA
Sutures	3-0 or 4-0 silk	5-0 or 6-0 monofilaments
Suture removal	7 days post-operatively	2–3 days post-operatively
Healing success at 1 year	40–90 %	85–97 %

satisfying both mechanical and biological concepts to produce predictable outcomes compared to traditional techniques. The endodontist can easily incorporate these techniques and concepts into their everyday practice enhancing available treatment strategies for the management of periradicular disease.

13.4 Anaesthesia and Haemostasis

1. Premedication with an NSAID such as ibuprofen 400 mg can be given to the patient 1 h preoperatively in patients that have no contraindications. A pre-surgical rinse of chlorhexidine can be recommended for 1 day preoperatively and for 1 min prior to commencing surgery. The protocol can be continued post-operatively until sutures are removed.
2. The administration of local infiltration of lidocaine 1:50,000 epinephrine is injected in the surgical site (2–3 cartridges). The injection is given slowly and steadily to allow time for diffusion of the fluid and avoid accumulation in the submucosa. A further infiltration is given in small increments directly in the region of the intended flap site resulting in tissue blanching. One must avoid injecting into the skeletal muscle in the area; otherwise, there will be an activation of the B-adrenergic receptors resulting in vasodilation and increased haemorrhage after flap reflection.
3. Block infiltrations can be administered using lidocaine to obtain a sustained level of anaesthesia during surgery. For posterior mandibular teeth, an inferior alveolar nerve block is supplemented with a mental block. Posterior surgeries involving maxillary teeth can be supplemented with posterior superior and middle superior alveolar nerve blocks and infraorbital blocks depending on the tooth in question. Anterior maxillary teeth can be supplemented with nasopalatine blocks.

13.5 Flap Design

A number of basic flap designs exist including envelope, triangular, rectangular, semilunar, Ochsenbein-Luebke and papillary base preservation flap. Maxillary palatal root access requires a palatal flap to be elevated with separate design features. It is critical that tissue incision, reflection and retraction are performed in a way that allows for healing by primary intention. Soft tissue manipulation should avoid tearing, severing, trauma and desiccation. The following principles are discussed broadly in relation to the specific types of flap designs, which can be selected:

1. **Incisions**

   All incisions are continuous in nature and penetrate through the mucosa, underlying periosteum down to cortical bone. The exception to this rule is when making the split thickness incision in relation to the papillary preservation flap. These sharp incisions to the bone ensure unfavourable tearing of tissues, and damage to marginal gingivae is reduced.

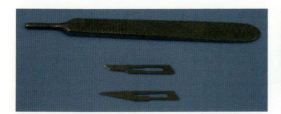

Fig 13.4 Clinical photograph showing scalpel holder and blades number 15 and 11 useful for intrasulcular and vertical relieving incision

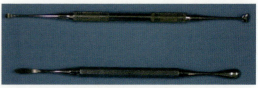

Fig 13.5 Clinical photograph showing the molt elevator (*above*) and Howarth periosteal elevator (*below*) used to reflect the flap once incision has been made

Vertical incisions should not extend near muscle attachments or highly vascular areas such as beyond the submucosa. The vertical incision is made originating at the line angle of the most anterior tooth of the flap and drawn parallel to the long axis of the adjacent roots. Horizontal incisions should follow the contour of the labial surface of teeth with particular attention being paid to the intrasulcular or interproximal areas. The papilla needs to be excised completely, and both buccal and palatal/lingual incisions are made to ensure this (Fig. 13.4).

Care must be excised when placing incisions in areas of bony prominence such as the canine region and areas of the jaws where bony architecture is irregular. Flap design and placement of relieving incisions must take these factors into account to minimize tearing and possible postoperative complications such as flap dehiscence, scarring and gingival recession.

2. Reflection

Reflection of the soft tissues should be carried out purposefully, slowly and with care to avoid accidental slippage. One should start in the area of the vertical relieving incision using an appropriate elevator (Molt no. 4 or Howarth's periosteal elevator). One must ensure that periosteum has been identified and the elevator is placed under this layer and is in contact with the underlying bone at all times. A piece of gauze can be useful to protect the soft tissues, as you reflect pushing against the bone and the gauze, not the flap. The sharp convex end of the elevator is used to carefully reflect the flap.

Care must be taken in regions of bony prominences, irregularities, concavities and areas of fenestrations where risk of tearing is high (Fig. 13.5).

3. Retractor placement

A suitable retractor (Minnesota) should be selected to protect the soft tissue flap and also prevent slippage of instruments that can cause further damage to soft tissues by tearing or crushing. The retractor, in turn, allows the operator to have a clear field of vision to the periapex of the tooth, which is unimpeded by the reflected flap. It may be useful to run a small round bur in a horizontal direction creating a small depression/groove in the bone above the root apex and the pathological defect where the retractor can rest in a firm secure position avoiding slippage. One must remember that whenever the flap is repositioned, it is worthwhile covering with a damp gauze soaked in saline to prevent drying out and shrinkage (Figs. 13.6 and 13.7).

Triangular/Rectangular Flap

The triangular flap design (Fig. 13.8) comprises a horizontal incision extending to several teeth and distal to the involved tooth and one vertical relieving incision placed mesially. If access is difficult, then the triangular flap can be converted to a rectangular one by placing an additional vertical relieving incision. This type of flap can be used for periapical surgery, root resorption, cervical resorption, perforation and resection of short roots. The main advantage of this type of flap is minimal disruption of the vascular blood supply of the reflected tissues and ease of repositioning. Healing following sulcular marginal incisions may lead to varying amounts of recession. Complete elevation of the papilla is technically difficult, especially in narrow interproximal areas. Frequently the most coronal portion of the papilla will be separated from the body of the papilla and left behind. Separated tissue fragments often necrotize during the healing

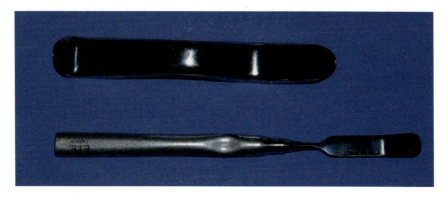

Fig 13.6 Clinical photographs showing Minnesota retractor (*above*) and Carr retractor (*below*)

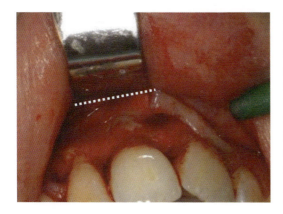

Fig 13.7 Retractor placement and potential site for groove where retractor could sit above root apex and pathological defect preventing trauma to soft tissues during procedure

phase resulting in loss of papilla height. The risk of gingival recession is of particular concern in patients with thin gingival biotypes and high lip lines ("gummy smiles").

Submarginal Flap

Often referred to as the Ochsenbein-Luebke flap (Fig. 13.9), it is similar to the rectangular flap except the scalloped horizontal incision is placed within the attached gingivae. This flap was used to prevent recession in aesthetically demanding cases. The disadvantages of this flap include risk of scar formation, possibility of incisions in close proximity to the bony cavity resulting in wound dehiscence and loss of attachment. This type of flap is now considered historical.

Papillary Preservation Flap

For a papillary based flap (Fig. 13.10), a split thickness incision is made; the first is a shallow cut perpendicular to the gingival margin. It is meant to sever the epithelium and connective tissue to a depth of approximately 1.5 mm from the surface of the gingivae. This is carried out in a curved line connecting one side of the papilla to the other. The second incision traces the first but is more vertical to alveolar bone. This cut will result in a split thickness flap at the apical portion of the papilla base. Intrasulcular incisions are made in the remaining cervical aspects of the surgical sites and vertical relieving incision either side of the surgical site or papilla to be reflected. The use of a microsurgical blade is essential for the execution of this type of flap.

This incision allows preservation of the entire papilla, thus eliminating any substantial loss of papilla height as a result of the surgical or healing process. A thick and flat gingival biotype is ideal to ensure optimal recession free healing post-operatively.

Envelope Flap

A simple horizontal intrasulcular incision is made following the labial contour of the teeth. No vertical incisions are made allowing ease of repositioning (Fig. 13.11). This type of flap design is only useful in case of cervical resorption defects, cervical perforations and periodontal procedures. Due to limited access and visibility, this type of flap is not indicated in periradicular surgery.

Semilunar Flap

This type of flap (Fig. 13.12) has been indicated when carrying out surgical trephination or where aesthetic crowns are at risk of gingival recession from the proposed surgery.

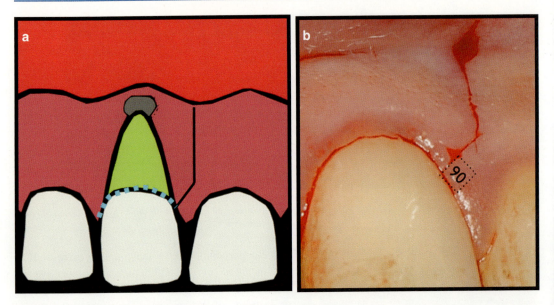

Fig 13.8 (**a, b**) Triangular flap design

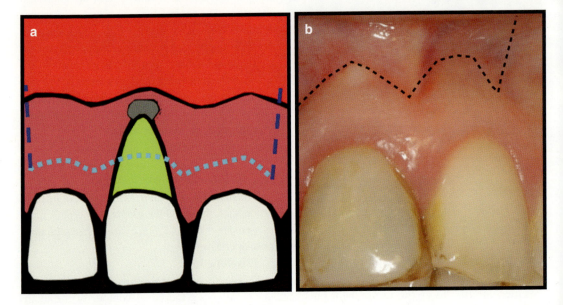

Fig 13.9 (**a, b**) Submarginal or Ochsenbein-Luebke flap

The flap itself expedites surgery by reducing incision and reflection times, maintains the integrity of the gingival attachment and eliminates potential crestal bone loss. Disadvantages include limited access and visibility, difficulties repositioning, increased incidence of postoperative scarring, predisposition to stretching and tearing of the flap and difficulties exposing the lesion in its entirety. Again this flap is mentioned from a historical point of view and is now somewhat obsolete in cases of peri-radicular surgery (Table 13.3).

13.6 Osteotomy

An initial assessment has been made from a parallel preoperative view as to the distance where the pathological defect lies in relation to the crown of the tooth (Fig. 13.13). This measurement is trans-

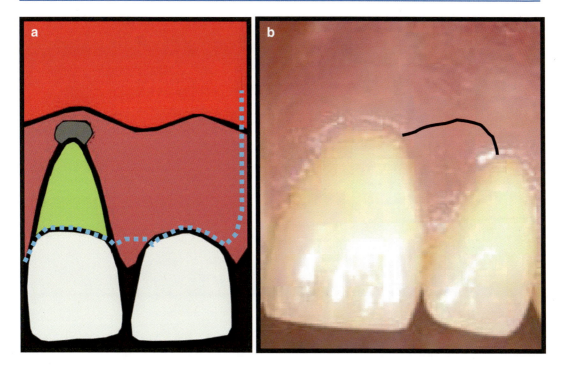

Fig 13.10 (**a**, **b**) Papillary base flap

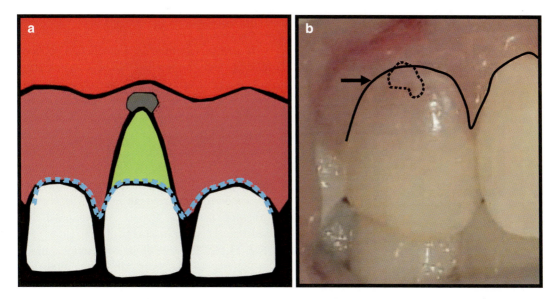

Fig 13.11 (**a**, **b**) Envelope flap. *Black arrow* signifies contour of gingival sulcus which incision line will follow

ferred to the mouth and the area explored for any pathological perforation of the cortical bone. If the soft tissue lesion has perforated the buccal plate, then osseous entry is simple.

Where an intact cortical plate is present, the area can be probed with an explorer to locate any area, which is reduced in density. Where the underlying soft tissue pathology is present but has not breached the cortical plate often, a thin amount of the bone may be present which is easily penetrated with a probe and removed using curettes (Fig. 13.14). Some authors have recommended

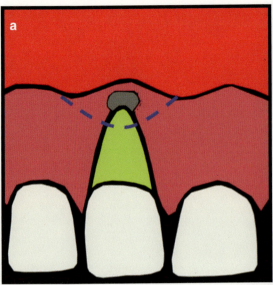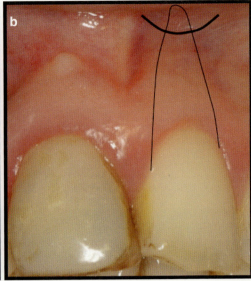

Fig 13.12 (**a**, **b**) Semilunar flap

Table 13.3 General points to consider regarding incisions and flap design

Firm continuous incisions should be made to sound bone
An incision should not cross an underlying bony defect
The vertical incision should be in the concavities between bone eminences
The vertical incision should not extend into the mucobuccal fold
The termination of the vertical incision at the gingival crest must be at the mesial or distal line angle of the tooth
The base of the flap must be at least equal to the width of its free end
The flap should offer adequate access and have an adequate blood supply
The flap must be of adequate size and fully reflected
The edges must lie on the sound bone
The flap should be protected throughout the surgical procedure with care not to cause further trauma to the soft tissues

drilling a small depression in the cortical bone and placing some radiopaque material such as softened gutta-percha, which can aid in orientation once a periapical radiograph is taken. The osteotomy is then extended in the appropriate direction.

Initial osteotomy should expose the apical portion of the root surface which is used as a guide to the apex. The osteotomy site is enlarged to expose the apical 3 mm of the root, which is to be resected.

It is important to make a distinction between root tip and surrounding bone. The operating microscope is useful for this purpose. Note root tissue is often more yellow and darker than adjacent bone. Unlike the bone, which is softer, it is not possible to indent with a probe and it does not bleed. The outline of the root also has a periodontal ligament, which can be stained using methylene blue dye (Fig. 13.15).

Osteotomy is carried out slowly with copious irrigation using an Impact Air 45 handpiece with an H161 Lindemann bone cutter bur (Fig. 13.16). The size of the osteotomy is based on access to the root tip with ultrasonic instruments freely within the bony crypt. Traditional peri-radicular surgery without the use of a microscope resulted in large osteotomies resulting in slower healing. The use of a dental microscope has resulted in smaller osteotomies – approximately 5 mm in diameter will be sufficient in most cases.

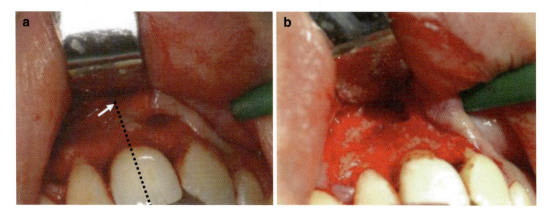

Fig 13.13 Clinical photographs showing (**a**) approximate measurement of estimated apex of the tooth (*white arrow*) based on preoperative radiographs and measurement of root length and (**b**) retractor sitting above pathological defect

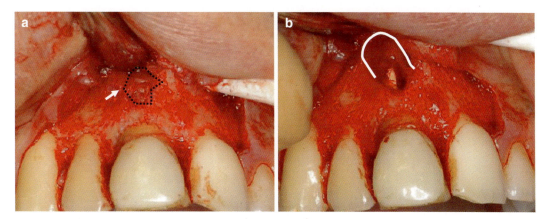

Fig 13.14 Clinical photographs showing (**a**) cortical plate intact but easily penetrable with a probe. *White arrow* signifies area overlying the apex where the bone is intact but thin. (**b**) Following removal of this layer of cortical bone exposed underlying pathology

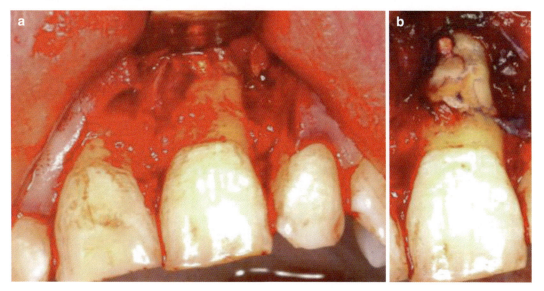

Fig 13.15 Clinical photographs demonstrating (**a**) exposed root surface and (**b**) following methylene blue staining. The dye is useful to confirm the periphery of the root as outlined with the periodontal ligament space and also for identifying root fractures as seen in this case

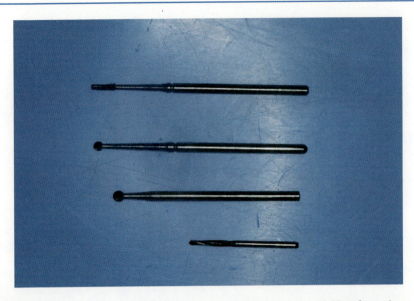

Fig 13.16 Clinical photograph showing typical burs used for surgical bone removal. Note fissure bur and round bur used for osteotomies and the Lindemann H161 bur at the *bottom* which is useful for root resection

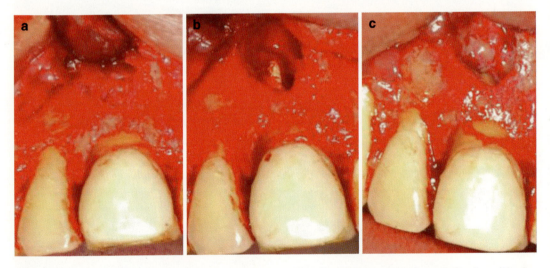

Fig 13.17 Clinical photographs showing (**a**) pre-osteotomy and (**b**) following osteotomy. Note hemorrhage within crypt due to granulation tissue still attached and (**c**) following complete removal of granulation tissue allowing visualization of the root apex

13.7 Peri-radicular Soft Tissue Curettage

Peri-radicular curettage alone does not eliminate the causative factors for a persistent lesion in most cases. However, it is an essential part of the procedure to remove the bulk of the diseased tissue, which surrounds the apex of the tooth. Removal of this tissue will allow unimpeded access for resection and retrograde obturation (Fig. 13.17).

Curettes (Fig. 13.18) can be used to completely remove the lesion from within the bony crypt. Occasionally the entire lesion cannot be removed until the root has been resected allowing further access to the most posterior aspect of the crypt. Granulation tissue is often responsible for

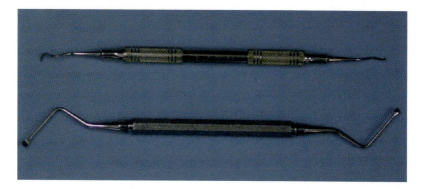

Fig 13.18 Clinical photograph showing currettes useful for periradicular curretage procedures and soft tissue removal in the bony crypt

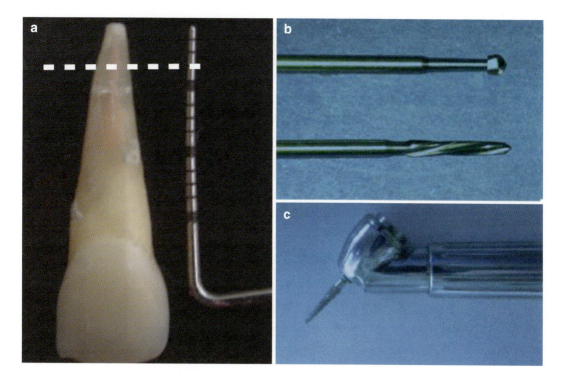

Fig 13.19 Clinical photographs showing (**a**) 3 mm of root resection perpendicular to long axis of the tooth, (**b**) surgical round bur and Lindemann bur, and (**c**) Impact Air 45 handpiece

haemorrhage within the crypt, and upon successful removal, haemostasis should be achieved.

13.8 Root-End Resection

Once the bony crypt is free of granulation tissue, the root tip can be easily identified allowing root-end resection to proceed. 3 mm of the root apex is resected at near perpendicular to the long axis of the root (Fig. 13.19). This is carried out with a Lindemann bur using the Impact Air 45 handpiece. Methylene blue stain is useful to identify the periphery of the periodontal ligament surrounding the resected root surface indicating complete resection using micro-mirrors under magnification.

The extent of the apical root resection is based on the findings that removing 3 mm of

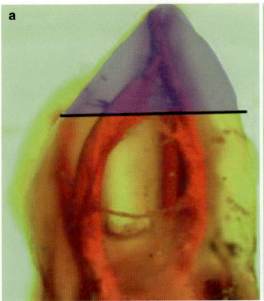 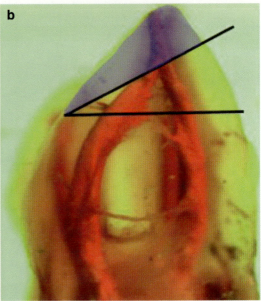

Fig 13.20 Clinical photograph of a cleared tooth showing (**a**) 0° perpendicular resection angle removing 98 % of apical ramifications and 93 % lateral canals compared to (**b**) traditional 45° resection angles. Note the volume of treated canal space by resection (*shaded areas*)

the apical root end reduces apical ramifications by 98 % and lateral canals by 93 % (Fig. 13.20).

This ideal length of resection must be balanced with the concept of a favourable crown-root ratio in order to remove apical ramifications responsible for persisting disease.

The angle or bevel of resection is also paramount to the clinical objective of ensuring all apical anatomy responsible for failure has been addressed. Traditional surgery where a dental operating microscope is not used will be more accommodating to a long bevel during preparation simply due to convenience.

This long bevel (angles of 30–45 or more) not only results in an increased length of resection but also inadequate removal of tooth structure, possible perforation of the lingual aspect of the root end due to spatial disorientation, less chance of inclusion of lingual anatomy during resection and increased leakage from dentinal tubules. A combination of any of these factors can account

for a less than desirable outcome leading to the possibility of failure.

A surgical microscopic technique, on the other hand, allows the root-end resection angle or bevel to be kept as short or as perpendicular to the long axis of the tooth as possible to facilitate the goal of complete resection, exposing all apical ramifications and root-end preparation without compromise and enhanced success.

The bevel angle of the resection is ideally perpendicular to the long axis of the root to ensure that fewer dentinal tubules are exposed preventing excess leakage (Fig. 13.21).

In resected root surfaces of maxillary permanent molars, mandibular molars or lower incisors, additional canal anatomy may be present on the lingual aspect, which has not been addressed during conventional endodontic treatment. A shorter bevel allows the clinician to identify this feature more readily facilitating further isthmus preparation and cleaning not achievable with a long bevel and its shortcomings.

13.9 Retrograde Preparation and Ultrasonic Instruments

Root-end preparation is completed using a variety of ultrasonic tips confining it to a depth of 3 mm within the long axis of the root canal resulting in a thoroughly cleaned and shape preparation. The ultrasonic tip is used in a light brushing motion slowly penetrating to the desired depth removing gutta-percha on withdrawal, which has been softened from the frictional heat generated (Fig. 13.22).

In mandibular incisors or mesiobuccal roots of maxillary molars following resection, there may be two canals connected by an isthmus (Fig. 13.23).

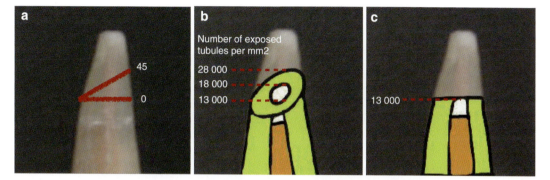

Fig 13.21 Diagrammatic representation of (**a**) number of dentinal tubules exposed according to angle of resection. (**b**) Note a long bevel of 45° results in a greater number of exposed tubules compared to (**c**) near perpendicular resection

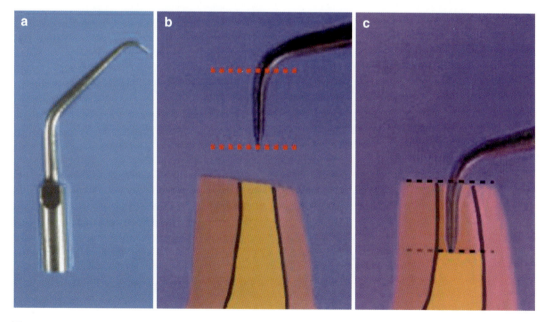

Fig 13.22 Clinical photographs and diagrammatic representation showing (**a**) ultrasonic tip used for root end preparation. (**b**) Note tip length approximately 3 mm and (**c**) placement of tip into root end to this depth creates retrograde filling space

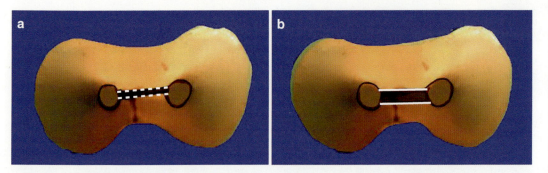

Fig 13.23 Diagrams showing (**a**) unprepared isthmus on an MB root and (**b**) following ultrasonic preparation

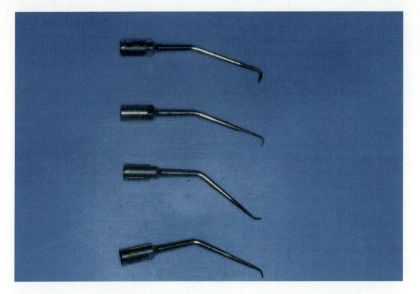

Fig 13.24 Clinical photographs showing various ultrasonic tips typically used for retrograde preparation. Note the tip is typically 3 mm in length; the ideal distance root end preparation is carried out following resection of the root

This groove between the canals can harbour necrotic material, which should be debrided. An ultrasonic tip used at low power can follow this groove connecting the two canals (Fig. 13.23), cleaning effectively without causing any detrimental damage to the tooth. The surgical operating microscope again is a prerequisite to ultrasonic preparation minimizing damage to the root end.

The appropriate ultrasonic tip is selected according to ease of access and visibility during retrograde preparation (Fig. 13.24).

Micro-mirrors are useful when inspecting the resected root surface to check that the resection is complete (Fig. 13.25). These mirrors come in a variety of shapes and sizes with diameters ranging from 1 to 5 mm. When using the surgical operating microscope, it is now possible to check for complete tissue removal, inspection of facial walls, ultrasonic retrograde preparation and filling material placement with ease.

13.10 Retrograde Obturation

Over the last century, every type of restorative material has been considered, at some time or another, for the purpose of a root-end filling material. The selection of an ideal root-end filling is based on principles, which fulfil a number of requirements (Table 13.4), which allow for healing.

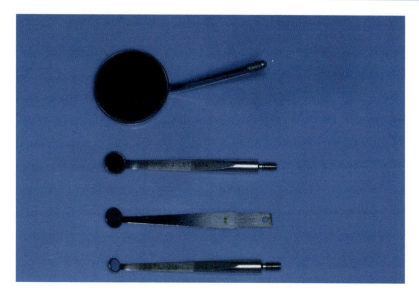

Fig 13.25 Clinical photograph showing normal standard dental mirror head (*above*) and micro-surgical mirrors (*below*). The micro-surgical mirrors are used in conjunction with the dental operating microscope under indirect vision. The compactness of the mirror head allows for a closer approach to the most inaccessible areas under examination

Table 13.4 Requirements of an ideal root-end filling material

Biocompatible promoting cementogenesis
Bactericidal and bacteriostatic
Moisture compatible and insoluble in tissue fluids
Ability to seal the root-end preparation
Ease of manipulation and placement with an adequate working time
Be radiopaque or easily discernible on radiographs
Does not discolour tooth structure or surrounding tissues

Traditionally amalgam has been used for many years as a root-end filling material. As dentists we are familiar with amalgam and its popularity was based on the fact that it was relatively inexpensive, easy to use and radiopaque and previously thought of as acceptable from a healing outcome perspective.

Clinical research has since contributed to its demise in popularity in relation to a root-end filling material. Questions have been raised as to its inability to seal effectively, handling difficulties and mercury content that does very little to promote tissue regeneration. The risk of amalgam corrosion, scatter and dispersion of particles into the surrounding tissues during manipulation and insertion is also a significant drawback. Potential discolouration and tattooing (tissue argyria) of the surrounding soft tissues can often result in areas where aesthetics is a concern (Fig. 13.26). Clinical follow-up studies have confirmed poor outcomes when using amalgam retrograde fillings and its use can no longer be supported.

Zinc oxide-eugenol cements such as IRM and Super EBA have demonstrated favourable results, in terms of healing, when used as root-end filling materials. Studies have shown that although regeneration is not possible, healing by repair does occur. Ease of manipulation of these types of material within an environment where moisture is an issue supports its use. Concerns have been raised with the potential for eugenol leaching, resulting in cytotoxicity, although this appears to be transient.

Mineral trioxide aggregate (MTA) developed at Loma Linda University, California, USA, has been shown to be biocompatible and encourage hard tissue deposition of cementum (cementogenesis) and excellent healing in randomized prospective clinical studies confirming its use as a root-end filling material. Its major disadvantages include cost, difficulty in manipulation, placement and setting properties. In a surgical field where moisture is a key concern, this can

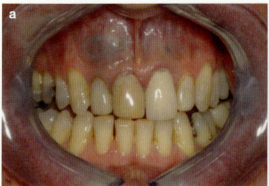
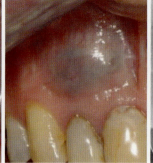
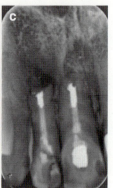

Fig 13.26 Clinical photographs and radiograph showing failed endodontic re-surgery. Amalgam retrograde fillings were placed. Note (**a**) and (**b**) typical amalgam tattoo and tissue argyria and (**c**) amalgam scatter in surrounding tissues, long bevel, and incomplete root resections associated with teeth 11 and 12

make the placement of MTA difficult although conversely it also encourages its setting.

Composite resins such as Retroplast have been shown to be clinically effective as root-end filling materials. Maintaining a dry field is a prerequisite when placing any composite, and this is probably its greatest disadvantage. The use of this type of material also is dependent on root-end cavity design based on a saucer-type preparation with a concave root-face preparation, which makes adhesion of the composite more amenable.

Diaket (a polyvinyl resin) has been advocated as a root-end filling material with favourable biocompatibility and regeneration similar to MTA. When the powder/liquid is mixed in a ratio of 2:1 the resultant consistency, handling and manipulation are far superior compared to MTA.

13.11 Closure and Suturing

Prior to closure of the wound and re-approximation of the tissue, flap compression is recommended. Firm pressure is applied with wet saline gauze for 5–10 min to reduce the coagulum to a thin fibrin clot between cortical bone and soft tissues providing optimal re-approximation and wound healing by primary intention.

Inadequate wound closure of an endodontic case can lead to delayed healing, wound dehiscence, scarring, gingival recession and ultimately an aesthetically unfavourable outcome. When selecting an appropriate suture material for closure of the surgical site, consideration must be given to the site of the flap and potential tension it may be under. The aim of sutures is to provide adequate tensile strength for proper repositioning of the soft tissues to their original position with the least amount of tension until healing has reached a stage whereby wound separation is unlikely to occur. The suture itself will induce a foreign body-type reaction, and delayed removal will increase the risk of infection and fibrous scarring. Nevertheless the suture material should not be removed early, and in situations where the wound may be under tension due to muscle attachments or frenal attachments, it may be prudent to leave the suture in for longer. Ideally sutures should be removed 3–5 days postoperatively when adequate wound strength has been achieved.

Suture materials available for wound closure include non-absorbable (synthetic) and absorbable (natural or synthetic) (Table 13.5). When there is a need to place buried intradermal sutures and when closing wide gaping wounds, absorbable sutures such as Vicryl are useful. Sutures can be further classified according to monofilament, multifilament or braided. The latter elicit a greater inflammatory tissue response.

Suture needles most frequently used in endodontic surgery are curved needles that range in shape from ¼ to 5/8 of a circle. A cutting needle of 11–13 mm in length with a 3/8 circle shape is most frequently used in dentistry.

Needle size denotes the diameter of the suture material. The smaller the diameter of the suture material, the less trauma potentially that may occur with the tissues to be sutured. Microsurgical wound closure requires non-absorbable suture material (such as monofilament polypropylene suture Prolene) from 5-0 to 8-0 in size.

Simple interrupted sutures are individually placed and tied to re-approximate the relieving incision during flap repositioning. A vertical mattress suture can be useful for papillary reattachment (Fig. 13.29). The total number of suture used is dependent on the type of flap selected and the minimal number needed to secure the flap in position. Remember that the sutures should not act as ligatures but keep the tissues in position without undue tension until wound strength is achieved.

Intra-oral suturing techniques require three main instruments: the needle holder (used to grab onto the suture needle) (Figs. 13.27 and 13.29), toothed tissue forceps (used to gently hold the tissues and grab the needle) (Figs. 13.28 and 13.29) and the suture scissors (used to cut the stitch from the rest of the suture material). Microsurgical instruments such as the Castroviejo microsurgery needle holder are useful when using 6-0–8-0 sutures (Fig. 13.27).

Sutures can be removed as early as 2–3 days or up to 7 days post-operatively (Fig. 13.30). Sutures are placed to ensure soft tissue reattachment occurs in the correct position. If adequate wound strength has not been achieved and sutures are removed too early, then the flap can detach leading to further post-operative complications. The use of monofilament

Table 13.5 Absorbable and non-absorbable suture materials commonly used in dento-alveolar surgery

A. *Absorbable sutures*
Surgical gut
Polyglactin 910 Vicryl (Ethicon)
Polyglycolic acid Dexon
Polyglyconate Maxon
Polydioxanone PDS II
B. *Non-absorbable sutures*
Silk suture
Nylon suture Ethilon
Polyester fibre Dacron
Polypropylene Prolene

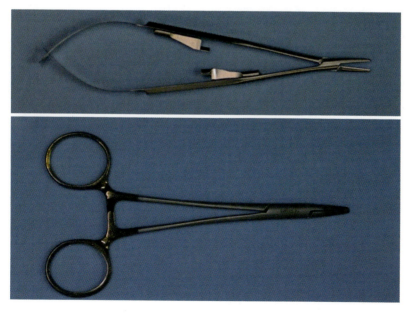

Fig 13.27 Clinical photographs showing Castroviejo microsurgical needle holder (*above*) and normal needle holder (*below*)

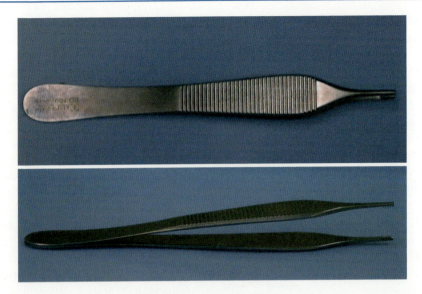

Fig 13.28 Clinical photograph showing single-toothed Adson, 7.6 cm (3 in.)

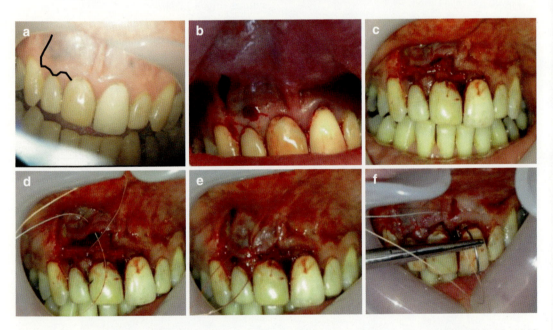

Fig. 13.29 Clinical photographs demonstrating intraoral sutures for repositioning a papillary preservation flap. Note (**a**) preoperative view demonstrating papillary incisions and vertical relieving incisions. (**b**) Perioperative view of papillary preservation flap. (**c**) Postsurgical completion and flap repositioning. A damp gauze was placed over the flap for 10 min with compression prior to suturing. (**d**) and (**e**) 5.0 interrupted suture to reposition papilla in 11 and 12 region. (**f**) and (**g**) Interrupted suture used to reposition midline papilla between 11 and 21. (**h**) Suturing complete using minimal number of sutures to reposition the flap. Interrupted sutures were also used for closure of the vertical relieving incision

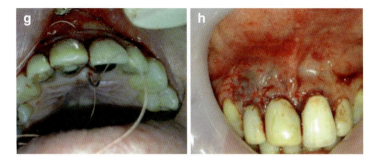

Fig. 13.29 (continued)

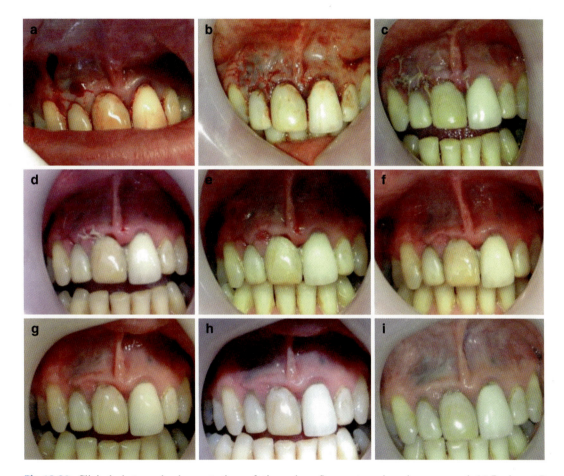

Fig 13.30 Clinical photographs demonstrating soft tissue healing for a papillary preservation flap over a 6-month duration. Note (**a**) perioperative view of papillary flap incision and (**b**) postsurgical view at day 0 with sutures in place. (**c**) Review at 3 days. (**d**) Review at 5 days. Some sutures have been removed. (**e**) Review at 7 days. All sutures have been removed. (**f**) Review at 14 days. (**g**) Review at 28 days. (**h**) Review at 3 months. (**i**) Review at 6 months. Note minimal gingival recession and scarring in overlying mucosa

sutures such as 5-0 or 6-0 polypropylene sutures further reduces inflammation due to the accumulation of plaque often associated with larger braided sutures in more traditional techniques. Soft tissue healing can be observed at 5 days, 28 days and 6 months to monitor whether any post-operative complications such as scarring or recession have occurred (Fig. 13.30).

13.12 Surgical Complications

Pain, bleeding, swelling, ecchymosis (bruising), lacerations, paraesthesia and sinus complications are all possible surgical sequelae depending on the site of surgery, patient and clinician. All patients should be given both verbal and written post-operative instructions as to the aftercare following surgical endodontics (Fig. 13.31). Patients are advised on diet and fluid intake. Oral hygiene is important during the early post-surgical period. The patient can be advised to use a chlorhexidine

mouthwash both preoperatively and 24 h postoperatively. The patient is advised to avoid brushing the teeth for the first 24 h to reduce any risk of flap trauma. Cotton swabs can be gently used to remove food debris using chlorhexidine. 24 h after surgery, the patient is advised to brush with care the remaining teeth and only the incisal or occlusal surface of the teeth in direct relation to the surgical site.

Pain

Mild pain is to be expected after surgical endodontics. Long-acting anaesthetics such as

INSTRUCTIONS TO BE FOLLOWED
AFTER ENDODONTIC SURGERY

TODAY:
1) As soon as possible, apply ice packs to your face - apply for one minute, off for a few seconds. Apply for a period of 15 minutes, rest for 15 minutes, then apply for another 15 minute period only.
2) Take medication as prescribed - tablets for pain are to be taken only as required.
3) Nothing to eat or drink for 2 hours (apart from water with the tablets) then have only food that is cool and soft for the rest of the day.

AVOID ALCOHOL AND REFRAIN FROM SMOKING

4) Keep quiet - no strenuous exercise.
5) No tooth brushing today.
6) Do not attempt to lift the lip to examine the surgery site at any time.

TOMORROW:
1) Rinse mouth for the first time after breakfast with warm salt and water solution. (Add half a tablespoon of salt to a cup of warm water).
                *Repeat after each meal and before bed.
2) Cold to warm (but not hot) food and drink can be taken.
3) Brush teeth normally, but avoid actual surgery site.

AFTER SUTURE REMOVAL:
1) For one week, rinse mouth with fairly hot salt-water solution after each meal and before bed.
2) Cold or hot foods can be taken.
3) Brush teeth normally, but avoid actual surgery site.

EXPECT SORENESS, SOME SWELLING AND BRUISING. SOME LIGHT BLEEDING ON THE FIRST DAY IS NORMAL.

Fig 13.31 Postoperative written instructions that can be given to the patient following endodontic surgery to minimize any complications

bupivacaine (Marcaine) can be injected into the surgical site at the end of the procedure to control pain for up to 8 h. Preemptive analgesics using non-steroidal anti-inflammatory agents are taken preoperatively. The patient is advised to continue with pain medication for the first 48 h and up to the first week if indicated.

Haemorrhage

Post-operative haemorrhage is often a rare complication that can occur. Light oozing from the surgical site is expected, and the patient is warned that this can occur for several hours after surgery and is normal. The patient is advised to avoid spitting or rinsing for 24 h. If minor bleeding occurs during the first 24 h, then the patient is instructed to apply a 2×2 in. gauze pad, which has been moistened with sterile water with moderate finger pressure for at least 10–15 min. If the bleeding cannot be stopped by this simple measure, then the patient should return to the endodontic office immediately. The patient is also advised against any strenuous activity including exercise and alcohol for 1–2 days post-operatively to reduce any blood pressure increases, which may inadvertently result in a greater chance of bleeding.

Swelling

Swelling is common post-operative sequelae and can often be of concern to the patient. The patient can be instructed to apply an ice pack with firm pressure over the surgical site. The ice pack is applied for approximately 20 min and then removed for 20 min. This regime is continued for 6–8 h post-operatively and initiated in the surgery prior to dismissal. The pressure and reduction in tissue temperature slows the blood flow to the surgical site promoting coagulation and counteracting rebound haemorrhage. Cold compression also has analgesic effects by reducing peripheral nerve endings and is advised to reduce post-operative bleeding and swelling. Continuous application is to be advised again since this will be counterproductive increased blood flow and consequently increased risk of bleeding.

Ecchymosis

The discolouration of the oral soft tissues due to the extravasation and subsequent breakdown of blood in the subcutaneous tissues can be alarming for the unadvised patient. The patient should be advised that any post-operative ecchymosis has no bearing on the success or outcome of the case. Moist heat application is useful to reduce ecchymosis and should be started 18–24 h post-operatively. The patient can be instructed to wet a towel with hot water and apply to the face every 30 min. The patient must be warned against heat application until 18–24 h since this will result in bleeding and swelling.

Lacerations

Careful handling of the soft tissues and prevention of retractor slippage are essential to avoid tearing or perforation of the flap. Overstretching of the lips should be avoided to prevent lacerations of the commissures. Care must be excised when placing incisions to ensure that only the surgical site is purposely cut.

Paraesthesia

Transient paraesthesia or the abnormal sensation of burning, itching or numbness can commonly occur due to localized inflammatory swelling. The most common nerves affected are the inferior alveolar nerve (after mandibular molar surgery) and mental nerve (after premolar surgery). As long as the nerve has not been severed, sensation will usually return in the coming weeks and months, and the patient should be reassured that sensation would return to normal eventually.

Sinus Complications

Posterior maxillary surgery carries the risk of breaching the maxillary sinus and perforation of the schneiderian membrane. If a breach is evident at time of surgery, then the clinician should ensure that no foreign material enters the sinus. Primary surgical closure should allow for uneventful healing in the coming weeks. The patient should be instructed to avoid blowing their nose that can increase the likelihood of an oral-antral communication being formed. Prophylactic antibiotics can be administered and anticongestants may be recommended.

13.13 Clinical Cases

Case 1 Foreign body reaction to Gutta-Percha

Tooth 21 had been root treated and obturated with gutta-percha and sealer following a complicated crown fracture sustained from a traumatic injury. The tooth was subsequently restored with a post and core restoration. The patient presented at specialist practice with a persistent fistula. Radiographic examination revealed a peri-radicular radiolucency with a radiopaque material at the centre of the lesion. A gutta-percha sinus-tracing radiograph confirmed the fistula was related to this material (Fig. 13.32e, f). A papillary preservation flap was made with a single relieving incision at the mucogingival margin of tooth 22. The flap was carefully elevated, reflected and retracted. The buccal cortical plate was fenestrated with evidence of gutta-percha within the soft tissue lesion (Fig. 13.32a, b). The periapical tissue was curetted. An apicectomy was performed with a Lindemann bone cutter in an Impact Air 45 handpiece. The resected root apex was examined and prepared with an ultrasonic tip. A well-mixed MTA retrograde filling was placed into the cavity and condensed with micropluggers. Excess MTA was removed with a curette and the resected root surface cleaned with a moist cotton wool pellet. The flap was repositioned using 5-0 monofilament sutures (Fig. 13.32d). The patient returned for suture removal 5 days later. The buccal sinus had resolved at 1- and 6-month review appointments.

Case 2 Surgical apicectomy of a tooth with a post crown restoration

A 34-year-old fit and healthy patient was referred for endodontic management of tooth 21. The patient had sustained a traumatic injury to the tooth whilst surfing as a teenager. The tooth had been treated with conventional root canal treatment, gutta-percha

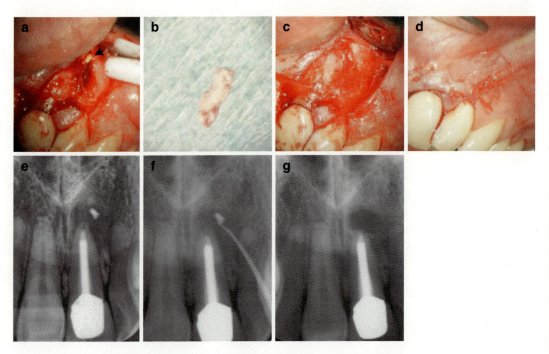

Fig 13.32 Clinical photographs and radiographs demonstrating failed endodontic treatment due to foreign body reaction related to a gutta-percha fragment (possibly from an overfill). Note (**a**) intraoperative view following papillary preservation flap reflection and retraction. (**b**) Removed gutta-percha. (**c**) Following curettage of soft tissue lesion. (**d**) Closure using 5.0 monofilament sutures. (**e**) Preoperative radiograph demonstrating orthograde root filling and post crown restoration. (**f**) Note sinus tracing radiograph associated with extruded gutta-percha piece. (**g**) Posttreatment radiograph showing removal of fragment, apicectomy, and retrograde MTA filling

orthograde filling and subsequent post crown restoration. The patient had been aware of pain and tenderness overlying the tooth. Radiographic examination revealed a well-fitting post crown restoration with orthograde root filling. A peri-radicular radiolucency was evident. A papillary preservation flap was made and tissues retracted and reflected to reveal an extensive buccal cortical plate fenestration. Periapical curettage was carried out and the lesion sent for biopsy. Root resection was carried out and retrograde preparation completed using ultrasonics. MTA was used as a retrograde filling. The surgical site was closed with 5-0 monofilament sutures. The patient was reviewed a week later for suture removal. Review examination at 6 months revealed the patient

remained asymptomatic. Radiographic examination revealed bony infilling with an intact periodontal ligament space associated with the periapex of tooth 21 (see Fig. 13.33). Histopathology confirmed a diagnosis of periapical granuloma.

Case 3 Endodontic retreatment, treatment and surgical apicectomy of teeth 31 and 41

A fit and healthy 29-year-old patient was referred for conventional endodontic retreatment of tooth 41 and treatment of tooth 31. Clinical examination revealed obvious buccal tenderness overlying the periapices of teeth 31 and 41. Tooth 31 was unrestored. Tooth 31 responded negatively to both electric pulp testing and thermal

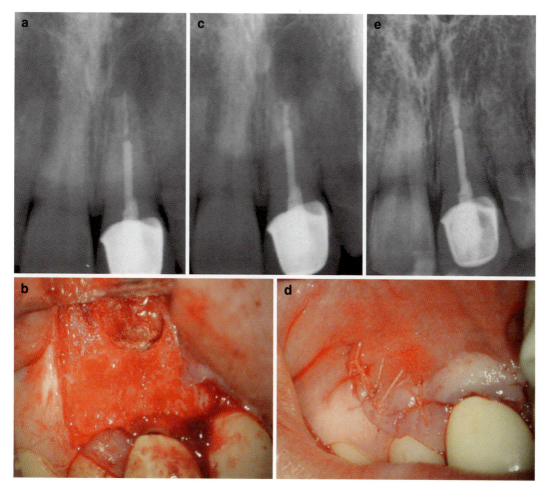

Fig 13.33 Clinical radiographs and photographs showing (**a**) preoperative view with existing periradicular area, (**b**) surgical osteotomy site exposing root end of tooth 21, (**c**) following root resection and MTA retrograde filling placement, (**d**) 5.0 sutures used for closure, and (**e**) 6-month review radiograph demonstrating healed case

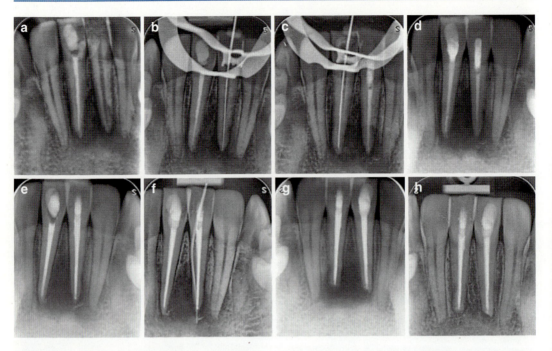

Fig 13.34 Clinical radiographs showing (**a**) preoperative view of suboptimal root treated 41 and non-vital 31. (**b**) and (**c**) Root canal instrumentation of 31 and 41. (**d**) Intracanal calcium hydroxide dressing which was placed for a period of 3 months. (**e**) Post-treatment radiograph demonstrating well-obturated canals. (**f**) 4-month post-treatment radiograph demonstrating sinus tracing related to periapex of tooth 31. (**g**) Immediate postsurgical radiograph demonstrating root resections and retrograde MTA fillings. (**h**) 6-month review radiograph demonstrating complete healing

stimulus (CO2 snow). Radiographic examination revealed previous endodontic treatment of tooth 41 (deemed suboptimal). An extensive peri-radicular radiolucency was associated with the periapices of teeth 31 and 41. Non-surgical root canal treatment and retreatment of teeth 31 and 41 were carried out. Intra-canal dressings of calcium hydroxide were used for an extended period of 3 months prior to completion of obturation. 4 months post treatment, the patient presented with a draining fistula, which was related to the periapex of tooth 31. Periapical surgery was carried out. Soft tissue lesion was curetted and sent for histopathological examination (confirmed as periapical granuloma). Root resection was carried out and retrograde preparation completed using ultrasonics. MTA was used for root-end fillings. The site was sutured and patient reviewed a week later for suture removal. The patient healed uneventfully and was reviewed at 6-month follow-up. Radiographic examination revealed intact periodontal ligament spaces associated with the periapices of teeth 31 and 41 (see Fig. 13.34).

Case 4 Endodontic retreatment and re-surgery of teeth 11 and 12

A 62-year-old nervous patient was referred for endodontic management of teeth 11 and 12. The patient presented with pain and swelling in relation to these teeth. Past history revealed the patient had undergone conventional root canal treatment and apicectomy on two occasions. Clinical examination revealed a fluctuant swelling in relation to teeth 11 and 12. Tissue argyria was evident with an amalgam tattoo. Radiographic examination confirmed previous orthograde root fillings and retrograde amalgam fillings in both teeth. A long bevel resection was evident with a peri-radicular lesion associated with the periapex of tooth 12. Non-surgical root canal retreatment was undertaken in both teeth. Amalgam retrograde fillings were deemed intact. Both teeth were obturated using a warm vertical compaction technique using AH Plus cement. Surgery was carried out under oral sedation.

A papillary preservation flap with a single distal relieving incision was made. The flap was

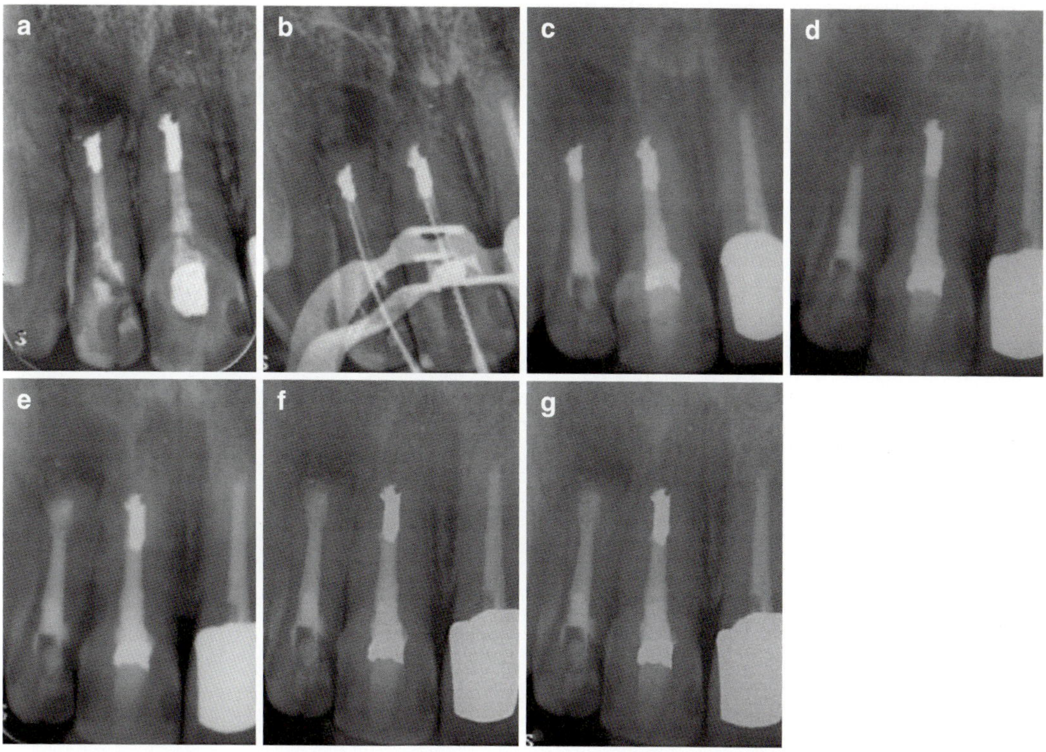

Fig 13.35 Clinical radiographs showing (**a**) preoperative view of teeth 11 and 12. The patient had previously undergone root canal treatments and surgical apicectomy and re-apicectomy. (**b**) Conventional re-treatment and (**c**) obturation of both teeth using a warm vertical compaction technique. (**d**) Surgical re-apicectomy showing removal of retrograde amalgam filling in tooth 12 without further amalgam scatter. (**e**) Postsurgical radiograph demonstrating MTA retrograde filling. (**f**) 6-month review radiograph showing bony infilling. (**g**) Further 6-month review show-ing further reduction in lesion size. The patient remained asymptomatic with no tenderness in the overlying soft tissues. This case will require careful follow-up and radiographic monitoring to ensure peri-apical healing continues. A persistent radiolucency and asymptomatic tooth may indicate the presence of peri-apical scar tissue that requires no further intervention. Previous surgery on two occasions and near through and through lesion extending from labial to palatal direction increases the likelihood of scar formation

reflected and retracted to confirm a buccal cortical plate fenestration overlying tooth 12. Soft tissue curettage was carried out to reveal a bony crypt with near through and through lesion extending palatally. Haemostasis within the crypt was achieved using epinephrine pellets.

The amalgam retrograde filling was removed using ultrasonics. A damp piece of cotton wool gauze was placed posteriorly within the crypt to prevent amalgam scatter. The resected root was inspected and a perpendicular bevel created using a Lindemann bone cutter in an Impact Air 45 handpiece. The resected root apex was examined under the dental operating microscope and retrograde preparation completed using ultrasonics. An MTA retrograde filling was placed and condensed with micropluggers. The root end was cleaned with a moistened cotton wool pellet. The flap was repositioned and sutured using 5-0 monofilament synthetic sutures. The patient returned for suture removal a week later with no post-operative complications. The patient was reviewed at 6 months and 12 months to assess periapical healing (see Figs. 13.26, 13.29, 13.30 and 13.35).

Case 5 Endodontic retreatment and apicectomy of teeth 31 and 41

A fit and healthy 22-year-old nurse was referred to the UCL Eastman Dental Institute for endodontic retreatment of teeth 31 and 41. Radiographic examination revealed an extensive peri-radicular radiolucency associated with both periapices. A postgraduate endodontic student undertook conventional root canal retreatment of both teeth, and only one canal was located in both teeth (Fig. 13.36).

The patient was reviewed in the department by myself 12 months later with obvious pain and tenderness in relation to both teeth. A decision was made to carry out surgical apicectomy. A full mucoperiosteal flap was raised with a single relieving incision in the 43 region. Care was taken to identify the right mental nerve and ensure that the incision was well away. The flap was reflected and retracted accordingly, and a large soft tissue lesion within a bony crypt was evident (Fig. 13.37).

Extensive buccal cortical bone was destroyed. Periapical curettage was carried out, and soft tissue was sent for histopathological diagnosis (confirmed as periapical granuloma) (Fig. 13.38).

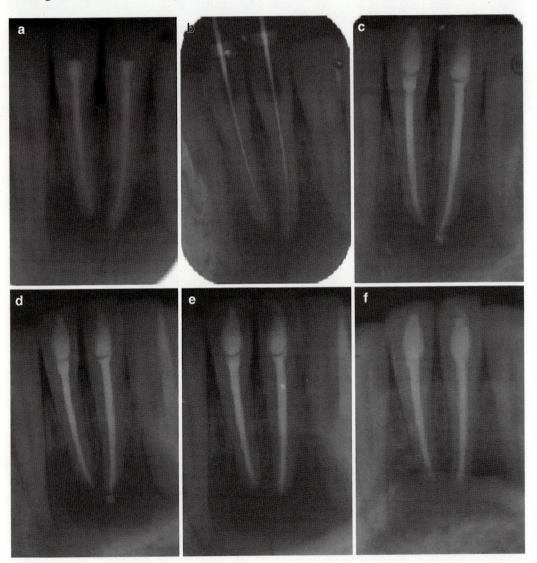

Fig 13.36 Clinical radiographs demonstrating endodontic re-treatment and surgical apicectomy carried out by post graduate endodontic students. Note (**a**) pre-operative view of teeth 31 and 41 demonstrating an extensive peri-radicular radiolucent lesion in relation to these teeth despite non surgical root canal therapy. (**b–c**) Conventional re-treatment. Note overfill surplus material associated with tooth 31. (**d**) The patient was seen 12 months later for further review. At this time she was complaining of ongoing pain and tenderness in relation to these teeth. A decision was made to carry out further endodontic surgery. (**e**) Immediately post-apicectomy. Surgical curettage, root resection, root end-preparation using ultrasonics and retrograde filling with MTA was carried out. (**f**) 9-month follow up demonstrating complete healing of teeth 31 and 41

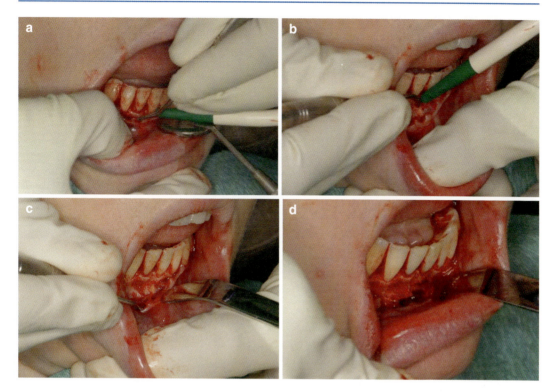

Fig 13.37 (**a-d**) Clinical photographs demonstrating full mucoperiosteal flap reflection and retraction revealing underlying buccal cortical plate destruction and extensive soft tissue lesion within the bony crypt

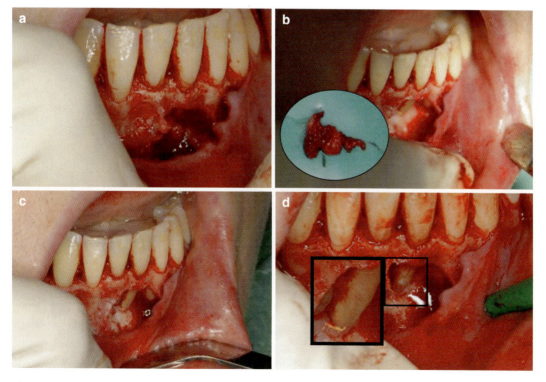

Fig 13.38 Clinical photographs demonstrating (**a**) and (**b**) soft tissue curettage. Insert lesion was sent for histopathology confirming periapical granuloma. (**c**) and (**d**) Bony crypt with overfilled root filling prior to root resection

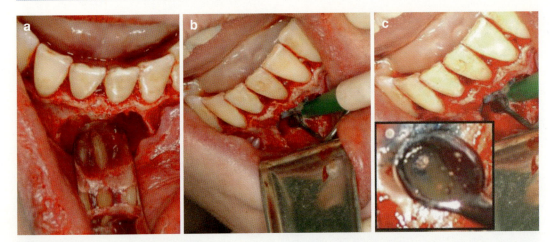

Fig 13.39 (a-c) Clinical photographs demonstrating resected root surfaces stained with methylene blue dye and examined under high magnification (×16) to check for signs of root fracture and additional missed/untreated canal anatomy or isthmuses. No additional anatomy was seen

The crypt was irrigated with saline and haemostasis achieved using epinephrine pellet technique. Root resections were carried out and retrograde ultrasonic preparation. The resected root surfaces were dried and stained with methylene blue dye. High magnification (X16) was used to inspect the resected root surfaces for any fractures and additional canals and isthmuses. No additional anatomy was noted (Fig. 13.39).

A well-mixed MTA retrograde filling was placed in both teeth followed by condensing with appropriate micropluggers. Excess MTA was removed using a moist cotton wool pellet. Final irrigation of the crypt was carried out using saline. The flap was repositioned and closure was carried out with monofilament synthetic 5-0 sutures. The patient returned for suture removal after 72 h. The patient returned three days later with failure of flap. Due to lower lip musculature, the flap had failed to heal. Further suturing was carried out and the patient returned a week later for suture removal. The patient healed uneventfully with no long-term consequences. The patient was reviewed at 9 months at which time she had begun fixed orthodontic appliance therapy. Radiographic examination revealed complete bony infill and healing with the absence of both clinical and radiographic signs and symptoms. An intact periodontal ligament space could be seen with both periapices of teeth 31 and 41 (Fig. 13.40).

Case 6 Through and through surgery of tooth 12

A fit and healthy 49-year-old female patient was referred for endodontic retreatment of tooth 12. At the consultation appointment, the patient reported pain and tenderness associated with the tooth and increasing mobility. She recalled this tooth had undergone root canal treatment in her teenage years after an impacted canine tooth was extracted. Clinical examination revealed obvious tenderness in the overlying alveolar mucosa on the labial aspect. Grade I mobility was noted with a normal periodontal profile. Radiographic examination confirmed previous endodontic treatment in tooth 12. A peri-radicular radiolucency was noted with obvious root foreshortening (Fig. 13.41). Treatment options were discussed and a decision was made to embark upon root canal retreatment of tooth 12.

The coronal restoration was dismantled and gutta-percha root filling identified. Root filling material was removed using a chloroform wicking technique. A large open apex was confirmed and a stainless steel hand file #140 could be passed through the apex. Minimal canal preparation was carried out and irrigation using 1 % sodium hypochlorite solution. An intra-canal dressing of calcium hydroxide was placed for a 6-week period. At the review appointment, the patient was still aware of tenderness overlying the periapex of tooth 12. A decision was made to carry out a surgical through and through approach combining

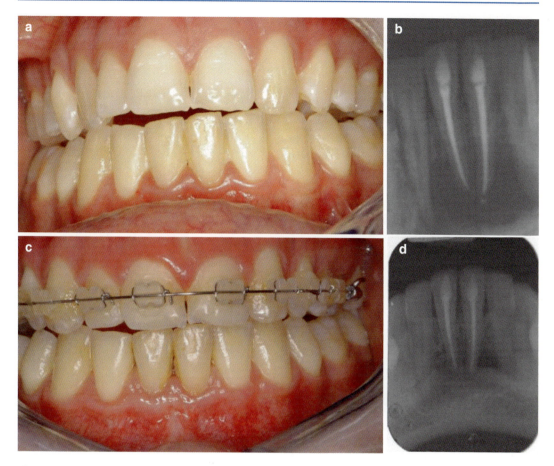

Fig 13.40 Clinical photographs and radiographs demonstrating (**a**) and (**b**) preoperative views and (**c**) and (**d**) postoperative views. Note complete healing observed after a 9-month period post apicectomy

periapical curettage with orthograde obturation of the large canal space with an irregular open apex. Normally a through and through treatment approach is indicated when exudation into the root canal cannot be controlled by non-surgical chemo-mechanical debridement. In this case a surgical approach using flap elevation would allow for periapical curettage and offer better control when completing obturation of the root canal system.

At time of surgery, the patient had taken pre-emptive analgesics 1 h preoperatively. The temporary coronal restoration was dismantled. A papillary preservation flap design was used with a single distal relieving incision in the 14 region. Following flap elevation the bony crypt was identified and soft tissue curettage carried out. The existing canal medicament was removed, and irrigation of the root canal system was performed using chlorhexidine solution. The canal

was dried using paper points. An orthograde MTA root filling was placed using the MAP system at the apex, and a flat plastic instrument was placed in the bony crypt overlying the root apex to prevent gross extrusion of MTA into the bony cavity. The MTA was allowed to set, and then the remaining root canal system was obturated with thermoplasticized injection gutta-percha (Obtura). The access cavity was then sealed with a double temporary restorative material using IRM and glass ionomer cement. The flap was repositioned and closure carried out with 5-0 Vicryl sutures. The patient was reviewed a week later and sutures were removed. Soft tissues were healing well, and the patient was followed up at 4 weeks at which time she remained asymptomatic. Further follow-up was arranged at 12 months to assess bony healing (see Figs. 13.41, 13.42 and 13.43).

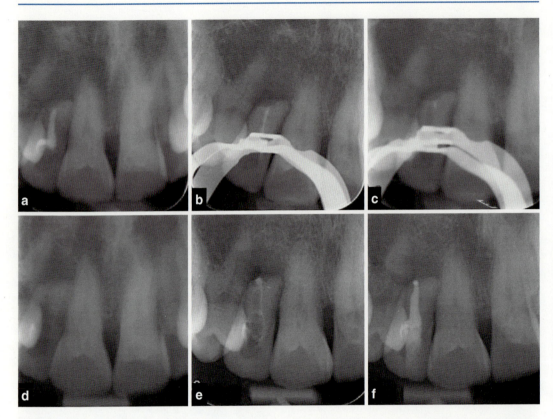

Fig 13.41 Clinical radiographs demonstrating nonsurgical root canal treatment and surgical through and through approach of tooth 12. Note (**a**) preoperative view demonstrating previous root filling in tooth 12. Note periradicular infection and foreshortened root apex of tooth 12. (**b**) and (**c**) Removal of gutta-percha using a chloroform wicking technique. (**d**) Apical foramen size was estimated greater than size #140. An intracanal medicament of calcium hydroxide was placed for 6 weeks. At the review appointment pain, tenderness and mobility were still evident with tooth 12. A decision was made to adopt a surgical approach combining a through and through approach to complete endodontic treatment. (**e**) MTA orthograde filling placement. (**f**) Completed root filling using AH Plus cement and gutta-percha (Elements Obturation)

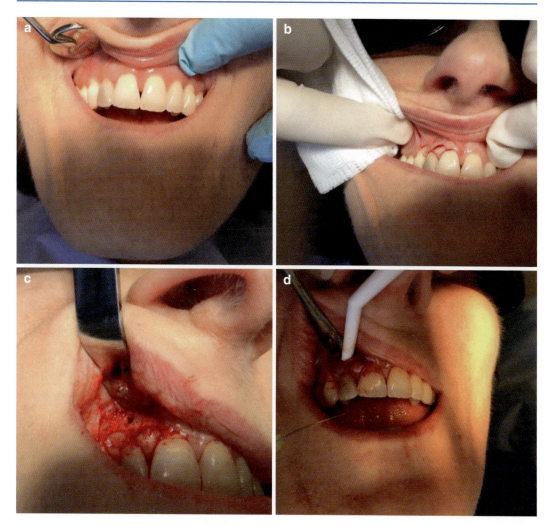

Fig 13.42 Clinical photographs demonstrating surgical through and through approach to complete obturation of canal system. Note (**a**) preoperative view demonstrating thick and flat gingival papillae ideal for use of a papillary preservation flap. (**b**) Incision of papillary preservation flap with one distal relieving incision. (**c**) Following flap reflection, bony crypt identified. Soft tissue curettage was carried out and apex of 12 identified. (**d**) Canal irrigation is carried out with chlorhexidine to ensure all remnants of calcium hydroxide dressing material have been removed

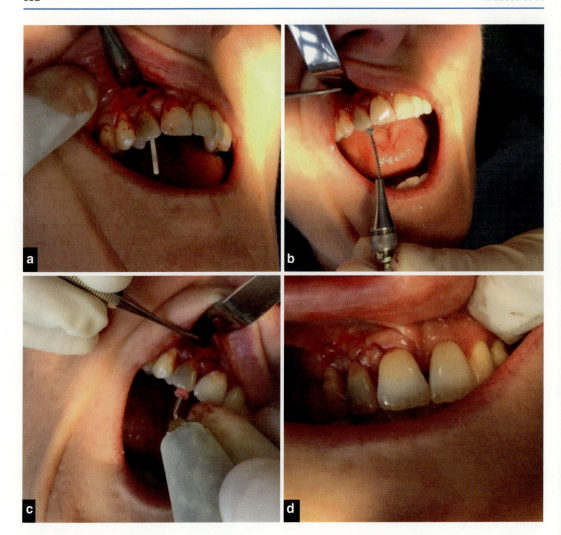

Fig 13.43 Clinical photographs demonstrating surgical through and through approach to manage endodontic re-treatment of tooth 12. Note (**a**) canal is dried with paper points prior to obturation procedure. (**b**) Orthograde MTA placement is completed using the MAP system. Excess MTA is prevented from overfilling by placement of a flat plastic instrument over the root end. (**c**) Once MTA has set, the remaining canal space is obturated with gutta-percha using Obtura. (**d**) After a temporary double seal coronal restoration of IRM and GIC is placed, the flap is repositioned and sutured using 5.0 Vicryl sutures

Clinical Hints and Tips when Carrying Out Surgical Endodontics

- **Clinical assessment**
  A thorough extra-oral and intra-oral examination should be undertaken, in particular noting mouth opening, swelling, sinus tracts, quality of cast restoration (marginal adaptation, history of decementation), periodontal status (the presence of isolated pocketing), occlusal relationship and sensibility and percussion testing.

- **Radiological assessment**
  Long cone parallel periapical view of the tooth should be obtained showing entire lesion and at least 3 mm beyond the radiolucent lesion. The use of limited volume conebeam CT scan is particularly useful in pre-surgical assessment to determine the exact location of root apex/apices and to evaluate the proximity of adjacent anatomical structures and their relationship to the planned surgery.

- **Referral**
  Appropriate referral should be made to a suitably trained colleague.

- **Preoperative medication**
  Uses of preemptive analgesics such as NSAIDS are proven to be effective for pain management. Prophylactic administration of antibiotics routinely for patients is not indicated unless medical history indicates necessity. Routine use of a chlorhexidine mouth rinse to reduce plaque formation is useful.

- **Anaesthesia**
  The use of a local anaesthetic with a vasoconstrictor is not only useful for allowing pain-free surgery but also to manage haemostasis at the surgical site.

- **Magnification**
  The use of microsurgical techniques and the dental operating microscope improves visualization and control of the surgical site and should be the standard of care.

- **Soft tissue management**
  Appropriate flap selection should be based on a number of factors including gingival biotype, size of peri-radicular lesion, status and type of coronal restoration and adjacent anatomical structures. The use of a semilunar flap is contraindicated due to difficulty with determining the exact size of the periapical lesion and increased risk of scarring. All relieving incisions should be placed on sound bone. After flap reflection the flap should be protected at all times with retractors resting on sound bone and the use of wet gauze to prevent desiccation. Following reflection of the mucoperiosteal flap, any bleeding tags of tissue from the surgical site should not be removed to facilitate healing at time of repositioning.

- **Hard tissue management**
  A preoperative assessment of the length of the root and its axis should be made to ensure that osteotomy is carried out at the appropriate site when the cortical plate is intact. The use of appropriate burs using a reverse-air handpiece cooled with copious sterile saline or water is essential to prevent risk of air emphysema at the surgical site.

- **Peri-radicular curettage**
  The majority of inflammatory soft tissue should be removed and sent for histopathological examination. If there is risk of damaging adjacent anatomical structures, then leaving tissue may be appropriate.

- **Root-end resection**
  Root resection should be carried out as close to 90° to the long axis of the tooth as possible to ensure adequate access to apical anatomy and minimize exposure of dentinal tubules. Removal of at least 3 mm of the root end using copious irrigation should ensure removal of the majority anatomical anomalies in the apical 1/3rd of the root. Root resection will be dictated by favourable root-crown ratio, and this must be taken into account prior to resection. Application of methylene blue sterile dye is indicated to help visualize apical anatomy and potential cracks and fractures that may be present.

- **Retrograde cavity preparation**
  Root-end preparation should be at least 3 mm in length and in the long axis of the tooth following pulp space morphology. The use of ultrasonic tips at appropriate power settings under direct or indirect vision using micro-mirrors and the dental operating microscope reduces risk of damage.
- **Retrograde filling**
  The use of an appropriate biologically compatible root-end filling material should be used to ensure an adequate apical seal that is well tolerated by the surrounding tissues. Amalgam is no longer recommended.
- **Bony crypt management prior to closure**
  Prior to closure the bony crypt should be carefully debrided and irrigated to ensure all haemostatic agents, root-end filling materials, debris and any gauze have been removed which can cause a potential foreign body reaction and delayed/unfavourable healing. A post-operative radiograph should be taken to assess the final root-end filling prior to closure.
- **Repositioning of flap and suturing**
  The soft tissue flap should be repositioned and reapposed with appropriate sutures that allow primary closure. Immediately following closure with sutures, the tissues should be firmly compressed for at least 5 min with a damp gauze to reduce the possibility of a blood clot forming between flap and the bone that can lead to potential delayed wound healing.
- **Post-operative care**
  Appropriate post-operative pain management includes the use of a long-acting local anaesthetic and the use of either NSAIDS or paracetamol with or without codeine. Application of cold compresses with an appropriate ice pack for the first 6 h may be useful to reduce post-operative swelling. Maintenance of good oral hygiene and the use of post-operative chlorhexidine mouth rinses may be beneficial to ensure good soft tissue healing. Both verbal and clear

written instructions should be given to the patient. Sutures should be removed when adequate wound strength has been achieved (72–96 h) to prevent infection by wicking. In areas under tension, sutures may be left in for up to 7 days before removal. The patient should be followed up 1 week and 4 weeks for soft tissue assessment and 6 months for a radiological review to determine bony healing. Further reviews may be required until evidence of healing is noted.

References

1. European Society of Endodontology. Quality guidelines for endodontic treatment: consensus report of the European Society of Endodontology. Int Endod J. 2006;39:921–30.
2. Kakehashi S, Stanley HR, Fitzgerald RJ. The effects of surgical exposures of dental pulps in germfree and conventional laboratory rats. J South Calif Dent Assoc. 1966;34:449–51.
3. Bergenholtz G. Micro-organisms from necrotic pulp of traumatized teeth. Odontol Revy. 1974;25:347–58.
4. Sundqvist G. Bacteriological studies of necrotic dental pulps. Umea University Odontological Dissertation No.7. Umea: University of Umea; 1976.
5. Friedman S, Mor C. The success of endodontic therapy – healing and functionality. J Calif Dent Assoc. 2004;32(6):493–503.
6. Nair PNR. Pathogenesis of apical periodontitis and the cause of endodontic failures. Crit Rev Oral Biol Med. 2004;15:348–81.
7. Sjogren U, Happonen RP, Kahnberg KE, Sundqvist G. Survival of Arachnia propionica in periapical tissue. Int Endod J. 1988;21:277–82.
8. Nair PNR, Sjogren U, Krey G, Sundqvist G. Therapy-resistant foreign-body giant cell granuloma at the periapex of a root-filled human tooth. J Endod. 1990;16:589–95.
9. Nair PNR, Sjogren U, Schumacher E, Sundqvist G. Radicular cyst affecting a root-filled human tooth: a long-term post-treatment follow-up. Int Endod J. 1993;26:225–33.
10. Cohen S. Treatment choices for negative outcomes with non-surgical root canal treatment: non-surgical retreatment vs. surgical retreatment vs. implants. Endod Top. 2005;11:4–24.
11. Friedman S. Considerations and concepts of case selection in the management of post-treatment endodontic disease (treatment failure). Endod Top. 2002;1:54–78.
12. Del fabbro M, Taschieri S, Testori T, Francetti L, Weinstein RL. Surgical versus non-surgical endodon-

tic re-treatment for periradicular lesions (Review). Cochrane Database Syst Rev. 2007;3:CD005511.

13. Torabinejad M, Corr R, Handysideds R, Shabahang S. Outcomes of nonsurgical re-treatment and endodontic surgery: a systematic review. J Endod. 2009;35:930–7.

14. Martin MV, Nind D. Use of Chlorhexidine gluconate for preoperative disinfection of apicoectomy sites. Br Dent J. 1987;162:459–61.

15. Lindeboom JA, Frenken JW, Valkenburg P, van den Akker HP. The role of preoperative prophylactic antibiotic administration in periapical endodontic surgery: a randomized, prospective double-blind placebo-controlled study. Int Endod J. 2005;38(12):877–81.

16. Dionne RA, Campbell RA, Hall DL, Cooper SA, Buckingham B. Suppression of postoperative pain by preoperative administration of ibuprofen in comparison to placebo, acetaminophen, and acetaminophen plus codeine. J Clin Pharmacol. 1983;23:37–43.

17. Carr G. Microscopes in endodontics. J Calif Dent Assoc. 1992;11:55–61.

18. Kim S, Pecora G, Rubenstein R. Color atlas of microsurgery in endodontics. Philadelphia: WB Saunders; 2001. p. 21–2.

19. Pecora G, Andreana S. Use of the dental operating microscope in endodontic surgery. Oral Surg Oral Med Oral Pathol. 1993;75:751–8.

20. Rubenstein R. Magnification and illumination in apical surgery. Endo Top. 2005;11:56–77.

21. Hargreaves K, Khan A. Surgical preparation: anaesthesia and haemostasis. Endo Top. 2005;11:32–55.

22. Velva rt P, Peters CI. Soft tissue management in endodontic surgery. J Endod. 2005;31:4–16.

23. Velva rt P. Surgical retreatment. In: Bergenholtz G, Horsted-Bindslev P, Reit C, editors. Textbook of Endodontology. Oxford: Blackwell Munksgaard; 2003. p. 311–26.

24. Velva rt P, Ebner-Zimmermann U, Ebner JP. Papilla healing following sulcular full thickness flap in endodontic surgery. Oral Surg Oral Med Oral Pathol Oral Radiol Endod. 2004;98:365–9.

25. Velva rt P. Papilla base incision: a new approach to recession free healing of the interdental papilla after endodontic surgery. Int Endod J. 2002;35:453–60.

26. Harrison JW, Jurosky KA. Wound healing in the tissues of the periodontium following peri-radicular surgery – 2. The dissectional wound. J Endod. 1991;17:544–52.

27. Peters LB, Wesselink PR. Soft tissue management in endodontic surgery. Dent Clin North Am. 1997;41:513–28.

28. Mckenzie WS, Rosenberg M. Iatrogenic subcutaneous emphysema of dental and surgical origin: a literature review. J Oral Maxillofac Surg. 2009;67:1265–8.

29. Yacker MJ, Klein M. The effect of irrigation on osteotomy depth and bur diameter. Int J Oral Maxillofac Implants. 1996;11:634–8.

30. Calderwood RG, Hera SS, Davies JR, Waite DE. A comparison of the healing rate of bone after the

production of defects by various rotary instruments. J Dent Res. 1964;43:207–16.

31. Guttmann JL, Harrison JW. Surgical Endodontics. Boston: Blackwell Science; 1991. p. 203–77.

32. Arens DE, Torabinejad M, Chivian N, Rubenstein RA. Practical lessons in endodontic surgery. Chicago: Quintessence; 1988. p. 79–87.

33. PittFord TR. Surgical treatment of apical periodontitis. In: Orstavik D, Pitt Ford RT, editors. Essential endodontology. Prevention and treatment of apical periodontitis. Oxford: Blackwell Sciences; 1988. p. 278–307.

34. Khoury F, Hensher R. The bony lid technique for the apical root resection of lower molars. Int J Oral Maxillofac Surg. 1987;16:166–70.

35. Nevins A, Ruden S, Pruden P, Kerpel S. Metastatic carcinoma of the mandible mimicking periapical lesion of endodontic origin. Endod Dent Traumatol. 1988;4:238–9.

36. Hutchinson IL, Hooper C, Cooner HS. Neoplasia masquerading as periapical infection. Br Dent J. 1990;168:288–94.

37. Abott P. Unusual periapical pathosis – adenoid cystic carcinoma. Aust Endod J. 2001;27:73–5.

38. Selim HA, el Deeb ME, Messer HH. Blood loss during endodontic surgery. Endod Dent Traumatol. 1987;3:33–6.

39. Kim S, Rethnam S. Haemostasis in endodontic microsurgery. Dent Clin North Am. 1997;41:499–511.

40. Jeonsonne BG, Boggs WS, Lemon RR. Ferric sulfate haemostasis: effect on osseous wound healing. II. With curettage and irrigation. J Endod. 1993;19:174–6.

41. Lemon RR, Steele PJ, Jeansonne BG. Ferric sulfate hemostasis: effect on osseous wound healing. Left in situ for maximum exposure. J Endod. 1993;19:170–3.

42. Tidmarsh BG, Arrowsmith MG. Dentinal tubules at the root ends of apicected teeth: a scanning electron microscopic study. Int Endod J. 1989;22(4):184–9.

43. Vertucci F. Root canal anatomy of human permanent teeth. Oral Surg Oral Med Oral Pathol. 1984;58:589.

44. Torabinejad M, Handysides R, Khademi AA, Bakland LK. Clinical implications of the smear layer in endodontics: a review. Oral Surg Oral Med Oral Pathol Oral Radiol Endod. 2002;94:658–66.

45. Fogel HM, Peikoff MD. Microleakage of root end materials. J Endod. 2001;27:456–8.

46. Oynick J, Oynick T. A study of a new material for retrograde fillings. J Endod. 1978;4:203–6.

47. Dorn SO, Gartner AH. Retrograde filling materials: a retrospective success-failure study of amalgam. EBA and IRM. J Endod. 1990;16:391–3.

48. Jesslen P, Zetterqvist I, Hemidahl A. Long term results of amalgam verses glass ionomer cement as apical sealant after apicoectomy. Oral Surg Oral Med Oral Pathol Oral Radiol Endod. 1995;79:101–3.

49. Chong BS, Pitt Ford TR, Hudson MB. A prospective clinical study of mineral trioxide aggregate and IRM when used as root-end filling materials in endodontic surgery. Int Endod J. 2003;36:520–6.

50. Rubenstein RA, Kim S. Short term observations of the results of endodontic surgery with the use of a surgical operating microscope and Super EBA as a root end filling material. J Endod. 1999;25:43–8.

51. Rubenstein RA, Kim S. Long term follow-up of cases considered healed one year after apical microsurgery. J Endod. 2002;28:378–83.

52. Regan JD, Gutmann JL, Witherspoon DE. Comparison of Diaket and MTA when used as root-end filling materials to support regeneration of the periradicular tissues. Int Endod J. 2002;35:840–7.

53. Rud J, Munksgaard EC, Andreasen JO, Rud V, Amussen E. Root filling with composite and a dentine bonding agent: I-IV. Tandlaegebladet. 1989;93: 156–160, 195–197, 223–229, 267–273, 343–345, 401–405.

54. Velvart P, Peters CI, Peters OA. Soft tissue management: suturing and wound closure. Endo Top. 2005;11:179–95.

55. Friedman S. The prognosis and expected outcome of apical surgery. Endo Top. 2005;11:219–62.

Intentional Replantation

14

Bobby Patel

Summary

Intentional replantation is an accepted endodontic treatment procedure in which a tooth is extracted and treated outside the oral cavity and then inserted into its socket to correct an obvious clinical or radiographic endodontic failure. Key prognostic factors to increase the likelihood of success include limiting the extra-oral time as short as possible and minimal trauma to the periodontal ligament and cementum. A team of two dentists should ideally work in tandem to prevent prolonged treatment time. The use of elevators is contraindicated, and the beaks of the forceps should not go beyond the cement-enamel junction. The tooth should be kept moist at all times with the use of an appropriate medium during the extra-oral period. Conventional apicectomy techniques including root resection, retrograde preparation and retrograde filling should be carried out. The use of MTA or Super EBA should be routinely used to ensure good marginal adaptation and biocompatibility ensuring promotion of new cementum deposition to the retro-filled surface.

Clinical Relevance

With correct case selection, it can be a reliable treatment modality in an effort to maintain the natural dentition. It is a suitable treatment option when non-surgical retreatment or peri-radicular surgery is unfeasible. For successful intentional replantation, an atraumatic extraction technique is crucial. Clinicians should be aware of adeverse outcomes including tooth fracture, peri-cemental damage, infection, external root resorption and ankylosis. It is important to realize that intentional replantation should be the treatment of last choice, selected only when all other options of treatment have been exhausted. Replantation can be a treatment of choice in cases in which a surgical approach can be difficult.

14.1 Review of the Literature

Intentional replantation consists of a technique whereby a tooth is intentionally extracted and replanted into its socket immediately after sealing

B. Patel, BDS MFDS MClinDent MRD MRACDS
Specialist Endodontist, Brindabella Specialist Centre,
Canberra, ACT, Australia
e-mail: bobbypatel@me.com

© Springer International Publishing Switzerland 2016
B. Patel (ed.), *Endodontic Treatment, Retreatment, and Surgery*,
DOI 10.1007/978-3-319-19476-9_14

Table 14.1 Indications and contraindications for intentional replantation

Indications
Failure of conventional endodontic therapy
If conventional root canal treatment, retreatment and surgical treatments have failed and are deemed impossible to perform
Anatomical limitations
Proximity of the intended tooth to nerves (mandibular or mental) or anatomical structures (maxillary sinus) are at risk of damage from the procedure
Surgical access
Surgical access of mandibular molars may be difficult due to dense buccal bone (external oblique ridge) or lingually displaced roots
Tooth factors
Root canal obstructions and restorative or perforation root defects that may be present and are inaccessible to non-surgical or surgical approaches
Contraindications
Root anatomy
Long curved or divergent roots are more prone to fracture during the extraction procedure
Periodontal disease
Teeth with poor periodontal support and tooth mobility are not good candidates for intentional replantation
Vertical root fracture
Teeth where a crack or vertical root fracture has been confirmed following extraction are not good candidates for replantation

the apical foramina [1]. Historically the profession has seen intentional replantation as a treatment option of last resort [2–4]. Others indicate that it is a reliable and predictable procedure and should be more often considered as a treatment modality in our efforts to maintain the natural dentition [5]. Contraindications are few but include teeth with flared or severely curved roots, poor periodontal support and vertically fractured teeth [5]. This procedure is particularly useful where surgical access may be difficult (such as lower molar surgery) or where anatomical structures are at risk (mental foramen, mandibular canal proximity) [6] (Table 14.1).

It is well documented that avulsed teeth recover optimal function under ideal conditions following replantation. Periodontal ligament cells can be damaged mechanically during extraction/replantation or biologically/chemically during the extra-oral period. Studies have shown that periodontal ligament cells can easily be damaged under stressful

conditions such as variable pH, osmotic pressure and dehydration [7–10]. Favourable healing of the periodontal ligament is dependent on how many viable cells are preserved on the root surface [7, 8]. Where the periodontal ligament is damaged, then the potential for surface resorption, inflammatory resorption and replacement resorption (ankylosis) is increased. This type of resorption is a well-known complication of replanted teeth, which adversely affects the long-term outcome [9, 10].

It can be extrapolated from avulsed teeth that optimal periodontal healing is seen when a tooth is immediately replaced in its socket. This ensures minimal damage to periodontal ligament cells reducing adverse effects during the healing period [11–14].

Success rates of intentionally replanted teeth are reported to range from 52 to 95 % [6, 8, 15, 16].

A key to a successful outcome is based on a safe extraction method without causing cracks or root fractures. This is also one of the prerequisites for successful intentional replantation [5]. Orthodontic extrusion and the use of an atraumatic extraction technique have been proposed to ensure a fracture-free safe extraction [17].

14.2 Technique

The objectives of extraction with replantation are to remove the tooth intentionally from its socket, carry out normal surgical root-end procedures extra-orally and replant the tooth. This indication is relevant when non-surgical root canal treatment is not possible or has not been successful and when surgical endodontics is not advisable.

The treatment procedure (Fig. 14.1) should, ideally, be carried out by two operators.

1. The extraction procedure is carried out with minimal trauma. During the extraction scraping or denudation of the periodontal ligament (PDL), the cementum should be avoided. Damage to either can increase the chances of root resorption ensuing postoperatively and inadvertently reducing the prognosis for success. Only the apical part of the socket can be aspirated or curetted with care (Fig. 14.1).

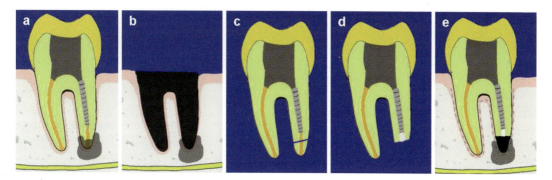

Fig. 14.1 Diagrams representing (**a**) preoperative view showing the tooth with periradicular lesion close to inferior dental nerve (contraindication to conventional surgery) and fractured post preventing conventional endodontic re-treatments. (**b**) Post extraction of the apical portion of the socket can be curetted ensuring minimal trauma to the remaining socket walls, (**c**) root resection, (**d**) retrograde filling placement, and (**e**) repositioning

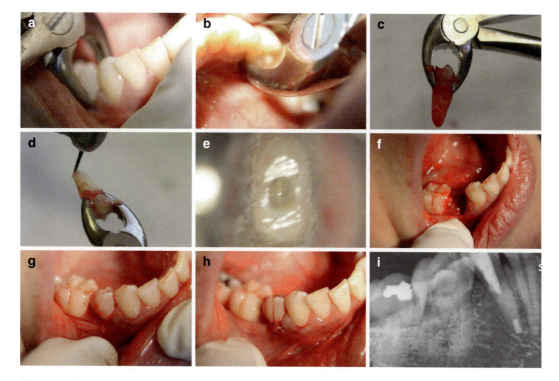

Fig. 14.2 Clinical photographs and radiographs demonstrating (**a–c**) extraction with minimal trauma, (**d, e**) root resection, (**f–h**) reimplantation, and (**i**) postoperative radiograph demonstrating repositioned tooth

2. Minimal pressure is exerted during the extraction. Care is taken to ensure that the beaks of the forceps are placed on the crown at all times and do not reach beyond the cement-enamel junction. The author has found that placing a rubber band around the handle of the forceps after extraction helps to apply a constant pressure on the crown thereby preventing slippage of the forceps or damaging the tooth. Also the handling of the tooth during the extra-oral period is markedly easier for both root resection and replantation purposes (Fig. 14.2).

3. Throughout the extra-oral dry period, when the tooth is resected, prepared for retrograde

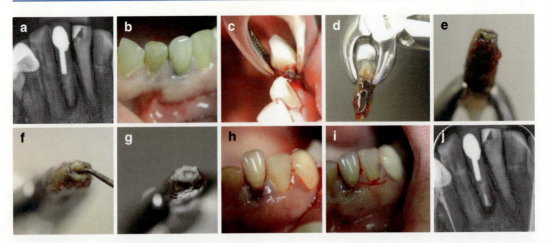

Fig. 14.3 Clinical photographs and radiographs demonstrating (**a**) preoperative radiograph and (**b**) clinical photograph of tooth 31 with post crown restoration in place. Note failed endodontic treatment, (**c, d**) atraumatic extrac-tion, (**e–g**) root resection, retrograde preparation and MTA filling, (**h–i**) replantation and suturing, and (**j**) postoperative radiograph

filling, retrograde filling placement and reimplantation, care is taken to avoid desiccation of the periodontal ligament. Extra-oral time should be as brief as possible. Efficient cutting of the root end and ultrasonic preparation are carried out with effective coolant spray. The periodontal ligament is also kept moist using physiological saline throughout the procedure.

4. Root resection is carried out with a high-speed turbine using copious amounts of water. Resection is carried out with a 0° bevel. Retrograde preparation is carried out with ultrasonics using conventional tips. A retrograde root filling of mineral trioxide aggregate (MTA) is placed (3 mm depth) (Fig. 14.3).

5. The tooth is then repositioned in the socket with minimal trauma. Following repositioning the clinician should press gently on the buccal and lingual plates. The patient can bite on cotton wool roll to help stabilize the tooth and aid in repositioning. Splinting is not usually advocated although temporary splinting using sutures in a figure of 8 can be used. Prolonged splinting (semi-rigid or rigid) is contraindicated since this does not allow for physiological mobility increasing the risk of replacement resorption and ankylosis of the root (Fig. 14.2).

14.3 Outcome

The main reason for failure in replanted teeth is root resorption, specifically surface resorption, ankylosis or replacement resorption (Fig. 14.4). Based on the literature, when the periodontal ligament cells have not been damaged during extraction and replacement of the tooth, if the tooth has been out of the mouth a minimal amount of time and the periodontal ligament has been kept moist, the prognosis is excellent. On the other hand, where damage to the periodontal ligament cells has been considerable, either because of trauma or dehydration, resorption of the root of the tooth will more likely occur.

14.4 Clinical Cases

Case 1 Failed non-surgical root canal treatment of tooth 46 due to additional untreated canal

A 24-year-old public servant was seen in specialist practice with a fluctuant swelling in the right mandibular area. Clinical examination revealed the first lower right molar was mobile and tender to touch. The radiograph revealed an extensive radiolucency associated with the mesial root. Conventional root canal

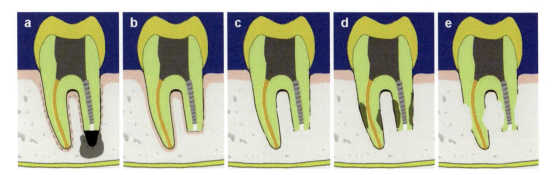

Fig. 14.4 Clinical diagrams showing outcome of intentional reimplantation. (**a**) Persistent periradicular disease, (**b**) normal periodontal ligament space (healed case), (**c**) surface resorption, (**d**) extensive root resorption, and (**e**) replacement resorption

treatment was undertaken. Access preparation was completed and four canals located. Canal preparation was completed using 1 % NaOCl solution. An intra-canal dressing of calcium hydroxide was placed for a period of 4 weeks. A buccal sinus had developed. A decision was made to carry out further intra-canal irrigation with adjunctive solutions including chlorhexidine and sonic irrigation. Access cavity was reassessed for any missed anatomy with particular reference to the distal root. Canal sizes were increased further. An intra-canal dressing was left in the tooth for a further 6 weeks. At the review appointment, the buccal sinus had failed to resolve. Treatment options were discussed with the patient, and surgical apicectomy was not considered due to anatomical constraints and patient preference. The tooth was subsequently obturated using a warm vertical compaction technique using gutta-percha and AH plus cement. A decision was made to extract the tooth, check for root fractures and replant it after performing an extra-oral root resection and retrograde filling (Figs. 14.5 and 14.6). Following extraction an additional apical foramen was confirmed in the distal root, which had been untreated (Fig. 14.6). The patient was reviewed 1 month, 3 months, 6 months, 12 months, 24 months and 48 months later. The periapical radiograph at 48 months demonstrates good healing with no peri-radicular rarefactions (Fig. 14.7). The tooth remains asymptomatic.

Case 2 Failed non-surgical root canal therapy of tooth 46 due to complex C-shaped anatomy

A 68-year-old well-controlled hypertensive patient was referred for endodontic management of tooth 46. Clinical examination revealed tooth 46 was missing (extracted in her early teens). Tooth 47 was mesially tilted and had a draining sinus in the overlying alveolar buccal mucosa. Radiographic examination revealed a gutta-percha sinus tracing associated with the peri-apex of tooth 47. A fused root was noted. Endodontic treatment was carried out. The tooth had a C-shaped canal system noted with confluence of the mesial canals in the apical 1/3rd. Chemomechanical preparation was carried out with supplemental ultrasonic irrigation using sodium hypochlorite solution. The patient had an inter-appointment intra-canal medicament of calcium hydroxide placed for 4 weeks followed by a review appointment. The draining sinus had resolved. The tooth was obturated using a warm vertical compaction technique using AH Plus cement and gutta-percha. The patient returned to her general dental practitioner for placement of a permanent cast restoration. The patient was then seen 2 years later for severe pain in the area. An extensive peri-radicular radiolucency was noted with the peri-apex of tooth 47. A well-fitting ceramic crown restoration had been placed with good marginal integrity. Treatment options were discussed including conventional retreatment through the existing crown and surgical apicectomy. The patient, who was very apprehensive in the dental setting, had decided to consider

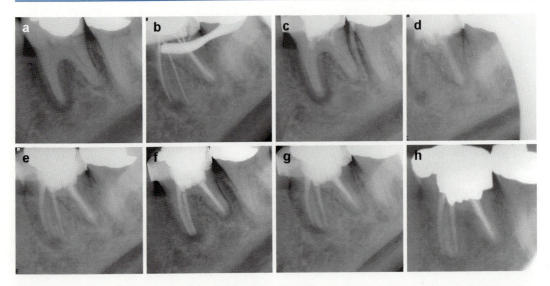

Fig. 14.5 Clinical radiographs demonstrating (**a**) preoperative view, (**b**) master apical files, (**c**) sinus tracing demonstrating distal root involvement, (**d**) inter-appointment antibacterial dressing showing placement in distal root, (**e**) postoperative obturation, (**f**) immediately following intentional replantation, (**g**) 12-month follow-up, and (**h**) 42-month follow-up. Note the tooth has been restored with a Nayyar amalgam core and amalgam cuspal coverage restoration

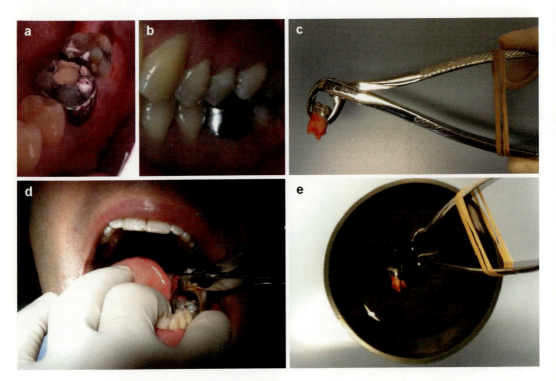

Fig. 14.6 Clinical photographs showing (**a**, **b**) preoperative view of tooth 46. (**c**, **d**) Extracted tooth 46 (note forceps beaks are not allowed to slip below the cementoenamel junction) and (**e**) sterile saline solution used to prevent the tooth from dehydrating during extra-oral surgical root resection and retrograde preparation and filling procedures

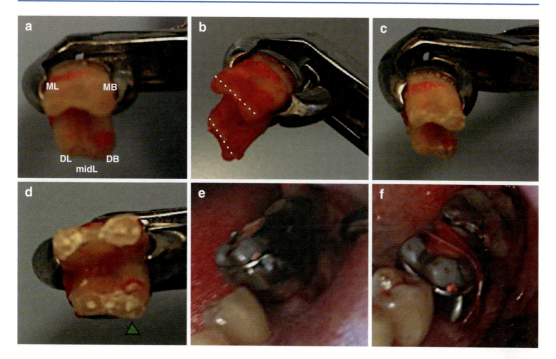

Fig. 14.7 Clinical photographs demonstrating (**a, b**) complex anatomy of mesial and distal roots (note bulbosity and intentional extruded gutta-percha associated with the disto-lingual canals), (**c, d**) resected mesial and distal roots (note MTA retrograde filling and untreated DB canal) (*green triangle*), (**e**) replantation of tooth 46, and (**f**) temporary splint using 3.0 Vicryl sutures. *ML* mesiolingual, *MB* mesio-buccal, *DB* disto-buccal, *DL* disto-lingual, *midL* mid-lingual

extraction. A third option of intentional reimplantation was discussed as a treatment of last resort. Tooth 47 was extracted with an atraumatic extraction technique. The entire extra-oral period was 15 min, and the tooth was kept moist at all times using physiological saline solution. Root resection was carried out confirming C-shaped anatomy. Ultrasonic preparation was carried out and retrograde MTA filling placed. The tooth was reimplanted and no splint was indicated. The patient was reviewed at 1 week and 4 weeks. At the 4-week period, her symptoms had improved significantly and the tooth was functional once again. The patient was reviewed at 6 months, 12 months, 24 months and 48 months. The tooth remained asymptomatic and the peri-radicular radiolucent lesion had resolved. An intact periodontal ligament space was noted with no evidence of root resorption or ankylosis both clinically and radiographically (Figs. 14.8, 14.9 and 14.10).

Case 3 Blocked MB canal in tooth 47 due to extensive buccal restoration obstructing canal space

A 65-year-old fit and healthy family friend was referred for endodontic management of tooth 47. The patient had seen his general dental practitioner for an extensive buccal restoration which involved the mesiobuccal root canal. Clinical examination revealed tooth 47 had an extensive coronal restoration with an overlying buccal glass ionomer restoration. Radiographic examination confirmed a bulbous root associated with tooth 47 with a peri-radicular radiolucent lesion. Non-surgical endodontic treatment was carried out revealing three canals. Patency was achieved in the ML and D canals. The MB canal could only be negotiated in the coronal aspect. The middle 1/3rd was blocked by the overlying buccal root restoration. Single visit endodontic treatment was completed using rotary Ni-Ti files and sodium hypochlorite irrigation. The canals

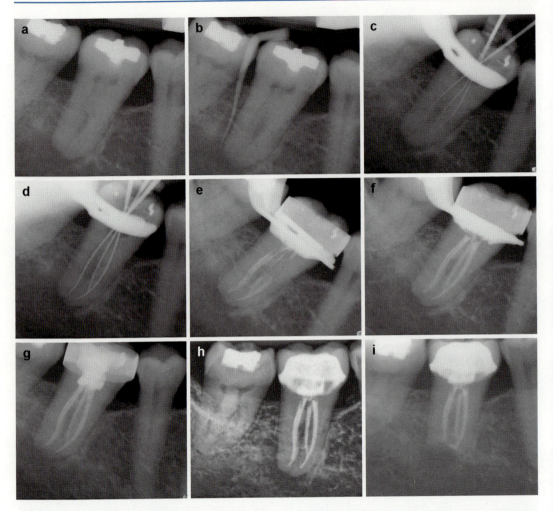

Fig. 14.8 Clinical radiographs showing endodontic management of tooth 47. Note (**a**, **b**) preoperative views demonstrating draining sinus associated with periapex of tooth 47. Fused single root anatomy may indicate a C-shaped canal system. (**c**, **d**) Initial and master apical file sizes showing confluent root canal system with increased complexity due to C-shaped anatomy. (**e**) Mid-fill radiograph demonstrating lateral sealer extrusion. (**f**) Final obturation completed using warm vertical compaction. (**g**) Double seal temporary restoration placed and patient referred back to general dental practitioner. (**h**) Patient seen 2 years later having had a cast ceramic restoration placed. Note extensive periradicular radiolucency that has not improved. The patient was experiencing severe pain with the tooth. (**i**) Immediately following intentional reimplantation procedure

Fig. 14.10 Clinical radiographs of follow-up following intentional reimplantation procedure for tooth 47. Risks include ankylosis, root resorption, infection, and failure. Note (**a**) 6-month review showing significant reduction in the periapical radiolucency. Complete healing was not evident. There appears to be no signs of root resorption at this stage. (**b**) A 12-month follow-up. (**c**) A 24-month follow-up. (**d**) A 48-month follow-up. Note an intact periodontal ligament space is associated with the periapex of the tooth

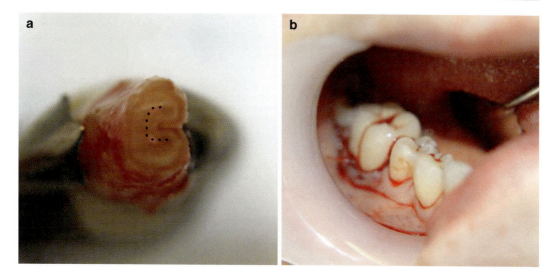

Fig. 14.9 Clinical photographs demonstrating extracted tooth 47 during intentional reimplantation procedure. Note (**a**) following root resection demonstration untreated isthmus between the mesial and distal canals. This was probably the cause of persistent infection and pain resulting in failure. Note the C-shaped root system. (**b**) Clinical picture showing tooth replanted into occlusion. No sutures were required due to minimal mobility once reimplanted

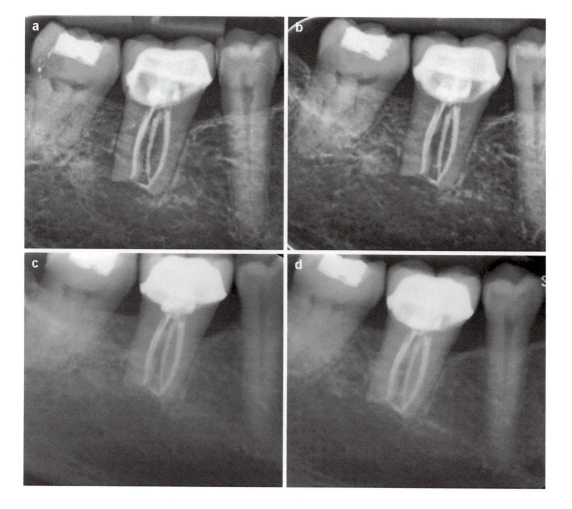

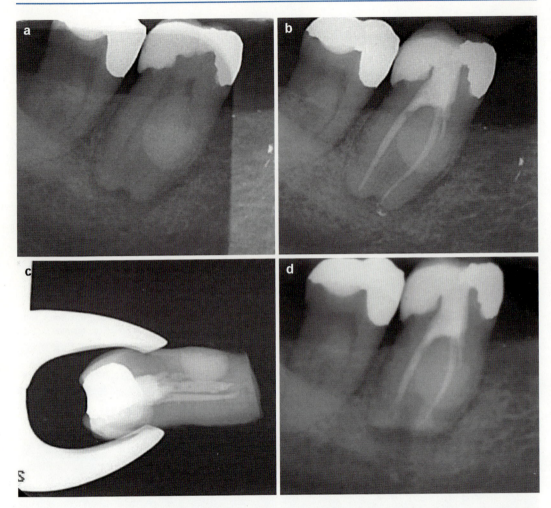

Fig. 14.11 Clinical radiographs demonstrating (**a**) preoperative view of tooth 47. Note extensive buccal restoration overlying the MB root. A periradicular radiolucency was noted. (**b**) Single-visit nonsurgical endodontic treatment using a warm vertical compaction technique using AH Plus cement. Note sealer extrusion associated with the ML canal. The MB canal could only be negotiated in the coronal 1/3. (**c**) Extracted tooth demonstrating retrograde preparation and filling prior to reimplantation. (**d**) Reimplanted tooth 47. Both nonsurgical endodontic treatment and reimplantation was carried out at the same visit. Total time for reimplantation was 15 min

were obturated using a warm vertical compaction technique. The tooth was restored with a double temporary Zinc-oxide Eugenol/glass ionomer restoration (Fig. 14.11).

A decision was made to carry out an intentional reimplantation procedure at the same visit. The tooth was extracted with no complications. An apical 3 mm root resection was carried out and retrograde preparation completed. Biodentine was used as a retrograde filling material (Fig. 14.12). The tooth was bathed in saline throughout the procedure. Radiographic examination was carried out to check the retrograde filling procedure prior to reimplantation. Prior to reimplantation curettage of the socket was carried out with care not to disturb the socket walls. The tooth was gently repositioned in the socket and a temporary suture sling placed (Fig. 14.13). The patient reported no symptoms that evening and the tooth has been placed on long-term review. This case highlights the option of intentional reimplantation as a treatment of last resort. The tooth was compromised and the patient was not considering a dental implant

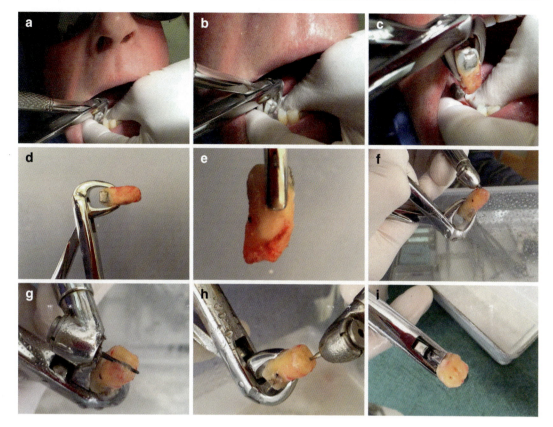

Fig. 14.12 Clinical photographs demonstrating intentional reimplantation procedure for tooth 47. Note (**a–c**) atraumatic extraction of the tooth. (**d, e**) Mesial and buccal views of the tooth. (**f, g**) Apical 3 mm root resection procedure. (**h**) Retrograde preparation and (**i**) completed root resection and retrograde preparation

following extraction. Surgical apicectomy was deemed to be risky given the position of the tooth in the arch and the compromised non-surgical treatment and overall restorative prognosis. The patient fully understood the risks associated with such a procedure but was keen to try and retain the tooth if possible.

Case 4 Failed non-surgical root canal treatment of tooth 37 due to complex anatomy and root perforation

A fit and healthy 38-year-old patient was referred for endodontic management of tooth 37. The patient had undergone root canal treatment with another dental practitioner 12 months previously followed by cast cuspal coverage restoration. Her chief complaint at examination was of a gumboil and swelling in relation to this tooth which had been present for several weeks. Clinical examination confirmed tooth 37 had a ceramic crown restoration in place. A buccal sinus was noted with 8 mm + probing profile on the mid-buccal aspect. Radiographic examination confirmed previous root canal treatment had been carried out. Three canals appeared to be obturated with the appearance of an overfill apically and unusual mid-root anatomy. A gutta-percha sinus-tracing radiograph was tracked to this area (Fig. 14.14).

A provisional diagnosis of failed root canal therapy was made with suspected mid-root perforation. After a lengthy discussion, treatment options were discussed including non-surgical root canal retreatment, surgical apicectomy, intentional reimplantation or extraction. Risks and benefits were discussed including cost estimates and prognosis. The patient agreed to an intentional reimplantation procedure and fully

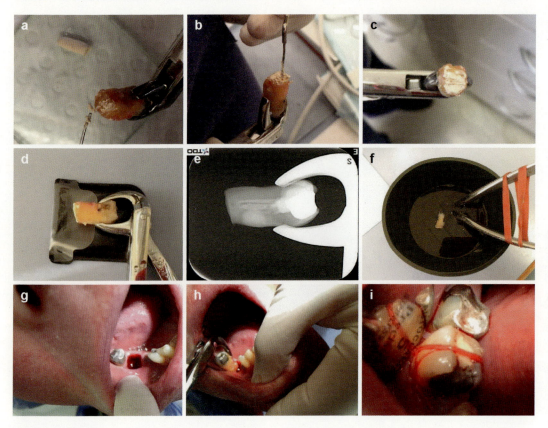

Fig. 14.13 Clinical photographs and radiograph demonstrating intentional reimplantation procedure for tooth 47. Note (**a–c**) retrograde filling of the tooth using Biodentine. (**d**, **e**) Radiographic assessment of root resection and retrograde filling procedure. (**f**) Saline bath used to prevent drying of the periodontal ligament cells throughout the procedure. (**g**, **h**) Manual repositioning of the tooth back into the socket. (**i**) Suture sling used to stabilize the tooth following reimplantation

understood the inherent risks involved including possible crown decementation; root fracture; post-operative sequelae including pain, swelling, root resorption and ankylosis; and failure of treatment. At the next appointment, tooth 37 was atraumatically extracted. During the extraction procedure, the crown decemented. On visual inspection a C-shaped root form was confirmed with overextended gutta-percha at the apex. An additional gutta-percha cone was noted from a suspected mid-root perforation. 3 mm of root apex was resected, and ultrasonic preparation of the C-shaped canal system was carried out with ultrasonics. MTA was placed as a retrograde filling. The overextended gutta-percha point was carefully removed from the mid-root perforation, and a further MTA filling was placed overlying the perforation site. The tooth was reimplanted atraumatically. The crown was temporarily recemented with Tempbond and occlusion checked (Fig. 14.15). The patient was advised a soft diet, analgesics and further review appointments scheduled at 1 week, 4 weeks and 6 months.

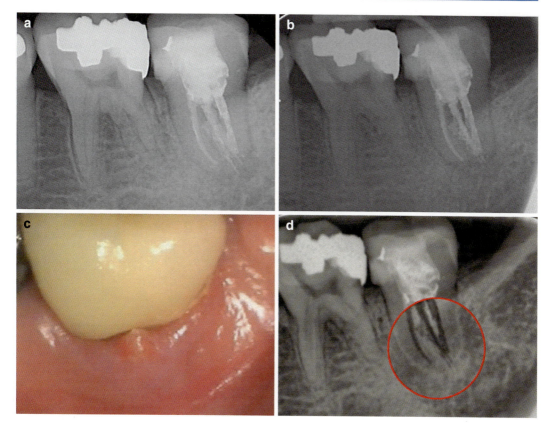

Fig. 14.14 Clinical photograph and radiographs demonstrating intentional reimplantation procedure for tooth 37. Note (**a**) preoperative view demonstrating cast restoration and endodontic treatment that had been carried out 12 months previously. (**b**) A gutta-percha sinus tracing radiograph was tracked to the mid-root level of tooth 37. (**c**) Clinical photograph demonstrating overlying buccal swelling and sinus in the attached mucosa. (**d**) Radiographic appearance of the mid-root level adjusted using digital x-ray software to provide further contrast (*red circle*) demonstrating unusual obturation. The patient was informed of the possibility of either a root fracture in this area or iatrogenic root perforation

Clinical Tips and Tricks

- The use of intentional replantation is reserved for those clinical cases which are not amenable to root canal treatment, retreatment or surgery.
- Due to the risk of root resorption and possibly ankylosis, the patient must be warned against this technique if they were to consider a dental implant in the future.
- Two operators should ideally work together, one as the oral surgeon extracting and replanting the tooth and the other as the endodontist performing surgical apicectomy extra-orally.
- Preservation of periodontal ligament cell viability on the root surface is a prerequisite for success. Minimal trauma during extraction, extra-oral manipulation and replantation with prevention of dehydration will aid in this.
- Careful follow-up for 1 month, 3 months, 6 months and yearly for 5 years should be recommended to ensure no root resorption ensues.

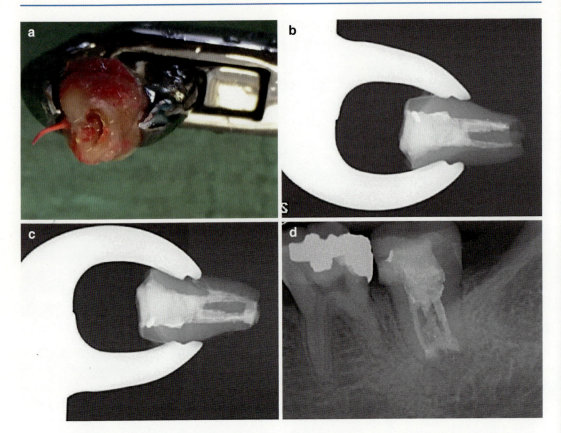

Fig. 14.15 Clinical photograph and radiographs demonstrating intentional reimplantation procedure for tooth 37. Note (**a**) clinical view of extracted tooth 37 confirming C-shaped root anatomy and overextended gutta-percha in a suspected mid-root perforation. (**b**) Radiographic appearance following apical root resection and ultrasonic preparation. (**c**) The overextended gutta-percha was removed and both the apical root end and mid-root perforation were sealed with MTA. A radiograph was taken to confirm retrograde obturation and mid-root perforation repair. (**d**) Post reimplantation radiograph with recemented coronal cast restoration using TempBond

References

1. Grossman LI. Endodontic practice. 11th ed. Philadelphia: Lea & Febiger. 1988. p. 334
2. Cohen S, Burns R. Pathways of the pulp. 4th ed. St. Louise: CV Mosby; 1987. p. 607–8.
3. Grossman L, Ship I. Survival rate of replanted teeth. Oral Surg. 1970;29:899–906.
4. Weine F. The case against intentional replantation. J Am Dent Assoc. 1980;100:664–8.
5. Peer M. Intentional replantation – a last resort treatment or a conventional treatment procedure? Nine case reports. Dent Traumatol. 2004;20:48–55.
6. Bender IB, Rossman LE. Intentional replantation of endodontically treated teeth. Oral Surg Oral Med Oral Pathol. 1993;76:623.
7. Bakland LK. Endodontic considerations in dental trauma. In: Ingle I, Bakland LK, editors. Endodontics. 5th ed. Hamilton: BC Decker Inc; 2002. p. 795–843.
8. Andreasen JO, Borum MK, Jacobsen HL, Andreasen FM. Replantation of 400 avulsed permanent incisors. 4 Factors related to periodontal ligament healing. Endod Dent Traumatol. 1995;11(2):76–89.
9. Andreasen JO. Analysis of topography of surface and inflammatory root resorption after replantation of mature permanent incisors in monkeys. Swed Dent J. 1980;4:135–44.
10. Andreasen JO. Analysis of pathogenesis and topography of replacement resorption (ankylosis) after replantation of mature permanent incisor teeth in monkeys. Swed Dent J. 1980;4:231–40.
11. Andreasen JO. A time-related study of periodontal healing and root resorption activity after replantation of mature permanent incisors in monkeys. Swed Dent J. 1980;4:101–10.
12. Andreasen JO. Periodontal healing after replantation and autotransplantation of tooth in adult monkeys. Int J Oral Surg. 1981;10:54–61.
13. Andreasen JO. Relationship between cell damage in the periodontal ligament after replantation and

subsequent development of root resorption. Acta Odontol Scand. 1981;39:15–25.33.

14. Andreasen JO, Kristerson L. The effect of limited drying or removal of the periodontal ligament. Periodontal healing after replantation of mature incisors in monkeys. Acta Odontol Scand. 1981; 39:1–13. [PubMed Link] Links

15. Madison S. Intentional replantation. Oral Surg Oral Med Oral Pathol. 1986;62:707–9.

16. Messkoub M. Intentional replantation: a successful alternative for hopeless teeth. Oral Surg. 1991;71:743–7.

17. Choi Y-H, Bae J-H. Clinical evaluation of a new extraction method for intentional replantation. JKACD. 2011;36:211–7.

Traumatic Injuries

15

Gursharan Minhas and Bobby Patel

Summary

Traumatic dental injuries occur in both young children and adults. Initial emergency management, correct diagnosis, treatment planning and follow-up are essential to ensure a favourable outcome. Treatment procedures are aimed at minimising undesired consequences, which may lead to early loss of the tooth, and also alveolar bone loss, which may have a negative impact on future replacement options. Treatment planning often involves a multidisciplinary approach, and an early endodontic opinion should be sought for the best possible outcome.

Clinical Relevance

Traumatic dental injuries can be classified according to trauma affecting the hard dental tissues, the pulp, the periodontal tissues, the supporting bone, gingivae and oral mucosa. The most favourable outcome of any traumatic dental injury is healing of the pulp and surrounding tissues. The outcome of dental trauma depends on a number of factors including type and severity of injury, timeliness of care and quality of treatment provided. Adherence to trauma guidelines will produce more favourable outcomes, including significantly lower complication rates. Appropriate follow up visits are essential to ensure prompt treatment of complications that can arise several months or even years after the initial injury. The clinician should be aware of types of injuries that can occur and the best possible treatment directed at ensuring optimal healing and retention of the tooth. It is the dentist's professional duty of care to provide appropriate emergency treatment to stabilise the condition prior to making the decision whether to refer to a specialist or not. Good record-keeping is mandatory since a proportion of trauma cases can often lead to legal proceedings for compensation and/or criminal convictions related to the injury sustained.

G. Minhas, BDS BSc MSc MFDS MOrth FDSOrth
Specialist Orthodontist, The Royal Surrey County Hospital, Hampshire, UK

Hampshire Hospitals NHS Foundation Trust, Basingstoke, UK

B. Patel, BDS MFDS MClinDent MRD MRACDS (✉)
Specialist Endodontist, Brindabella Specialist Centre, Canberra, ACT, Australia
e-mail: bobbypatel@me.com

© Springer International Publishing Switzerland 2016
B. Patel (ed.), *Endodontic Treatment, Retreatment, and Surgery*,
DOI 10.1007/978-3-319-19476-9_15

15.1 Overview of Traumatic Injuries

The World Health Organization classification of dental trauma modified by Andreasen was first described in 1972 but has since undergone various modifications making a clear distinction between various dental hard tissue and periodontal tissue injuries. It includes injuries to the dental hard tissue, supporting structures, gingiva and oral mucosa allowing anatomical, therapeutic and prognostic considerations to be derived from the classification system [1].

There are eight types of dental hard tissue injuries described dependent on the tooth structures involved and six types of periodontal tissue injuries described dependent on the force and direction of the impact (Table 15.1) [1–3].

The most commonly observed injury to the dental hard tissues involves uncomplicated crown fractures of the maxillary anterior teeth [4]. Crown fractures account for up to 76 % of the dental trauma reported to the permanent dentition. This consists of enamel infraction, enamel fracture, uncomplicated crown fracture, complicated crown fracture and crown-root fractures [4].

Table 15.1 The WHO classification of dental trauma modified by Andreasen

Dental hard tissue injury
Enamel infraction
Enamel fracture
Enamel-dentine fracture (uncomplicated crown fracture)
Enamel-dentine-pulp fracture (complicated crown fracture)
Crown-root fracture without pulp exposure
Crown-root fracture with pulp exposure
Root fracture
Alveolar fracture
Periodontal tissue injury
Concussion
Subluxation
Extrusion luxation (partial avulsion)
Lateral luxation
Intrusion luxation (central dislocation)
Avulsion

Of the periodontal tissue injuries, luxation injuries were consistently found to be the most frequent dental trauma involving the periodontal tissue in studies followed by subluxation. Almost one-third (31.6 %) of teeth suffered a combination of tooth fracture and luxation injury. Furthermore, two-thirds of all combination injuries were observed amongst teeth with minor luxation injuries such as concussion and subluxation [5–8].

The avulsion of permanent teeth is considered to be one of the most serious dental injuries to occur and is seen in 0.5–3 % of all dental traumas. In the worst case scenario the tooth is lost or extracted due to the complications following replantation. The loss of an upper central incisor has a significant effect on dental and facial aesthetics due to the prominence of the maxillary teeth, and this can affect an individual's self-esteem and general social interaction [9, 10].

Infraction injuries are microcracks in the enamel (incomplete enamel fracture without loss of tooth structure). They can be relatively common as a direct result of impact trauma to a tooth requiring no immediate treatment. Pulpal complications are considered to be rare. Pulpal necrosis has been reported in 1.6 % of teeth with enamel infraction and concomitant enamel fracture, whilst 2.3 % of teeth with enamel infraction and concomitant enamel-dentine fracture developed pulpal necrosis. Interestingly, when enamel infraction occurred in isolation, 3.5 % developed necrosis. This has been attributed to the traumatic impact being dissipated through the pulp rather than transfer of energy directly to the supporting tissues resulting in loss of tooth structure. The rate of pulpal necrosis for enamel infraction with a concomitant injury from a concussion or luxation injuries has been shown to range from 14.7 to 60.0 %. Furthermore, the state of root development has been found to be associated with the risk of developing pulpal necrosis (more common in a mature fully developed closed apex teeth). Pulp treatment is rarely indicated and only carried out following definitive signs and symptoms of irreversible pulpitis or pulpal necrosis with infection. The clinician should bear in mind that reactions to pulp sensibility testing in traumatised teeth are lowered immediately following trauma requiring longer observation times before a definitive decision can be made regarding the likely status of the pulp. As with all traumatic injuries, further follow-up after the initial injury is advised [1, 4, 11–14].

Enamel fractures without the exposure of the dentine result in the loss of the enamel structure. The mesial or distal corners of the maxillary central incisor teeth usually sustain this type of injury. Since loss of tooth structure is confined to enamel, patients are asymptomatic not requiring emergency treatment. Pulp survival following enamel fractures has been found to be high (>99 %). However, when there is a concomitant luxation injury, the chances of pulp survival can decrease to 33.3 %. The stage of root development is associated with the potential of pulpal healing following enamel fractures. The risk of pulpal necrosis in teeth that suffered enamel fracture with incomplete root development and open apices was 1.0 % compared to the risk of 2.5 % in teeth with complete root development and closed apices [5–8, 11–15].

When an enamel-dentine fracture without pulpal involvement occurs, the treatment objective is to maintain pulp vitality and restore aesthetics and function. Direct dentine exposure can result in discomfort from temperature changes. Additionally, the enamel-dentine fracture may result in a near pulpal exposure. Emergency treatment prior to definitive restoration includes protection of the exposed dentine. When the fractured crown is retained, bonding and reattachment is considered more aesthetically desirable than the use of tooth-coloured restorative materials. The prognosis of pulpal healing has been reported to range from 94.0 to 100 %. Both extent of dentine exposure and presence of a concomitant injury affecting the periodontal tissues can have an adverse effect on pulp survival. In enamel-dentine fractured teeth with a concomitant luxation injury, 16.8–69.9 % have been reported to develop pulpal necrosis [1, 11–16].

The treatment of the enamel-dentine fracture involving the pulp (complicated crown fracture) is aimed at removing the possibility of bacterial ingress into the pulp, thereby allowing the pulp time to recover and repair. Various treatment modalities including direct pulp capping, partial pulpotomy and pulpectomy have been recommended depending on extent of pulpal exposure and the time elapsed between injury and treatment provided.

In young patients with immature (developing) teeth, it is advantageous to try and maintain pulp vitality by either pulp capping or partial pulpotomy procedures. Pulp capping is indicated when a small exposure is present and can be treated shortly after the dental trauma occurs. When the pulp is more severely exposed and there has been a time delay, then the extent of pulpal inflammation may result in irreversible damage of the superficial layer of the pulp. If an enamel-dentine-pulp fracture occurred, the removal of a minimum of 2 mm of pulp beneath the exposure is required to remove the inflamed pulp. This has given rise to the procedure known as 'partial pulpotomy'. Alternative levels of pulpal amputation are recommended based on the extent of pulpal inflammation as determined clinically by the presence of pulpal haemorrhage following a dental trauma. In instances where pulpotomy cannot be performed due to the magnitude of pulpal inflammation, pulpectomy is indicated. Following pulpal therapy, the fractured tooth can be restored in a similar manner to an enamel-dentine fracture. The long-term prognosis of the enamel-dentine-pulp-fractured tooth depends on the presence of other concomitant injuries, time elapsed between pulp exposure and treatment, bacterial infection and the stage of root development. Long-term studies of enamel-dentine-pulp fractures treated with partial pulpotomy and using calcium hydroxide showed a success rate of 87.5 % after a follow-up period of 7.5–11 years. The teeth that did not recover required endodontic treatment due to a new injury or for aesthetic purposes [1, 14, 17–20].

Crown-root fractures involve the enamel, dentine and part of the root (cementum) surface of the tooth. The fracture line invariably passes subgingivally often exposing the pulp requiring endodontic therapy if the tooth is to be retained. The treatment of a crown-root fracture is challenging and further complicated by the extent of the subgingival fracture often requiring a multidisciplinary approach. Treatment options include periodontal surgery to expose crown margins, restorative management only with extension of the margins of the restoration below the level of the gingival margin, orthodontic extrusion, intentional replantation (surgical repositioning), autotransplantation, root submergence (decoronation), extraction and replacement or orthodontic space closure. Treatment of crown-root fractures can be complex and time consuming, but often teeth with these types of fractures can be saved. In an adult patient, implant replacement is sometimes a viable alternative. In the case of a growing patient with a tooth that is not restorable, root submergence (decoronation) may be indicated to preserve the bone and allow for normal alveolar development prior to implant placement when growth is complete [21–28].

Root fractures are relatively uncommon, making up 0.5–7.7 % of dental trauma. The maxillary permanent central incisors are most frequently affected (up to 80 % of cases). They involve the cementum, dentine and the pulp and can present with or without clinical signs of luxation of the coronal fragment. The fracture can appear radiographically as a single line or multiple lines across the root in the apical, middle or coronal 1/3. Radiographic diagnosis of root fractures requires multiple views at different vertical angles to obtain a three-dimensional image. Root fractures can occur in either the cervical, middle or apical portion of the tooth.

Many root fractures heal without intervention in one of three modalities: hard tissue interposition, interposition of the bone and periodontal ligament or interposition of the periodontal ligament alone. In the past, rigid splints were used for an extended period of time (up to 4 months); however, no additional benefits were found with regard to pulpal or periodontal healing. The prognosis of root-fractured teeth appears to be multifactorial related to the position of the root fracture, the stage of root development, presence of bacterial infection and the type of healing pattern that occurs. Pulpal necrosis of the coronal fragment has been reported in up to 25 % of teeth with root fractures. Pulp canal obliteration (partial or complete) may occur in up to 70 % of cases. Obliteration of the apical root canal is commonly seen in cases of calcified tissue healing. When interposition of either the connective tissue or the connective tissue and bone occurs between the fragments, obliteration occurs more likely in both apical and coronal fragments. Interestingly, treatment delays showed no significant effect on the frequency and type of healing after accounting for factors such as root development and the extent of displacement. Root-fractured teeth should be splinted for up to 4 weeks initially and then reviewed. In cases where the root fracture has occurred, coronally extended splinting times may be necessary to ensure adequate stabilisation and healing occurs. Follow-up will be required to monitor pulpal status and fracture healing [29–46].

Jaw fractures can involve the base of the mandible or maxilla and often the alveolar process. Tooth involvement is common in mandibular and maxillary fractures and may require additional endodontic management. Nonsurgical treatment of bone fractures involves immobilisation, which for the facial bones is achieved with either maxillomandibular fixation (MMF) using dental fixed arch bars or direct internal fixation using screws and plates. Associated tooth injuries are difficult or impossible to treat during immobilisation, so that some treatment is necessary beforehand (e.g. coverage of exposed dental areas, temporary filling of crown fractures, repositioning of luxated teeth and endodontic treatment if the pulpal vascular supply is lost in the accident). Teeth in the line of a mandibular fracture should not be extracted as a first-aid measure unless they impair repositioning of the jaw fragments [47–54].

Luxation injuries represent the majority of dental trauma in the primary teeth and are the second most common type of injury sustained in the permanent dentition. The extent of injuries to the periodontal tissues is largely determined by the resilience of the underlying periodontal structures. Periodontal injuries often result in displacement of the affected tooth. Treatment of the displaced tooth aims to reduce the amount of dislocation from the tooth socket by repositioning. Common endodontic complications include pulp necrosis with infection, pulp canal calcification, ankylosis and root resorption. Factors that affect the prognosis of luxated teeth include the degree of displacement, delayed treatment time, root maturation and concomitant crown fractures. Most cases of pulp necrosis in luxated teeth become evident with the first 4 months. Root resorption often occurs within the first 6 months after injury and can develop quite rapidly, particularly in immature teeth. Hence, frequent follow-up examination is recommended. In some cases, pulp necrosis may appear at a much later date, and therefore long-term follow-up is also essential.

Concussion and subluxation injuries result from disturbances and/or laceration of the periodontal ligament fibres with very little disturbance to the neurovascular supply. These teeth display little displacement from the bony socket and therefore repositioning and splinting is seldom prescribed. Marked tenderness to percussion but no abnormal loosening or displacement of the traumatised tooth characterises a concussion injury to the supporting structures. Reported frequency of pulpal necrosis ranges from 3 %, and 2–7 % may undergo further pulp canal calcifications. Subluxation injuries are characterised by abnormal loosening of the tooth but without any displacement. Teeth are tender to percussion, and there may be some bleeding in the gingival crevice. Prognosis for subluxation injuries is generally good. Reported frequency of pulp necrosis ranges from 6 to 26 %. Pulp canal calcification has been reported to occur in 9–12 % of cases and progressive root resorption in less than 2 % [1, 6, 55–59].

Extrusive luxation of the tooth presents as a displaced tooth extruded from its socket. Emergency treatment requires repositioning and splinting. A delay in treatment usually results in difficulty in correct repositioning due to an established blood clot. In teeth that suffered an extrusive luxation injury, 26–80 % developed pulpal necrosis. The stage of root development significantly influenced the risk of pulpal necrosis development, with immature roots having a risk of 5.9 % compared with 56.5 % for teeth with complete root development. Root resorption, mainly in the form of inflammatory or surface resorption, was consistently observed in 5.5–9.4 % of extruded teeth [1, 6–8, 60–64, 91].

A lateral luxation injury is associated with a comminution or fracture of the alveolar socket. The tooth may be immobile as the injury crushes the bony socket walls. Emergency treatment for a laterally luxated tooth involves separation of the displaced tooth from the bony lock, repositioning the tooth and then stabilisation for at least 4 weeks. In laterally luxated teeth, the risk of developing pulpal necrosis was found to be between 33 % and 58 % and is related to the stage of root development. When the roots are immature, the risk of developing pulpal necrosis is reported to be 4.7 % compared to the risk of 65.1 % for mature roots. External root resorption is reported in 27 % of laterally luxated teeth and is predominantly surface resorption. The risk of developing inflammatory resorption is relatively low (0.8 %) [1, 5, 7, 8, 63–66, 91].

Intrusive luxation injuries result in a tooth being displaced in an axial position into the alveolar bone. This type of injury results in compression of the periodontal ligament and is accompanied by comminution or fracture of the alveolar socket. The emergency management of an intruded tooth may involve passive repositioning with spontaneous re-eruption or active repositioning with orthodontically guided eruption or surgical repositioning. For intruded teeth with immature root development, spontaneous eruption is preferred. For patients above 17 years of age, active repositioning with surgical or orthodontic intervention is recommended. The type of repositioning depends on the stage of root development and also on the extent of intrusion. For teeth with up to 3 mm of intrusion, passive repositioning is recommended; for 3–7 mm intrusion cases, orthodontic repositioning is preferred; for more than 7 mm of intrusion, surgical intervention is recommended. Of all the periodontal injuries, intrusive luxations are considered to be the most severe due to both the disruption of the vascular supply and the damage to the periodontal ligament cells. Pulpal necrosis is observed in 44–96 % of intruded teeth. Additionally, root resorption is found in up to 80 % of intruded teeth, of which 40 % resulted in replacement resorption [67–73, 91].

Avulsion or exarticulation occurs when a traumatic injury totally displaces a tooth from the socket resulting in potential for periodontal ligament damage and alveolus fracture. Although the prognosis for an avulsed tooth must always be guarded, replantation as soon as possible followed by a brief period of flexible splinting and endodontic therapy has been shown to be the most effective method of treatment. The shortest extra-oral period (less than 15 min), the minimum manipulation of the tooth surface and the socket and the use of an appropriate storage medium (milk, saliva and Hanks' balanced salt solution) have been identified as important factors that minimised subsequent root resorption.

The most common reason for unfavourable long-term survival of avulsed teeth is root resorption. A number of factors have been identified as being important in the prevention and management of root resorption associated with avulsed teeth including the stage of root development, the viability of the periodontal ligament cells and amount of damage sustained, the tooth storage conditions and the duration of time prior to replantation (extra-alveolar drying time).

The best outcome for a tooth avulsion is when the tooth can be replanted within a few minutes after the accident. The prognosis of a replanted avulsed tooth depends on the survival of both the periodontal ligament cells and the pulp. A large percentage of teeth that are replanted within 15 min will result in viable periodontal ligament cells and potential for reattachment within a few weeks. The extra-oral alveolar time has been shown to have detrimental effects on the survival of the periodontal ligament cells (approximately 20 min), and an inadequate storage medium often results in replacement resorption. If an avulsed tooth is left dry for more than 1 h, the odds of periodontal ligament cell survival are very poor. Despite the risk of ankylosis and replacement resorption, it may still be worthwhile replanting the tooth, particularly in a young patient, where several more years of use may be attained before eventual loss of the tooth [1, 10, 74–90].

Transient apical breakdown is a process that can develop as a result of certain traumatic injuries (subluxation, extrusion and lateral luxation) to teeth and their supporting tissues. Radiographically, a periapical radiolucency develops with the affected tooth that resolves without complication and does not require any endodontic intervention. The incidence of transient apical breakdown is relatively low and was reported to be 4.2 % of luxated cases. The condition was associated with either a pronounced radiolucency appearing spontaneously within a short time after injury or with a persistent expansion of the periodontal ligament space progressing over an extended period. During follow-up periods, the radicular and bony conditions either had returned to normal or showed evidence of surface resorption and/or root canal obliteration without further complications [60].

Pulp canal obliteration (calcification of the root canal) is a common sequel following luxation injuries to permanent teeth, particularly teeth that have been injured before their root formation has been completed. Clinically, a yellowish discolouration of the crown may be observed. Pulp canal calcification is also a common occurrence in root-fractured teeth occurring principally in the region of the fracture and in the apical fragment. It may also occur in teeth associated with alveolar and jaw fractures. In most traumatised teeth that have pulps undergoing calcification, the hard tissue is deposited longitudinally along the dentinal walls of the pulp canal. This gradually diminishes the pulp in size until it can barely be observed radiographically. Endodontic treatment is not indicated unless there is evidence of irreversible pulpitis or pulpal necrosis. Pulp necrosis and infection may occur up to 20 years following injury. Assessment of the status of the pulp is difficult since these teeth do not usually respond to thermal pulp sensibility testing. Most, however, do respond to electrical stimulus, and therefore electric pulp sensibility testing is the desirable method for assessing the status of the pulp in calcified teeth [92–94].

Root resorption is a common sequel to dental trauma and may be caused either directly by the traumatic incident or indirectly through subsequent infection. The three most common types of resorption following trauma include surface resorption, replacement root resorption and inflammatory root resorption. Surface resorption is believed to be a self-limiting response to a localised injury to the periodontal ligament or cementum. In traumatised teeth, this type of resorption occurs more commonly in the apical portion of the root and may be seen as a shallow rounding of the external root shape. Replacement root resorption, generally associated with luxated or replanted avulsed teeth, results in the replacement of tooth structure by the bone and can be recognised radiographically by the diffuse nature of the resorption defect and the disappearance of the periodontal space adjacent to the area of the resorption. This progressive type of resorption has a very poor prognosis. Irreversible damage to the periodontal ligament leads to a fusion between the dentine and bone with progressive replacement of the dentine by the bone.

Inflammatory root resorption occurs as a result of a necrotic and infected pulp, which can be recognised radiographically by the development of radiolucency in the bone adjacent to the resorptive defect. Removal of the infected pulp tissue, dressing with an anticlastic medicament and subsequent filling of the root canal with gutta-percha will usually halt the resorptive process [92, 95, 96].

The management of dental traumatic injuries would be incomplete without a discussion of the need to fully assess a patient with dental injuries including dental hard and soft tissues and injuries to supporting tissues and to the patient as a whole. All traumatic dental injuries need to be followed up over time. Follow-up procedures include a clinical examination, a radiographic assessment and pulp sensibility testing [97]. Recommendations for follow-up examinations for injuries are in accord with those recommended by the International Association of Dental Traumatology [1, 14, 15, 20, 27, 44, 51, 58, 60, 63, 73, 90].

Routine radiographic examinations for preoperative, perioperative and postoperative monitoring of complications and healing of dental trauma cases should include a parallel periapical radiograph with the central beam projected through the tooth in question and a lateral angulation from either the mesial or distal aspect of the tooth. The latter allows enhanced visualisation of root fractures that may not be noted when the beam is aimed centrally [98, 99].

Splinting of teeth with luxation injuries, avulsions and root fractures is often necessary to stabilise a tooth in position and to assist in periodontal and pulpal healing. A non-rigid flexible splint has been shown to be the most desirable. An ideal splint should amongst other things be easily fabricated in the mouth without additional trauma; be passive, allow for physiological mobility; be non-irritating to the soft tissues, not interfere with the occlusion; allow endodontic access; and be easily cleaned and easily removed. Recommended splinting times are up to 2 weeks for most avulsion and luxation injuries unless they occur in association with alveolar fractures; up to 4 weeks for lateral luxation injuries, alveolar fractures and root fractures; and up to 4 months for cervical-third root fractures. Many dental injuries do not occur singly. Thus, these splinting times cannot be rigorously applied. In general, splinting times have to be adjusted to accommodate the more major injuries [100–102].

There is limited evidence for the adjunctive use of systemic antibiotics for luxation injuries and no current evidence that antibiotic coverage improves the outcome for root-fractured teeth. The use of intra-canal antibiotics and corticosteroids immediately after replantation appears to halt the progression of inflammatory root resorption, although replacement resorption still occurs to some extent. Antibiotic coverage may be warranted by the patient's medical health and/ or injuries sustained, and the decision to provide any coverage lies with the individual practitioner in line with current guidelines [54, 103, 104].

Pulp sensibility testing immediately after trauma is an unreliable means of predicting the true status of the pulp. A negative response is often a common finding immediately after the pulp has suffered trauma. Teeth that initially give a negative response may prove to respond positively in the coming months. Endodontic treatment is only indicated for those teeth in which pulp necrosis has occurred. At least two signs and symptoms (clinical and/or radiographic) are necessary to make the diagnosis of a necrotic pulp. Responses to sensibility testing need to be followed up over time before a definitive diagnosis of pulp necrosis is made [105, 106].

Treatment planning for the management of traumatic injuries should be based on sound biological principles that form the basis of current guidelines. Careful adherence to treatment protocols with these goals in mind should allow for optimal healing and retention of the tooth where possible [107].

15.2   Initial Management and First Aid

Initial management of any trauma should consider the general wellbeing of the patient and any loss of consciousness; acute bleeding, respiratory problems or neurological signs/symptoms may indicate life-threatening conditions requiring urgent medical attention. Often the patient presenting with dental trauma in your office will be stable, showing normalisation of vital functions. The secondary survey starts with the initial history taking and should include general patient details, general medical health of the patient, past tetanus status and questions related to the injury (when, where and how the injury occurred). It is highly pertinent that all information should be obtained in chronological order with contemporaneous notes recorded including time and date of the trauma. This is particularly relevant when an assault is alleged resulting in legal ramifications or insurance matters related to trauma at school or the workplace. It is important for the clinician to calm

and reassure the often-distressed patient prior to any initial examination.

Extra-orally simple visual inspection can assess facial symmetry, swelling, facial muscle movements (cranial nerve VII) and mouth opening and deviation (including maximal interincisal distance). Clear draining fluid from either the nose or ears may indicate cerebrospinal fluid, which indicates severe cranial damage. Palpation noting any marked tenderness, bony steps, mobility/crepitus and facial sensation abnormalities (cranial nerve V) can give further clues to any underlying facial bone fractures. Numbness of the lower lip in the context of a facial trauma can be highly suggestive of a mandibular fracture. Numbness of the cheek, nose, upper lip or maxillary teeth may indicate a complex fracture involving the orbitozygomatic complex. Numbness of the maxillary teeth alone may indicate an orbital floor fracture affecting branches of the middle to anterior superior alveolar dental nerve.

Dental injuries can often result in facial or lip lacerations that may require suturing or referral to an appropriate specialist (Figs. 15.1 and 15.2). Before examination of the mouth, a thorough facial examination should have been carried out including assessment of frontal, naso-orbital, nasal, middle-third, zygomatic, orbital and mandibular fractures. Inability to open the mouth, limited opening or deviation may all indicate mandibular or temporomandibular joint fractures. Mandibular fractures will usually be associated with painful, limited opening, and if a condyle is involved, then the jaw may deviate towards the side of the fracture. A deranged occlusion may also indicate a fracture of the mandible or zygoma until proven otherwise. Appropriate referral to an oral maxillofacial surgeon may be required.

Intra-oral examination should include assessment of the crowns of the teeth (checking for signs of possible fracture or pulp exposure), displaced teeth (luxation injuries) and missing teeth, occlusion disturbances and abnormal mobility of individual or groups of teeth and surrounding soft

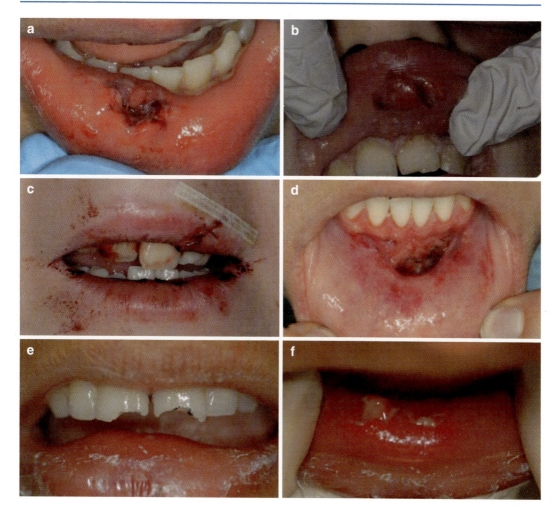

Fig. 15.1 Clinical photographs demonstrating soft tissue lacerations associated with traumatic injuries. Note: (**a, b**) lacerations affecting lips – simple resorbable sutures can be used for primary closure. Deep sutures may be required for muscle repair. (**c**) Laceration affecting the upper lip with vermillion border involvement. Correct suturing will be required to align vermillion border with appropriate skin sutures. (**d**) De-gloving injury affecting the alveolar mucosa. (**e, f**) Uncomplicated maxillary central incisor crown fractures embedded in the lower lip (Pictures courtesy of Drs K Dang, A Timmermann, and D Felman)

tissues (including degloving injuries). All missing teeth and fragments should be accounted for (Figs. 15.1 and 15.2).

Radiographic assessment will be invaluable in the diagnosis and management of dental trauma. Extra-oral plain film radiography or cone beam computer tomography is indicated when suspected facial fractures including jaw and condylar fractures are suspected. Soft tissue radiographic assessment is indicated when tooth fragments or foreign objects might have been embedded into the lips. Pretreatment radiographs are essential to determine the size of pulp chamber, the stage of root development and the appearance of the periodontal ligament and presence of any root fractures. Parallel periapical radiographs are also essential to monitor any changes in the pulp space, resorption and calcifications that may indicate future therapeutic intervention.

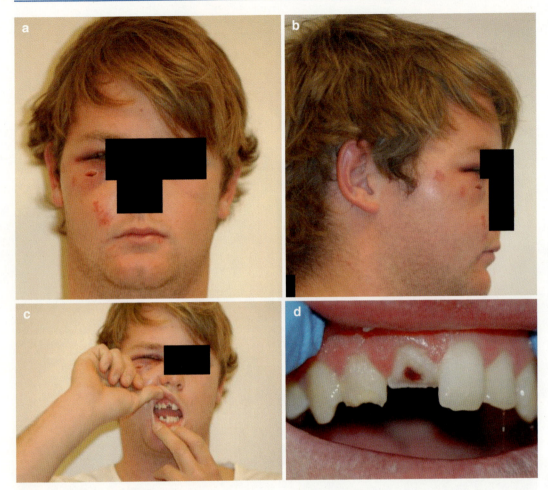

Fig. 15.2 Clinical photographs demonstrating soft tissue lacerations associated with traumatic injuries. Note: (**a, b**) facial laceration affecting right infraorbital area with swelling and bruising. (**c, d**) Intraoral injury. A complicated crown fracture affecting tooth 11; an uncomplicated crown fracture associated with tooth 12 (Pictures courtesy of Dr K Dang, A Timmermann, and D Felman)

15.3   Crown Fractures

Enamel infraction

Clinical and radiographic findings

An incomplete fracture (crack) of the enamel has occurred without loss of tooth structure (Fig. 15.3). The use of indirect light or transillumination or dyes may help visualise the craze line. Clinical examination reveals no abnormal tenderness to percussion or palpation. Radiographic appearance reveals no abnormalities.

Treatment objectives

Often no treatment is usually indicated. In cases of marked infraction, etching and sealing with a composite resin may prevent future discolouration of the fracture line.

General prognosis

Pulpal complications are rare.

Recommended follow-up

No further follow-up is generally needed.

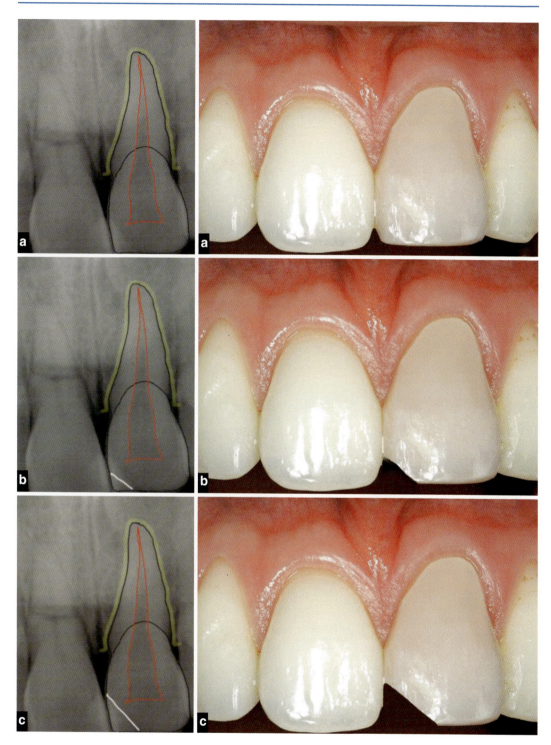

Fig. 15.3 Diagrams representing the different types of crown/root fractures that may present following a traumatic injury. (**a**) Enamel infraction requiring no treatment. (**b**) Uncomplicated crown fracture – enamel only. Reattachment of the tooth fragment or tooth colored restoration will protect the underlying pulp. (**c**) Uncomplicated crown fracture – enamel and dentine. Dentinal tubule exposure can result in sensitivity and pulpal inflammation if left untreated

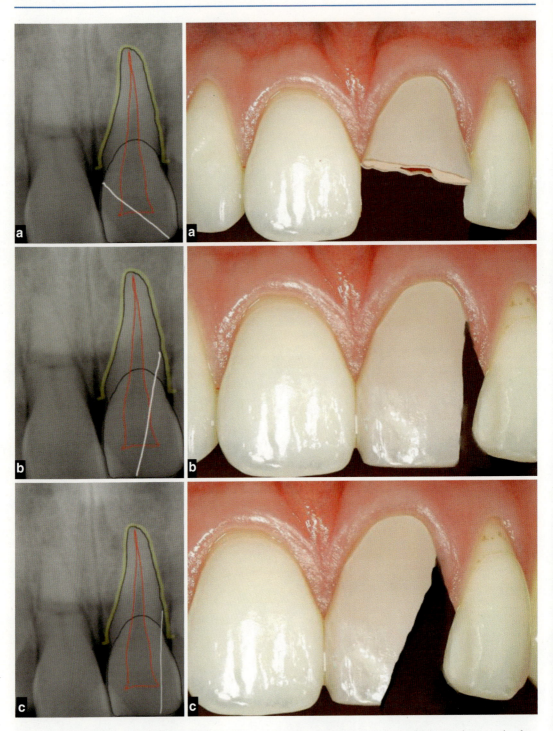

Fig. 15.4 Diagrams representing the different types of crown/root fractures that may present following a traumatic injury. (**a**) Complicated crown fracture – enamel, dentine, and pulp. Treatment options include either pulp preservation procedures (direct pulp capping or Cvek pulpotomy) or pulpectomy procedures. Pulp preservation should be attempted in immature teeth with incomplete root development. Conversely, in mature teeth with extensive loss of tooth structure, root canal therapy is sagacious before cast restoration. (**b**) Complicated crown-root fracture – enamel, dentine, and pulp. (**c**) Uncomplicated crown-root fracture – enamel and dentine only

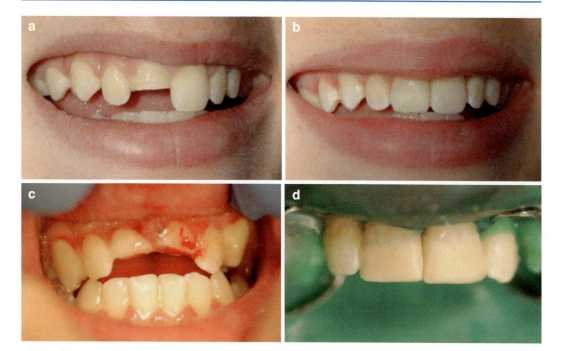

Fig. 15.5 Clinical photographs demonstrating uncomplicated crown fractures. Note (**a**, **b**) uncomplicated crown fracture affecting tooth 11 restored with composite resin restoration. (**c**, **d**) Uncomplicated crown fractures affecting teeth 11 and 21 with appropriate restorations (Pictures courtesy of Drs K Dang and A Timmermann)

Enamel fracture (uncomplicated)

Clinical and radiographic findings

Clinical findings reveal loss of tooth structure confined to enamel (Fig. 15.3). Clinical examination reveals the tooth exhibits no abnormal pain or tenderness. Normal mobility is noted and pulp sensibility testing is normal. Radiographic examination of the soft tissues (lips) may be recommended to rule out the presence of any tooth fragments or foreign material potentially displaced into the lips. Two periapical films should be taken with either a mesial or distal tube shift to rule out the presence of any underlying root fractures.

Treatment objectives

The aim of any proposed treatment is to maintain pulp vitality and restore aesthetics and function. Minor fractures or rough margins/edges should be smoothed. If the tooth fragment is available, then re-bonding may be possible using composite resin and the acid-etch technique. When unavailable, restoration with a composite resin restoration will achieve the desired aesthetic outcome.

General prognosis

Overall prognosis is good although any concomitant periodontal injury sustained can have an adverse affect on outcome.

Recommended follow-up

Due to the unpredictability of dental trauma, pulp vitality testing should be carried out both immediately after the occurrence of the injury and again in 6–8 weeks and 1 year.

Enamel-dentine fracture (uncomplicated)

Clinical and radiographic findings

Crown fractures involving enamel and dentine without pulpal exposure are called uncomplicated crown fractures (Figs. 15.3 and 15.5). Clinical examination reveals loss of tooth structure confined to enamel and dentine with potential exposure of dentinal tubules that can lead to pulpal inflammation. Radiographic examination confirms enamel-dentine loss. Soft tissue radiographic examination of the lips may be indicated to ensure no fragments are present. Presence of root fractures should also be assessed using two parallel periapical radiographs with mesial or distal cone shift technique.

Treatment objectives

The aim is to preserve the vitality of the underlying pulp by sealing the exposed dentinal tubules and restore aesthetics and function for the patient. If the tooth fragment is available, it may be possible to reattach the fragment; otherwise, direct application of dentine bonding agents and the use of bonded tooth-coloured restorations will be effective. Reattachment of the tooth fragment requires isolation of the tooth under rubber dam. Both the tooth fragment and fractured tooth should be cleaned with pumice and water prior to reattachment. Accuracy of fit should be checked prior to the use of acid-etch technique according to manufacturer directions and type of bonding system used. Cases where exposed dentine encroaches to within 0.5 mm of the underlying pulp (determined by visible pink pulp tissue beneath the exposed dentine) will require application of an indirect pulp capping material.

General prognosis

The survival of the pulp and formation of tertiary dentine (reactionary) or pulpal necrosis depend on a number of factors including residual dentine thickness, age of the patient, concomitant periodontal injury and the length of time between trauma and treatment intervention. The overall prognosis for these types of fractures is generally good.

Recommended follow-up

Periodic evaluation is necessary to determine pulpal status and whether pulp necrosis has developed. The patient should be reviewed 6–8 weeks following treatment and at 1 year.

Crown fracture (complicated)

An enamel-dentine fracture with pulp exposure.

Clinical and radiographic findings

Crown fractures involving enamel, dentine and pulp are known as complicated crown fractures (Fig. 15.4 and 15.6). The degree of pulpal involvement can range from a pinpoint exposure to complete coronal pulp exposure. Clinically the exposed pulp may be sensitive to stimuli. Radiographic examination confirms pulpal involvement.

Treatment objectives

Following pulp exposure, bacterial contamination precludes any healing and repair unless the exposure is treated and protected. The initial reaction to pulpal exposure is haemorrhage at the site followed by a superficial inflammatory response. The longer the pulp is exposed before adequate protection, the greater the risk of either destructive (necrosis) or proliferative changes (pulpal polyp). Treatment modalities include direct pulp capping procedures, partial pulpotomy (Cvek), and full pulpotomy or pulpectomy procedures. Vital pulp therapy procedures in young patients with immature developing, thin, weak roots offer the potential for continued root development. Conversely in the fully developed permanent dentition, pulpectomy procedures may offer a better chance of success rather than risking the development of apical periodontitis following direct pulp capping or pulpotomy procedures.

General prognosis

Overall prognosis of attempts to maintain pulp vitality as opposed to complete pulpectomy procedures is dependant on any underlying concomitant periodontal injury sustained, age of the pulp exposure and stage of root development (incomplete versus complete). Treatment modalities aimed at preserving pulp tissue may result in either failure in the future or degenerative pulp changes such as pulpal calcification.

Recommended follow-up

Periodic evaluation both clinically and radiographically should be carried out at 6–8 weeks and 1 year following treatment. Pulp preservation treatments should be assessed for continued pulp vitality ensuring necrosis has not developed.

Crown-root fracture

An enamel, dentine and cementum fracture with or without pulpal exposure.

Clinical and radiographic findings

Enamel, dentine and cementum fracture is present with or without pulpal exposure (Fig. 15.4). The crown fracture will extend below the gingival margin. Clinical examination reveals percussion tenderness. The coronal tooth fragment may be mobile, attached to the gingivae and displaced with or without pulpal exposure. Radiographic examination may reveal a radiolucent oblique line often detected following the use of more than one film using different angulations (horizontal or vertical).

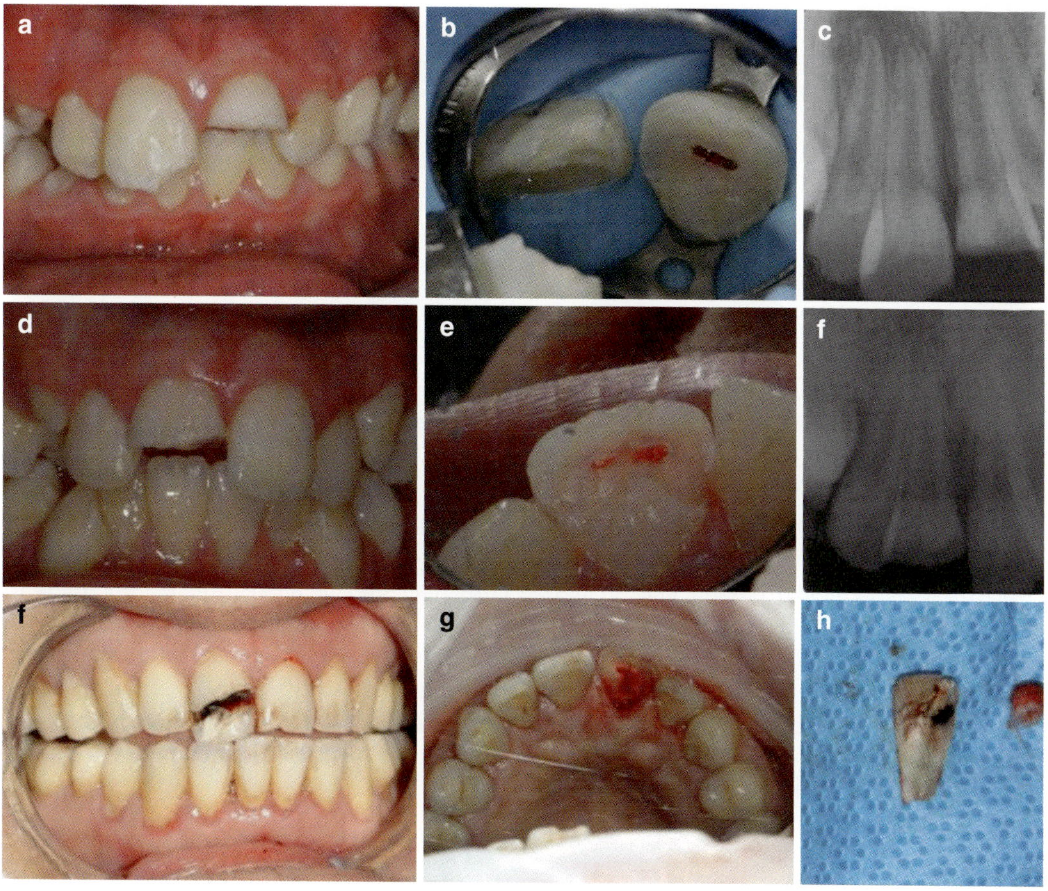

Fig. 15.6 Clinical photographs and radiographs demonstrating complicated crown fractures (enamel-dentine-pulp injuries). Note: (**a–c**) complicated crown fracture affecting tooth 21. (**d–f**) Complicated crown fracture affecting tooth 21. (**f–h**) Complicated crown fracture affecting tooth 21 (Pictures courtesy of Drs K Dang, A Timmermann, and D Felman)

Treatment objectives

Depending on the extent of the fracture, several different treatment options are available. Emergency treatment requires stabilisation of the coronal fragment. Definitive treatment depends on the extent of the fracture. The most conservative approach includes removal of the coronal fragment followed by supragingival restoration. Fragment removal and gingivectomy may be indicated if the fracture extends below the gum. Root canal treatment will often be required prior to further crown lengthening and post and core restoration. Following removal of the fractured coronal fragment and endodontic stabilisation, the apical root may be extruded using either a surgical approach or orthodontics prior to restoration. Sufficient root length must be available after extrusion to support a post-retained crown. If the remaining tooth structure is deemed unrestorable, then either root submergence or extraction and prosthodontics replacement can be carried out. The former is acceptable in cases where implants are planned in the future and alveolar ridge preservation is desirable.

General prognosis

The long-term success in either no pulp or pulp involvement will be dependant on the restorative outcome and ability to maintain a coronal seal. Due to the loss of significant tooth structure and restorability issues, the prognosis is deemed to be guarded.

Recommended follow-up

6–8 weeks and 1 year initially

15.4   Root Fractures

Root fracture

Clinical and radiographic findings

Horizontal or oblique root fractures involving the dentine, cementum and pulp. They can be sub-classified according to the location of the fracture line (apical, middle or coronal) (Fig. 15.7).

Clinical findings reveal a mobile coronal segment attached to the gingivae that may be displaced. Bleeding may be evident in the gingival sulcus and the tooth may or may not be tender to percussion. Initial sensibility testing may be negative indicating transient or permanent nerve damage. Monitoring of the pulp status is recommended. Clinically if some time has elapsed since injury and presentation, then transient crown discolouration may be evident (grey/red). Multiple radiographs exposed at different angulations may be required to confirm the presence of a root fracture. Either a horizontal or oblique fracture involving the root of the tooth may be evident with possible separation of root fragments. Often fractures that are in the horizontal plane in the cervical 1/3 can be detected using a regular 90° angle film with the central beam through the tooth. If the plane of the fracture is more oblique (as in apical or middle 1/3 root fractures), then additional film angulations will be necessary to visualise the fracture line.

Treatment objectives

If the coronal fragment is displaced, then it should be repositioned with a non-rigid semi-flexible splint for 4 weeks. Coronal 1/3 fractures may require additional splinting for up to 4 months to allow for healing of the periodontal ligament. If the fracture line is in the apical 1/3 and there is no mobility and the tooth remains asymptomatic, then no treatment will be indicated. Repositioning of fragments should be confirmed radiographically ensuring correct anatomical apposition to allow for optimal healing of both periodontal ligament and neurovascular supply whilst maintaining form, function and aesthetics. If pulpal necrosis develops, then root canal treatment of the coronal segment to the fracture line is indicated (Fig. 15.8).

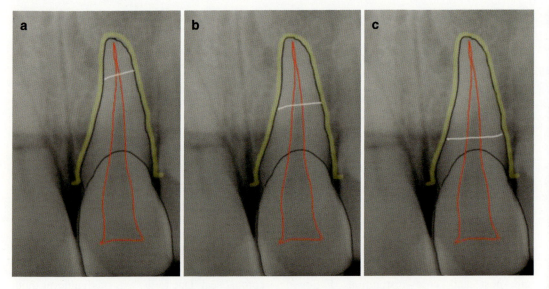

Fig. 15.7 Diagrams representing the different types of root fractures that may present following a traumatic injury. (**a**) Root fracture in the apical 1/3, (**b**) root fracture in the middle 1/3, and (**c**) root fracture in the coronal 1/3

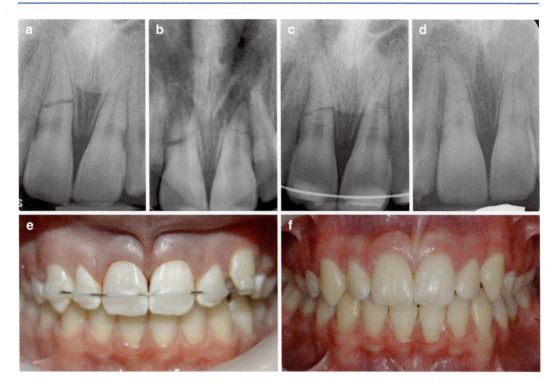

Fig. 15.8 Clinical photographs and radiographs demonstrating middle 1/3 root fracture of tooth 11 and 21 and its management. Note (**a**) preoperative parallel view of the anterior maxillary teeth. Discernible fracture line evident in tooth 11. (**b**) Vertical tube shift revealing additional fracture line in tooth 11. (**c**) Repositioning of fractured segments with a semirigid splint. (**d**) The splint was removed following a period of 2 months. The patient was reviewed a further 6 months later. Note pulp canal obliteration seen in both teeth. Good alignment of the fractures has occurred. Both teeth remain vital responding to thermal stimulus (CO_2 snow) and electric pulp testing. Clinically the teeth were firm with no tenderness to palpation or percussion. The patient was placed on long-term review to monitor pulpal status. (**e**) Clinical photograph of splint in place and (**f**) following splint removal (Pictures courtesy of Drs K Dang and A Timmermann)

General prognosis

Healing of fractures when repositioned occurs by either hard calcified tissue, interposition of connective tissue, interposition of the connective tissue and bone or interposition of granulation tissue. Middle-third fractures are considered to have the best prognosis, whereas fractures located close to the gingival crevice (coronal 1/3) have the poorest outcome. Pulp necrosis in root-fractured teeth is attributed to displacement of the coronal fragment and mature root development. In young patients with immature root formation, positive pulp sensibility testing at the time of injury and approximation of fractured segments to within 1 mm have been found to be advantageous to both pulpal healing and hard tissue repair at the fracture site.

Recommended follow-up

Splinting periods range from 4 weeks to 4 months depending on location of the fracture line. Recommended follow-up should be carried out at 6–8 weeks and 4-month, 6-month and 12-month periods after initial treatment. During the healing period within the first year, the pulpal status should be assessed, bearing in mind that false-negative responses may be possible for up to 3 months. The radiographic appearance of healing of the fracture with hard calcified tissue results in a discernible line with close contact of the fragments. Healing with interproximal connective tissue results in fractured fragments separated by a narrow radiolucent line with rounding of the fracture edges. Healing with interproximal bone and connective tissue results in fragments separated by an obvious bony bridge. No healing with inflammatory interproximal tissue results in a widened fracture line with/without a developing radiolucency.

15.5   Alveolar Process Fractures

Clinical and radiographic findings

Alveolar process fractures are classified as either closed fractures or comminution (crushing or compression) that involves the socket walls (Fig. 15.9). Clinical examination may confirm segment mobility and dislocation with several teeth moving together. A deranged occlusion may be evident. The use of horizontal tube-shift radiographs with an additional panoramic radiograph may be helpful in determining the course and position of the fracture line.

Treatment objectives

The displaced segment should be repositioned to reduce the fracture followed by stabilisation by splinting for 4 weeks. Any gingival lacerations should be sutured. Fracture stabilisation should be carried out as soon as possible

to reduce the chance of pulpal necrosis of teeth. Teeth involved in the fracture line should not be routinely extracted since they help in stabilisation (Figs. 15.10 and 15.11).

General prognosis

Teeth involved in the fracture line should be pulp tested and followed up to assess whether vitality is maintained.

Recommended follow-up

Due to the risk of pulp complications associated with teeth in the fracture line, careful follow-up is recommended at 6–8-week and 4-month, 6-month and 12-month periods after initial treatment.

15.6   Luxation Injuries

Tooth luxation injuries from least to most severe are concussion, subluxation, extrusive luxation, lateral luxation and intrusion (Fig. 15.12). With the exception of concussion injuries, luxation injuries frequently result in pulpal necrosis requiring root canal treatment. The fundamental basis of all treatment modalities is to reposition the tooth in the correct position to allow for optimal healing. Prognostic factors for pulpal survival include

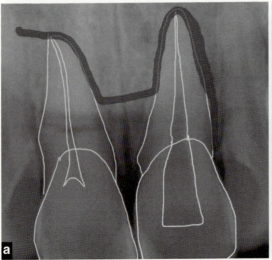
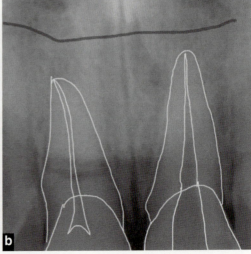
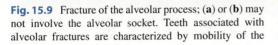

Fig. 15.9 Fracture of the alveolar process; (**a**) or (**b**) may not involve the alveolar socket. Teeth associated with alveolar fractures are characterized by mobility of the alveolar process; several teeth typically will move as a unit when mobility is checked. Occlusal interference is often present

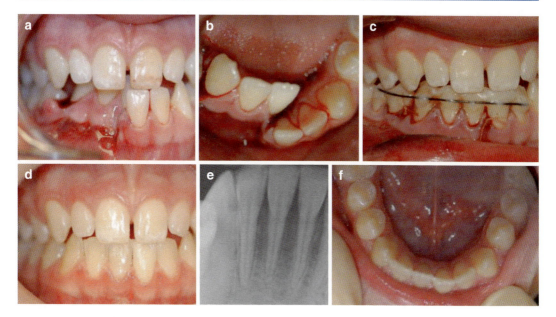

Fig. 15.10 Clinical photographs and radiographs demonstrating dentoalveolar fracture in regions 41, 42, and 43. Note: (**a**, **b**) preoperative views demonstrating deranged occlusion with obvious dentoalveolar fracture. (**c**) Rigid splinting in position. (**d–f**) 4 months have elapsed since splint placement. Occlusion is restored and splint has been removed. Teeth 41, 42, and 43 remain vital with no signs of pulp necrosis (Pictures courtesy of Drs K Dang and A Timmermann)

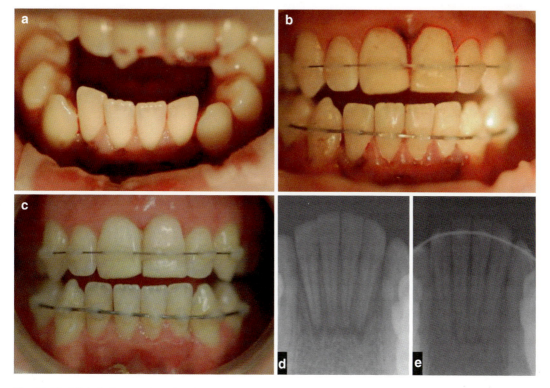

Fig. 15.11 Clinical photographs and radiographs demonstrating dentoalveolar fracture in the lower anterior region extending from 42 to 32. Note: (**a**) preoperative view demonstrating displaced anterior segment with deranged occlusion. (**b**) Rigid splint fixation used to realign lower anterior teeth. (**c**) Splint in position at 3-month review. (**d**) Preoperative lower occlusal radiograph demonstrating periapical appearance due to alveolar segment displacement. (**e**) Following rigid splinting after 3-month interim period. Pulpal sensibility testing using electric pulp testing and thermal stimulus indicate teeth remain vital (Pictures courtesy of Drs K Dang and A Timmermann)

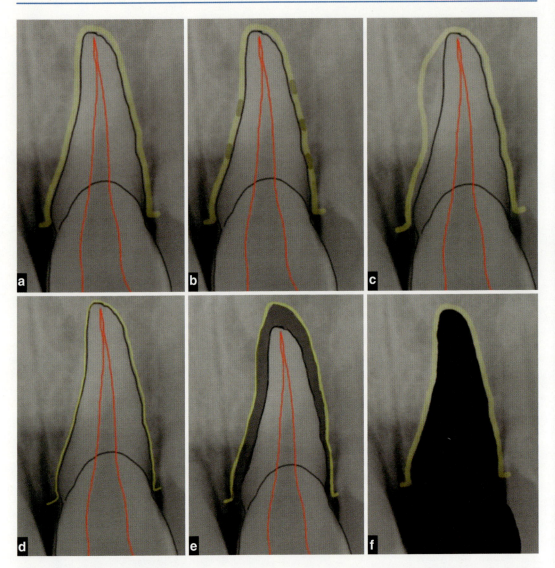

Fig. 15.12 Diagrams representing traumatic dental injuries sustained to the tooth supporting structures (periodontal injury). Note: (**a**) concussion, (**b**) subluxation, (**c**) lateral luxation, (**d**) intrusion, (**e**) extrusion, and (**f**) avulsion

the stage of root development (immature vs. mature) or size of apical foramen (wide open apex vs. closed fully developed), length of the pulp, age of the patient, type of injury sustained, bacterial contamination of the periodontal ligament and pulp and optimal repositioning of displaced teeth.

Trauma and severity related to the type of injury sustained ultimately affect both the blood supply and neurovascular bundle at the apical foramen. Teeth with immature root development with large apical foramina have a greater potential for recovery compared to mature fully

developed teeth where pulpal revascularisation (regrowth of new blood vessels and vital cells into the severed pulp) may be limited.

In luxation injuries, stabilisation may be necessary to reposition the tooth in its correct position. This should be done in a gentle manner without excessive forces to ensure further trauma is kept to a minimal and when carried out the sooner after the injury, the better. Current concepts regarding splinting of traumatised teeth (luxation injuries, root fractures and avulsions) are to use a splint that permits some mobility of the injured tooth/teeth. The splint is termed non-rigid and functional which allows for healing of damaged periodontal ligament fibres with less resorption compared to traditional rigid splints of the past. Orthodontic wires bonded to crowns of teeth using composite are sufficient for most cases.

In immature teeth with incomplete root development, the treatment objectives are to promote pulpal healing, revascularisation and continued root development. Initially displaced teeth with pulpal injuries may have temporary ischaemia and subsequent coagulation necrosis, which would account for negative sensibility testing in the first few months. Provided the teeth are protected from bacterial invasion, then the potential for revascularisation and restoration of pulp vitality is possible. Maintenance of pulp vitality for immature teeth is essential for continued root development, and current treatment modalities should be applied to safeguard this concept.

Concussion

Injury to the tooth-supporting structures has occurred without abnormal loosening or displacement of the tooth (Fig. 15.12).

Clinical and radiographic findings

Concussion is the mildest form of injury to the periodontal ligament characterised by sensitivity to percussion only. The periodontal ligament absorbs the injury resulting in inflammation. No abnormal loosening or displacement of the tooth is evident. Pulp sensibility testing will be normal. Radiographic examination reveals no abnormalities. Two baseline radiographs should be taken with different-angled views to rule out the possibility of other injuries to the tooth itself.

Treatment objectives

Concussion injuries do not require any immediate treatment as such. The aim of treatment is to optimise periodontal healing and maintain pulp vitality. The patient is instructed to rest the tooth as much as possible with a soft diet for up to 1 week.

General prognosis

The overall prognosis should be good. Teeth should be monitored for development of pulpal necrosis confirmed by sensibility testing, colour changes and radiographic appearance.

Recommended follow-up

Pulp status should be monitored at 4 weeks, 6 weeks and 12 months following initial presentation.

Subluxation

Clinical and radiographic findings

Injury to the tooth-supporting structures has occurred with abnormal loosening but without any tooth displacement (Fig. 15.12). Pulp sensibility testing should be normal and no radiographic abnormalities should be seen.

Treatment objectives

The treatment objectives are to optimise healing of the periodontal ligament and maintain pulp vitality. Tooth stabilisation with a flexible splint for up to 2 weeks may be required with recommended soft diet for up to 1 week (Fig. 15.13).

General prognosis

General prognosis should be good. There is a greater risk of pulp necrosis in fully developed teeth due to associated injuries at the apex of the tooth.

Recommended follow-up

The patient should be periodically followed up at 4 weeks, 6–8 weeks and 12 months following initial treatment.

Extrusive luxation

Clinical and radiographic findings

Partial displacement of the tooth has occurred axially from the socket (partial avulsion). The periodontal ligament is usually torn. Clinically the tooth will appear elongated with excessive mobility (Figs. 15.12 and 15.14). Pulp sensibility testing is likely to give negative results. Radiographic examination reveals an increased periodontal ligament space apically.

Treatment objectives

To promote healing of the periodontal ligament and neurovascular supply, repositioning of the tooth as soon as possible followed by stabilisation with a flexible splint for up to 2–3 weeks is recommended (Fig. 15.14). In mature teeth with closed apices, the risk of pulpal necrosis is high. Root canal treatment should be considered when signs and symptoms of pulpal necrosis ensue.

General prognosis

In mature teeth with closed apices and complete root development, the risk of pulp necrosis and pulp canal obliteration is high.

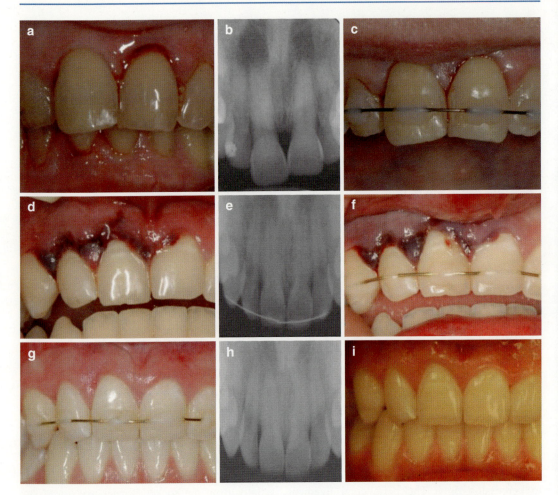

Fig. 15.13 Clinical photographs and radiographs demonstrating subluxation injuries. Note: (**a–c**) subluxation associated with tooth 21. Note tell-tell sign of bleeding at the gingival margin indicating subluxation injury. No discernible features usually noted on the radiograph. A semirigid splint is placed for 7–10 days to allow for patient comfort and uneventful healing to take place. (**d**) Subluxation injuries to teeth 21, 11, 12, and 13. (**e**) Post-splint radiograph as a baseline record. (**f**) Semirigid splint placed for 10 days. (**g**) Prior to splint removal. (**h**, **i**) Radiographic and clinical examination at 6 months post trauma (Pictures courtesy of Drs K Dang and A Timmermann)

Recommended follow-up

The patient should be reviewed at 4-week, 6–8-week, 6-month and 12-month periods following initial treatment. Radiographic follow-up will also be required to ensure that external inflammatory root resorption has not occurred.

Lateral luxation

Clinical and radiographic findings

Displacement of the tooth has occurred in a direction other than axially. The periodontal ligament is torn and contusion or fracture of the supporting alveolar bone occurs (Fig. 15.12). Clinically the tooth has been displaced laterally with the crown either in a palatal or buccal direction, and the tooth may be locked in this new position. The tooth may be nonmobile with no tenderness to percussion. A high metallic sound may be evident on percussion testing indicating ankylosis. Alveolar fracture may also be present. Pulp sensibility testing is likely to be negative. Radiographic findings indicate an increase in the periodontal ligament space with displacement of the apex towards or through the labial bone plate.

Treatment objectives

Repositioning of the tooth is desired as soon as possible, and stabilisation of the tooth in its

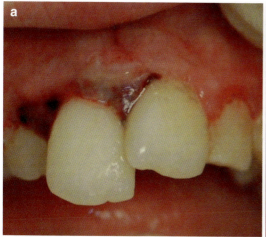
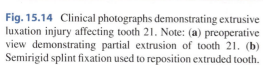
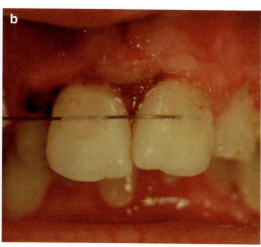

Fig. 15.14 Clinical photographs demonstrating extrusive luxation injury affecting tooth 21. Note: (**a**) preoperative view demonstrating partial extrusion of tooth 21. (**b**) Semirigid splint fixation used to reposition extruded tooth. The splint will be removed at 4–6 weeks, and provided there is no excessive mobility, the tooth will be monitored for signs of pulpal necrosis (Pictures courtesy of Drs K Dang and A Timmermann)

anatomically correct position using a flexible splint for 2–4 weeks is recommended in order to facilitate optimal healing of the periodontal ligament and neurovascular supply whilst maintaining aesthetic and functional integrity. Repositioning should be done with firm digital pressure using minimal excessive forces. Occasionally a displaced tooth may require disimpaction and extrusion to free itself from the apical lock in the cortical bone. The use of forceps to disengage the tooth from the bony lock may be required if digital manipulation is unsuccessful. Pulp status is monitored and root canal treatment commenced if signs and symptoms indicate pulp necrosis (Fig. 15.15).

General prognosis

Common healing complications include pulp necrosis and pulp canal obliteration especially in mature teeth with closed apices and fully developed roots. Development of external inflammatory root resorption or replacement resorption can occur.

Recommended follow-up

Due to pulpal complications, clinical monitoring of pulp status and radiographic follow-up will be required at 4-week, 6–8-week, 6-month and 12-month periods following initial treatment.

Intrusion

Clinical and radiographic findings

Apical displacement of the tooth has occurred into the alveolar bone. The tooth is driven into the socket, compressing the periodontal ligament and commonly causing a crushing fracture of the alveolar socket (Fig. 15.12). Clinical examination revealed the tooth in question may appear shortened or missing. The tooth is often nonmobile and non-tender to percussion. Radiographic findings confirm the tooth has been displaced apically, and the periodontal ligament space does not appear to be continuous. The cement-enamel junction of the intruded tooth will appear to be located more apically when compared to the adjacent non-injured tooth.

Treatment objectives

The tooth should be repositioned in the correct anatomical position followed by stabilisation using a flexible splint for a 2–4-week period. Teeth with incomplete wide-open apices should be allowed to undergo passive repositioning by spontaneous re-eruption. If the intrusion is greater than 7 mm, then either surgical or orthodontic repositioning may be required. Teeth that have undergone complete root development and intrusion of less than

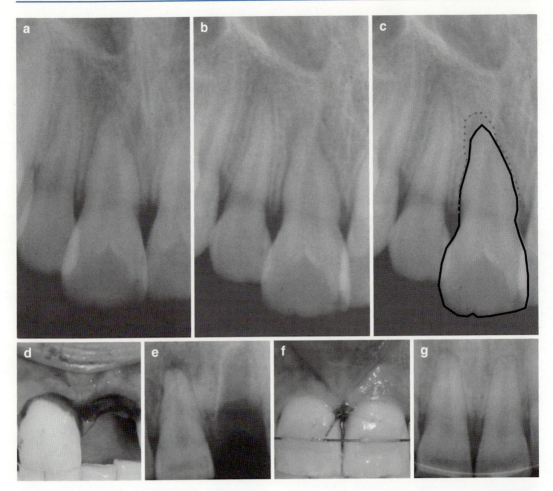

Fig. 15.15 Clinical radiographs demonstrating lateral luxation injury affecting tooth 21. Note: (**a**) long-cone parallel periapical of tooth 21 and (**b**) vertical tube shift to check for any root fractures. (**c**) A peri-radicular radiolucency is evident surrounding the periapex of the tooth confirming a lateral luxation injury. The tooth will need to be ideally manually repositioned. Occasionally the tooth may require surgical repositioning with forceps to disengage the tooth. Complete root development has occurred indicating that the chance of pulp survival is diminished. Follow-up will be required to ascertain whether the pulp survives. (**d–g**) Lateral luxation injury to tooth 11 and avulsion injury of tooth 21. Tooth 21 has been replanted and 11 repositioned into correct position prior to semirigid fixation (Pictures courtesy of Drs K Dang and A Timmermann)

3 mm should be allowed to undergo active eruption with no intervention to minimise further pulp and periodontal ligament damage. If no movement has occurred after 2–4 weeks, then orthodontic or surgical repositioning will be required before ankylosis develops. If tooth intrusion is greater than 7 mm, then surgical repositioning will be indicated. After surgical repositioning, the tooth may require additional stabilisation with a flexible splint for a further 4–8 weeks. Mature teeth that have sustained

intrusion injuries have a high chance of pulp necrosis developing. In particular, teeth that have undergone surgical repositioning will often require pulpectomy procedures 2–3 weeks after repositioning (Fig. 15.16).

General prognosis

In mature teeth with closed apices and fully developed roots, there is considerable risk of developing pulpal necrosis, pulp canal obliteration and progressive root resorption (external inflammatory and replacement resorption).

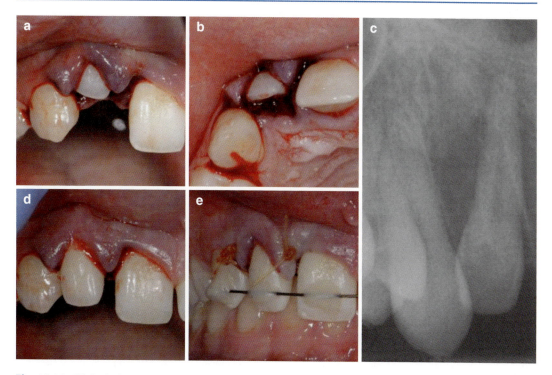

Fig. 15.16 Clinical photographs and radiograph demonstrating intrusive luxation injury affecting tooth 12. Note: (**a**, **b**) preoperative views demonstrating partial intrusion of tooth 12. (**c**) Periapical radiograph showing intruded lateral incisor tooth. (**d**) Repositioned tooth and (**e**) semirigid splint fixation used. The splint will be removed at 4–6 weeks, and provided there is no excessive mobility, the tooth will be monitored for signs of pulpal necrosis (Pictures courtesy of Drs K Dang and A Timmermann)

Recommended follow-up

Due to the high risks of pulp necrosis developing, close monitoring and follow-up are recommended. The patient should be reviewed at 4 weeks, 6–8 weeks, 6 months and 12 months thereafter following initial treatment.

15.7   Avulsion Injuries

Complete displacement of the tooth has occurred out of the socket. The periodontal ligament is severed and fracture of the alveolus may occur (Figs. 15.17, 15.18, and 15.19).

Immediate management at site of injury/ telephone advice

An avulsed permanent tooth is one of the few real emergency situations in dentistry, and all dentists should have prior knowledge as to the management of such cases. Immediate management of an avulsed tooth includes the following points:

1. If a tooth is avulsed, check whether it is a permanent or primary tooth. Primary teeth should not be replanted due to risk of damaging the permanent successor.
2. Find the tooth and pick it up by the crown (the white part) and avoid touching any part of the root.
3. If the tooth is dirty, wash it briefly (maximum time 10 s) under cold running water prior to repositioning.
4. Try to encourage the patient/guardian to replant the tooth. Once the tooth is back in place, ask the patient to bite on a handkerchief to hold it in position.
5. If this is not possible, for example, in an unconscious patient, then place the tooth in a glass of milk or another suitable storage medium and bring it with the patient to the emergency clinic. The tooth can also be transported in the mouth, keeping it inside the lip or cheek if the patient is conscious. If the

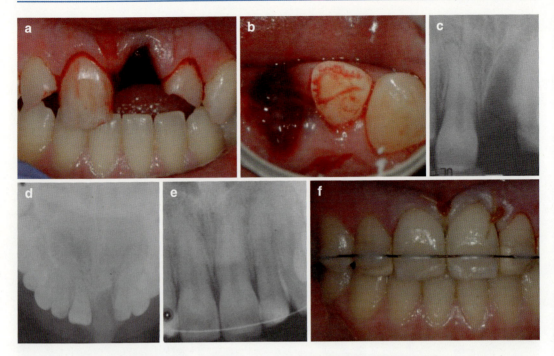

Fig. 15.17 Clinical photographs and radiographs demonstrating uncomplicated crown fractures associated with teeth 11, 12, and 22 and avulsion injury associated with tooth 21. Note: (**a**, **b**) uncomplicated crown fractures and avulsion injury to anterior maxillary dentition. (**c**, **d**) Preoperative parallel periapical and standard maxillary occlusal film to check for any undiagnosed root fractures. (**e**) Avulsed tooth replanted and (**f**) semirigid splint place. Root development is completed in this adult patient. The tooth will require endodontic therapy. Long-term sequelae include root resorption and ankylosis of the tooth (Pictures courtesy of Drs K Dang and A Timmermann)

patient is very young, it is advisable to get the patient to spit in a container and place the tooth in it due to the risk of ingestion or inhalation of the tooth. Avoid storage in water.
6. If there is access at the place of accident to special storage or transport media (e.g. tissue culture/transport medium, Hank's balanced salt solution (HBSS) storage medium or saline), such media can preferably be used.
7. Seek emergency dental treatment immediately.

Treatment guidelines for avulsed permanent teeth

The management of avulsion injuries is related to root maturation (open or closed apex) and whether the periodontal ligament (PDL) cells have survived. The condition and viability of the cells is dependent on the extra-oral time the tooth has remained out of the mouth (extra-oral dry time) and the storage medium used.

After an extra-oral dry time of 60 min or more, all PDL cells can be considered non-viable. For this reason, it is very important to assess from the patient's history the extra-oral dry time and type of storage medium used.

Prior knowledge of the extra-oral dry time and storage medium used will aid the clinician in assessing the condition of the PDL cells, thereby classifying the avulsed tooth into *viable* (the tooth has been replanted immediately or after a very short time at the place of accident), *viable but compromised* (the tooth has been kept in a suitable storage medium (e.g. tissue culture, HBSS, saline, milk or saliva) and the total dry time has been less than 60 min) or *non-viable* (where the extra-oral dry time has been more than 60 min regardless if the tooth was stored in additional medium or not). The goal for replanting immature teeth (incomplete root development) in children is to allow for possible revascularisation of the pulp space.

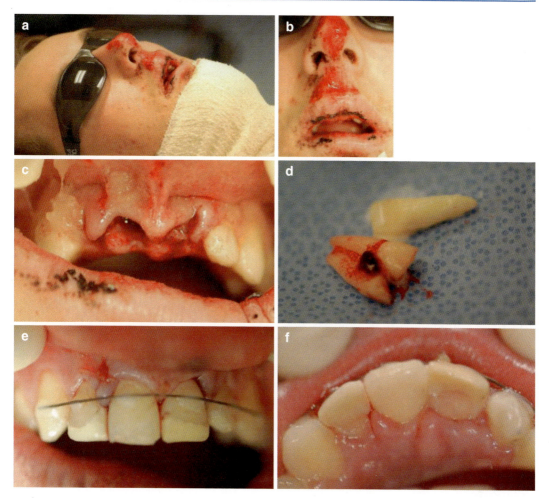

Fig. 15.18 Clinical photograph showing multiple avulsed teeth in the upper anterior maxillary arch following a road traffic accident. Note: (**a**, **b**) extraoral views showing abrasions to mid-face. The patient had had a primary and secondary survey carried out revealing no underlying bony fractures. (**c**) Intraorally the patient had avulsed teeth 11, 12, and 21. (**d**) Avulsed teeth had been found at the scene of the accident and placed in milk. (**e**, **f**) Repositioned teeth with semirigid fixation. The teeth have a guarded long-term prognosis and will require endodontic intervention and long-term follow-up to ensure that no external replacement root resorption occurs (Pictures courtesy of Drs K Dang and A Timmermann)

The advantage of revascularisation in this situation lies in the possibility of continued root development and reinforcement of the dentinal walls by hard tissue deposition allowing further strengthening and reduced long-term propensity to root fracture. If that does not occur, root canal treatment may be recommended (see endodontic considerations). Replantation of adult mature teeth with closed apices has often been seen as a temporary measure with the risk of ultimately succumbing to root resorption. However there are many cases where teeth have survived, maintaining their integrity and function. It is therefore advisable that all teeth deemed viable should be replanted. Furthermore teeth that are deemed non-viable can be replanted with the knowledge that the risks of failure are greater (Figs. 15.17 and 15.18).

Treatment guidelines for avulsed permanent teeth with incomplete or complete root development and PDL cells are deemed viable.

If the tooth has already been replanted before the patient's arrival at the clinic, then leave the tooth in place. The site of injury is cleaned with water spray, saline or chlorhexidine. Gingival lacerations are sutured. The correct anatomical position of the replanted tooth is verified both clinically and radiographically prior to stabilisation with a flexible splint for up to 2 weeks. Systemic antibiotics may be administered. The patient's tetanus protection is checked and patient instructions are given including soft diet for up to 1 week. Root canal treatment may be initiated 7–10 days after replantation and prior to splint removal. Follow-up is always recommended.

Treatment guidelines for avulsed permanent teeth with incomplete or complete root development and PDL cells are deemed viable but compromised.

The root surface and apical foramen are cleaned with saline, and the tooth is soaked in saline, thereby removing contamination and dead cells from the root surface. Following local anaesthesia (see anaesthesia), the socket is irrigated with saline and examined for any alveolar socket fracture. If there is a fracture of the socket wall, reposition it prior to replanting the tooth. Replantation is carried out slowly with slight digital pressure without the use of any excessive force. Gingival lacerations are sutured, if present. The normal position of the replanted tooth is verified both clinically and radiographically prior to flexible splint application for up to 2 weeks. Administer systemic antibiotics and tetanus protection if required. The patient is given postoperative instructions (see Patient instructions). Root canal treatment is initiated 7–10 days after replantation and before splint removal (see Endodontic considerations). The tooth is followed up appropriately (see follow-up procedures).

Treatment guidelines for avulsed permanent teeth with incomplete or complete root development and PDL cells are deemed non-viable

Delayed replantation has a poor long-term prognosis. The periodontal ligament will be necrotic and is not expected to survive. The goals in delayed replantation are to restore aesthetics and function and to maintain alveolar bone contour. However, the expected outcome is ankylosis and resorption of the root resulting in eventual tooth loss. The technique for delayed replantation includes the removal of all attached non-viable soft tissue carefully using gauze. The procedure can be carried out mechanically with curettage or chemically using 17 % EDTA, citric acid or sodium hypochlorite solution. In an attempt to prevent or arrest osseous replacement of the tooth, treatment of the root surface with fluoride prior to replantation has been suggested (2 % sodium fluoride solution for 20 min). Emdogain consisting of hydrophobic enamel matrix proteins derived from porcine-developing embryonic enamel has also been used. It should be pointed out that the use of either treatment should not be seen as an absolute prerequisite in preventing/arresting osseous replacement. Root canal treatment to the tooth can be carried out prior to replantation or later (see endodontic considerations). Following administration of local anaesthesia (see anaesthesia), the socket is irrigated with saline and inspected for fracture of the socket wall (requiring repositioning if present). The tooth is replanted, and gingival lacerations are sutured, if present. Correct position of the replanted tooth is verified clinically and radiographically prior to stabilisation of the tooth with a flexible splint (for up to 4 weeks). Administration of systemic antibiotics (see antibiotics) and tetanus protection is advised (see Tetanus).

Careful follow-up is required, and good communication is necessary to ensure that both the patient and parent understand the likely outcome. Decoronation may be necessary later when more than 1 mm of infraposition is seen.

Anaesthesia

Patients and parents will often be advised to consider replanting the tooth at the place of accident without any local anaesthesia. When the patient is seen in the dental setting where anaesthesia is readily available, normal techniques should be considered. Traumatic

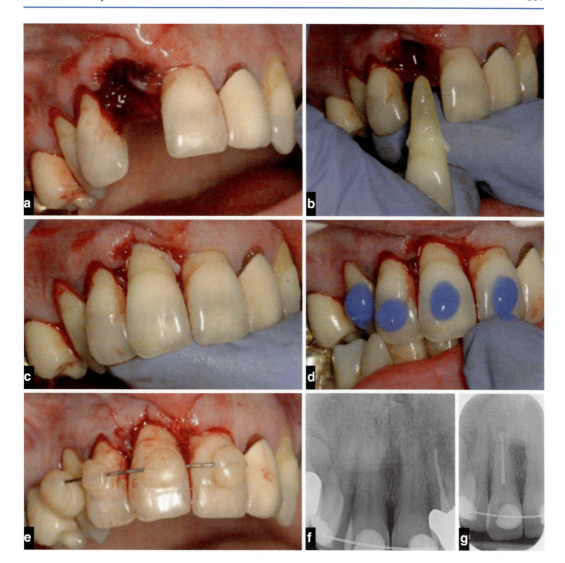

Fig. 15.19 Clinical photographs and radiograph showing management of avulsion injury in a fully developed permanent tooth 11 (extraoral dry period ideal). Note: (**a**) preoperative view showing avulsed tooth 11. (**b**) Tooth 11 is reimplanted with digital pressure. (**c**) Reimplanted 11. (**d**) Acid etch is applied to teeth prior to (**e**) flexible composite wire splint attachment. (**f**) Radiograph is taken to check position of replanted tooth 11. The patient is advised a soft diet, appropriate oral hygiene (chlorhexidine mouthwash), and oral antibiotics (100 mg doxycycline bd. 7 days provided not pregnant). (**g**) Root canal treatment is commenced 7–10 days later with an intracanal dressing of Ledermix and then calcium hydroxide (if resorption present) (Pictures courtesy of Ms Serpil Djemal)

dental injuries often present with concomitant injuries of the soft tissues including lacerations, which require suturing and therefore prior adequate anaesthesia. Concern is sometimes raised whether there are risks of compromising pulpal healing by using vasoconstrictor in the anaesthesia. No strong evidence is currently available for omitting vasoconstrictor.

Antibiotics

The use of systemic antibiotics as an adjunctive therapy in the management of avulsed permanent incisors (open or closed apices) has been recommended. The first choice is tetracycline (doxycycline twice daily for seven days). In many countries, systemic tetracycline use is not recommended for patients under 12 years of age due to the risk of discolouration in the developing permanent dentition. Penicillin (amoxicillin) can be given as an alternative to tetracycline (Fig. 15.19). Caution is also advised in pregnant patients and concomitant use of antibiotics and oral contraceptives.

Tetanus status

The patient should be advised to see their general medical practitioner for evaluation of need for a tetanus booster if the avulsed tooth has contacted soil or tetanus coverage is uncertain.

Splinting of replanted teeth

Splinting of luxated teeth is not only recommended to maintain the repositioned tooth in its correct anatomical position but also ensure that the patient is comfortable during the follow-up period as well as improve function. Current evidence supports short-term, flexible splints for stabilisation of replanted teeth. Studies have shown that for ideal periodontal and pulpal healing to occur the luxated tooth should not be completely rigid but allowed slight motion and the splinting time should not be overly extended. To date there is no specific type of splint related to healing outcomes. The splint should be placed on the buccal surfaces of the maxillary teeth and mandibular teeth to enable lingual access for endodontic procedures and to avoid occlusal interference. Various types of splints are available including resin, composite and wire, orthodontic brackets and titanium mesh. Acid-etch bonded composite splints using orthodontic wire have been widely used to stabilise teeth because fabrication in the dental setting is relatively straightforward. Furthermore, they allow good oral hygiene and are well tolerated by the patients (Fig. 15.19).

Patient instructions

To ensure satisfactory healing and the potential for optimal outcome, the patient must understand both aftercare instructions including home care advice and the need for follow-up evaluation. Patients/parents should be advised with regard to:

1. Avoiding participation in contact sports during the healing period; furthermore, a custom-made mouthguard would be advisable in the future.
2. Soft diet is recommended for up to 2 weeks to prevent further trauma to the dentition.
3. The patient is advised to brush teeth with a soft toothbrush after each meal.
4. The use of chlorhexidine (0.1 %) mouth rinse twice a day for 1 week is advisable. The patient should be warned of the possibility of staining of teeth.

Endodontic considerations

When root canal treatment is indicated, then the ideal time to begin treatment is 7–10 days post replantation. Calcium hydroxide is recommended as an intra-canal medication for up to 1 month followed by root canal filling with an acceptable material. Alternatively if an antibiotic-corticosteroid paste is chosen to be used as an anti-inflammatory, anticlastic intra-canal medicament, it may be placed immediately or shortly following replantation and left for at least 2 weeks. If the antibiotic in the paste is tetracycline, there is a risk of tooth discoloration.

If the tooth has been dry for more than 60 min before replantation, then the root canal treatment may be carried out extra-orally prior to replantation. The canal should be dressed with calcium hydroxide medicament to promote disinfection of the root canal and prevention of inflammatory root resorption. The dressing can be left in place for a longer follow-up period during which time the tooth can be assessed as to whether replacement root resorption has progressed.

In teeth with wide-open apices (immature incompletely developed roots), which have been replanted immediately or kept in appropriate storage media prior to replantation, pulp revascularisation may be possible. The risk of infection-related root resorption should be weighed up against the potential for pulp space revascularisation.

Follow-up procedures

Replanted teeth should be monitored both clinically and radiographically after 4 weeks, 3 months, 6 months, 1 year and yearly thereafter. Percussion tenderness, palpation tenderness, colour, mobility, periodontal probing profile and sensibility test testing (electric pulp testing and thermal stimulus) and appropriate parallel periapical radiographs should be recorded at review appointments.

Loss of tooth

Dental traumatic injuries including avulsion injuries often affect maxillary central incisors and often occur before the age of 18 years. Replantation of avulsed teeth gives rise to complications including replacement root resorption (ankylosis) and external inflammatory resorption. Whilst appropriate endodontic therapy is effective in the treatment of external inflammatory resorption, replacement resorption cannot be arrested or repaired. Replacement resorption occurs due to the absence of vital periodontal ligament resulting in normal osteoclastic activity causing bone remodelling and tooth resorption. Under normal bone remodelling, the root is continuously resorbed and replaced with the bone. In an adult mature tooth, no clinical signs and symptoms exist other than a metallic sound in response to percussion testing. In immature teeth as growth continues, the ankylosed tooth will result in infraocclusion. Treatment options include either decoronation aimed at preserving the tooth in situ where continued alveolar growth is expected (immature teeth) or extraction and prosthodontic replacement (mature teeth). Restoring teeth in growing patients poses a unique set of problems associated with aesthetic and function. One must bear in mind that the ideal replacement of a missing tooth with a solitary implant by virtue of osseointegration will result in ankylosis and infraocclusion in the growing patient. Often an interdisciplinary approach is recommended depending on the treatment plan proposed. Options for replacement of an unsuccessful avulsed tooth lost prematurely include replacement with autotransplantation, use of a single-tooth implant prosthesis, orthodontic closure of the space or space maintenance using a removable denture, resin-bonded bridge or fixed bridgework. Crown and bridgework should be avoided in the growing patient where similar to alveolar growth the gingival margin continues to mature to the cement-enamel junction resulting in exposed roots and unsightly aesthetics at the gingival margin if early treatment is provided before gingival maturation has occurred (age 18+).

Treatment Summary for an Avulsion Injury

Clinical and Radiographic Findings

- Clinical and radiographic findings reveal either the tooth is not in the socket or the tooth has already been replanted.
- Radiographic evidence will confirm the tooth is not intruded when the tooth has not been found.

Treatment Objectives

- To replant the tooth into its anatomically correct position as soon as possible to optimise healing of the periodontal ligament and neurovascular supply whilst maintaining aesthetics and function.
- Stabilisation using a flexible splint for 2 weeks.
- Tetanus prophylaxis and antibiotic coverage should be considered.
- Treatment strategies are aimed at avoiding inflammation that may occur as a result of the tooth's attachment damage and/or pulpal inflammation.
- Choice of treatment is related to the *maturity of the root* (open or closed apex) and *the condition of the PDL cells* (viable or non viable). The condition of the cells is dependent on the storage medium and the time out of the mouth. Note the extra-alveolar dry time is critical for survival of the cells. After a dry time of 60 minutes or more all PDL cells are non-viable. For this reason, the dry time of the tooth, before it was replanted or placed in a storage medium, is very important to assess from the patient's history.
- *The PDL cells are most likely viable.* The tooth has been replanted immediately or after a very short time at the place of accident. Initiate root canal treatment in mature teeth 7–10 days after replantation and before splint removal. In immature teeth (not fully developed) it may be worthwhile waiting for possible revascularization of the pulp space. If this does not occur then root canal treatment will be necessary.
- *The PDL cells may be viable but compromised.* The tooth has been kept in storage medium

(e.g. tissue culture medium, HBSS, saline, milk or saliva and the total dry time has been less than 60 min). In mature teeth initiate root canal treatment 7–10 days after replantation and before splint removal. In immature teeth you must weigh up the potential of possible revascularization against the risk of infection related root resorption. Such resorption can be very rapid in children and so careful follow up will be required with the possibility of endodontic intervention where necessary.

- *The PDL cells are non-viable.* The total extra-oral dry time has been more than 60 min. The PDL will be necrotic and not expected to heal. Non-viable soft tissue is carefully removed. In both mature and immature teeth root canal treatment can be done either on the tooth prior to replantation or 7-10 days after replantation and splint removal. In order to slow down osseous replacement of the tooth, treatment of the root surface with fluoride prior to replantation has been suggested (2% sodium fluoride solution for 20 min) but it should not be seen as an absolute recommendation.
- Consider decoronation procedures when clinical infraposition of the tooth appear and/or clinical and radiographic findings of anyklosis are present.

General Prognosis

- Pulp necrosis, external inflammatory root resorption, ankylosis and replacement resorption are common healing complications.

Recommended Follow-Up

- Splinting 2–4 weeks depending on extra-oral dry time period
- General follow up should be at 4 weeks, 6–8 weeks, 6 months, 1 year and yearly up to 5 years.
- In immature teeth where revascularization is being monitored teeth should be reviewed every 4weeks with appropriate pulp testing and radiographs.

References

1. DiAngelis AJ, Andreasen JO, Ebeleseder KA, Kenny DJ. Trope International Association of Dental Traumatology guidelines for the management of traumatic dental injuries: 1. Fractures and luxations of permanent teeth. Dent Traumatol. 2012;28:2–12.
2. Andreasen JO, Andreasen FM, Skeire A, Hjørting-Hansen E, Schwartz O. Effect of treatment delay upon pulp and periodontal healing of traumatic dental injuries, a review article. Dent Traumatol. 2002;18:116–28.
3. Flores MT, Andersson L, Andreasen JO, Bakland LK, Malmgren B, Barnett F, Bourguignon C, DiAngelis AJ, Hicks ML, Sigurdsson A, Trope M, Tsukiboshi M, von Arx T. Guidelines for the management of traumatic dental injuries. I. Fractures and luxations of permanent teeth. Endod Top. 2006;14:102–18.
4. Ravn JJ. Dental injuries in Copenhagen school children, school years 1967–1972. Community Dent Oral Epidemiol. 1974;2:231–45.
5. Lauridsen E, Hermann NV, Gerds TA, Ahrensburg SS, Kreiborg S, Andreasen JO. Combination injuries 1. The risk of pulp necrosis in permanent teeth with concussion injuries and concomitant crown fractures. Dent Traumatol. 2012;28:364–70.
6. Lauridsen E, Hermann NV, Gerds TA, Ahrensburg SS, Kreiborg S, Andreasen JO. Combination injuries 2. The risk of pulp necrosis in permanent teeth with subluxation injuries and concomitant crown fractures. Dent Traumatol. 2012;28:371–8.
7. Lauridsen E, Hermann NV, Gerds TA, Kreiborg S, Andreasen JO. Combination injuries 3. The risk of pulp necrosis in permanent teeth with extrusion or lateral luxation and concomitant crown fractures without pulp exposure. Dent Traumatol. 2012;28:379–85.
8. Lauridsen E, Hermann NV, Gerds TA, Kreiborg S, Andreasen JO. Pattern of traumatic dental injuries in the permanent dentition among children, adolescents, and adults. Dent Traumatol. 2012;28:358–63.
9. Day PF, Duggal MS. Interventions for treating traumatised permanent front teeth: avulsed (knocked out) and replanted. Cochrane Database Syst Rev. 2010;(1):CD006542. doi:10.1002/14651858.CD006542.pub2.
10. Andersson L, Andreasen JO, Day PF, Heithersay G, Trope M, DiAngelis AJ, Kenny DJ, Sigurdsson A, Bourguignon C, Flores MT, Hicks ML, Lenzi AR, Malmgren B, Moule AJ, Tsukiboshi M. International association of dental traumatology guidelines for the management of traumatic dental injuries: 2. Avulsion of permanent teeth. Dent Traumatol. 2012;28:88–96.

11. Stålhane I, Hedegård B. Traumatized permanent teeth in children aged 7–15 years. Part II. Swed Dent J. 1975;68:157–69.
12. Ravn JJ. Follow-up study of permanent incisors with enamel cracks as a result of an acute trauma. Scand J Dent Res. 1981;89:213–7.
13. Moorrees CF, Fanning EA, Hunt EE. Age variation of formation stages for ten permanent teeth. J Dent Res. 1963;42:1490–502.
14. Andreasen FM, Andreasen JO. Crown fractures. In: Andreasen JO, Andreasen FM, Andersson L, editors. Textbook and color atlas of traumatic injuries to the teeth. 4th ed. Oxford: Blackwell; 2007. p. 280–305.
15. Andreasen JO, Andreasen FM, Bakland LK, Flores MT. Crown fracture without pulp exposure. In: Traumatic dental injuries. A manual. Oxford: Blackwell/Munksgaard Publishing Company; 2003. p. 28–9.
16. Robertson A. A retrospective evaluation of patients with uncomplicated crown fractures and luxation injuries. Endod Dent Traumatol. 1998;14:245–56.
17. Cvek M. A clinical report on partial pulpotomy and capping with calcium hydroxide in permanent incisors with complicated crown fracture. J Endod. 1978;4:232–7.
18. Fuks AB, Bielak S, Chosak A. Clinical and radiographic assessment of direct pulp capping and pulpotomy in young permanent teeth. Pediatr Dent. 1982;4:240–4.
19. Fuks AB, Gavra S, Chosack A. Long-term follow up of traumatized incisors treated by partial pulpotomy. Paediatr Dent. 1993;15:334–6.
20. Andreasen JO, Andreasen FM, Bakland LK, Flores MT. Crown fracture with pulp exposure. In: Traumatic dental injuries. A manual. Oxford: Blackwell/Munksgaard Publishing Company; 2003. p. 30–1.
21. Kahnberg K-E. Surgical extrusion of root fractured teeth – a follow-up study of two surgical methods. Endod Dent Traumatol. 1988;4:85–9.
22. Kahnberg K-E, Warfvinge J, Birgersson B. Intraalveolar transplantation (I). The use of autologous bone transplants in the periapical region. Int J Oral Surg. 1982;11:372–9.
23. Kahnberg K-E. Intraalveolar transplantation of teeth with crown-root fractures. J Oral Maxillofac Surg. 1985;43:38–42.
24. Warfvinge J, Kahnberg K-E. Intraalveolar transplantation of teeth. IV. Endodontic considerations. Swed Dent J. 1989;13:229–33.
25. Tegsjö U, Valerius-Olsson H, Olgart K. Intra-alveolar transplantation of teeth with cervical root fractures. Swed Dent J. 1978;2:73–82.
26. Calişkan MK, Türkün M, Gomel M. Surgical extrusion of crown-root-fractured teeth: a clinical review. Int Endod J. 1999;32:146–51.
27. Andreasen JO, Andreasen FM, Bakland LK, Flores MT. Crown-root fracture. In: Traumatic dental injuries. A manual. Oxford: Blackwell/Munksgaard Publishing Company; 2003. p. 32–3.
28. Andreasen JO, Andreasen FM. Crown-root fractures. In: Andreasen JO, Andrasen FM, Andersson L, editors. Textbook and color atlas of traumatic injuries to the teeth. 4th ed. Oxford: Blackwell; 2007. p. 314–66.
29. Majorana A, Pasini S, Bardellini E, Keller E. Clinical and epidemiological study of traumatic root fractures. Dent Traumatol. 2002;18:77–80.
30. Molina JR, Vann WF, McIntrye JD, Trope M, Lee JY. Root fractures in children and adolescents: diagnostic considerations. Dent Traumatol. 2008;24:503–9.
31. Andreasen FM, Andreasen JO, Bayer T. Prognosis of root fractured permanent incisors – prediction of healing modalities. Endod Dent Traumatol. 1989;5:11–22.
32. Andreasen FM, Andreasen JO. Resorption and mineralization processes following root fracture of permanent incisors. Endod Dent Traumatol. 1988;4: 202–14.
33. Andreasen JO, Andreasen FM, Mejàre I, Cvek M. Healing of 400 intra-alveolar root fractures. 1. Effect pre-injury and injury factors such as sex, age, stage of root development, fracture type, location of fracture and severity of dislocation. Dent Traumatol. 2004;20:192–202.
34. Andreasen JO, Andreasen FM, Mèjare I, Cvek M. Healing of 400 intra-alveolar root fractures. 2. Effect of treatment factors such as treatment delay, repositioning, splinting type and period antibiotics. Dent Traumatol. 2004;20:203–11.
35. Cvek M, Tsilingaridis G, Andreasen JO. Survival of 534 incisors after intra-alveolar root fracture in patients aged 7–17 years. Dent Traumatol. 2008;24: 379–87.
36. Andreasen JO, Hjørting-Hansen E. Intraalveolar root fractures: radiographic and histologic study of 50 cases. J Oral Surg. 1967;25:414–26.
37. Cvek M. Treatment of non-vital permanent incisors with calcium hydroxide. IV. Periodontal healing and closure of the root canal in the coronal fragment of teeth with intra-alveolar fracture and vital apical fragment. A follow-up. Odontol Revy. 1974;25:239–46.
38. Cvek M, Andreasen JO, Borum MK. Healing of 208 intraalveolar root fractures in patients aged 7–17 years. Dent Traumatol. 2001;17:53–62.
39. Cvek M, Mejàre I, Andreasen JO. Healing and prognosis of teeth with intra-alveolar fractures involving the cervical part of the root. Dent Traumatol. 2002;18:57–65.
40. Welbury RR, Kinirons MJ, Day P, Humphreys K, Gregg TA. Outcomes for root-fractured permanent incisors: a retrospective study. Pediatr Dent. 2002; 24:98–102.

41. Jacobsen I, Zachrisson BU. Repair characteristics of root fractures in permanent anterior teeth. Scand J Dent Res. 1975;83:355–64.

42. Wölner-Hanssen AB, von Arx T. Permanent teeth with horizontal root fractures after dental trauma. A retrospective study. Schweiz Monatsschr Zahnmed. 2010;120(3):200–12.

43. Andreasen JO, Andreasen FM, Bakland LK, Flores MT. Root fracture. In: Traumatic dental injuries. A manual. Oxford: Blackwell/Munksgaard Publishing Company; 2003. p. 34–5.

44. Andreasen FM, Andreasen JO, Cvek M. Root fractures. In: Andreasen JO, Andreasen FM, Andersson L, editors. Textbook and color atlas of traumatic injuries to the teeth. 4th ed. Oxford: Blackwell; 2007. p. 337–71.

45. Andreasen JO, Ahrensburg SS, Tsilingaridis G. Root fractures: the influence of type of healing and location of fracture on tooth survival rates -an analysis of 492 cases. Dent Traumatol. 2012;28:404–9.

46. Andreasen JO, Ahrensburg SS, Tsilingaridis G. Tooth mobility changes subsequent to root fractures: a longitudinal clinical study of 44 permanent teeth. Dent Traumatol. 2012;28:410–4.

47. Roed-Petersen B, Andreasen JO. Prognosis of permanent teeth involved in jaw fractures. A clinical and radiographic follow-up study. Scand J Dent Res. 1970;78:343–52.

48. Oikarinen K, Lahti J, Raustia AM. Prognosis of permanent teeth in the line of mandibular fractures. Endod Dent Traumatol. 1990;6:177–82.

49. Andreasen JO. Fractures of the alveolar process of the jaw. A clinical and radiographic follow-up study. Scand J Dent Res. 1970;78:263–72.

50. Andreasen JO, Andreasen FM, Bakland LK, Flores MT. Fracture of the alveolar process. In: Traumatic dental injuries. A manual. Oxford: Blackwell/Munksgaard Publishing Company; 2003. p. 36–7.

51. Andreasen JO. Injuries to the supporting bone. In: Andreasen JO, Andreasen FM, Andersson L, editors. Textbook and color atlas of traumatic injuries to the teeth. 4th ed. Oxford: Blackwell; 2007. p. 489–515.

52. Andreasen JO, Jensen SS, Kofod T, Schwartz O, Hillerup S. Open or closed repositioning of mandibular fractures: is there a difference in healing outcome? A systematic review. Dent Traumatol. 2008;24:17–21.

53. Hermund NU, Hillerup S, Kofod T, Schwartz O, Andreasen JO. Effect of early or delayed treatment upon healing of mandibular fractures: a systematic literature review. Dent Traumatol. 2008;24:22–6.

54. Andreasen JO, Jensen SS, Schwartz O, Hillerup S. A systematic review of prophylactic antibiotics in the surgical treatment of maxillofacial fractures. J Oral Maxillofac Surg. 2006;64:1664–8.

55. Bastone EB, Freer TJ, McNamara JR. Epidemiology of dental trauma: a review of the literature. Aust Dent J. 2000;45:2–9.

56. Miyashin M, Kato J, Takagi Y. Experimental luxation injuries in immature rat teeth. Endod Dent Traumatol. 1990;6:121–8.

57. Andreasen JO, Andreasen FM, Bakland LK, Flores MT. Concussion. In: Traumatic dental injuries. A manual. Oxford: Blackwell/Munksgaard Publishing Company; 2003. p. 38–9.

58. Andreasen FM, Andreasen JO. Concussion and subluxation. In: Andreasen JO, Andreasen FM, Andersson L, editors. Textbook and color atlas of traumatic injuries to the teeth. 4th ed. Oxford: Blackwell; 2007. p. 404–10.

59. Hermann NV, Lauridsen E, Ahrensburg SS, Gerds TA, Andreasen JO. Periodontal healing complications following concussion and subluxation injuries in the permanent dentition. A longitudinal cohort study. Dent Traumatol. 2012;28:386–93.

60. Andreasen FM. Transient apical breakdown and its relation to color and sensibility changes after luxation injuries to teeth. Endod Dent Traumatol. 1986;2:9–19.

61. Andreasen FM, Zhijie Y, Thomsen BL, Anderson PK. Occurrence of pulp canal obliteration after luxation in the permanent dentition. Endod Dent Traumatol. 1987;3:103–15.

62. Andreasen JO, Andreasen FM, Bakland LK, Flores MT. Extrusive luxation. In: Traumatic dental injuries. A manual. Oxford: Blackwell/Munksgaard Publishing Company; 2003. p. 42–3.

63. Andreasen FM, Andreasen JO. Extrusive luxation and lateral luxation. In: Andreasen JO, Andreasen FM, Andersson L, editors. Textbook and color atlas of traumatic injuries to the teeth. 4th ed. Oxford: Blackwell; 2007. p. 411–27.

64. Hermann NV, Lauridsen E, Ahrensburg SS, Gerds TA, Andreasen JO. Periodontal healing complications following extrusive and lateral luxation in the permanent dentition. A longitudinal cohort study. Dent Traumatol. 2012;28:394–402.

65. Elena C, Ferrazzini P, von Arx T. Pulp and periodontal healing of laterally luxated permanent teeth: results after 4 years. Dent Traumatol. 2008;24:658–62.

66. Andreasen JO, Andreasen FM, Bakland LK, Flores MT. Lateral luxation. In: Traumatic dental injuries. A manual. Oxford: Blackwell/Munksgaard Publishing Company; 2003. p. 44–5.

67. Andreasen JO, Bakland LK, Matras R, Andreasen FM. Traumatic intrusion of permanent teeth. Part 1. An epidemiological study of 216 intruded permanent teeth. Dent Traumatol. 2006;22:83–9.

68. Andreasen JO, Bakland LK, Matras R, Andreasen FM. Traumatic intrusion of permanent teeth. Part 2. A clinical study of the effect of preinjury and injury factors, (such as sex, age, stage of root development, tooth location, and extent of injury including number of intruded teeth) on 140 intruded permanent teeth. Dent Traumatol. 2006;22:90–8.

69. Andreasen JO, Bakland LK, Matras R, Andreasen FM. Traumatic intrusion of permanent teeth. Part 3.

A clinical study of the effect of treatment variables such as treatment delay, method of repositioning, type of splint, length of splinting and antibiotics on 140 teeth. Dent Traumatol. 2006;22:99–111.

70. Al-Badri S, Kinirons M, Cole BOI, Welbury RR. Factors affecting resorption in traumatically intruded permanent incisors in children. Dent Traumatol. 2002;18:73–6.

71. Chaushu S, Shapiro J, Heling J, Becker A. Emergency orthodontic treatment after the traumatic intrusive luxation of maxillary incisors. Am J Orthod Dentofacial Orthop. 2004;126:162–72.

72. Andreasen JO, Andreasen FM, Bakland LK, Flores MT. Intrusive luxation. In: Traumatic dental injuries. A manual. Oxford: Blackwell/Munksgaard Publishing Company; 2003. p. 46–7.

73. Andreasen FM, Andreasen JO. Intrusive luxation and lateral luxation. In: Andreasen JO, Andreasen FM, Andersson L, editors. Textbook and color atlas of traumatic injuries to the teeth. 4th ed. Oxford: Blackwell; 2007. p. 428–43.

74. Andreasen JO, Borum MK, Jacobsen HL, Andreasen FM. Replantation of 400 avulsed permanent incisors. I. Diagnosis of healing complications. Endod Dent Traumatol. 1995;11:51–8.

75. Andreasen JO, Borum MK, Jacobsen HL, Andreasen FM. Replantation of 400 avulsed permanent incisors. II. Factors related to pulp healing. Endod Dent Traumatol. 1995;11:59–68.

76. Andreasen JO, Borum MK, Jacobsen HL, Andreasen FM. Replantation of 400 avulsed permanent incisors. III. Factors related to root growth after replantation. Endod Dent Traumatol. 1995;11:69–75.

77. Andreasen JO, Borum MK, Jacobsen HL, Andreasen FM. Replantation of 400 avulsed permanent incisors. IV. Factors related to periodontal ligament healing. Endod Dent Traumatol. 1995;11:76–89.

78. Andreasen JO. Periodontal healing after replantation of traumatically avulsed human teeth. Assessment by mobility testing and radiography. Acta Odontol Scand. 1975;33:325–35.

79. Cvek M, Granath LE, Hollender L. Treatment of non-vital permanent incisors with calcium hydroxide. III. Variation of occurrence of ankylosis of reimplanted teeth with duration of extra-alveolar period and storage environment. Odontol Revy. 1974; 25:43–56.

80. Hammarström L, Blomlöf L, Feiglin B, Andersson L, Lindskog S. Replantation of teeth and antibiotic treatment. Endod Dent Traumatol. 1986;2:51–7.

81. Kling M, Cvek M, Mejare I. Rate and predictability of pulp revascularization in therapeutically reimplanted permanent incisors. Endod Dent Traumatol. 1986;2:83–9.

82. Pierce A, Lindskog S. The effect of an antibiotic/corticosteroid paste on inflammatory root resorption in vivo. Oral Surg Oral Med Oral Pathol. 1987;64: 216–20.

83. Trope M, Friedman S. Periodontal healing of replanted dog teeth stored in Viaspan, milk and Hank's balanced salt solution. Endod Dent Traumatol. 1992;8:183–8.

84. Bryson EC, Levin L, Banchs F, Abbott PV, Trope M. Effect of immediate intracanal placement of Ledermix Paste® on healing of replanted dog teeth after extended dry times. Dent Traumatol. 2002;18:316–21.

85. Chen H, Teixeira FB, Ritter AL, Levin L, Trope M. The effect of intracanal anti-inflammatory medicaments on external root resorption of replanted dog teeth after extended extra-oral dry time. Dent Traumatol. 2008;24:74–8.

86. Pohl Y, Filippi A, Kirschner H. Results after replantation of avulsed permanent teeth. I. Endodontic considerations. Dent Traumatol. 2005;21:80–92.

87. Pohl Y, Filippi A, Kirschner H. Results after replantation of avulsed permanent teeth. II. Periodontal healing and the role of physiologic storage and anti-resorptive-regenerative therapy. Dent Traumatol. 2005;21:93–101.

88. Pohl Y, Filippi A, Kirschner H. Results after replantation of avulsed permanent teeth. III. Tooth loss and survival analysis. Dent Traumatol. 2005;21:102–10.

89. Andreasen JO, Andreasen FM, Bakland LK, Flores MT. Avulsion. In: Traumatic dental injuries. A manual. Oxford: Blackwell/Munksgaard Publishing Company; 2003. p. 48–51.

90. Andreasen FM, Andreasen JO. Avulsions. In: Andreasen JO, Andreasen FM, Andersson L, editors. Textbook and color atlas of traumatic injuries to the teeth. 4th ed. Oxford: Blackwell; 2007. p. 444–88.

91. Andreasen FM, Pedersen BV. Prognosis of luxated permanent teeth – the development of pulp necrosis. Endod Dent Traumatol. 1985;1:207–20.

92. Oikarinen K, Gundlach KK, Pfeifer G. Late complications of luxation injuries to teeth. Endod Dent Traumatol. 1987;3:296–303.

93. Andreasen FM, Zhjie Y, Thomsen BL, Andersen PK. Occurrence of pulp canal obliteration after luxation injuries in the permanent dentition. Endod Dental Traumatol. 1987;3(3):103–15.

94. McCabe PS, Dummer PMH. Pulp canal obliteration: an endodontic diagnosis and treatment challenge. Int Endod J. 2012;45(2):177–97.

95. Trope M. Root resorption due to dental trauma. Endod Top. 2002;1(2):79–100.

96. Fuss Z, Tsesis I, Lin S. Root resorption–diagnosis, classification and treatment choices based on stimulation factors. Dent Traumatol. 2003;19(4): 175–82.

97. International Association of Dental Traumatology. URL: http://www.iadt-dentaltrauma.org. Accessed June 2013.

98. Cohenca M, Simon JH, Roges R, Moragy Y, Malfax JM. Clinical indications for digital imaging in dento-alveolar trauma. Part 1: traumatic injuries. Dent Traumatol. 2007;23:95–104.

99. Cohenca M, Simon JH, Roges R, Moragy Y, Malfax JM. Clinical indications for digital imaging in dento-alveolar trauma. Part 2: root resorption. Dent Traumatol. 2007;23(2):105–13.

100. Kahler B, Hithersay GS. An evidence-based appraisal of splinting luxated, avulsed and root fractured teeth, a systematic review. Dent Traumatol. 2008;241:2–10.
101. Hinckfuss S, Messer LB. Splinting duration and periodontal outcome of replanted avulsed teeth, a systematic review. Dent Traumatol. 2009;25(2):150–7.
102. Oikarinen K. Tooth splinting – a review of the literature and consideration of the versatility of a wire-composite splint. Endod Dent Traumatol. 1990;6(6):237–50.
103. Mohammadi Z, Abbott PV. On the local applications of antibiotics and antibiotic-based agents in endodontics and dental traumatology. Int Endod J. 2009;42(7):555–67.
104. Hinckfuss SE, Messer LB. An evidence-based assessment of the clinical guidelines for replanted avulsed teeth. Part II: prescription of systemic antibiotics. Dent Traumatol. 2009;25(2):158–64.
105. Peterson K, Söderström C, Kiani-Anaraki M, Levy G. Evaluation of the ability of thermal and electrical tests to register pulp vitality. Dent Traumatol. 1999;15(3):127–31.
106. Patel B. Clinical examination and Diagnosis. In: Mastering endodontics. Diagnosis, pathology & treatment planning. Springer: Cham; 2015
107. Bakland LK, Andreasen JO. Biological considerations in the management of traumatic dental injuries. Endod Top. 2014;30:44–50.

Root Resorption

Bobby Patel

Summary

A correct diagnosis and an understanding of the underlying aetiology and processes involved in root resorption are essential for both effective management and appropriate treatment strategies. Tooth resorption can be broadly classified according to physiological or pathological processes as either internal or external. Resorption may be further categorized as due to either trauma, infection or hyperplastic invasive causes. The stimulus for internal resorption and external peri-radicular inflammatory resorption is intra-pulpal infection. Non-surgical root canal treatment will aim to eliminate intra-pulpal bacteria and arrest the resorptive process. Root resorption related to pressure such as orthodontic tooth movement, impacted teeth or tumours can be arrested by removal of the pressure stimulus. In external cervical root resorption infection originates from the periodontal sulcus, which provides the stimulus for continued tooth resorption. Removal of the granulation tissue and adequate sealing are prerequisites for repair. External replacement resorption is a direct consequence of irreversible periodontal ligament cell damage often seen in severe tooth trauma or non-physiological extra-oral storage of an avulsed tooth. Ankylosis and replacement resorption will ensue with normal remodelling of the surrounding bone and tooth structure resulting in the eventual demise.

Clinical Relevance

Effective management of resorption requires a thorough understanding of the underlying cause including early recognition of the process and optimal treatment modalities that can be applied to ensure the elimination and prevention of such processes. Some transient trauma-induced resorptions require no treatment but careful monitoring. Trauma-induced resorption and invasive cervical tooth resorptions pose a unique set of challenges that may require specialist referral to ensure correct management. Occasionally, a multidisciplinary approach may be required with

B. Patel, BDS MFDS MClinDent MRD MRACDS
Specialist Endodontist, Brindabella Specialist Centre,
Canberra, ACT, Australia
e-mail: bobbypatel@me.com

© Springer International Publishing Switzerland 2016
B. Patel (ed.), *Endodontic Treatment, Retreatment, and Surgery*,
DOI 10.1007/978-3-319-19476-9_16

particular attention to replacement resorption and the eventual demise of the tooth requiring prosthodontic replacement.

16.1 Overview of Tooth Resorption

Resorption can be a physiological or pathological process, resulting in loss of dentine, cementum or bone through the continued action of osteoclastic cells. Under normal physiological processes, resorption may occur in the deciduous/mixed dentition resulting in the exfoliation of the primary teeth. In the adult dentition, resorption is predominantly pathological due to inflammation occurring subsequent to traumatic dental injuries, orthodontic treatment, periodontal treatment, bleaching procedures and chronic infections of the pulp [1].

In normal circumstances, the mineralized tissues of permanent teeth are resistant to resorption. The pre-cementum and periodontal ligament and predentine act as barriers to external and internal root resorption preventing binding of clastic cells. It has been postulated that anti-invasion factors in the periodontal tissues play a role in maintaining the integrity of the root. In cases where injury is to occur to these protective layers, osteoclastic binding can occur unimpeded, and in situations where inflammation persists, tooth resorption can ensue resulting in premature loss of the tooth without subsequent intervention [2–4].

Tooth resorption can be classified according to site, aetiology and type of resorptive process. A distinction is generally made between internal and external resorptions. External resorption can be further subdivided into external surface resorption, invasive cervical root resorption, inflammatory root resorption, ankylosis, replacement resorption and transient apical breakdown (Figs. 16.1 and 16.2) [1–3, 5–10].

Internal root resorption is usually asymptomatic and identified by chance on routine radiographic examination. If left untreated, it can result in the progressive destruction of intra-radicular dentine and dentinal tubules along the middle and apical thirds of the canal walls as a result of clastic activities. In the initial stages, this resorption defect is the result of inflamed necrotic coronal pulp tissue with the recruitment of clastic precursor cells through vital blood vessels usually present more apically. Treatment is aimed at severing the blood supply to the resorbing tissues by means of conventional root canal treatment. Extensive resorption can eventually lead to root perforation resulting in the formation of a sinus tract. Such lesions will result in extensive tooth loss and weakened tooth structure resulting in a poorer prognosis that may or may not be amenable to treatment. Radiographically, internal root resorption appears as a 'ballooning out' of the root canal. The resorption lesion is an oval or round radiolucency with smooth, well-defined margins that does not change position relative to the root canal when using parallax radiographs [11–13].

Transient apical breakdown can develop as a result of certain traumatic injuries to teeth and their supporting structures. Moderate injuries to the pulp including subluxation, extrusion, lateral luxation, orthodontic treatment and occlusal trauma can result in either a spontaneous periapical radiolucency or persistent progressive expansion of the periodontal ligament space over an extended period of time. In such cases, the injured tissue undergoes a spontaneous process of repair, usually returning to normal within 1 year. Therefore, no endodontic treatment is necessary [14, 15].

External surface resorption is a transient situation in which the root surface undergoes spontaneous destruction and repair as a direct consequence of localized and limited injury to the root surface or surrounding periodontium. Since the process is self-limiting, no treatment

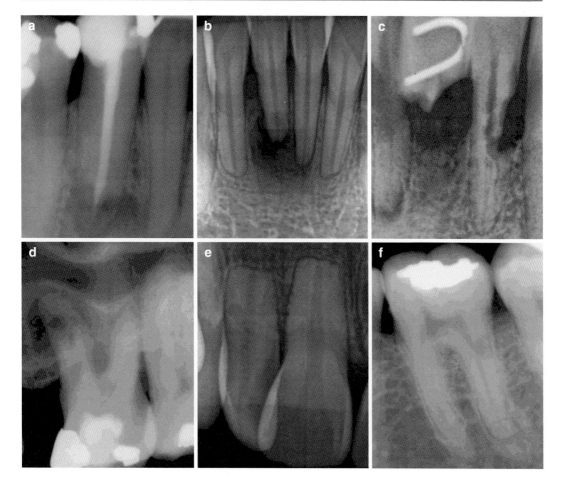

Fig. 16.1 Clinical radiographs demonstrating (**a**, **b**) external inflammatory root resorption associated with apical pathosis, (**c**) external replacement resorption, (**d**) internal root resorption, (**e**) orthodontic pressure root resorption, and (**f**) external invasive cervical root resorption

intervention is required with resultant superficial resorptive cavities healing with new cementum within 2–3 weeks or in cases of dentine involvement partial restoration of the root surface [2, 10, 16].

External inflammatory root resorption commonly occurs following traumatic injury to the tooth or following the application of pressure due to iatrogenic orthodontic stimulus or pathophysiological stimulus of impacted teeth or tumours. The resultant damage to the periodontal ligament cells on the root surface results in a denuded root surface, whereby loss of cementum allows direct communication with the internal root canal system and external root surface. A necrotic, infected pulp, bacteria and their by-products can then provide the continued stimulus leading to extensive and progressive resorption of the root surface [9, 16].

External invasive cervical root resorption is a relatively uncommon phenomenon whose true aetiology remains obscure and can potentially result in an often destructive and aggressive condition in any permanent tooth. Potential

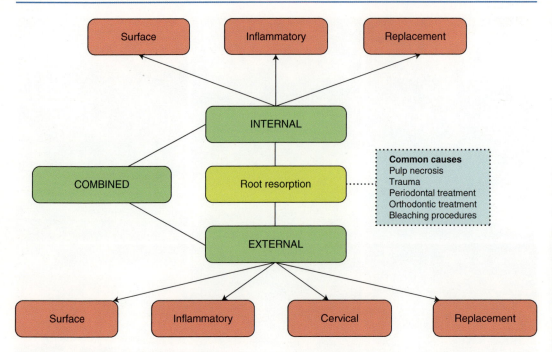

Fig. 16.2 Schematic classification of internal and external root resorption (based on classification proposed by Andreasen)

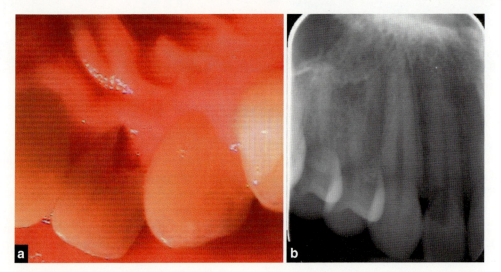

Fig. 16.3 (**a**) Clinical photograph and (**b**) radiograph showing extensive cervical root resorption affecting tooth 12. The patient reported a history of orthodontic treatment previously and possible trauma. (**c–f**) Clinical radiograph, photograph, CBCT scan, and maxillary reconstruction demonstrating external cervical root resorption affecting the labial aspect of tooth 12. This sixteen-year-old patient underwent fixed orthodontic appliance therapy. Following completion of orthodontic treatment and debanding, a pink spot lesion was noted with tooth 12. A parallel periapical radiograph confirmed an irregular lucency in the cervical aspect of tooth 12. CBCT scan confirmed a Heithersay class II/III lesion requiring nonsurgical root canal therapy combined with a surgical approach treating the lesion with 90 % TCA (trichloroacetic acid solution) and repair with glass ionomer cement

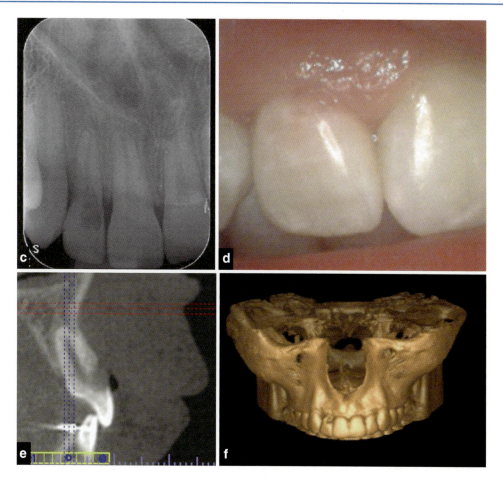

Fig. 16.3 (continued)

predisposing factors cited as causes include dental trauma, orthodontic treatment, intracoronal bleaching, periodontal therapy and idiopathic origin. The resorptive process is characterized by invasion of the cervical region of the tooth by fibrovascular tissue derived from the periodontal ligament, which will eventually invade the pulp space resulting in extensive destruction of sound tooth structure (see Fig. 16.3). The pulp survives and withstands invasion until late due to inherent protection provided by predentine and odontoblasts making early diagnosis difficult unless there are chances of radiographic findings. Treatment, where indicated, is aimed at inactivation of all resorbing tissue and the reconstitution of the resorptive defect either by placement of a suitable filling material or by the use of biological systems. The radiographic appearance of external cervical root resorption depends on the severity of the lesion. Early lesions may appear as poorly defined borders of mixed radiolucency in the cervical region of the tooth.

The root canal walls should be visible and running vertically through the radiolucent defect, indicating that the lesion lies on the external surface of the root.

The parallax technique may be helpful to detect and determine the location (palatal or labial) of the external cervical root resorption lesions [17–22].

Ankylosis and replacement resorption are commonly seen in teeth associated with luxation injuries and in particular avulsed teeth with an extended extra-oral dry time. Cementum and root dentine are resorbed by osteoclasts with subsequent replacement by alveolar bone deposited by osteoblasts. These teeth are lost usually 3–7 years after initiation of the root resorption process [23–25].

Timely intervention is essential for optimal management of dental resorption based on appropriate diagnosis from both clinical and radiographic findings. Intraoral radiographs do not provide an indication of the true three-dimensional lesion size with potential for underestimation of true extent and risks associated with management thereof. Cone beam computed tomography (CBCT) technology has been specifically designed to produce three-dimensional scans of the maxillofacial skeleton and has been successfully used to evaluate the true nature and severity of resorption lesions in the endodontic literature.

Effective management and treatment strategies must be applied according to the type of resorptive process responsible and dependent on lesion size, site and nature. Non-surgical and/or surgical treatment modalities must be weighed up against alternative approaches including extraction for teeth deemed to have poor prognoses (see Figs. 16.3, 16.4 and 16.5) [15, 20, 26, 27].

16.2 Internal Inflammatory Root Resorption

For internal root resorption to occur, the outermost protective odontoblast layer and predentine of the canal wall must be damaged, resulting in exposure of the underlying mineralized dentine to odontoclasts. Pulp canal necrosis and infection provide the inflammatory stimulus to sustain the process. Various aetiologies including dental trauma, caries, excessive heat generation during restorative procedures, use of cytotoxic materials

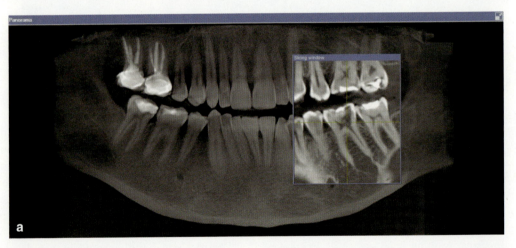

Fig. 16.4 Cone beam CT scans demonstrating external cervical root resorption in tooth 36. Note: (**a**) panoramic, (**b**) axial, and (**c**) cross-sectional views. Intraoral radiographs do not indicate the true dimensions of the lesion. The resorptive defect may spread within the tooth in all directions, and this may not be reflected in either the size or position of the radiolucency seen on standard radiographs. The recent advent of three-dimensional imaging has provided the endodontist with previously unavailable tools providing greater geometric accuracy in diagnosing and managing resorptive lesions. This case demonstrates how the CBCT scan allowed determination of the nature and extent of the resorptive lesion and confirmation that nonsurgical management would suffice

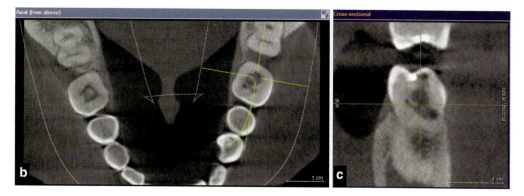

Fig. 16.4 (continued)

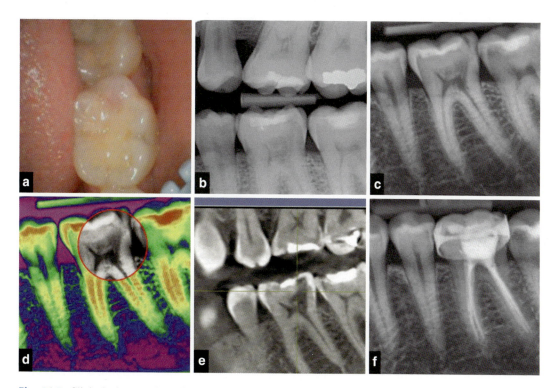

Fig. 16.5 Clinical photograph, radiographs, and cone beam CT scans showing management of external cervical root resorption in tooth 36. Note: (**a**) clinical intraoral photograph showing "pink spot" visible beneath the crown distally. (**b–d**) Conventional digital radiography showing irregular radiolucent lesion in cervical aspect of tooth. Cervical resorption lesion (*red circle*). (**e**) Cone beam CT scan of tooth 36. (**f**) Completed nonsurgical root canal treatment and treatment of the resorptive lesion using TCA

in vital teeth such as calcium hydroxide pulpotomies and orthodontic tooth movements have been cited in the literature as potentially responsible for potential damage to the internal canal wall. The process has been described as either transient or progressive.

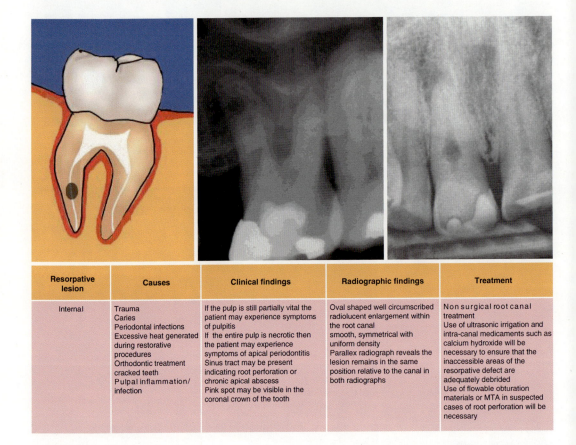

Resorpative lesion	Causes	Clinical findings	Radiographic findings	Treatment
Internal	Trauma Caries Periodontal infections Excessive heat generated during restorative procedures Orthodontic treatment cracked teeth Pulpal inflammation/ infection	If the pulp is still partially vital the patient may experience symptoms of pulpitis If the entire pulp is necrotic then the patient may experience symptoms of apical periodontitis Sinus tract may be present indicating root perforation or chronic apical abscess Pink spot may be visible in the coronal crown of the tooth	Oval shaped well circumscribed radiolucent enlargement within the root canal smooth, symmetrical with uniform density Parallex radiograph reveals the lesion remains in the same position relative to the canal in both radiographs	Non surgical root canal treatment Use of ultrasonic irrigation and intra-canal medicaments such as calcium hydroxide will be necessary to ensure that the inaccessible areas of the resorpative defect are adequately debrided Use of flowable obturation materials or MTA in suspected cases of root perforation will be necessary

Clinically, the early stages of internal resorption are usually asymptomatic. Partial pulp necrosis may result in signs and symptoms of pulpitis. Eventually, when the entire root canal system becomes necrotic, the patient may develop apical periodontitis and symptoms thereof. Sinus tracts may be present indicating either root perforation or chronic apical abscess. A pink discolouration may be visible within the crown of the tooth although this 'pink spot' may be pathognomonic of external invasive cervical root resorption. The radiographic appearance is that of an oval or circular well-circumscribed symmetrical radiolucency associated with the root canal. The radiolucency has a uniform density and will remain in the same position relative to the canal when using the parallax radiographic technique (Fig. 16.6).

Once internal root resorption has been diagnosed, the prognosis of the tooth is dependent on whether the lesion communicates with the external surface of the root making non-surgical root canal treatment difficult due to risk of extrusion through the perforation between internal and external root surfaces. Non-surgical root canal treatment is recommended in cases where the lesion is confined within the canal, without breaching the external root surface, and where the tooth is deemed restorable.

Root canal systems have complex morphology that can harbour bacteria, by-products and remnants of necrotic pulp tissue in nonvital teeth. Teeth with internal root resorption pose a unique challenge as a result of actively resorbing balloon-sized lesions that contain inflamed bleeding pulpal and granulation tissues that are inaccessible

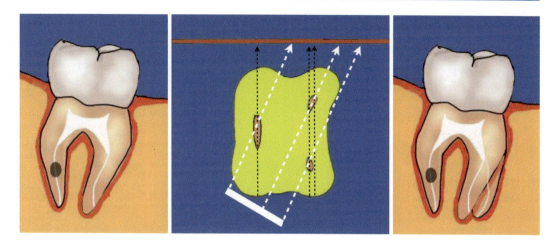

Fig. 16.6 Clinical diagrams demonstrating the parallax radiographic technique used to determine whether the resorptive lesion is internal or external. A second radiograph taken at a different angle often confirms the nature of the resorptive defect. Both external root resorption and external invasive cervical root resorption will move in the same direction as the X-ray tube shift if they are lingually/palatally positioned. They will move in the opposite direction to the tube shift if they are buccally positioned. Internal resorptive lesions on the other hand should remain in the same position relative to the canal in both radiographs

to direct mechanical instrumentation techniques. As a result, adjunctive use of ultrasonic instrumentation and intra-canal antibacterial medicaments should be used to improve disinfection and debridement of the internal resorptive defects. Thermoplastic gutta-percha techniques are ideal when used to seal and fill the resorptive defect provided the root canal wall has not been perforated. In cases of perforation, an alternative technique using mineral trioxide aggregate may need to be utilized due to enhanced biocompatibility important at the restorative-tooth interface (Fig. 16.7).

16.3 Surface Resorption

This type of self-limiting resorption is transient and is often induced following some traumatic injuries or orthodontic treatment. It results in damage to the underlying cementum with shallow resorption of the root contour with involvement of a small amount of underlying dentine that will heal uneventfully with reparative cementum in the absence of underlying infection. Radiographic observations may reveal only subtle changes in the root morphology with no signs of any radiolucency associated with superimposed infections. The lamina dura and periodontal membrane remain intact.

16.4 Pressure Resorption

This type of resorption is commonly induced by the pressure of a crypt of an underlying unerupted/erupting tooth, by some neoplasms and more commonly due to orthodontic treatment. The resorption is often extensive and easily observable radiographically.

Tumours such as cysts, ameloblastomas, giant cell tumours and fibro-osseous lesions are frequently associated with slow growth and expansion whereby the underlying pathological process is responsible for activation of the resorptive process. Usually, the tooth will remain asymptomatic unless the process is close to the apical foramen with the possibility of disturbing the blood supply. Treatment strategies are aimed at removing the underlying cause usually by surgical means, which remove the pressure and arrest the process.

Apical root resorption during tooth movement can result in significant shortening of the roots directly due to continued pressure during orthodontic tooth movements. Teeth will remain

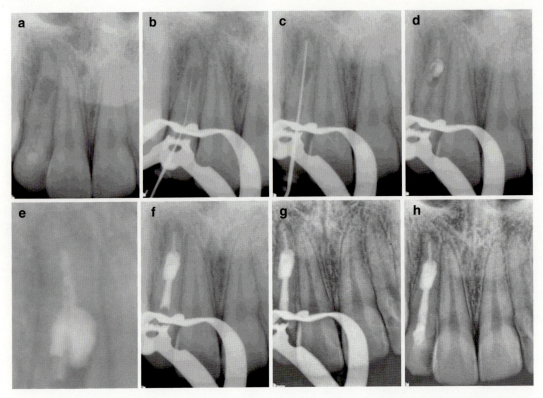

Fig. 16.7 Clinical radiographs demonstrating management of internal root resorption associated with tooth 12. Note: (**a**) preoperative radiograph demonstrating internal well-circumscribed radiolucency associated with the apical 1/3 of the root. (**b**, **c**) IAF and MAF files confirming working lengths. Following chemo-mechanical debridement, use of sodium hypochlorite solution, and adjunctive ultrasonic agitation, a calcium hydroxide dressing was placed for a further two weeks. At the obturation appointment, the patient remained asymptomatic. (**d**) Cold lateral compaction with gutta-percha and AH plus cement was used in the apical 1/3 followed by warm vertical condensation using System B. Note partial filling of the resorptive lesion (**e**). (**f**, **g**) The remainder of the canal was filled using Obtura. (**h**) A temporary coronal restoration of IRM and glass ionomer cement was placed to ensure adequate seal prior to permanent restoration with the corresponding general dental practitioner

asymptomatic, and provided the underlying forces used to tooth movement are not heavy, the pulp remains vital. No treatment is required, and provided the underlying cause is removed, this non-infective resorption will become inactive and uncomplicated repair can occur.

16.5 External Inflammatory Root Resorption

This type of external root resorption is often seen radiographically as an extensive peri-radicular radiolucency associated with an extensive inflammatory response to endodontic pathosis. It is also indicative of an infection superimposed on a traumatic injury commonly seen in both avulsion and luxation injuries. The initiating stimulus for this type of resorption is damage to the underlying protective cementum resulting in surface resorption and exposure of the adjacent dentine with direct communication with the root canal system. Superimposed infection as a result of pulpal necrosis prevents normal reparative cementum to be replaced sustaining the resorptive process due to unimpeded passage of bacteria and bacterial by-products from within the tooth. An inflammatory response persists including the activation of clastic cells resulting in both tooth and bone resorption.

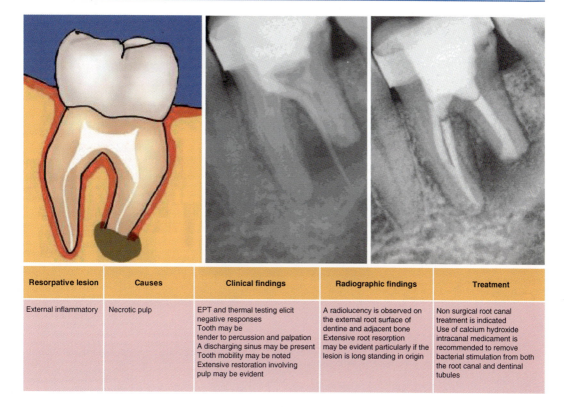

Resorpative lesion	Causes	Clinical findings	Radiographic findings	Treatment
External inflammatory	Necrotic pulp	EPT and thermal testing elicit negative responses Tooth may be tender to percussion and palpation A discharging sinus may be present Tooth mobility may be noted Extensive restoration involving pulp may be evident	A radiolucency is observed on the external root surface of dentine and adjacent bone Extensive root resorption may be evident particularly if the lesion is long standing in origin	Non surgical root canal treatment is indicated Use of calcium hydroxide intracanal medicament is recommended to remove bacterial stimulation from both the root canal and dentinal tubules

Clinical examination may reveal no abnormalities unless the infection is acute in nature demonstrated by the tooth becoming tender to touch or an overlying swelling or discharging sinus. Radiographic examination may result in bowl-like radiolucencies in both the tooth and adjacent bone that if allowed to progress will result in eventual destruction and replacement. Treatment strategies to halt progression of this type of resorption include provision of effective non-surgical root canal treatment including chemo-mechanical preparation to remove irritants from within the root canal system. Smear layer removal including the sequential use of 17 % EDTA, 1 % sodium hypochlorite and a final rinse with EDTA has been shown to be an effective treatment modality to ensure diffusion of intra-canal medicaments such as Ledermix paste through the dentine to the external surface of the tooth. The corticosteroid and antibacterial components of Ledermix have been shown to exert beneficial effects on clastic cells responsible for the resorptive processes that occur. Following initial use of this anticlastic agent, conventional calcium hydroxide medicament can be placed to influence hard tissue deposition on the resorbed tooth surface prior to completion of endodontic treatment.

16.6 Ankylosis and Replacement Resorption

Progressive replacement of tooth structure by alveolar bone can ultimately result in tooth loss. This type of process follows the death of viable periodontal ligament cells due to either severe compression or drying of the cells usually seen in severe traumatic injuries such as luxation, intrusion and avulsion. An interface devoid of viable periodontal ligament cells between bone and dentine results in normal remodelling processes associated with skeletal bone turnover at the expense of dentine. Ankylosis occurs with total loss of mobility with a characteristic high-pitched metallic percussion sound. At this stage, there is no loss of root dentine or cementum. Eventually progressive replacement of tooth structure by surrounding bone occurs resulting in the eventual demise of the tooth.

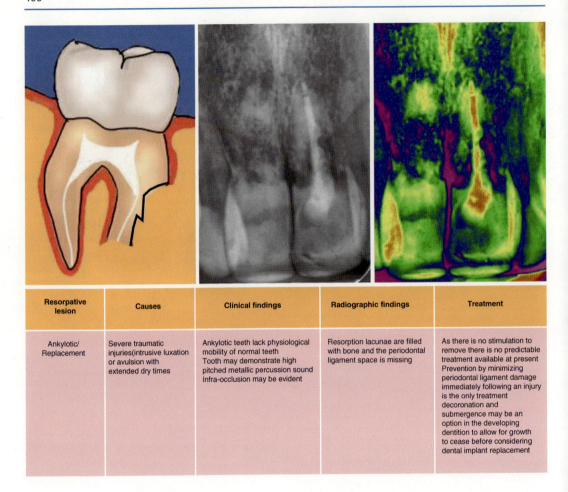

Resorpative lesion	Causes	Clinical findings	Radiographic findings	Treatment
Ankylotic/ Replacement	Severe traumatic injuries(intrusive luxation or avulsion with extended dry times	Ankylotic teeth lack physiological mobility of normal teeth Tooth may demonstrate high pitched metallic percussion sound Infra-occlusion may be evident	Resorption lacunae are filled with bone and the periodontal ligament space is missing	As there is no stimulation to remove there is no predictable treatment available at present Prevention by minimizing periodontal ligament damage immediately following an injury is the only treatment decoronation and submergence may be an option in the developing dentition to allow for growth to cease before considering dental implant replacement

From a clinical management point of view, the replacement resorption process usually proceeds at a slow rate and in some cases taking years to reach a stage where intervention is required. In the mature dentition, alternative prosthodontic replacement options will need to be considered. In the developing dentition, ankylosis can severely disrupt arch integrity with infra-occlusion of the ankylosed tooth that becomes more obvious as skeletal growth continues. In cases of ankylosis with advanced replacement resorption, the procedure of decoronation and submergence has been recommended to allow for continued alveolar growth and uncomplicated transition to implant therapy once growth has stopped.

16.7 Invasive External Cervical Root Resorption

Progressive external resorption with persistent inflammation may be localized at the cervical level whereby resorbing tissues invade the hard tissues of the tooth in an uncontrolled destructive fashion. Numerous terms have been used to describe these phenomena including odontoclastoma, peripheral cervical resorption, extracanal invasive resorption, peripheral inflammatory root resorption and sub-epithelial external root resorption. Hiethersay who preferred the term invasive cervical root resorption, which is both invasive and aggressive, has described this form of external root resorption at length. In the absence of treatment, this type of resorption leads to progressive and destructive replacement of tooth structure. Resorption of coronal dentine and enamel often creates a clinically obvious pinkish colour in the crown of the tooth as highly vascular resorptive tissue becomes visible through the underlying thin residual dentine. Exploration with a probe may reveal a sub-gingival, supra-crestal non-carious cavity. In other instances, it may only become obvious as an incidental finding following routine radiographic examinations. The pulp remains vital in most cases with symptoms of pulpitis developing on the late stages of the disease where severe progression and advancement of the resorptive process have occurred. Several potential predisposing factors have been identified including dental trauma, orthodontic treatment, intracoronal bleaching, periodontal therapy and idiopathic aetiology. Total removal or inactivation of the resorptive tissue is essential to safeguard against reoccurrence. The high predisposition for reoccurrence is due to the invasive nature of the resorptive tissue responsible whereby small infiltrative channels are often created within the underlying dentine, which may interconnect with the surrounding periodontal ligament in positions more apical to the main resorptive defect. Unless all the tissue is inactivated, the possibility of progression remains.

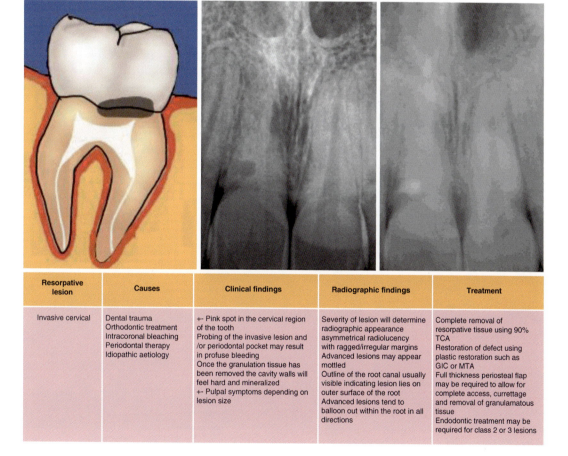

Resorptive lesion	Causes	Clinical findings	Radiographic findings	Treatment
Invasive cervical	Dental trauma Orthodontic treatment Intracoronal bleaching Periodontal therapy Idiopathic aetiology	+- Pink spot in the cervical region of the tooth Probing of the invasive lesion and /or periodontal pocket may result in profuse bleeding Once the granulation tissue has been removed the cavity walls will feel hard and mineralized +- Pulpal symptoms depending on lesion size	Severity of lesion will determine radiographic appearance asymmetrical radiolucency with ragged/irregular margins Advanced lesions may appear mottled Outline of the root canal usually visible indicating lesion lies on outer surface of the root Advanced lesions tend to balloon out within the root in all directions	Complete removal of resorpative tissue using 90% TCA Restoration of defect using plastic restoration such as GIC or MTA Full thickness periosteal flap may be required to allow for complete access, currettage and removal of granulamatous tissue Endodontic treatment may be required for class 2 or 3 lesions

Management and prognosis vary according to the extent and severity of the lesion, location and accessibility, whether there is concomitant pulpal involvement and overall restorability of the tooth in question. Hiethersay has classified invasive cervical root resorption according to the extent of the lesion within the tooth. Class I lesions are small resorptive lesions near the cervical aspect of the tooth with only a shallow penetration into the dentine. Class 2 lesions represent a well-defined invasive resorptive lesion that has penetrated close to the coronal pulp chamber but shows little or no extension into the underlying radicular dentine. Class 3 lesions represent deeper invasion of the dentine extending into the coronal third of the root. Class 4 lesions are extensive large invasive resorption defects that have extended beyond the coronal third of the root canal. Careful case selection is important and only classes 1–3 are amenable to treatment. Class 4 lesions should be left untreated provided they remain asymptomatic; otherwise, extraction is the only viable option.

Treatment should involve surgical exposure of the lesion and curettage of the inflammatory tissue followed by placement of an adequate seal by utilizing restorative materials such as glass ionomer cement. Occasionally, non-surgical access may be possible although this increases the risk of failure due to the nature and position of the resorptive tissues involved. Both non-surgical and surgical treatment strategies should be directed at removal of all resorptive tissue facilitated by using topical application of 90 % trichloroacetic acid (TCA) solution. The effect of TCA is to cause coagulation necrosis rendering the resorptive tissue avascular reducing the potential for reoccurrence. Pulpal exposure following curettage of resorptive tissue requires additional non-surgical root canal therapy.

Surgical management involves periodontal flap reflection, curettage and restoration of the defect. Periodontal reattachment may not be expected with glass ionomer cement, and there is some evidence to suggest the use of ProRoot MTA might be more beneficial in such cases.

The patient should be re-examined at regular intervals with careful clinical and radiographic assessments to determine whether the process has been arrested (Fig. 16.8).

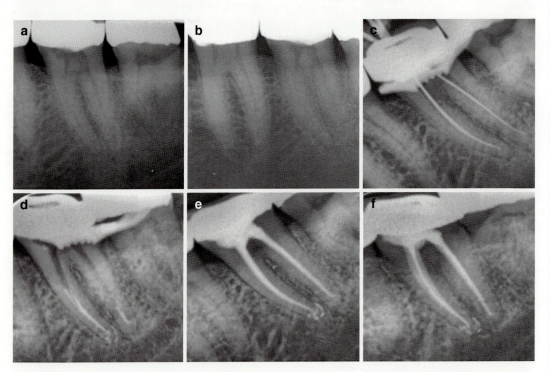

Fig. 16.8 (**a**) and (**b**) Clinical radiographs demonstrating external cervical root resorption associated with tooth 46. The patient was experiencing symptoms of pulpitis suggesting pulpal involvement of the lesion. Clinically the lesion could not be probed from both buccal and lingual aspects. A decision was made to access the tooth through the existing cast restoration to determine the extent of the lesion and whether it was amenable to non-surgical treatment. Following access through the crown, the defect could be visualized under the dental operating microscope and illumination, confirming granulation tissue mesial to the mesial root canals. Following curettage and TCA application pulp exposure was confirmed. (**c–f**) Non-surgical root canal treatment was performed over two appointments. A coronal glass ionomer cement restoration was placed to seal the mesial resorptive defect

16.8 Clinical Cases

Case 1 Non-surgical root canal treatment of tooth 36 demonstrating external inflammatory root resorption

A fit and healthy 33-year-old patient was referred for endodontic treatment of tooth 36. The patient had recalled the tooth had had a cast restoration (ceramic Cerec crown) placed 4 months earlier. The patient reported ongoing pain and discomfort exacerbated with biting/chewing and temperature sensitivity, which culminated in severe pain. The general dental practitioner had carried out an emergency pulp extirpation through the existing crown to help alleviate pulpal symptoms.

Radiographic examination confirmed prior endodontic access. A peri-radicular radiolucency was noted with both mesial and distal root apices. An oval radiolucency was also noted in the middle third of the mesial root (see Fig. 16.9).

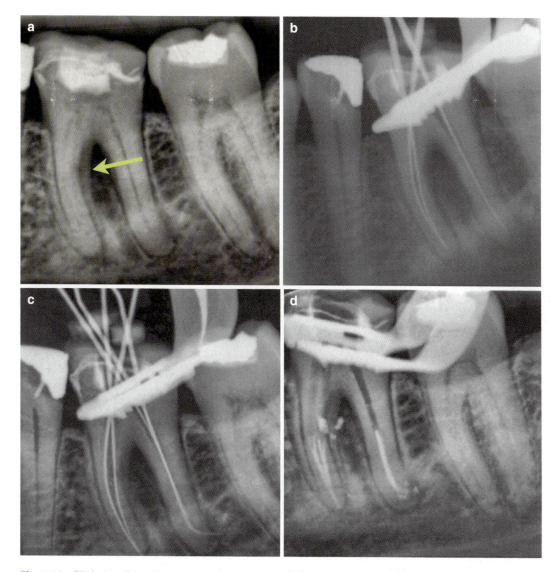

Fig. 16.9 Clinical radiographs demonstrating external root resorption due to pulpal infection. Note: (**a**) preoperative radiograph demonstrating an irregular radiolucency in the middle 1/3 of the root (*yellow arrow*). (**b**, **c**) IAF and MAF files. (**d**) Mid-fill radiograph following warm vertical compaction using AH plus cement and System B. Note: sealer extrusion noted at mid-root level in the mesial root showing internal/external communication due to root resorption

Access preparation was refined and chemo-mechanical preparation completed using 1 % sodium hypochlorite solution. Confluence was noted in the MB and ML and DB and DL canals in the apical third and patency was maintained in all canals. An acute apical curvature was noted in the distal canal (see Fig. 16.9). An interim dressing of calcium hydroxide was placed for 4 weeks. At the second appointment scheduled for obturation, the patient was completely asymptomatic.

Obturation was completed using a warm vertical compaction technique using AH Plus cement.

Following cone fit placement using AH Plus cement and 4 % tapered gutta-percha cones, appropriate-sized System B pre-fitted pluggers were used to carry out the downpack. A mid-fill radiograph was taken to assess apical obturation prior to backfill with gutta-percha root filling material. Sealer extrusion was noted in the middle third of the mesial root (see Fig. 16.9). Following the backfill procedure, an irregular oval-shaped root filling was confirmed in the mesiolingual canal (Fig. 16.10). A temporary double-seal IRM/glass ionomer restoration was placed in the coronal access cavity.

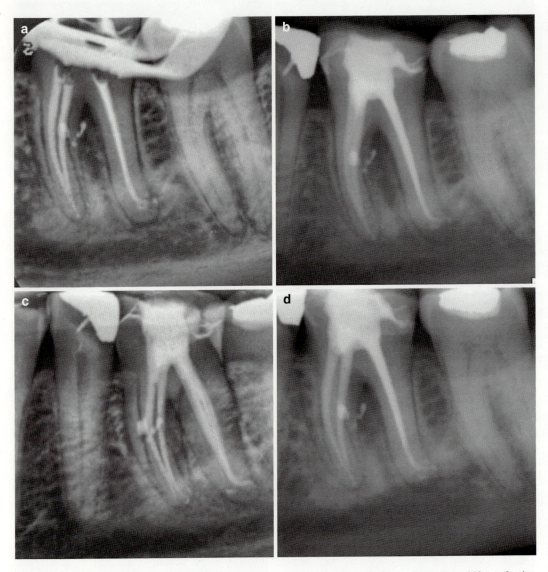

Fig. 16.10 Clinical radiographs demonstrating external root resorption due to pulpal infection. Note: (**a**) backfill following warm vertical compaction using gutta-percha and Obtura. (**b–d**) External root resorption lesion demonstrated by mesial to distal cone shift confirming communication between the internal root canal and external root surface

The patient was warned of the possibility of post-operative sequelae including pain and sensitivity related to the sealer extrusion. The patient was reviewed a week later and patient remained asymptomatic. The patient was advised to return to their general dental practitioner for placement of a permanent coronal restoration in the tooth.

Case 2 Non-surgical root canal treatment of tooth 27 demonstrating external cervical inflammatory root resorption

A 48-year-old patient suffering from well-controlled hypertension was referred for endodontic management of tooth 27. The general dental practitioner had noted an irregular radiolucency associated with the mesial aspect. A provisional diagnosis of caries was made and an attempt to restore the tooth. During the removal of caries, the general dental practitioner noted granulation tissue in the mesial defect. The patient was referred for endodontic opinion with the suspicion of cervical root resorption.

Access cavity was prepared confirming 4 canals. MB1 and MB2 canals were confluent. Chemomechanical preparation was completed uneventfully. Mesially, granulation tissue was noted with bleeding tags of tissue. TCA was applied to cotton wool pledgets and placed in the mesial defect. Granulation tissue was excavated with repeated TCA dressings applied until hard tissue was evident. A further application of TCA was applied prior to restoration of the defect. A resin-modified glass ionomer was placed in the mesial defect and light cured in increments. An intra-canal dressing of calcium hydroxide was placed and the patient reviewed 4 weeks later. Obturation of the four canals was completed using a warm vertical compaction technique. The patient was referred to his general dental practitioner for permanent cuspal coverage restoration of the tooth.

Long term, the patient was made aware of the possibility of continuation of the resorptive process and the need for periodic monitoring to assess whether the lesion had been truly arrested (see Figs. 16.11 and 16.12).

Case 3 Non-surgical and surgical root canal treatment of tooth 24 demonstrating external cervical inflammatory root resorption

A fit and healthy 51-year-old female patient was referred for an opinion regarding tooth 24. The general dental practitioner had taken routine bitewing radiographs at a periodic examination, which revealed radiolucency in the cervical region of the tooth. Previous bitewings taken 4 years ago did not reveal any pathology. The tooth was asymptomatic at time of consultation.

The dentist was concerned that there may be internal root resorption associated with the tooth. Clinical examination revealed tooth 24 was unrestored. No previous history of trauma or orthodontic treatment was noted. Tooth 24 had a positive response to thermal stimulus (CO_2 snow) (diminished and delayed compared to control tooth). Electric pulp testing was positive.

Radiographic examination revealed an irregular radiolucency in the cervical aspect of the tooth. A second radiograph with a mesial tube shift was taken confirming the lucency had moved. Clinically, a defect was noted on the palatal aspect of the tooth below the gingival margin. A cone beam CT scan was obtained confirming a radiolucent lesion below the cement-enamel junction on the palatal aspect of tooth 24 (see Fig. 16.13). The radiolucency was very close to the palatal root. A provisional diagnosis of external cervical root resorption was made. The patient was seen for surgical exploration of the area and warned of the possibility that root canal treatment would be required in addition to the management of the cervical resorptive lesion. A palatal envelope flap was raised confirming granulation tissue in the cervical aspect. The granulation tissue was curetted and TCA was applied. The palatal root canal was involved (see Fig. 16.14).

An endodontic access cavity was prepared under rubber dam application. Two canals were located and chemomechanically prepared. The palatal canal was temporarily sealed with gutta-percha to prevent restorative material blocking coronal access. The dam was removed and haemostasis was gained in the cervical defect using cotton wool pellets soaked in anaesthetic solution. The cervical resorptive defect was restored with glass ionomer cement. The tooth was reaccessed under rubber dam and following irrigation with sodium hypochlorite solution, an interim dressing of calcium hydroxide was placed with temporarily sealing of the access cavity (see Fig. 16.15).

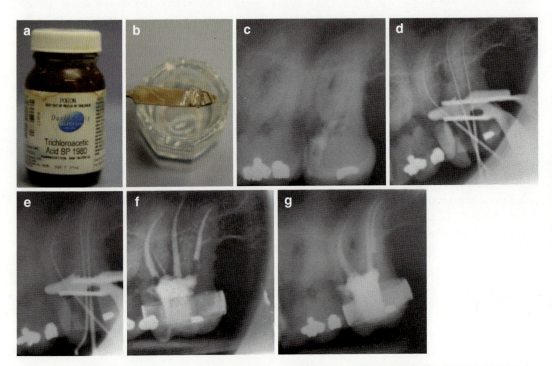

Fig. 16.11 Clinical photographs and radiographs demonstrating non-surgical management of invasive cervical root resorption associated with the mesial aspect of tooth 27. Due to difficulties with surgical access, a decision was made to attempt to treat the lesion non-surgically. The patient was made aware that the long-term prognosis was guarded. (**a, b**) Ninety per cent TCA used for topical application to aid in coagulation necrosis of the invasive resorptive tissue. (**c**) Pre-operative radiograph demonstrating the extent of the mesial lesion cervically. (**d**) IAF following access preparation. (**e**) MAF preparation completed. The lesion was treated with TCA at the same appointment and then an intra-canal calcium hydroxide dressing was left in place for 3 weeks. (**f**) Post obturation. (**g**) Post-operative view demonstrating completed case and mesial lesion restoration

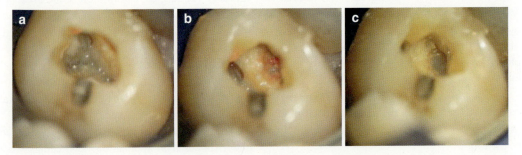

Fig. 16.12 Clinical photographs showing nonsurgical management of invasive cervical root resorption associated with tooth 27. (**a**) Following access refinement confirming the presence of MB1, MB2, DB and P canals, ultrasonic refinement was carried out mesially to reveal (**b–d**) the resorptive lesion. (**e–h**) Curretage was carried out using application of 90% TCA. (**i**) After several applications of TCA and curettage no further bleeding was evident from within the resorptive cavity and probing confirmed hard mineralized tissue. Complete removal of the resorptive granulation tissue was noted. The mesial defect was restored with resin-modified glass ionomer cement. Non-surgical root canal treatment was completed

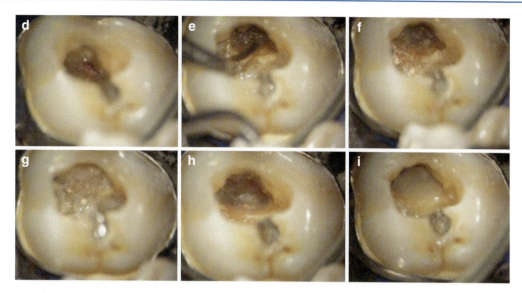

Fig. 16.12 (continued)

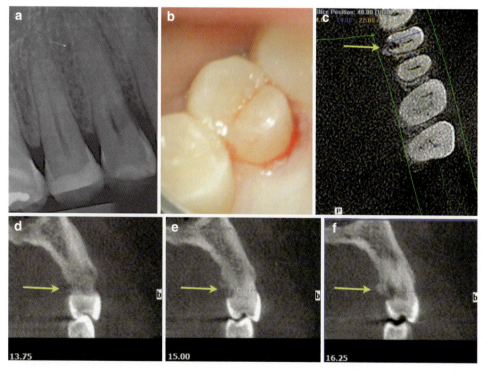

Fig. 16.13 Clinical radiographs and photographs demonstrating invasive cervical root resorption in tooth 24. Note (**a**) preoperative intraoral conventional radiograph showing irregular radioluceny associated with the cervical aspect of tooth 24. Clinically the patient exhibited no symptoms with the area of concern noted on chance radiographic finding by the referring dentist. (**b**) Clinical examination revealed no obvious abnormalities with the crown and the defect could not be probed. (**c–f**) CBCT images reveal the true nature of the lesion including degree of palatal root involvement (*yellow arrows*). Past history revealed no etiological factors such as orthodontic treatment, periodontal treatment, or trauma. A decision was made to raise a palatal mucoperiosteal flap to gain access to the lesion for complete currettage using 90 % TCA. The patient was warned that if pulpal involvement was noted at time of surgery, then nonsurgical endodontic treatment would be required

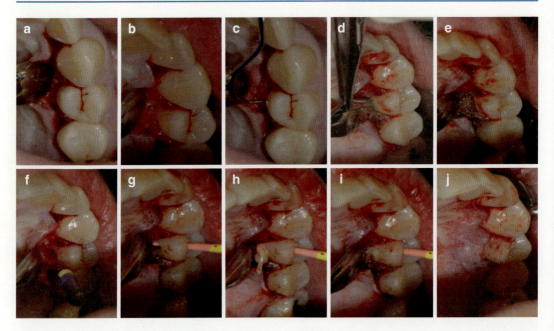

Fig. 16.14 Clinical photographs showing step-by-step surgical management of cervical invasive root resorption of tooth 24. Note (**a**, **b**) palatal mucoperiosteal envelope flap to reveal (**c**) resorpative lesion. (**d**, **e**) Curettage of lesion using 90 % TCA. (**f**) Following curettage of the lesion, involvement of the palatal root canal was confirmed using a 10K file. Non-surgical root canal treatment was initiated and chemo-mechanical debridement completed using 1 % sodium hypochlorite solution under rubber dam preparation. (**g**, **i**) The rubber dam was removed to allow unobscured access to the palatal lesion. A gutta-percha cone was placed in the palatal root canal to prevent restorative material blocking the canal. (**j**) Glass ionomer cement was placed in the palatal defect and following setting of the material the surgical site was closed using Vicryl sutures. The root canal system was reaccessed under rubber dam and an interim intra-canal calcium hydroxide dressing was placed. The tooth was temporarily sealed and the patient rebooked for completion of obturation 4 weeks later. The patient was reviewed at 1 week for suture removal and to ensure soft tissue healing was uneventful

The surgical site was closed using resorbable 5.0 sutures and the patient reviewed at 1 week and 4 weeks. The resorbable sutures were removed at the 1-week period and the patient healed uneventfully. The root canals were obturated using a warm vertical compaction technique using AH Plus cement. The patient was referred back to her general dental practitioner for placement of a cast cuspal coverage restoration. Further follow-up appointments were made, and the patient was warned of the possibility of further progression of the lesion and long-term possibility of a localized periodontal defect associated with the sub-gingival restoration (see Figs. 16.13, 16.14 and 16.15).

Case 4 Non-surgical and surgical root canal treatment of tooth 46 demonstrating external inflammatory root resorption and internal root resorption

A fit and healthy 43-year-old Australian defence force member was referred for endodontic management of tooth 46. The patient was aware of some localized gum swelling and pain in relation to this tooth. Clinical examination revealed tooth 46 had been restored with a cast gold full-crown restoration with good marginal integrity. The patient reported a history of cracked tooth syndrome in relation to this tooth prior to crown cementation. A draining sinus was noted in the overlying buccal mucosa and a 5 mm + probing profile was evident in the mid-buccal furcation region. Radiographic assessment revealed an extensive peri-radicular radiolucency associated with the periapex of tooth 46. A gutta-percha sinus tracing radiograph confirmed involvement of tooth 46. A well-circumscribed radiolucent lesion was noted in the coronal third of the distal root (see Fig. 16.16).

Access cavity was prepared through the gold crown restoration revealing a necrotic pulp.

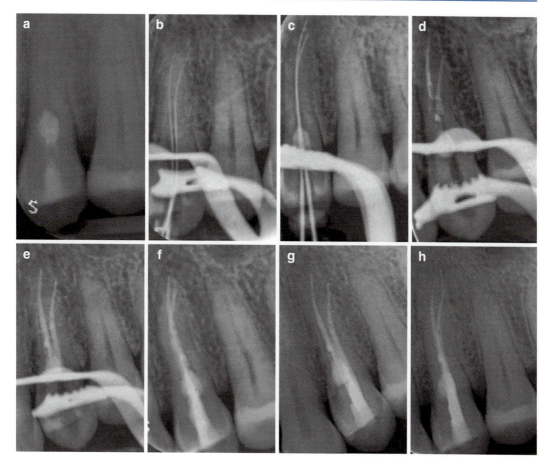

Fig. 16.15 Clinical radiographs demonstrating surgical and nonsurgical management of tooth 24. (**a**) Invasive resorptive lesion repaired with glass ionomer cement following surgical access and curettage. (**b**) IAF and (**c**) MAF preparation following surgical access of tooth 24. (**d**) Mid-fill and (**e**) backfill using warm vertical compaction using AH plus cement and gutta-percha. (**f–h**) Postoperative radiographs demonstrating root canal obturation and resorptive lesion repair. Note parallax views demonstrating the defect moving in the same direction of the X-ray tube (palatal). The patient was placed on a 6 monthly recall

Ultrasonic troughing was carried out to remove pulp stones in the floor of the pulp chamber. No visible crack lines or fracture was evident internally. Initial access preparation revealed three canals (MB, ML and DL). A small #10 K file was used to explore the DL canal system confirming an internal resorptive defect in the coronal third (Fig. 16.16). The file could not negotiate any apical anatomy beyond the resorptive lesion. An initial apical file radiograph was taken to confirm working lengths in the MB and ML canals (Fig. 16.17). Further ultrasonic troughing was carried out to reveal an additional DB canal. The DB canal could be negotiated to full working length with patency.

Chemomechanical preparation of the MB, ML, DB and DL canals was carried out using rotary files and 1 % sodium hypochlorite solution. Additional supplemental sonic irrigation was carried out using the EndoActivator. A master apical file radiograph was taken (Fig. 16.17). An intracanal medicament of calcium hydroxide was placed with a double temporary coronal seal of IRM and glass ionomer cement. The patient was scheduled for a review appointment 4 weeks later to reassess whether the draining sinus had healed.

At the review appointment, the buccal sinus had resolved and the patient had remained asymptomatic. A further appointment was scheduled for obturation of the tooth.

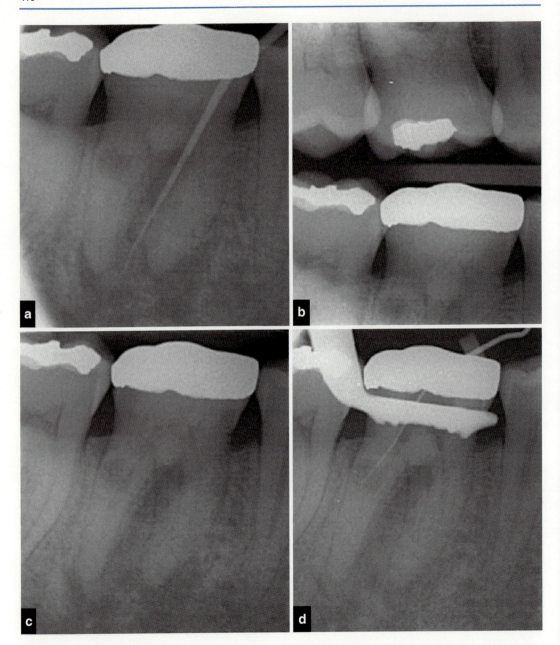

Fig. 16.16 Clinical radiographs demonstrating (**a**) preoperative gutta-percha sinus tracing radiograph confirming involvement of tooth 46. (**b**) Parallel bitewing radiograph showing well-circumscribed radiolucent lesion in the distal root. (**c**) Parallel periapical confirming extensive peri-radicular radiolucency and well-circumscribed radiolucent lesion in the distal root. A provisional diagnosis of chronic apical periodontitis with suppuration was made with internal root resorption. (**d**) Initial apical file placement in the DL canal confirmed associated resorptive lesion. The apical portion of the DL canal beyond the resorptive lesion could not be negotiated

Tooth 46 was obturated using AH Plus cement and gutta-percha technique. The DL canal was obturated using the 'squirt' technique. A final rinse of 1 % sodium hypochlorite solution and 17 % EDTA was used followed by drying of the canals. A very small amount of AH Plus sealer was introduced into the DL canal with paper points. A size #20 needle was used to express

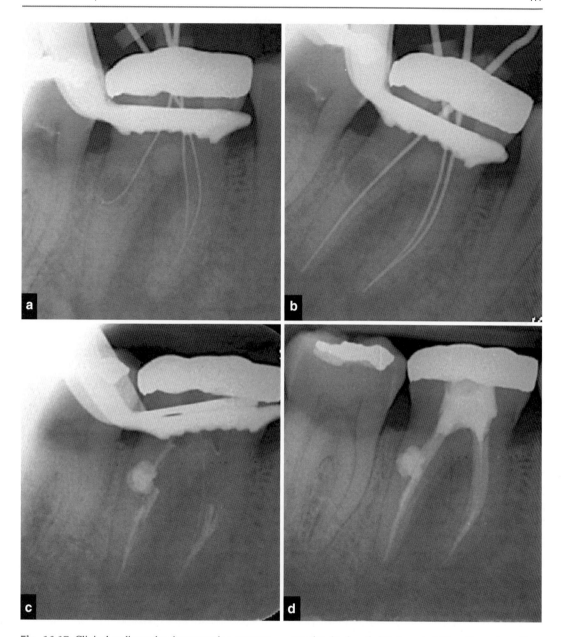

Fig. 16.17 Clinical radiographs demonstrating management of internal root resorption in tooth 46. Note: (**a**) initial apical file radiograph demonstrating negotiation of the mesial canals. The DL canal could only be partially instrumented. Once the file entered the resorptive lesion, it was impossible to negotiate any apical anatomy that may have been present. (**b**) Further ultrasonic troughing was carried out to reveal an additional DB canal which could be negotiated to length. Master apical file radiograph confirming working lengths in the DB, MB, and ML canals. (**c**) Mid-fill radiograph demonstrating apical gutta-percha fillings and obturation of the DL canal. The "squirt" technique was used to obturate the DL canal using the Obtura extruder gun and gutta-percha. (**d**) Final radiograph following completion of obturation and placement of a temporary IRM/glass ionomer cement double-seal temporary restoration

gutta-percha from the Obtura extruder into the DL canal. An appropriate-sized plugger was then used to further compress the gutta-percha ensuring minimal shrinkage. The DB, MB and DL canals were obturated using a warm vertical compaction technique. Master cones were coated with minimum AH Plus sealer and seated to working lengths. Downpacking was carried out with an appropriate 6 % tapered System B tip to within 5 mm of the apex. A mid-fill radiograph was taken to assess the apical gutta-percha fillings and DL canal obturation (Fig. 16.17). The remaining canal spaces in the MB, ML and DB canals were backfilled using gutta-percha and Obtura. The access cavity was temporized with IRM and glass ionomer cement. A final postoperative radiograph was taken (Fig. 16.17). The patient was referred back to his general dental practitioner for placement of a permanent coronal restoration. Further review appointments were scheduled to ensure continued healing was taking place.

Clinical Hints and Tips for Managing Root Resorption

- The stimulation factor for internal root resorption and external peri-radicular inflammatory root resorption is intra-pulpal infection. Adequate root canal treatment aimed at removing intra-pulpal bacteria will arrest the resorption process.
- Root resorption related to pressure during orthodontic treatment or an impacted tooth or tumour is managed by removal of the pressure stimulation factor.
- Replacement root resorption and ankylosis have no predictable treatment and cannot be arrested. The long-term prognosis is poor and tooth replacement is inevitable.
- In cervical root resorption, infection originates from the periodontal sulcus, which stimulates the pathological process. Removal of granulation tissue from the resorption lacuna and sealing is necessary for repair. Class 1 and 2 lesions (Hiethersay classification) are amenable to treatment. Classes 3 and 4 have a guarded/poor prognosis resulting in the likely demise of the tooth.

References

1. Darcey J, Qualtrough A. Resorption: part 1. Pathology, classification and aetiology. Br Dent J. 2013;214(9):439–51.
2. Fuss Z, Tsesis I, Lin S. Root resorption – diagnosis, classification and treatment choices based on stimulation factors. Dent Traumatol. 2003;19:175–82.
3. Gunraj MN. Dental root resorption. Oral Surg Oral Med Oral Pathol Oral Radiol Endod. 1999;88:647–53.
4. Lindskog S, Hammarström L. Evidence in favour of anti-invasion factor in cementum or periodontal membrane of human teeth. Scand J Dent Res. 1980;88:161–3.
5. Andreasen JO. External root resorption: its implications in dental traumatology, paedodontics, periodontics, orthodontics and endodontics. Int Endod J. 1985;18:109–18.
6. Tronstad L. Root resorption – aetiology, terminology and clinical manifestations. Endod Dent Traumatol. 1988;4:241–52.
7. Feiglin B. Root resorption. Aust Dent J. 1986;31:12–22.
8. Ne RF, Witherspoon DE, Gutmann JL. Tooth resorption. Quintessence Int. 1999;30:9–26.
9. Trope M. Root resorption due to dental trauma. Endod Topics. 2002;1(1):79–100.
10. Heithersay GS. Management of tooth resorption. Aust Dent J. 2007;52(s1):S105–21.
11. Calişkan M, Tűrkűn M. Prognosis of permanent teeth with internal resorption. Endod Dent Traumatol. 1997;13:75–81.
12. Haapasalo M, Endal U. Internal inflammatory root resorption: the unknown resorption of the tooth. Endod Topics. 2006;14:60–79.
13. Patel S, Ricucci D, Durak C, Tay F. Internal root resorption. A review. J Endod. 2010;36(7):1107–21.
14. Andreasen FM. Transient apical breakdown and its relation to color and sensibility changes after luxation injuries to teeth. Endod Dent Traumatol. 1986;2:9–19.
15. Cohenca N, Karni S, Rotstein I. Transient apical breakdown following tooth luxation. Dent Traumatol. 2003;19(5):289–91.
16. Andreasen JO. Relationship between surface and inflammatory resorption and changes in the pulp after replantation of permanent incisors in monkeys. J Endod. 1981;7(7):294–301.
17. Heithersay GS, Wilson DF. Tissue responses in the rat to trichloracetic acid-an agent used in the treatment of invasive cervical resorption*. Aust Dent J. 1988;33(6):451–61.
18. Hiethersay GS. Clinical, radiologic and histopathologic features of invasive cervical resorption. Quintessence Int. 1999;30:27–37.
19. Hiethersay GS. Invasive cervical resorption. Endod Topics. 2004;7:73–92.
20. Patel S, Dawood A. The use of cone beam computed tomography in the management of external cervical resorption lesions. Int Endod J. 2007;40(9):730–7.
21. Patel S, Kanagasingam S, Pitt Ford T. External cervical resorption: a review. J Endod. 2009;35(5):616–25.

22. Schwartz RS, Robbins WJ, Rindler E. Management of invasive cervical resorption: observation from three private practices and a report of three cases. J Endod. 2010;36(10):1721–30.

23. Hammarström L, Pierce A, Blomlöf L, Feiglin B, Lindskog S. Tooth avulsion and replantation – a review. Endod Dent Traumatol. 1986;2:1–8.

24. Hammarström L, Blomlöf L, Lindskog S. Dynamics of dentoalveolar ankylosis and associated root resorption. Endod Dent Traumatol. 1989;5:163–75.

25. Andreasen JO. Analysis of pathenogenesis and topography of replacement resorption. Swed Dent J. 1980;4:231–40.

26. Patel S, Dawood A, Wilson R, Horner K, Mannocci F. The detection and management of root resorption lesions using intraoral radiography and cone beam computed tomography–an in vivo investigation. Int Endod J. 2009;42(9):831–8.

27. Darcey J, Qualtrough A. Resorption; part 2. Diagnosis and management. Br Dent J. 2013;214:493–509.

Restoration of the Endodontically Treated Tooth

17

John Cho, Robert Fell, and Bobby Patel

Summary

Endodontically treated teeth have often lost a considerable amount of tooth structure due to caries, endodontic therapy and/or previous restoration, which may increase the propensity for tooth fracture. It is therefore accepted that endodontically treated teeth are weaker and often require special restorative consideration to not only increase long-term survival but also to prevent further bacterial ingress by means of coronal leakage that can contribute to failure. A plethora of materials can be utilised by the clinician ranging from simple Nayyar amalgam cuspal coverage restorations to complex cast restorations. Occasionally a post may be indicated where remaining coronal tooth structure is minimal and retention of core material is required. Several post designs are available including prefabricated or custom-made. Of paramount importance to the longevity of the restored endodontically treated tooth is the presence of an adequate ferrule between core or post and core and crown margin. This ferrule effect provides additional bracing to protect the integrity of the root.

Clinical Relevance

Prior to embarking on complex endodontic treatment, the restorative needs of the individual tooth must be assessed. Dismantling of the restoration not only ensues that sound tooth structure remains but also allows the clinician to visualise the future restorative needs in his/her mind's eye. Following completion of endodontic treatment, a suitable permanent coronal restoration must be placed for protection against catastrophic fracture and further bacterial ingress from the oral cavity. Core build-up materials and post and core restorations are discussed in relation to anterior and posterior

J. Cho, BDS (Hons), MDSc (Prosthodontics)
University of Sydney, Canberra, ACT, Australia

R. Fell, BDS, DClinDent, FRACDS, FRACDS
Specialist Periodontist, Canberra, ACT, Australia

B. Patel, BDS MFDS MClinDent MRD MRACDS (✉)
Specialist Endodontist, Brindabella Specialist Centre,
Canberra, ACT, Australia
e-mail: bobbypatel@me.com

© Springer International Publishing Switzerland 2016
B. Patel (ed.), *Endodontic Treatment, Retreatment, and Surgery*,
DOI 10.1007/978-3-319-19476-9_17

teeth including indications, techniques, advantages and disadvantages. Careful appraisal of individual teeth according to morphology, remaining tooth structure, position in the arch and ideal preparation prerequisites is discussed to ensure longevity of the tooth following root canal therapy.

17.1 Overview of Coronal Leakage and Contemporary Methods of Restoring Teeth

The primary goal of restorative treatment following endodontic therapy is well accepted with the aim of restoring teeth to maintain form and function as well as providing a complete seal to prevent recontamination and introduction of bacteria within the decontaminated root canal system [1–3]. Exposure of gutta-percha to saliva within the pulp chamber can result in apical migration of bacteria within days [4]. The restoration of the endodontically treated tooth is a subject that has been discussed widely in the dental literature, and the understanding of this topic remains complex and controversial [5]. In the last 20 years, a plethora of materials and techniques have become available to the clinician with the emergence of adhesive approaches that have increased the clinicians' repertoire, aimed at tooth structure preservation that is critical to the survival of endodontically treated teeth [6]. The choice of final restoration must be judged on the best scientific evidence available rather than an empirical approach that can often lead to failure.

Any tooth undergoing endodontic treatment must take into account both restorative and periodontal factors that may affect the long-term prognosis. The clinical decision making process to retain any tooth must form part of a comprehensive overall treatment plan formulated with the patient and taking into consideration not only local tooth factors but also its overall strategic value and a cost/benefit analysis compared with alternative replacement options (Figs. 17.1 and 17.2).

Historically it was thought that the dentine of endodontically treated teeth was significantly different when compared to their vital counterparts with factors such as moisture content and loss of collagen cross-linking being attributed to the demise of root treated teeth and their propensity to fracture [7, 8]. These findings were disputed and did not support the conclusion that endodontically treated teeth are more brittle [9, 10]. It is in fact the loss of both structural integrity associated with access preparations [11] and impairment of neurosensory feedback mechanisms following pulp tissue removal [12] that may lead to a higher occurrence of fractures associated with endodontically treated teeth. The anterior and posterior teeth are subjected to masticatory loads in normal function (laterally and vertically) with increased cuspal deflection when endodontic access cavities have been prepared [5, 13]. Taken together, these studies would suggest that the definitive restoration not only serves to provide an enhanced coronal seal and minimise future risk of micro-leakage and recontamination [14] but more importantly to prevent catastrophic fracture particularly when under heavy masticatory loading during normal function [15].

Endodontically treated teeth with intracoronal restorations are at higher risk of cuspal fracture [16–18]. In a 20-year retrospective analysis, the cumulative survival rate (retention of both cusps) and fracture pattern of 1639 endodontically treated posterior teeth were assessed. All teeth had an MO/DO or an MOD cavity restored with amalgam without cuspal overlay. The 20-year survival rate of teeth with an MO/DO cavity was markedly higher than teeth with an MOD cavity. Maxillary bicuspids with MOD restorations showed the lowest survival rate overall (28 % fractured within 3 years, 57 % were lost after 10 years and 73 % after 20 years) [17]. The loss of tooth structure in combination with an increased cavity depth due to endodontic access results in greater cuspal deflection compared to a vital tooth [13]. Bicuspid teeth (such as maxillary premolars) can be more prone to longitudinal root fractures where the mesiodistal dimension is narrow [19].

Endodontically treated teeth as abutments have also shown to be at greater risk of fracture [12]. In a retrospective clinical investigation

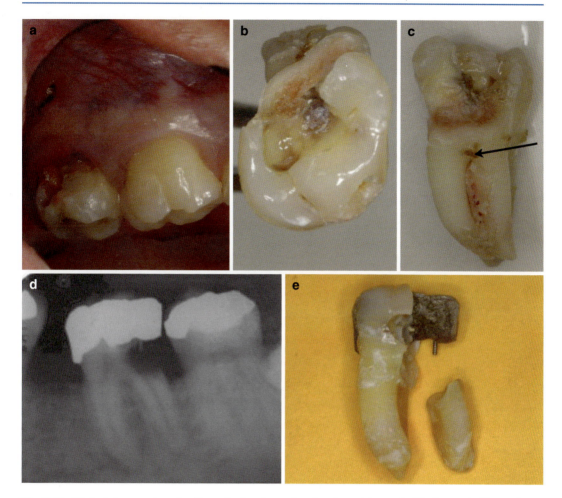

Fig. 17.1 Clinical photographs and radiographs showing pre-endodontic restorability and periodontal assessment considerations. Note: (**a–c**) tooth 17 presented with gross buccal caries extending subgingivally. A crown-lengthening procedure was not possible due to the extent of caries and future crown margin encroaching near the furcal region of the tooth (*black arrow*). The tooth was extracted. (**d–e**) A lower left first molar presented with gross secondary caries. The tooth was deemed unrestorable and extraction carried out. The decision to carry out complex endodontic treatment must take into account the long-term restoration and whether or not this is feasible

comparing 1273 endodontically treated teeth as abutments or crowns, it was found that the greatest failure rate was associated with pulpless teeth without a crown (24.2 %). A comparison also indicated that the failure rate of abutments when used for removable partial dentures (22.6 %) was twice that of fixed bridges (10.2 %). Overall success rate was found to be highest in endodontically treated teeth that had been restored with single crowns (94.8 %). Additional observations concluded that the presence of intra-coronal reinforcement did not appreciably increase the success rate for survival without coronal coverage.

Post placement had limited influence on the success rate of fixed partial denture abutments but interestingly significantly improved the success for partial denture abutment endodontically treated teeth. ParaPost and amalgam or resin composite cores had considerably greater success compared to tapered cast post and core restorations [20].

There is strong evidence to support the notion that the clinical longevity of an endodontically treated posterior tooth is significantly improved with a coronal cuspal coverage restoration [18, 20–22]. One retrospective study, using a

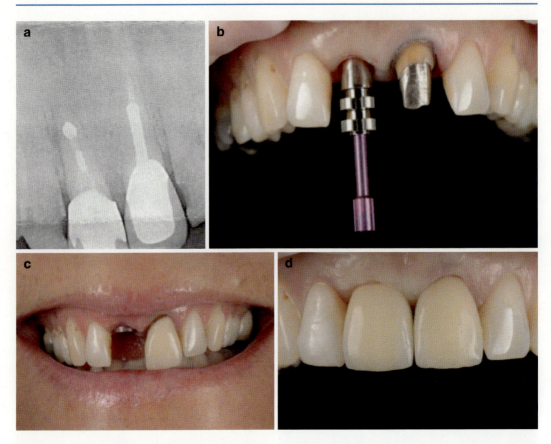

Fig. 17.2 Clinical radiographs and photographs demonstrating (**a**) failing endodontic treatment associated with tooth 11. The tooth had previously undergone periapical surgery and suboptimal orthograde root canal treatment. Treatment options were discussed with the patient, and a decision to replace the tooth with a single tooth implant was made. (**b–d**) The tooth was extracted and replaced with a single tooth implant. Tooth 21 had a cast restoration replaced to match the new implant abutment and provide optimal aesthetics

multivariant model and proportional hazard survival analysis, evaluated the effect of crown placement on endodontically treated teeth and their survival. Endodontically treated teeth without crowns were lost at a six times greater rate than teeth with crowns [22].

All endodontically treated teeth that require extra-coronal cuspal coverage restorations also require a coronal-radicular core restoration. The purpose of the core restoration with or without a post is to replace lost dentine and provide internal support and retention for the crown ensuring resistance against cervical tooth fracture. The presence of a circumferential ring of sound tooth structure (ferrule) at the crown-root interface is critical for the long-term success of the crowned endodontically treated tooth (Fig. 17.3).

A minimum ferrule of 1.5–2 mm is required between core and crown margin to provide a bracing or casing action to protect the integrity of the root. When a crown is placed with optimal ferrule, the crown and root function as one integrated unit dissipating occlusal forces to the underlying periodontium without undue stresses resulting in crown/post dislodgement or root/post fracture. In cases where an adequate ferrule is not present then due consideration must be given to either forced orthodontic eruption or surgical crown lengthening or extraction [23, 24].

The anchorage provided by a well-placed core utilising the pulp chamber can be sufficient to both reinforce and replace the remaining coronal tooth structure. In posterior molar teeth, a coronal-radicular core build-up using

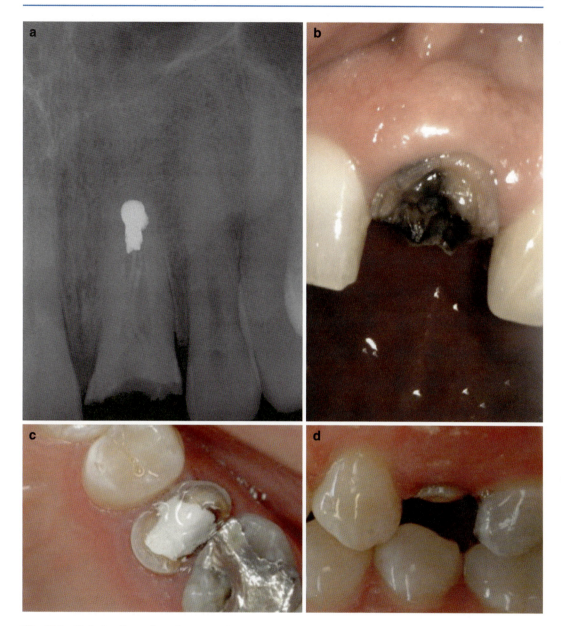

Fig. 17.3 Clinical radiographs and photographs showing limited coronal tooth structure and inadequate ferrule. Note: (**a, b**) tooth 21 has previously undergone root canal treatment and apicoectomy procedures. (**c, d**) Tooth 25 shows limited circumferential ring of sound tooth structure (ferrule). Both cases highlight the complexities involved when treatment planning cases for endodontic treatment. The cost/benefit of root canal procedures, crown lengthening, and complex post and core restorations must be outweighed against perhaps more predictable alternative prosthodontic replacement options

amalgam utilising the pulp chamber and 2 mm into each canal space has proved to be successful in clinical studies [25]. Additional retention can also be provided by the use of intra-dentinal pins [26], amalgapins [27] and dentinal slots and grooves [28]. With the advent of modern adhesive techniques, these types of retention methods have been superseded due to concerns of further weakening the tooth as a direct result of further coronal tooth structure loss [29].

Anterior teeth with minimal loss of tooth structure can be restored conservatively with a bonded restoration in the access opening without the use of a post [18]. The use of modern direct composites and resin bonding materials is at the forefront of contemporary minimally invasive aesthetic dentistry and will provide satisfactory aesthetic results restoring function and aesthetics, whilst preserving healthy tooth tissue [30]. Where there has been substantial tooth structure loss or in addition where the tooth is aesthetically displeasing, then crowning may be indicated. The primary disadvantage of using indirect conventional metal-ceramic crowns is the significant buccal surface tooth reduction (approximately 1.5–2 mm) that is required to accommodate both metal and ceramic core [31]. The use of all-ceramic crowns (e.g. Procera, Nobel Biocare, Zurich, Switzerland. Empress, Ivoclar Vivadent, Amherst, NY, USA. In-ceram, H.Rauter GmbH & Co. KG, Bad Säckingen, Germany) as an alternative to metal-ceramic restorations has been driven by both superior aesthetics and increased strength in thin sections resulting in a viable option for anterior and posterior teeth [32].

In posterior teeth, as discussed earlier, the longevity of the root canal therapy is dependent on the quality of the coronal restoration in terms of both tooth survival and potential fracture and prevention of coronal leakage and possible reinfection. Root canal treatment outcomes evaluated in a large-scale epidemiological study of more than one million patients showed that 85 % of teeth that had been extracted had no full coronal restoration. They also found a sixfold increase in failure rate in posterior teeth with no crowns compared with posterior teeth with crown restorations [33]. Prosthetic reconstruction of posterior endodontically treated teeth without adequate cuspal coverage using conventional amalgam has been shown to be not suitable [17]. The use of amalgam crown restorations, with a minimal 2 mm thickness of cuspal coverage, has shown a cumulative survival rate of 88 % after 100 months and a less expensive alternative to cast restorations [34, 35]. Their intended use may be particularly beneficial when the endodontic prognosis is

questionable and longer-term follow up is envisaged providing a relatively inexpensive and predictable interim restoration.

The use of tooth coloured direct composite restorations has also been evaluated for use in the restoration of root-filled teeth. Fibre posts with direct composite restorations in root-filled premolars with limited tooth structure loss have been shown to exhibit equivalent survival rates compared with premolars restored with crowns after 3 years [36]. The long-term survival of direct composite restorations, particularly in load-bearing areas, is questionable due to natural wear and tear resulting in either fracture or marginal discrepancies that can lead to reinfection and failure. In a longitudinal outcome study based on a systematic review, root-filled teeth restored with crowns had a 10-year survival rate of 81 %. Teeth restored with direct restorations (such as amalgam or composite) had a survival rate of 63 % [37]. The use of composite restorations in posterior teeth may be best served as a core material in preparation for future cast cuspal coverage restoration.

Cast gold partial restorations (onlay, three-quarter and seven-eighths) and full coverage crowns allow for the most conservative tooth preparation ensuring optimal preservation of residual tooth structure. They are useful in posterior teeth where aesthetic demands are not of paramount importance or where the patient exhibits parafunctional habits (bruxism) or there is limited inter-occlusal space. The reduction required for gold restorations can be as little as 0.7 mm in non-load-bearing areas and up to 1.5 mm in load-bearing areas [6]. Both metal-ceramic restorations and all-ceramic crowns have also been shown to be effective and again useful when aesthetics is of particular importance.

When insufficient coronal tooth structure exists to retain a core, then a post is a universally accepted treatment modality. Previously considered to provide further reinforcement, it is now widely recognised to help retain the core build-up albeit there is a greater risk of significantly weakening the root as result of post preparation [15, 38, 39]. The decision to place a post must be weighed up against the inherent risks associated with post preparation including procedural accidents such as perforations in the apical or mid-root of the tooth, increased risk of root fracture and treatment failure [40] (Fig. 17.4).

Posts can be categorised into metallic posts, prefabricated posts, zirconium and ceramic posts and non-metallic posts (fibre). Metallic and prefabricated post systems are conventionally more rigid in design compared to non-rigid fibre post systems. Metallic custom-cast post and core systems are constructed by making an impression of the post space (direct or indirectly) and fabrication of the post from precious or non-previous casting alloys in the laboratory. A systematic review demonstrated no superiority between cast posts over direct post and core restorations [41].

The disadvantage of a custom-cast post and core system includes increased cost and time involved for the patient. The main advantage of the custom-cast post designed to fit the tooth is the greater potential for tooth conservation. This is of particular importance in teeth with small thin tapered roots such as premolars, maxillary lateral incisors and mandibular molars which could be significantly weakened by further instrumentation necessary to fit a prefabricated post [42].

Prefabricated posts are typically made from stainless steel, nickel-titanium alloy or titanium and come in a variety of designs. They can be divided into tapered or parallel and active or passive. A tapered post is less retentive in comparison to a parallel post but helps to preserve dentine

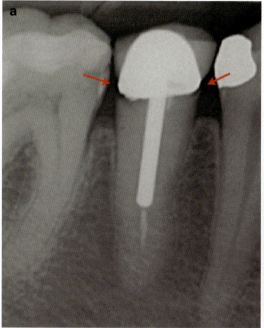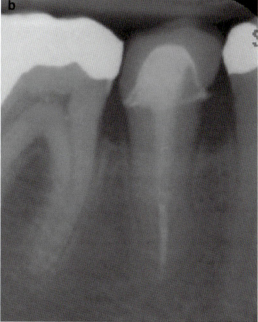

Fig. 17.4 Clinical radiographs demonstrating endodontic re-treatment, crown lengthening, and new post and core crown replacement for tooth 45. Note (**a**) preoperative radiograph showing parallel post-core restoration with defective margins (*red arrows*) and coronal microleakage. Clinically minimal ferrule height was confirmed following removal of crown and post. After initial removal of gutta-percha, chemo-mechanical preparation, and patency confirmation, the tooth was dressed with calcium hydroxide. The patient was referred to a periodontist to confirm that crown lengthening was feasible. Following completion of endodontic therapy, the patient returned to the periodontist for crown lengthening, followed by an interim 3-month healing period. (**b**) The patient was then seen for final fiber post, core, and permanent crown placement. Complex re-treatment occasionally requires a multidisciplinary approach. Provided all stages of treatment are executed correctly, then the long-term prognosis should be good. Careful planning with the patient is crucial from the outset including discussion of alternative prosthodontic replacement options. In this case the patient could have opted for a single-unit implant which would have been of similar expense

and reduces the amount of dentine that needs to be removed to accommodate the post [43]. Conversely the parallel post provides the greatest retention (particularly if the surface is grooved or roughened) but requires tooth structure to be sacrificed in order to accommodate the post. There has been concern with regard to the wedging effect when using tapered posts that may predispose to root fracture and loss of post retention. Passive posts are retained primarily by the frictional retention of the luting cement and induce less stress into the root compared to active posts, although are less retentive. Active posts imply that the threads of the post engage or screw into the walls of the canal.

Zirconium and ceramic post systems were developed in view of the aesthetic problems associated with metal posts and the possibility of visibility through translucent all-ceramic restorations. Disadvantages of these posts include greater rigidity and brittleness, greater tooth removal required as a consequence of thicker post diameters necessary to compensate for weakness and significantly more root fractures in vitro compared to fibre posts [44, 45]. In addition, retrieval of zirconium and ceramic posts is very difficult if endodontic retreatment is indicated requiring excessive removal of dentine and post removal by grinding the ceramic or zirconium post, which is both risky and tedious. Their use should be avoided if at all possible.

Non-rigid non-metallic prefabricated post systems consist of carbon fibre, glass fibre, quartz fibre and silicon fibre posts. The posts were manufactured for use in conjunction with highly aesthetic restorations whereby the post was bonded utilising resin luting cements incorporating composite cores. The first reinforced fibre posts were made with longitudinally arranged black carbon fibres embedded in an epoxy resin matrix that fell out of favour due to their dark colour. These were rapidly replaced by more aesthetically pleasing tooth coloured/white and translucent glass and quartz fibres. The main advantage of using a fibre post is that the mode of failure is generally more retrievable compared to other post systems.

Although the load to failure is greater in metallic posts, they result in significantly greater root fractures [45–47].

Post retention is dependent on several factors including post configuration, length, diameter, surface preparation and cementation. Post diameter is the least important factor and should be designed to conform to the pre-existing canal diameter without sacrificing further tooth structure, which further weakens the tooth (Fig. 17.5). Regarding post configuration, the active threaded post is the most retentive, followed by the passive parallel post. The passive tapered post is the least retentive [43, 48]. One must bear in mind that active threaded posts can induce stresses in the root dentine that may lead to crack initiation and predisposition to root fracture at a later time.

Increasing the length of the post increases the retention. The length of the post should at least equal the length of the clinical crown [21]. Short posts lead to greater stress in the coronal aspect of the canal increasing susceptibility to dislodgement or root fracture (Figs. 17.5 and 17.6). One study reported that two-thirds of the posts associated with vertically fractured endodontically treated teeth were extremely short, terminating in the cervical third of the root [49]. Ideal post length must be weighed up against anatomical and morphological factors such as apical root structure thickness and furcal concavities which may increase the risk of perforation and weakening of the tooth together with the need to maintain an apical seal (dictated by remaining gutta-percha) [50]. To avoid reinfection of the periapical region following post preparation, at least 4–5 mm of apical gutta-percha should be retained [50, 51]. Once the post has been prepared, the post should be cemented as soon as practically possible to reduce the potential for apical leakage and reinfection [52, 53].

The long-term success of post retained restorations is also dependent on the resistance form. Resistance refers to the ability of the post and tooth to withstand lateral and rotational forces and is provided by three factors: anti-rotation features, the presence of a ferrule [23, 24] and

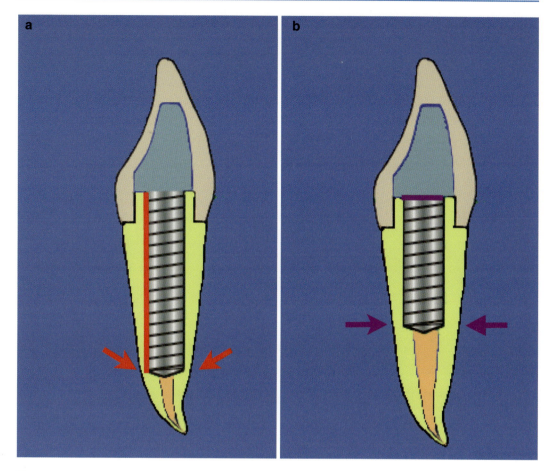

Fig. 17.5 Diagrammatic representation of (**a**) post length and (**b**) post diameter and their effect on post retention. Increasing the post length increases the retention of the post and the length should be at least equal to the length of the clinical crown. Post length must be weighed up against anatomical and morphological factors which may increase the risk of perforation (*red arrows*). Post diameter is the least important factor when designing an ideal post and should conform to the preexisting canal diameter without sacrificing further root structure and predisposing to fracture or perforation (*purple arrows*)

remaining tooth structure. Anti-rotation features such as slots or pins can be incorporated in the absence of significant vertical tooth height [18, 54]. A minimum crown height of at least 1.5 mm apical to the margin of the core is needed to provide significant resistance to fatigue failure of the cement seal [55].

The failure of endodontically treated teeth is usually not a consequence of endodontic treatment, but inadequate restorative therapy or periodontal reasons. Prior to the initiation of endodontic treatment, the restorability, occlusal function, periodontal health, biological width and crown-root ratio need to be assessed. Direct adhesive restorations, indirect bonded restorations and traditional full crowns are three therapeutic options for single posterior endodontically treated teeth. Posts may be utilised for retention of core material and to replace missing tooth structure. The amount of remaining sound tooth structure is the most significant factor in determining the most appropriate technique, material and type of restoration employed to restore the functional needs of the patient [56, 57].

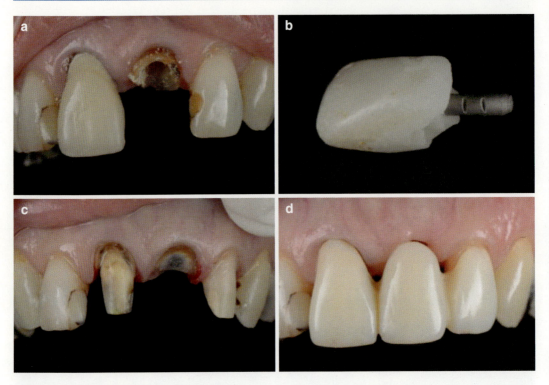

Fig. 17.6 Clinical photographs demonstrating a failed post and core restoration associated with tooth 21. Note: (**a**) limited coronal tooth structure with adequate ferrule and (**b**) short post length resulted in prosthodontic failure.

(**c–d**) The 21 was subsequently de-coronated and a temporary fixed-fixed tooth-supported FDP fabricated following its extraction

17.2   Core Materials

Amalgam

The use of amalgam as a material for core restorations of endodontically treated teeth has been advocated and practised since its earliest use as a conventional restorative material. In addition to its well-documented physical properties, its handling has allowed clinicians to utilise amalgam as a direct core material in situations where bonding would either be difficult or inappropriate for reasons of moisture control. Its inherent compressive strength has made it the material of choice for posterior load-bearing situations; whilst it had been used in anterior teeth prior to the advent of reliable resin bonding techniques, its colour (inherent as well as imparted) has obvious

drawbacks in the aesthetic zone. Also worth noting is its low strength in thin sections and under tensile forces; clinicians should therefore ensure that adequate resistance form is present when placing amalgam in smaller sections, and as such, adequate tooth preparation to ensure these parameters are fulfilled may result in further undermining and resultant weakening of residual tooth structure.

The Nayyar core has been the most prevalent application of amalgam as a core material, and this technique has been shown to provide a reliable seal for the endodontic obturation, as well as providing a stable foundation restoration for any overlying indirect restorations. In some cases, where the morphology of the residual tooth dictates (e.g. thin axial walls, inadequate cuspal height), the Nayyar core technique may be employed to build up a direct 'amalgam crown' which utilises the canal orifices and pulp chamber morphology to retain a single restoration from orifice to cusp tip. It should be noted, however, as with any technique, that the efficacy of amalgam as a core material is primary derived from the initial seal at the restoration-obturation interface; this is best achieved with a layer of barrier material, such as glass ionomer cement or Cavit, between the obturation material and the amalgam core. Pulp burs or post preparation drills may be utilised to prepare adequate width and depth of space to allow condensation of amalgam into orifices and chambers (Fig. 17.7).

Composite

The advent of reliable resin bonding techniques by Buonocore has led to the use of resins in various restorative situations, including as a core material. The primary obstacles for all resin restorations are inherent in these situations, as they often involve challenging moisture control and poor access for light penetration to photoactivators. However, improved handling characteristics and physical properties have resulted in composite resins being utilised more widely as a core material, not only in aesthetically sensitive sites but also posterior teeth where access may be more difficult. Enhanced packability (i.e. the ability for composite resin to be condensed by instrumentation) allows clinicians to place resins into smaller and more morphologically complex cavities. Reduced polymerisation shrinkage and smaller accompanying c-factors have also played a significant role in the suitability of composite resin materials for placement into previously inappropriate cavity configurations. In addition, the increased prevalence of dual- or self-curing resins has given clinicians greater flexibility in the range of situations in which these materials may be utilised with greater degrees of success, where light penetration may be less than optimal (e.g. deep orifices, posterior teeth). Despite advances in dentine bonding, clinicians should still be wary

of utilising resins at the obturation-restoration interface, as moisture control following preparation can often be difficult in these sites, and the use of a barrier material (such as GIC or Cavit) is still recommended (see Fig. 17.8).

Glass ionomer cement

Various forms of glass ionomer cement (GIC) have become available since the early introduction of the material, which have improved on the handling characteristics and mechanical properties of conventional GIC. These include metal-reinforced GIC, resin-modified (or hybrid) GIC and compomers. As with any core material, however, compressive strength and resistance to fracture under oblique loading situations is highly critical; to date, none of these variations or conventional forms of GIC appear to meet the criteria for satisfactory core restorations. The use of GIC as a lining material under other core materials is recommended due to its tight chemical seal with dentine under moist conditions.

Pins

The use of pins to facilitate the mechanical retention of restorative materials has been widely documented and practised. However, due to advances in the chemical adhesion of resin and glass ionomer materials to tooth structure, their use has been increasingly limited to scenarios in which mechanical retention is lacking for metallic (cast/indirect or condensed/direct) restorations. The use of pins has also been shown to increase susceptibility of surrounding tooth structure to fracture, especially in areas where the morphology of residual tooth structure is thin or undermined. As such, the use of pins should be avoided in canal orifice or peri-radicular areas, as residual dentine walls are often thin and significantly weakened. In addition, the use of amalgam in these situations most often does not require the auxiliary mechanical retention provided by pins as the divergent canal orifices and pulp chamber morphology should provide sufficient retentive form for the core.

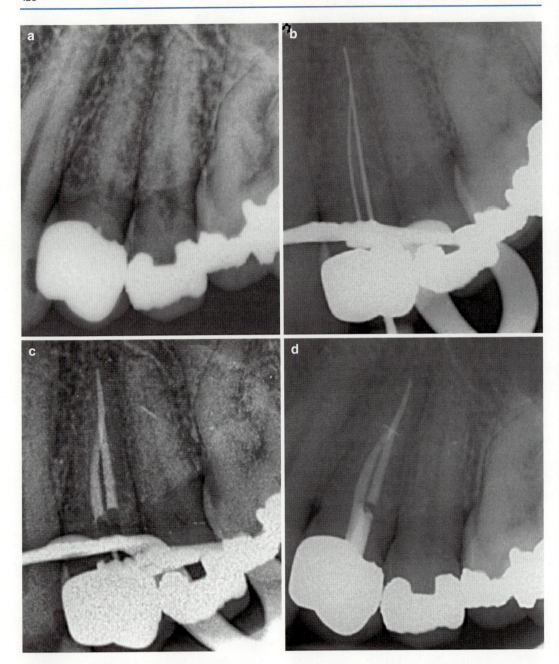

Fig. 17.7 Clinical radiographs demonstrating nonsurgical endodontic treatment of tooth 24 through a metal-ceramic crown restoration. Note: (**a**) preoperative view of tooth 24 demonstrating periradicular infection and calcified root canal system. (**b**) Following access cavity preparation through the crown, two canals were located which were confluent in the apical 1/3. Chemo-mechanical preparation was completed using sodium hypochlorite solution (1 %), and an interim calcium hydroxide dressing was placed for 3 weeks. (**c**) The canals were obturated using AH plus cement and warm vertical compaction technique. (**d**) The coronal pulp chamber and access cavity is sealed with a Nayyar core technique

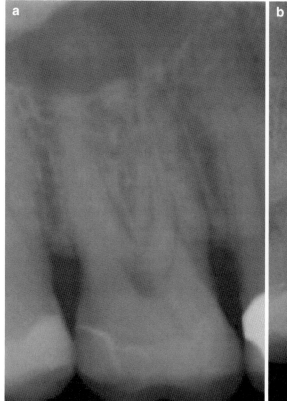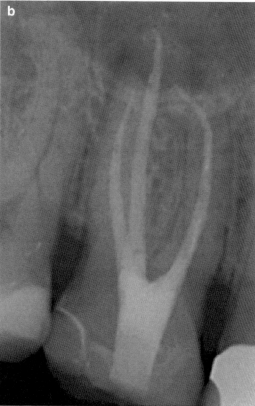

Fig. 17.8 Clinical radiographs demonstrating nonsurgical root canal treatment of tooth 26. Note: (**a**) preoperative radiograph showing ceramic onlay restoration. The tooth was non-vital with a periradicular radiolucency associated with the palatal root. (**b**) Completed endodontic treatment with a glass ionomer and composite core buildup

17.3   Full Cuspal Coverage Restorations

Amalgam

The use of amalgam as a definitive, cuspal coverage restoration in endodontically treated teeth is well documented. The historical use of amalgam as a conventional restorative material for large posterior restorations has led naturally to its employment in cuspal coverage situations for endodontically treated teeth. This is most conventionally performed as a single amalgam post-core-crown restoration, where amalgam is condensed from the prepared canal orifices all the way to the coronal cuspal aspect. As with all cuspal coverage restorations using amalgam, it is important to follow cavity preparation guidelines, especially with regard to adequate cuspal reduction to allow for sufficient bulk strength of amalgam over these sites. The direct amalgam crown is a particularly useful technique when the morphology of residual tooth structure indicates that further axial preparation will lead to significant weakening of the tooth, or loss of retention or resistance form. Its use should also be considered when previous restorations have deep gingival margins, which may then lead to encroachment of the biologic width with further gingival preparation for indirect restorations. The ability to visualise and prepare a deep gingival margin as well as the potential difficulties associated with tissue management, moisture control and accurate impression taking should also be considered, and in these situations, a direct amalgam crown may be more appropriate.

Gold

The main advantage of the cast gold restoration is its high strength in thin sections, which allows for minimal preparation of underlying teeth. In addition, the finer preparation margins allow for better adaptation and seal with mechanical burnishing of high-gold alloys against preparation margins. As such, in endodontically treated teeth which have already suffered significant loss of tooth structure, especially on the axial aspects, cuspal coverage utilising gold is of great value in preserving the remaining tooth structure. In addition, posterior sites with limited interarch (or inter-occlusal) space also benefit from the minimal occlusal reduction required for placement of cast gold restorations. Conversely, teeth that have minimal loss of existing structure other than the endodontic access cavity may also benefit from the maximal preservation of tooth material afforded by cast gold preparations. These less extensive preparations may take the form of partial onlays, three-quarter or seven-eigth crowns (partial veneers) which seek to provide protection of vulnerable cusps (with flexure widths of under 3 mm) without further preparation of more robust areas of the residual tooth; this in turns allows for less destruction of tooth structure and also preservation of buccal faces for aesthetic purposes. Cast gold restorations can also be luted onto tooth structure with most luting agents, excluding those which require photoactivation for polymerisation. As such, in sites where moisture control may be difficult, the placement of cast gold restorations utilising conventional GIC or zinc phosphate cements may be highly appropriate.

Ceramic

The use of all-ceramic restorations for the restoration of endodontically treated teeth is a relatively contemporary phenomenon, with the advent of stronger ceramic materials allowing clinicians to increase their restorative armamentarium in such situations. The move away from purely feldspathic porcelains to tougher, more resilient ceramic materials has led to the increasing use of these restorations in a wider range of clinical scenarios. More recently, the burgeoning technologies of computer-aided design (CAD) and computer-aided manufacture (CAM) have resulted in a plethora of ceramic materials being available for multiple clinical uses, including cuspal coverage restorations. Leucite-reinforced lithium disilicate, zirconia and alumina are the major material types currently available on the ceramic market. These materials boast physical properties which make their consideration in certain clinical scenarios appropriate; these include high compressive and flexural strength, low coefficient of thermal expansion and favourable optical properties. However, due to this diversity of materials and their properties, clinicians must exercise care in their selection of the appropriate material for each case, as their varying properties will have a significant influence on their success in each scenario. One of the main points to consider is the flexural strength of these restorations, especially in thin sections, which may be required at gingival margins. In addition, the suggested luting materials for these restorations are often resin-based, which requires absolute moisture control, which may be difficult to achieve in certain sites. Wear of opposing materials (restorative or natural tooth) should also be considered when employing ceramic restorations that may or may not be veneered by feldspathic porcelain or treated with glazing layers. The increased use of monolithic materials by clinicians and laboratories employing on-site CAD/CAM fabrication processes requires clinicians to be vigilant about achieving high surface smoothness by appropriate polishing protocols.

The CAD/CAM CEREC (computer-assisted CERamic REConstruction) system is used for electronically designing and milling restorations. Dentists who employ this technique can manufacture a restoration without the need for laboratory assistance, impressions or temporary restorations. The restoration can be designed in less than 5 minutes and milled in 10–12 minutes resulting in significant time and cost savings for the dental practice. A number of clinical studies of CEREC-manufactured restorations have reported ditching at the margins due to wear of the resin cement which could result in marginal leakage and failure of endodontic treatment (Fig. 17.9).

Adequate ferrule

The presence of an adequate ferrule is a foundational concept in the restoration of endodontically treated teeth. In engineering terms, a ferrule is a metal ring or band that provides stability and strength to a terminal end of a rod or joint. This banding effect allows for the distribution of forces from a working or loaded end to the supporting handle or rod without damage to the joint or handle. As such, the transfer of force is optimal when distributed circumferentially and is only as strong as the weakest point. For endodontically treated teeth, this idea of a re-enforcing ring is best captured by a ring of natural, healthy, robust tooth structure which forms the circumferential seat of an indirect restoration.

In general, ferrule should be completely circumferential (without exception), at least 2 mm high, and as thick as possible (minimum 1.0 mm) (Fig. 17.10). This ring of sound tooth structure is what allows for consistent and even distribution of loading forces onto a wider surface of tooth and minimises the concentration of force on one particular aspect of the restoration margin or underlying post or core restoration. Undue forces in these areas (especially down a post) can lead to premature tooth or root fracture, which is most often irretrievable and unrestorable.

17.4 Posts

Types

The primary purpose of the endodontic post is the provision of additional retention for the core restoration, regardless of material type. Much of the research to date has shown that past attempts to utilise posts to stiffen residual tooth structure, especially at the cervical region, were largely unsuccessful and this paradigm has since shifted to the preferred preservation of tooth structure and the utilisation of posts purely for core retention.

The large variety of posts available on the market today can be classified into several different categories: prefabricated/custom, active/passive, serrated/smooth, tapered/parallel, metal/carbon fibre/composite/ceramic and bonded/cemented (Figs. 17.11 and 17.12).

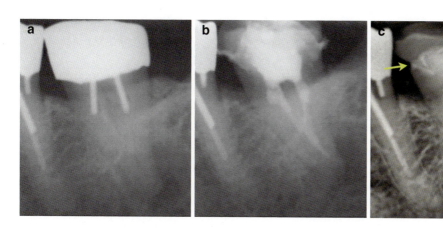

Fig. 17.9 Clinical radiographs demonstrating nonsurgical endodontic re-treatment of tooth 37. Note: (**a**) preoperative view demonstrating post retained full gold crown restoration with suboptimal root canal therapy and periradicular infection. (**b**) Post-treatment radiograph. The full gold crown restoration was dismantled, posts removed and endodontic re-treatment carried out. A double-seal IRM/GIC core restoration was placed and temporary crown re-cemented. The patient was advised to see her general dental practitioner for permanent cast cuspal coverage restoration. (**c**) A 12-month follow-up radiograph demonstrating periapical healing. A CEREC crown had been constructed. Note the marginal discrepancy mesially (*yellow arrow*) with composite cement that could potentially lead to failure

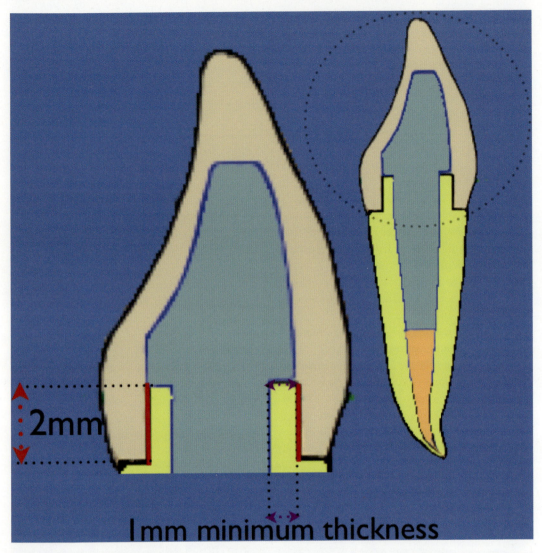

2mm

1mm minimum thickness

Fig. 17.10 Clinical diagram showing ferrule principle. Note: ferrule walls (*solid red lines*) almost parallel. Minimum height of ferrule wall should be at least 2 mm and minimum thickness of 1 mm to ensure adequate bracing of the crown to prevent catastrophic root fracture

In all of these key differences, each option must be carefully considered by the clinician to select the most appropriate type for each case. The increasing cost of precious alloys and higher patient demand for aesthetic restorations have led to the increased prevalence of prefabricated post types. The custom post (or cast post-core) also requires more clinical stages and is more susceptible to error at each stage; nevertheless, the cast post-core restoration is one of the best documented post types and has the advantage that it is the only post type which allows minimal preparation of the canal for post space, which is especially pertinent in cases where there is a paucity of residual radicular structure. The other key benefit of the cast post-core is the inherent cohesion between the post and core parts of the restoration; these two aspects are cast as the same restoration and, as such, afford the best union between the core and post.

A reliable method for fabricating a custom-cast post and core is direct fabrication of the pattern

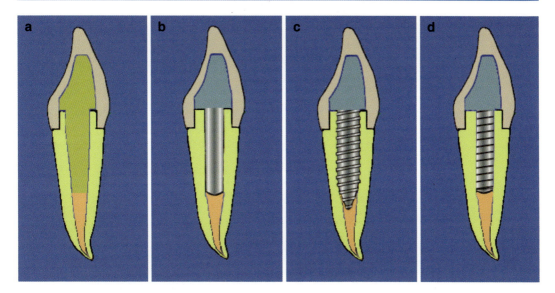

Fig. 17.11 Clinical diagrams showing (**a**) custom cast post and core design and (**b–d**) prefabricated post designs. Note: (**b**) tapered smooth, (**c**) tapered self-threading, and (**d**) parallel serrated

utilising an autopolymerising resin (Duralay self cure resin or GC Pattern Resin). The tooth is prepared for the crown after the existing restoration, any dental caries and weakened tooth structure are removed. A post space is created ensuring adequate length by removal of gutta-percha maintaining 4–5 mm of apical seal. The canal is lightly lubricated and the plastic dowel is checked for fit ensuring it extends to the full depth of the post space. A bead brush technique is used, and autopolymerising resin is added to the canal space, and the plastic dowel is seated completely. The resin is not allowed to set completely by loosening the dowel and re-seating it several times whilst it is still 'setting'. Once the resin has polymerised, the pattern is removed and inspected for any undercuts that are removed accordingly. The pattern post is again measured to verify correct post length and fit and ensuring it goes easily in and out of the canal without any interference. Additional resin is then added for the core. The final resin pattern post is then invested and cast in type II or type IV gold. Following casting the precious metal post can be cemented using zinc phosphate cement or GIC luting cement for intimate adaptation. A further impression is required for the overlying casting (see clinical case 3).

Alternatively the indirect method for fabrication of a custom post and core restoration is to take an impression of the post space using an elastomer and then the pattern can be fabricated on a die. The advantages of a custom post and core are less mechanical interfaces (i.e. post, tooth and core, crown) as opposed to three surfaces using prefabricated posts (i.e. post, tooth; core, crown; and post, core). Less mechanical interfaces means a greater chance of marginal adaptation with less discrepancies. The disadvantage, however, is that they are technically demanding and require greater chairside time (Fig. 17.13).

Conversely, all prefabricated post types require some degree of canal preparation to allow for a 'best-fit' post to be inserted into the space. This will require removal of radicular wall dentine and can result in a poor adaptation of the post to the canal if the most appropriate size post is not selected. The use of drills for the preparation of the post space is also a potentially hazardous stage, as maintaining parallelism along the path of the canal can be difficult. Nevertheless, the large range of materials and designs available for prefabricated posts has led to their increasing use in a variety of clinical situations. Regardless of the type of post used, it should be noted that these

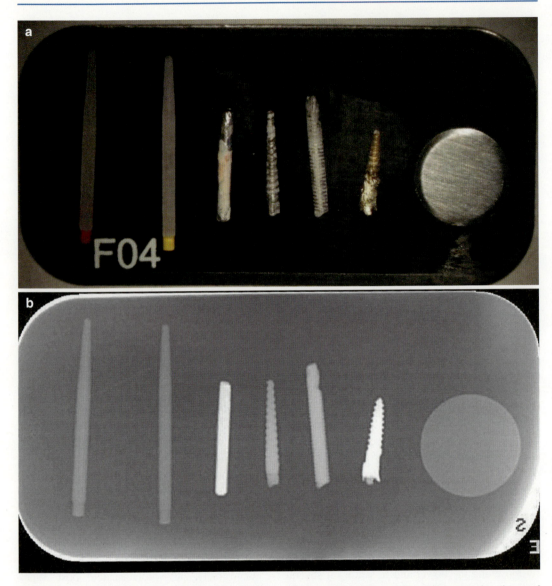

Fig. 17.12 Clinical photograph and radiograph demonstrating several types of posts and their respective radiodensities. Note: (**a**) shows fiber posts, smooth parallel, tapered serrated, smooth parallel serrated, and tapered self-threading screw post. (**b**) Fiber posts have the least radiopacities compared to prefabricated metal posts

are technique-sensitive procedures and, as such, care should be exercised in all stages of post placement. Those which require additional steps, such as flaring of post spaces, or bonding of resin-based luting cements, can be particularly challenging. The introduction, manipulation and control of etching agents, primers and bonding agents in constricted canal spaces is difficult in most situations, as is the photoactivation of luting agents with curing lights. Therefore, where

possible, conventionally cemented posts should be utilised in preference to bonded post types. In addition, the use of screw-type (active) posts should be avoided as these have been shown to introduce microfractures in dentine walls, which result in premature fatigue failure of tooth structure around active posts.

The defining feature of any successful post should be preservation of a maximal amount of residual tooth structure and adequate means

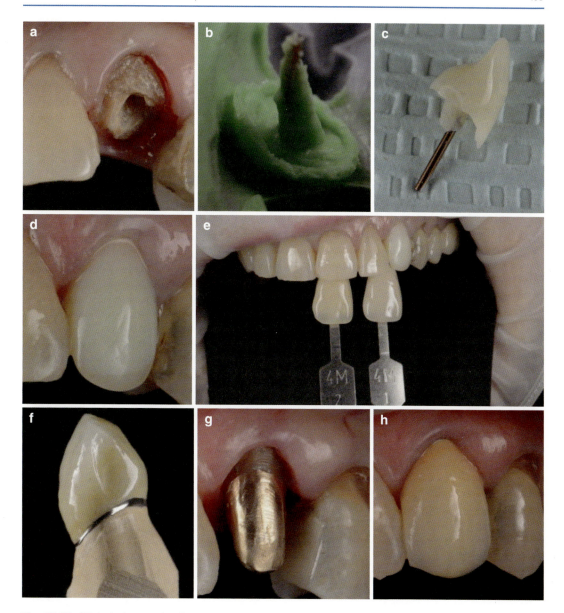

Fig. 17.13 Clinical photographs of post crown preparation in tooth 23 using the indirect method of fabrication. Note (**a**) pre-operative view showing minimal ferrule. (**b**) Following crown preparation an elastomeric impression is taken of the pre-prepared post space. (**c**) A temporary post crown is fabricated using a pre-fabricated parallel smooth post. (**d**) Temporary post crown restoration in place with good marginal adaptation to maintain coronal seal. (**e**) Shade selection. (**f**) Metal-ceramic crown on die and (**g**) custom fabricated gold post cemented in place. (**h**) Final permanent post core restoration with overlying metal-ceramic crown cemented in place

of adhesion (mechanical or chemical) to the overlying core material.

Post space preparation

The primary goal of post space preparation should be to preserve a maximal amount of resid-

ual tooth whilst creating the means for a close adaptation between the post and root. The integrity of the apical seal should also be maintained by preserving at least 4–5 mm of obturation material apical to the post space (Fig. 17.14). In addition, the use of a barrier seal above the obtu-

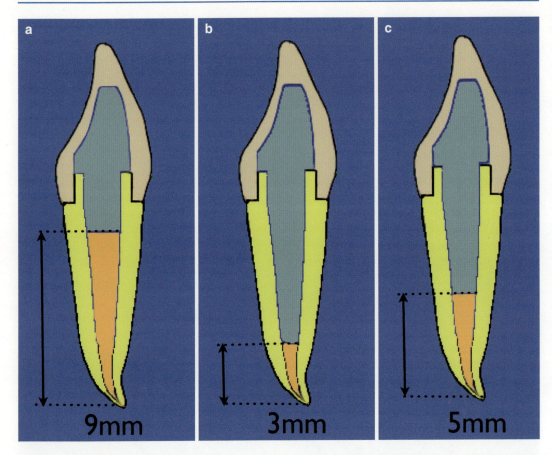

Fig. 17.14 Diagrammatic representation of ideal length of remaining root filling and post length. Note: (**a**) 9 mm of gutta-percha results in a short post with poor retention. (**b**) 3 mm of remaining gutta-percha increases the post length but compromises the apical seal. (**c**) Ideally 5 mm of gutta-percha ensures the apical seal is maintained with an adequate length of post

ration should be utilised to maximise the extent and effect of the coronal seal – this may take the form of CAVIT or GIC. Where a post is to be cemented using GIC, this barrier may not be necessary, provided that the GIC luting agent is introduced carefully into the most apical part of the preparation under the post. Post length should extend ½–¾ of the length of the root; however, in shorter roots, the minimum apical seal of 4 mm should be preserved at the cost of post length. No more than a single post is necessary for the retention of the core, and the most robust root with the widest canal space should be selected in multi-rooted teeth (palatal roots of maxillary molars, buccal roots of maxillary premolars, distal roots of mandibular molars).

Cementation

Several luting agents are available to the clinician including zinc phosphate, glass ionomer, polycarboxylate, resin-modified glass ionomer and resin cements. Zinc phosphate cement is often the cement of choice as it has an extended working time and high strength. The complete introduction of luting agent into a post space is critical in the successful seating of posts. Prior to this however, the prepared space should be debrided of the dentinal smear layer and proteinaceous debris with the application of appropriate conditioning agents, rinsing with ample water and appropriate drying. All of these processes can prove difficult in constricted spaces, and as such, auxiliary measures such as the use of long taper-tipped micro-applicator brushes and paper points may be required for these stages. The post should be smeared with an even layer of cement and thin coating of cement introduced into the post space. Once the post is inserted, it should be stabilised during the initial setting phase of the luting agent. Excess cement that extrudes past the coronal aspect of the post should be cleared in order to allow core material to come into intimate contact with the underlying tooth and post head.

17.5 Clinical Cases

Case 1 Non-surgical treatment of tooth 17 (distal bridge abutment) and permanent restoration with composite resin

A fit and healthy 42-year-old female patient was referred for endodontic management of tooth 17 in specialist endodontic practice. The patient had been aware of localised pain and gingival swelling in relation to the tooth. Tooth 17 was a distal bridge abutment with good marginal adaptation. Two draining sinuses were present in the overlying attached and alveolar mucosa. A narrow 7 mm probing profile was noted in the mid-buccal aspect of the tooth. Radiographic examination revealed a fused root with obvious peri-radicular infection. Gutta-percha points placed in the draining sinuses were tracked to the peri-apex of tooth 17. The patient was warned of the possibility of a root fracture, and a decision was made to embark upon non-surgical root canal therapy. Access cavity was prepared through the existing crown to reveal two necrotic canals. Chemomechanical preparation was completed using 1 % sodium hypochlorite solution. An interim calcium hydroxide dressing was placed and the patient reviewed at 4 weeks. At the review appointment, the sinuses had resolved and the pocketing was within normal limits. The patient returned for completion of endodontic treatment, and obturation was completed using a warm vertical compaction technique using AH plus cement. A double seal IRM/glass ionomer restoration was placed, and the patient returned to her general dental practitioner for placement of a composite core restoration (Fig. 17.15).

Case 2 Non-surgical retreatment of tooth 15 and permanent restoration with CEREC crown

A fit and healthy 24-year-old medical student was referred for endodontic retreatment of tooth 15. The patient had been experiencing pain and tenderness in relation to this tooth intermittently. Radiographic examination confirmed previous suboptimal root canal therapy in a single canal. An extensive peri-radicular infection was noted. A second untreated canal was suspected and the patient agreed to non-surgical root canal retreatment. Access cavity was prepared and previous root filling material removed using a chloroform wicking technique. A second untreated palatal canal orifice was located. Patency was achieved in both canals and chemomechanical preparation completed using 1 % sodium hypochlorite solution. An interim calcium hydroxide dressing was placed for 3 months. At the review appointment, the patient's symptoms had resolved and the tooth remained asymptomatic. The patient returned for completion of endodontic treatment. A warm vertical compaction technique using AH plus cement was used to obturate the canals. An interim double seal IRM/glass ionomer temporary restoration was placed. The patient was advised to proceed with permanent cast cuspal coverage restoration. At the 6-month review appointment, the tooth remained asymptomatic. The patient had had a CEREC crown placed. Radiographic examination revealed an intact periodontal ligament space associated with the peri-apex of tooth 15 (Fig. 17.16).

Case 3 Non-surgical retreatment of teeth 12 and 25 and permanent restoration with post crowns (direct Duralay method)

A 21-year-old fit and healthy male patient was referred for endodontic retreatment of teeth 12 and 25 at the Eastman Dental Hospital.

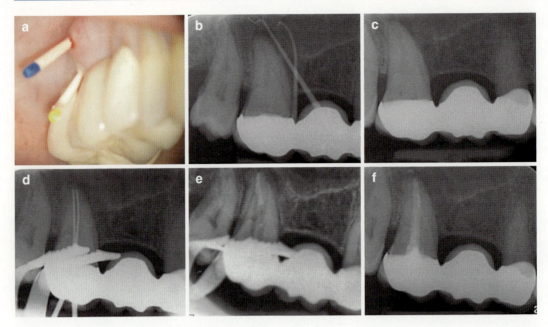

Fig. 17.15 Clinical photographs and radiographs showing nonsurgical endodontic treatment of tooth 17 (distal bridge abutment). Note: (**a**) gutta-percha points placed in the draining sinuses overlying the buccal aspect of tooth 17. (**b**) Gutta-percha sinus tract radiograph confirming association with tooth 17. (**c**) Preoperative parallel radiograph revealing calcified canal system and periradicular infection apically. (**d**) Following access preparation through the existing cast restoration, two necrotic canals were chemo-mechanically prepared using 1 % sodium hypochlorite solution. An intra-canal dressing of calcium hydroxide was placed and the patient reviewed at 4 weeks. (**e–f**) Following review the localized pocketing and sinuses had resolved. Obturation was completed using a warm vertical compaction technique using AH plus cement. A double temporary seal using IRM/glass ionomer cement was used. The patient returned to her general dental practitioner for placement of a permanent composite core restoration to prevent future reinfection

The patient's chief complaint was related to the dark appearance of tooth 12. The patient reported both teeth had undergone root canal treatment in his early teens, and following completion of treatment, the teeth had remained asymptomatic.

Clinical examination revealed tooth 12 had been restored with a composite restoration, which was stained. The clinical crown was discoloured with a yellow-grey appearance. Tooth 25 had an extensive MOD amalgam restoration.

Radiographic examination revealed tooth 12 had an overextended root filling beyond the radiographic apex. A non-corticated well-defined radiolucency was noted. Tooth 25 had a poorly condensed root filling noted with a widened periodontal ligament space at the peri-apex. The patient agreed to non-surgical root canal retreatment of both teeth (Fig. 17.17).

The overextended gutta-percha in tooth 12 was retrieved using a Hedström braiding technique. Chemomechanical debridement and preparation was uneventful. Nevertheless at the time of obturation, the coronal ½ of the crown fractured resulting in a further master apical file radiograph being taken to confirm the working length. After obturating the canal system, a post space was created using the ParaPost system by the hand (red), ensuring that at least 5 mm of apical gutta-percha remained. 2 mm of IRM was placed over the remaining gutta-percha and the tooth was temporised using a temporary post and TempBond cement. A putty impression of tooth 12 was made on the study cast. A temporary crown was constructed using bis-acryl resin (Integrity, Dentsply, Weybridge, UK) and cemented in place until a post and core were constructed using the direct Duralay technique.

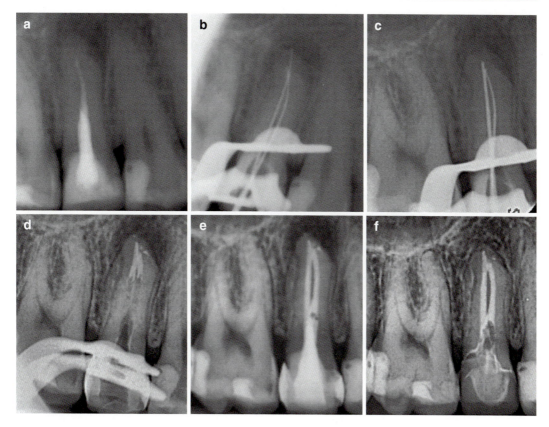

Fig. 17.16 Clinical radiographs demonstrating endodontic re-treatment of tooth 15. Note: (**a**) preoperative view showing single off-center canal obturated short of the apex. An extensive periradicular radiolucency was evident. A second untreated canal was suspect. (**b, c**) IAF and MAF radiographs. Following removal of previous root filling material using a chloroform wicking technique, two canals were chemo-mechanically prepared using 1 % sodium hypochlorite solution. Patency was maintained throughout the cleaning procedure and sonic irrigation was used to supplement canal cleaning. An interim dressing of calcium hydroxide was placed for 3 months. At the review appointment, the tooth remained asymptomatic. (**d–e**) The canals were obturated using a warm vertical compaction technique using AH plus cement. A double-seal temporary IRM/glass ionomer restoration was placed as a temporary measure. (**f**) The patient returned 6 months later and the tooth has been restored with a CEREC restoration. Radiographic examination confirmed an intact periodontal ligament space apically

Tooth 25 was asymptomatic but was being re-root treated on the grounds of technical revision of the existing root filling prior to a permanent cast restoration being provided. Restorability was judged to be possible with the provision of a cast post to retain any future core. Root canal retreatment was completed over two visits, and at the final visit after obturation, post space was created in both palatal and buccal canals. 2 mm of IRM was placed over the remaining root filling and the tooth temporised with IRM until crown preparation and post impression for a direct two-part sectional post and core.

Teeth 12 and 25 were prepared to receive a ceramo-metal crown. For the indirect post and core restoration of tooth 12, the margins were kept on natural tooth structure. A solid plastic ParaPost equivalent to the drill used for post preparation was verified for fit into the canal. In a Dappens dish, acrylic resin monomer and polymer were mixed to moderate viscosity (Duralay). The canal was lubricated with petroleum jelly and the orifice of the canal filled with acrylic resin. The pattern was coated with monomer and seated in the canal. The pattern was then pumped in and out during its setting phase (Fig. 17.19). After the

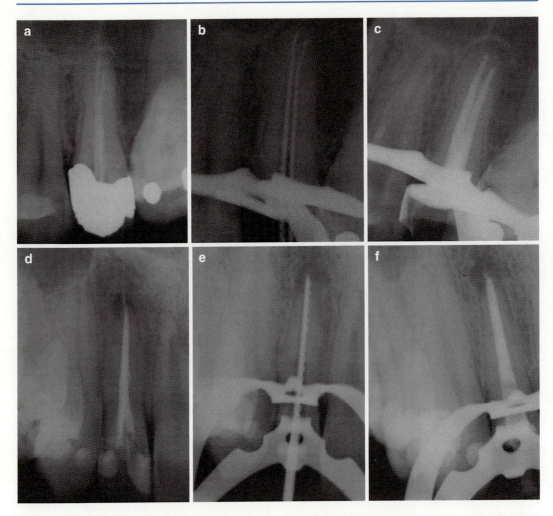

Fig. 17.17 Clinical radiographs demonstrating (**a–c**) nonsurgical endodontic re-treatment of tooth 25 and (**d–f**) nonsurgical endodontic re-treatment of tooth 12. Note: the MOD amalgam in the tooth was dismantled and restorability assessment confirmed that a post-crown restoration would need to be constructed. Tooth 12 was originally to be treated with a full ceramic crown restoration. However, during the chemo-mechanical preparation phase, the crown fractured. A post and core restoration would need to be fabricated to support the final cast restoration. Both teeth were treated using the indirect post and core method using Duralay

resin had polymerised, a second mix of acrylic resin was mixed and placed around the exposed part of the sprue and roughly moulded before final adjustments using fine sandpaper discs. In tooth 25, the palatal canal was employed for the dowel preparation using the Duralay technique described above. The buccal canal had an orthodontic wire seated of equivalent diameter to ParaPost drill used for post preparation. When the acrylic had become tough and doughy, the orthodontic wire was pumped in and out to ensure that it could be removed easily. The crown form was subsequently built up (Figs. 17.18 and 17.19).

For both teeth 12 and 25, a 4 mm wax sprue was attached to the facial surface of the Duralay pattern at an angle of about 45° (Figs. 17.18 and 17.19). The pattern was then sprayed with a wetting agent, and a layer of vacuum-mixed phosphate-bonded investment material (Cera-Fina, Whip Mix Corporation, Utah, USA) was applied with a brush to the external surface of the pattern. The sprued pattern was placed in a lined casting ring,

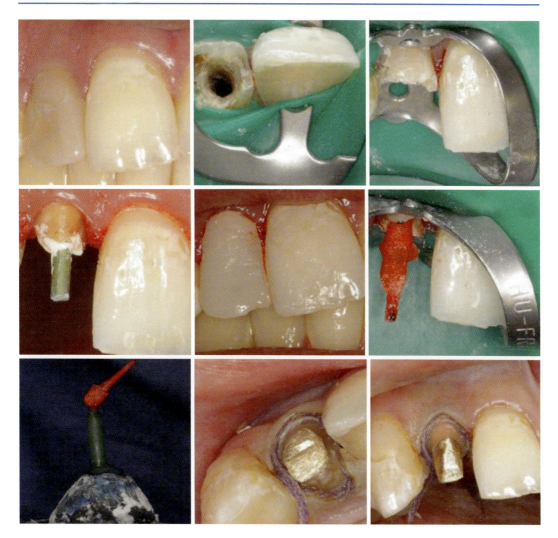

Fig. 17.18 Clinical photographs demonstrating direct post and core construction for tooth 12

which was then filled with investment material. The laboratory technician carried out the casting procedure. After extraction from the casting ring, the post and core were treated with a 50 mm glass bead 'sandblasting' to remove the oxide layer. The sprue was then removed and any casting imperfections were removed under a microscope.

The post and cores were tried in to assess fit. A periapical radiograph was taken to confirm seating of the post and core. The post and core restorations were cemented using zinc phosphate cement and the excess removed (Fig. 17.20). An overimpression was made from the diagnostic cast using Lab putty. Temporary crowns were constructed using bis-acryl resin (Integrity, Dentsply, Weybridge, UK) and cemented in place using TempBond cement prior to final definitive cast restoration construction.

Case 4 Non-surgical endodontic treatment tooth 47 and permanent restoration with full gold crown restoration

A fit and healthy 36-year-old patient was referred to the department of endodontics at the Eastman Dental Institute by his general dental practitioner (GDP) for root canal treatment of

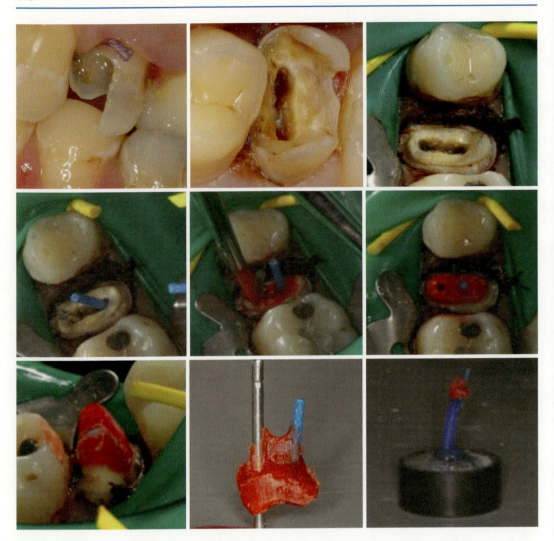

Fig. 17.19 Clinical photographs demonstrating direct sectional post and core construction for tooth 25

teeth 36 and 47. The patient attended his GDP who explained that both 36 and 47 were deeply carious and required endodontic therapy. The patient was aware of 'past endodontic failures' and given the strategic importance of these teeth preferred to be seen by a specialist if possible. The patient was an irregular attendee prior to registration with his GDP.

Soft tissue examination revealed a large hyperplastic discharging sinus associated with the mesial aspect of tooth 47. Tooth 47 had a fractured amalgam restoration with a mesial temporary dressing. Extensive caries was noted in tooth

36. Tooth 47 had a large carious lesion affecting the mesial pulp horn. The broad single root had an associated widening of the periodontal ligament.

Tooth 36 was extracted under local anaesthesia. The extraction site healed uneventfully. Endodontic treatment of tooth 47 was carried out over three visits with calcium hydroxide used as an inter-appointment dressing. Irrigation using 2.5 % sodium hypochlorite was used throughout treatment. Working lengths of all canals were estimated using an electronic apex locator and subsequently verified

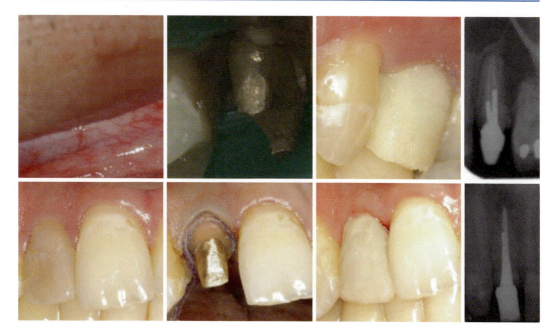

Fig. 17.20 Clinical photographs and radiographs demonstrating post-cementation of the post and core and temporary crown restorations in teeth 12 and 25

radiographically. Master apical file radiograph confirmed that the ML and D canals joined apically with the MB canal having a separate foramen. Obturation was completed with resolution of the sinus tract, using gutta-percha and Roth's® SEALER, with a combination of 'chloroform dip' and cold lateral compaction apically, followed by the 'energised spreading' technique coronally. The core was formed with IRM and amalgam (see Fig. 17.21).

Tooth 47 was subsequently prepared for a full gold crown restoration. A sectional silicone impression was taken of tooth 47 to aid in making a temporary restoration. The tooth was prepared and impressions were taken using light- and heavy-bodied President silicone impression material. A working cast was constructed, trimmed and mounted in the intercuspal position using a Duralay bonnet (Fig. 17.21).

The restoration was waxed up on the sectional cast and marginated on the respective die under magnification. The die was then sprued, invested and cast with type III gold (70 %). The fitting surface was examined under magnification to check

for casting errors and the restoration polished and occlusion checked. The restoration was then tried in the mouth, and the fit, margin and occlusion were checked prior to cementation with zinc phosphate (Fig. 17.21).

Case 5 Non-surgical retreatment of tooth 17 and permanent restoration with full-cast gold crown restoration

A 58-year-old fit and healthy accountant was referred for root canal retreatment of tooth 17 at the Royal London Dental Hospital. The patient had been experiencing intermittent localised pain and discomfort with the tooth, which had been previously treated, more than 15 years ago. Clinical examination revealed tooth 17 had been restored with a full gold crown restoration. Tooth 17 was non-functional (opposing bilateral free end saddle cobalt-chrome denture). Radiographic examination confirmed a marginal discrepancy associated with the coronal cast restoration. Gutta-percha root filling material was seen in the palatal canal (P) and silver point fillings in the

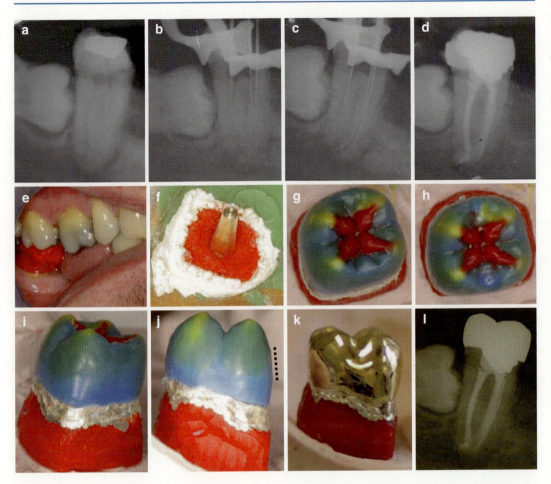

Fig. 17.21 Clinical radiographs and photographs demonstrating nonsurgical endodontic treatment of tooth 47 and full gold crown restoration. Note: (**a**) preoperative view of tooth 47 with fused root and periradicular infection. (**b**) IAF and (**c**) MAF radiographs demonstrating acute apical curvatures and confluence of canals. (**d**) Final obturation using warm lateral compaction technique. (**e**–**k**) Full gold crown preparation including laboratory wax up and casting. (**l**) Final full gold crown restoration cemented in place. Note: guide planes and rest seats were incorporated for lower partial denture

mesiobuccal (MB1) and distobuccal (DB) canals. A peri-radicular radiolucency was noted with the MB1 and P apices.

A sectional impression was taken of tooth 17, as a template for fabrication of the temporary crown. The crown, caries and access cavity restorative material were removed. The silver points were removed by engaging them with a 25 size Hedström file and then elevating the file in a clockwise motion with artery forceps, using the remaining coronal structure as a rest.

Following chemomechanical preparation, all canals were obturated with gutta-percha and Roth® Sealer; IRM® was used as a sub-coronal seal and the access cavity filled with amalgam (Fig. 17.22).

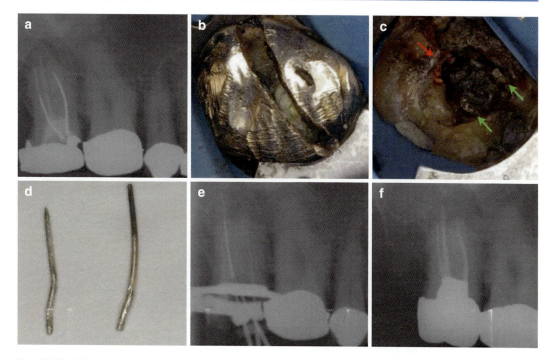

Fig. 17.22 Clinical radiographs and photographs demonstrating nonsurgical root canal re-treatment of tooth 17 and full gold crown restoration. Note: (**a**) preoperative view demonstrating defective cast restoration with overhang distally and mesial discrepancy. Note gutta-percha root filling and silver points in MB and DB canals. (**b**) Crown restoration sectioned. (**c**) Following dismantling of core underlying gutta-percha (*red arrow*) and silver points identified (*green arrows*). (**d**) Successful retrieval of silver points. (**e**) Master apical files in place and working lengths confirmed radiographically and by electronic apex locator. (**f**) Obturation completed and core and final cast cuspal coverage full gold crown restoration cemented in place

Following completion of root canal retreatment of tooth 17, clinical and laboratory work for construction of a cast restoration was conducted. The gold crown on tooth 16 had decemented. The crown was removed, amalgam core dismantled, caries removed and core replaced. The crown preparations on teeth 16 and 17 were refined and a master impression taken using light- and heavy-bodied silicone. A face bow record along with a lower alginate impression (denture in situ) was taken in order to mount the upper cast.

The silicone and alginate impressions were poured using vacuum-mixed Fuji-Rock®. The casts were trimmed and mounted in RCP using the face bow record on a Denar® semi-adjustable articulator.

The restorations were waxed up on the sectional cast and marginated on the dies under magnification. These were then sprued, invested and cast with type III gold (70 %) (Figs. 17.23, 17.24 and 17.25). The fitting surfaces were examined under magnification to check for casting errors and the crowns polished and the occlusion checked. The finished full gold crowns were tried in the mouth and the fit, margins and occlusion were checked. Zinc phosphate cement was then used to cement the castings in place (Fig. 17.22).

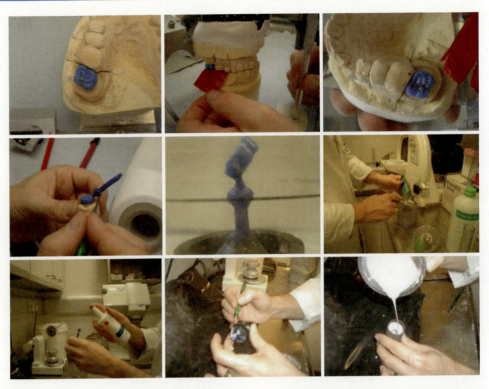

Fig. 17.23 Clinical photographs showing completed anatomic wax up of tooth 17 and laboratory stages for full gold crown construction

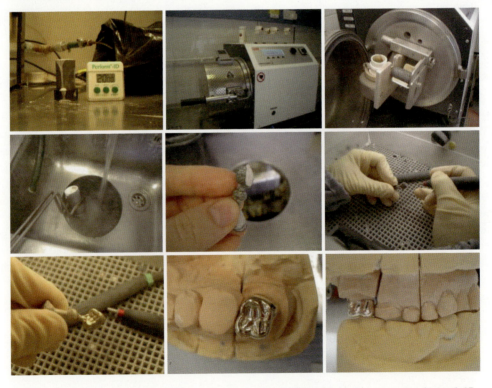

Fig. 17.24 Clinical photographs demonstrating laboratory stages for full gold crown construction for tooth 17

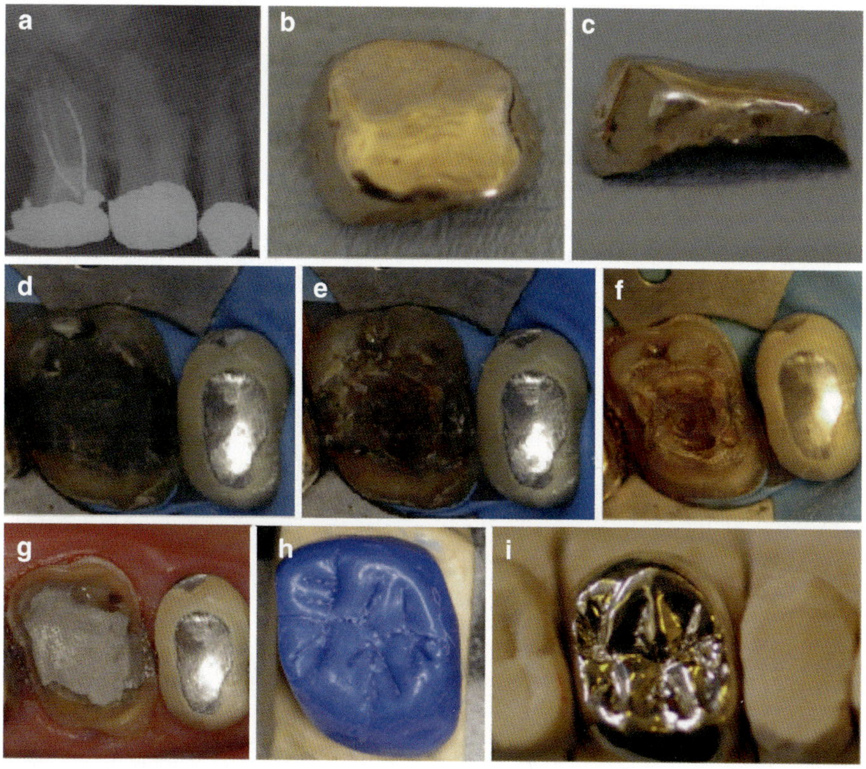

Fig. 17.25 Clinical radiograph and photographs showing full gold crown construction for tooth 16. Note: (**a**) Preoperative view of tooth 16. The pulpal status of this tooth was deemed to be vital. (**b, c**) Tooth 16 crown debonded. (**d–g**) Previous core removal, refinement of crown preparation, and replacement core. (**h**) Anatomic wax up of new crown. (**i**) Full gold crown construction completed, ready for definitive cementation

Clinical Hints and Tips for Restoring Endodontically Treated Teeth

- Restorability assessment should begin prior to initiating root canal therapy. Existing coronal restorations should be dismantled to allow the clinician to visualise remaining sound tooth structure and plan for the definitive restoration.

- During endodontic procedures and/or post space preparation, the loss of tooth structure should be minimised.

- Intact anterior teeth (incisors and canines) with conservative endodontic access and intact marginal ridges do not require coronal coverage restorations or posts. Composite resin restorations should be suitable to maintain coronal seal.

- Posterior endodontically treated teeth should be restored with cuspal coverage restorations. MOD onlay restorations, ¾ crowns, 7/8th crowns and full crown restorations can be placed depending on remaining tooth structure. Inlay restorations should be avoided.

- When preparing teeth for cuspal coverage restorations, ensure that parallel ferrule walls are present with a minimal 2 mm length in the apico-coronal direction. In addition, the thickness of remaining dentine should be no less than 1 mm on both the buccal/lingual and interproximal aspect.

- Posts are only indicated to retain the core build-up. They do not strengthen the tooth or root.

- Morphological structure and function must be considered when planning post placement to avoid iatrogenic perforation.

- Increased post length results in increased retention and resistance to fracture. Length of posts must be balanced against the risk of root thinning or perforation and minimal apical gutta-percha of 5 mm to maintain the apical seal. Minimum post length that extends into the root below the crown margin should be a length at least equal to the height of the crown.

- Dentine conservation is paramount when selecting a particular post, and a post diameter should be selected that requires minimal canal preparation. Increasing the diameter of the post does not increase the retention. Parallel post designs offer increased retention over tapered designs.
- The type of cement used appears to be of minimal importance in relation to retention and resistance of the post.
- Parallel passive, serrated, self-vented, prefabricated posts are recommended for small circular canals. Where concerns exist regarding thin roots, a tapered post design may be preferred.
- Custom-cast post and core restorations are recommended when coronal tooth structure loss is moderate to severe.

References

1. Siqueira JF, Rocas IN, Ricucci D, Hulsmann M. Causes and management of post-treatment apical periodontitis. Brit Dent J. 2014;216(6):305–12.
2. Ray HA, Trope M. Periapical status of endodontically treated teeth in relation to the technical quality of the root filling and the coronal restoration. Int Endod J. 1995;28:12–8.
3. Tronstad L, Asbjornsen K, Doving L, Paedersen I, Eriksen HM. Influence of coronal restorations on the periapical health of endodontically treated teeth. Endod Dent Traumatol. 2000;16:218–22.
4. Saunders WP, Saunders EM. Coronal leakage as a cause of failure in root canal therapy: a review. Endod Dent Traumatol. 1994;10:105–8.
5. Guttmann JL. The dentine-root complex: Anatomic and biologic considerations in restoring endodontically treated teeth. J Prosthet Dent. 1992;67(4): 458–67.
6. Mannocci F, Cowie J. Restoration of endodontically treated teeth. Brit Dent J. 2014;216(6):341–6.
7. Helfer AR, Melnick S, Schilder H. Determination of moisture content of vital and pulpless teeth. Oral Surg Oral Med Oral Pathol. 1972;34:661–70.

8. Rivera EM, Yamauchi M. Site comparisons of dentine collagen cross-linking from extracted human teeth. Arch Oral Biol. 1993;38:541–6.
9. Huang TG, Schilder H, Nathanson D. Effects of moisture content and endodontic treatment on some mechanical properties of human dentin. J Endod. 1992;18:209–15.
10. Sedgley CM, Messer HH. Are endodontically treated teeth more brittle? J Endod. 1992;18:332–5.
11. Reeh ES, Messer HH, Douglas WH. Reduction in tooth stiffness as a result of endodontic and restorative procedures. J Endod. 1989;15:512–6.
12. Randow K, Glantz P. On Cantilever loading of vital and non-vital teeth. Acta Odontol Scand. 1986;44: 271–7.
13. Pantivisai P, Messer HH. Cuspal deflection in molars in relation to endodontic and restorative procedures. J Endod. 1995;21:57–61.
14. Swanson K, Madison S. An evaluation of coronal micro-leakage in endodontically treated teeth. Part I: time periods. J Endod. 1987;13(2):56–9.
15. Schwartz RS, Robbins JW. Post placement and Restoration of Endodontically treated teeth: a literature review. J Endod. 2004;30(5):289–301.
16. Hansen EK. In vivo cusp fracture of endodontically treated premolars restored with MOD amalgam or MOD resin fillings. Dent Mater. 1988;4:169–73.
17. Hansen EK, Asmussen E, Christiansen NC. In vivo fractures of endodontically treated posterior teeth restored with amalgam. Endod Dent Traumatol. 1990;6:49–55.
18. Sorensen JA, Martinoff JT. Intra-coronal reinforcement and coronal coverage: a study of endodontically treated teeth. J Prosthet Dent. 1984;51:780–4.
19. Tamse A, Zilburg I, Halpern J. Vertical root fractures in adjacent maxillary premolars: an endodontic-prosthetic perplexity. Int Endod J. 1998;31(2):127–32.
20. Sorensen JA, Martinoff JT. Endodontically treated teeth as abutments. J Prosthet Dent. 1985;53:631–6.
21. Sorensen JA, Martinoff JT. Clinically significant factors in dowel design. J Prosthet Dent. 1984;52: 28–35.
22. Aqualina SA, Caplan DJ. Relationship between crown placement and the survival of endodontically treated teeth. J Prosthet Dent. 2002;87:256–63.
23. Sorensen JA, Engleman MJ. Ferrule design and fracture resistance of endodontically treated teeth. J Prosthet Dent. 1990;63:529–36.
24. Juloski J, Radovic I, Goracci C, Vulicevic ZR, Ferrari M. Ferrule effect: A literature review. J Endod. 2012;38:11–9.
25. Nayyar A, Walton RE. An amalgam coronal radicular dowel and core technique for endodontically treated posterior teeth. J Prosthet Dent. 1980;44:511–5.
26. Papa J, Wilson PR, Tyas MJ. Pins for direct restorations. J Dent. 1993;21:259–64.
27. Shavell HM. The amalgapin technique for complex amalgam restorations. J Calif Dent Assoc. 1980;8: 48–55.

28. Newsome PRH. Slot retention: an alternative to pins in the large amalgam restoration. Dent Update. 1988;15:202–7.
29. Tjan AHL, Munoz-Viveros CA, Valencai-Rave GM. Tensile dislodgment of composite/amalgam cores: dentin adhesives versus mechanical retention. J Dent Res. 1997;76:183.
30. Mackenzie L, Parmar D, Shortall AC, Burke FJ. Direct anterior composites: a practical guide. Dent Update. 2013;40:297–317.
31. Shillingburg HT Jr, Hobo S, Whitsett L, Jacobi R. Fundamentals of fixed prosthodontics. In: Chapter 10 Preparations for full veneer crowns. 3rd ed. Chicago, IL: Quintessence publishing Co, Inc.; 1997. pp. 138–154
32. Pjetursson BE, Sailer I, Zwahlen M, Hammerle CH. A systematic review of the survival and complication rates of all-ceramic and metal-ceramic reconstructions after an observation period of at least 3 years. Part I: single crowns. Clin Oral Implants Res. 2007;18 Suppl 3:73–85.
33. Salehrabi R, Rotstein I. Endodontic treatment outcome in a large patient population in the USA: an epidemiological study. J Endod. 2004;12:846–50.
34. Plasmans J, Creugers NH, Mulder J. Long-term survival of extensive amalgam restorations. J Dent Res. 1998;77:453–60.
35. Starr CB. Amalgam crown restorations for posterior pulpless teeth. J Prosthet Dent. 1990;63(6):614–9.
36. Mannocci F, Bertelli E, Sherriff M, Watson TF, Ford TR. Three-year clinical comparison of survival of endodontically treated teeth restored with either full cast coverage restorations or with direct composite restorations. J Prosthet Dent. 2002;88:297–301.
37. Stravropoulou AF, Koidis PT. A systematic review of single crowns on endodontically treated teeth. J Dent. 2007;35:761–7.
38. Robbins JW. Restoration of the endodontically treated tooth. Dent Clin N Am. 2002;46:367–84.
39. Ree M, Schwartz R. The Endo-restorative interface: current concepts. Dent Clin N Am. 2010;54:345–74.
40. Tsesis I, Fuss Z. Diagnosis and treatment of accidental root perforations. Endodontic Topics. 2006;13:95–107.
41. Heydecke G, Peters MC. The restoration of endodontically treated single rooted teeth with cast or direct post and cores: a systematic review. J Prosthet Dent. 2002;87:380–6.
42. Gluskin AH, Radke RA, Frost SL, Watanabe LG. The mandibular incisor: rethinking guidelines for post and core design. J Endod. 1995;21:33–7.
43. Standlee JP, Caputo AA, Hanson EC. Retention of endodontic dowels: effects of cement, dowel length, diameter and design. J Prosthet Dent. 1978;39:401–5.
44. Mannocci F, Ferrari M, Watson TF. Intermittent loading of teeth restored using quartz fiber, carbon-quartz fiber and zirconium dioxide ceramic root canal posts. J Adhes Dent. 1999;1:153–8.
45. Akkayan B, Gulmez T. Resistance to fracture of endodontically treated teeth restored with different post systems. J Prosthet Dent. 2002;87(4):431–7.
46. Ferrari M, Cagidiaco MC, Grandini S, De Sanctis M, Goracci C. Post placement affects survival of endodontically treated premolars. J Dent Res. 2007;86:729–34.
47. Ferrari M, Vichi A, Garcia-Godoy F. Clinical evaluation of fiber-reinforced epoxy resin posts and cast post and cores. Am J Dent. 2000;13:15B–8.
48. Nergiz I, Schmage P, Ozcan M, Platzer U. Effect of length and diameter of tapered posts on the retention. J Oral Rehabil. 2002;29:28–34.
49. Fuss Z, Lustig J, Katz A, Tamse A. An evaluation of endodontically treated vertical root fractured teeth: impact of operative procedures. J Endod. 2001;27:46–8.
50. Mattison GD, Delivanis PD, Thacker RW, Hansel KJ. Effect of post preparation on the apical seal. J Prosthet Dent. 1984;51:785–9.
51. Raiden GC, Gendleman H. Effect of dowel space preparation on the apical seal of root canal fillings. Endod Dent Traumatol. 1994;10:109–12.
52. Fox K, Gutteridge DL. An in-vitro study of coronal microleakage in root-canal treated teeth restored by the post and core technique. Int End J. 1997;30:361–81.
53. Fan B, Wu MK, Wesselink PR. Coronal leakage along apical root fillings after immediate and delayed post space preparation. Endo Dent Traumatol. 1999;15:124–7.
54. Newburg RE, Pameijer CH. Retentive properties of post and core systems. J Prosthet Dent. 1976;36:636–43.
55. Libman WJ, Nicholls JI. Load fatigue of teeth restored with cast post and cores and complete crowns. Int J Prosthodont. 1995;8:155–61.
56. Trushkowsky RD. Restoration of endodontically treated teeth: criteria and technique considerations. Quintessence Int. 2014;45(7):557–67.
57. Polesel A. Restoration of the endodontically treated posterior tooth. G Ital Endod. 2014;28:2–16.

Nonvital Bleaching

18

Sarita Atreya and Bobby Patel

Summary

The walking bleach technique with a mixture of sodium perborate (Bocasan) and distilled water is a technique recognized for intra-coronal bleaching. A well-condensed root filling must be present with the absence of any signs or symptoms that would indicate the presence of apical periodontitis. To prevent the potential for resorption, a cement barrier must be in place to prevent the passage of oxidizing agent into the dentinal tubules in the cervical aspect of the tooth.

Clinical Relevance

With correct case selection, it can be a reliable treatment modality in an effort to improve the appearance of a discoloured tooth with relatively low risk. The benefits must be weighed against the risk of external cervical root resorption often associated with a history of trauma. Furthermore sufficient cervical sealing and avoiding the use of the thermocatalytic method (hydrogen peroxide 30 % with heat) minimize this risk of resorption.

18.1 Overview of Nonvital Bleaching

It is of paramount importance that dental practitioners understand the aetiology of tooth discolouration in order to arrive at a correct diagnosis leading to selection of an appropriate treatment modality for any particular tooth discolouration. Tooth discolouration can be classified as extrinsic, intrinsic or a combination of both (see Table 18.1).

The discoloured anterior nonvital tooth has likely been weakened from a combination of previous trauma, endodontic therapy, dental caries and restorative treatment. Destructive alternative prosthodontic treatment options such as veneers or crowns are odds to further weaken the tooth lending it towards possible failure and extraction in the future.

Nonvital tooth bleaching is both useful and less detrimental in the treatment of traumatized discoloured anterior teeth. Different protocols

S. Atreya, BDS, MFDS RCS(ED)
ACT Health, Canberra, ACT, Australia

B. Patel, BDS MFDS MClinDent MRD MRACDS (✉)
Specialist Endodontist, Brindabella Specialist Centre,
Canberra, ACT, Australia
e-mail: bobbypatel@me.com

© Springer International Publishing Switzerland 2016
B. Patel (ed.), *Endodontic Treatment, Retreatment, and Surgery*,
DOI 10.1007/978-3-319-19476-9_18

Table 18.1 Causes of tooth discolouration

A. Extrinsic
- (i) Chromogenic diet (wine, coffee, tea)
- (ii) Tobacco
- (iii) Mouthrinses
- (iv) Plaque

B. Intrinsic
- *(i) Systemic causes*
  - Tetracycline staining
  - Metabolic disorders (fluorosis, dystrophic calcification)
  - Genetic (congenital erythropoietic porphyria, amelogenesis imperfecta, dentinogenesis imperfecta)
- *(ii) Local causes*
  - Pulp necrosis
  - Intrapulpal haemorrhage
  - Pulp tissue remnants after endodontic treatment
  - Endodontic materials
  - Coronal filling materials
  - Root resorption
  - Ageing
  - Trauma (calcific metamorphosis)

have been advocated for bleaching these teeth including the conventional walking bleach technique [1–3], the chairside power bleaching technique [3] and a modified home bleaching technique [4].

The bleaching agents commonly used for whitening root-filled teeth include hydrogen peroxide (concentrations ranging from 5 to 35 %) [5], carbamide peroxide (10 %) [6] and sodium perborate [1, 7–9].

Sodium perborate is an oxidizing agent available as powder (Bocasan). The walking bleach technique utilizes a paste formed by mixing sodium perborate and distilled water. This technique can lead to successful whitening of nonvital root-filled teeth reducing the risks of side effects [5].

Nonvital bleaching is proposed for endodontically treated teeth which have become discoloured as a result of pulpal necrosis [5], intrapulpal haemorrhage [10], pulp tissue remnants after endodontic treatment [11] and incomplete removal of filling materials and sealer remnants in the coronal access cavity [12].

The occurrence of external cervical root resorption is a serious complication following nonvital bleaching techniques, and its incidence ranges from 1 to 13 % [13–18]. External cervical root resorption can occur more frequently in those cases where higher concentrations of bleach were used, past history of trauma and use of the thermocatalytic method of bleaching (application of heat) [16–18].

The patient must be informed that although the option of nonvital bleaching is a relatively low-risk intervention, from a restorative point of view, it is prone to reversal and reoccurrence of discolouration in the long term [19].

To summarize in the walking bleach technique, the root filling should be completed first, and a cervical seal must be established. The bleaching agent is left in the tooth so that it can function as walking bleach until the next visit. The bleaching agent should be changed every 3–7 days for up to 3–4 visits [20].

18.2 Walking Bleach Technique

1. First the surface of the tooth is cleaned with pumice and the pretreatment tooth shade is recorded. The patient should be informed that the results of bleaching are not predictable and not guaranteed in all cases. Furthermore the patient is instructed as to the number of appointments and possible complications including cervical root resorption. Preoperative clinical photographs are helpful when demonstrating the change following bleaching to the patient.

2. Before commencing bleaching, a preoperative radiograph should be taken to assess the existing quality of the root canal filling and status of the peri-apical tissues. Under no circumstances should bleaching be undertaken if there are any concerns with regard to this. Root canal retreatment should be carried out when in doubt and the filling material allowed to set at least a week prior to commencing intra-coronal bleaching (Figs. 18.1 and 18.2).

3. Rubber dam should be used to isolate the tooth in question. The access cavity is prepared, and all coronal remnants of restorative material,

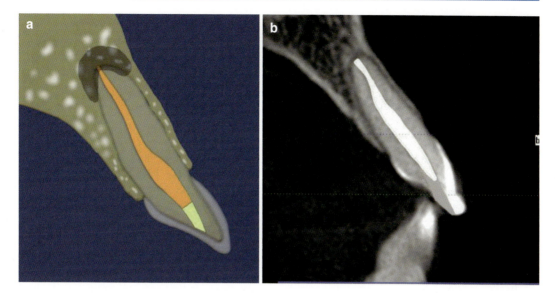

Fig. 18.1 Diagrammatic representation showing radiographic contraindications and indications prior to carrying out the non-vital walking bleach technique. Note: (**a**) obvious preexisting periradicular disease and (**b**) no pre-existing lucency. If there are any clinical and/or radiographic signs and symptoms correlated with apical periodontitis, then endodontic re-treatment should be carried out in the first instance

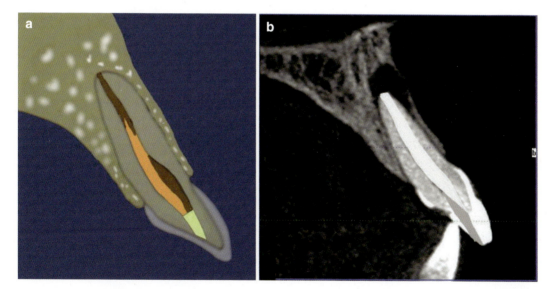

Fig. 18.2 Diagrammatic representation showing radiographic indications and contraindications prior to carrying out non-vital walking bleach technique. Note (**a**) Non-homogenous root filling, poor condensation and voids visible. The root filling terminates >2 mm from the radiographic apex and is deemed 'unacceptable' even though no peri-radicular pathology is present. Re-treatment is indicated prior to non vital bleaching procedures. (**b**) Although a well condensed root filling is present and deemed acceptable peri-radicular pathology is present. Re-treatment should be carried out prior to bleaching procedures

root filling materials and necrotic pulp tissue should be completely removed. In the anterior teeth, it is important to incorporate the mesial and distal pulp horns in the access cavity design and ensure that these areas are ultrasonically prepared to remove any remnants.

4. The root filling should be reduced 1–2 mm below the cement-enamel junction (CEJ). This can be determined by using a periodontal probe placed in the pulp cavity and comparing to external probing depths to the CEJ. The root filling should be sealed with a base (IRM or glass ionomer cement) of at least 2 mm to prevent diffusion of bleaching agents from the pulp chamber to the apical foramen. This sealing material should also reach the level of the CEJ to prevent leakage of bleaching products into the surrounding periodontium resulting in increased risk of external cervical root resorption. A radiograph can be taken to confirm that this step is correct (Figs. 18.3 and 18.4).

5. The pulp chamber is etched with 37 % phosphoric acid for 30–60 s, washed and dried. This allows opening of dentinal tubules for penetration of bleaching agent (Fig. 18.4).

6. Sodium perborate (Bocasan) is mixed with distilled water in a ratio of 2:1. The bleaching agent can be applied with a suitable carrier or plugger (Fig. 18.7).

7. A small piece of dry cotton wool is placed over the bleach and the cavity sealed with either IRM or glass ionomer cement. The patient is reviewed on a weekly basis and the process repeated until the tooth is slightly overbleached. Usually successful bleaching will become apparent by 2–4 visits.

8. Once bleaching has been completed, the access cavity should be restored with a resin composite which is bonded using an acid etch technique. Optimal time for bonding is usually 3 weeks following completion of bleaching. An interim dressing of calcium hydroxide is recommended during this time period to prevent any bacterial penetration and minimize further the risk of cervical root resorption (Fig. 18.5). A final postoperative clinical photograph should be taken to record colour changes achieved.

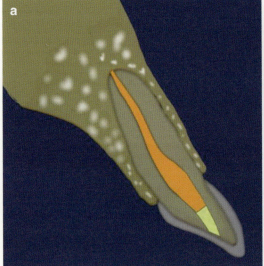
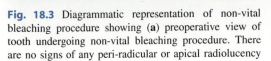
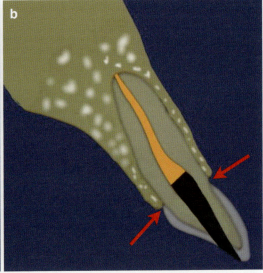

Fig. 18.3 Diagrammatic representation of non-vital bleaching procedure showing (**a**) preoperative view of tooth undergoing non-vital bleaching procedure. There are no signs of any peri-radicular or apical radiolucency and the existing root filling is well obturated. (**b**) The root filling material is cut back to below the level of the cement-enamel junction (CEJ) (*red arrow*)

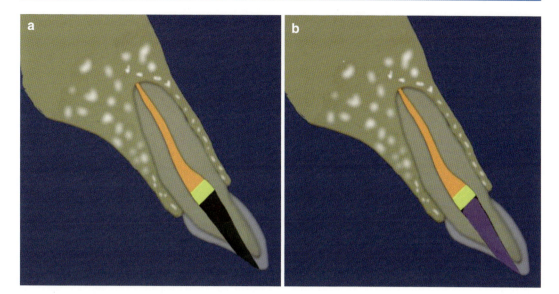

Fig. 18.4 Diagrammatic representation of the non-vital bleach technique showing (**a**) preexisting root filling cut 1–2 mm below the level of the CEJ (*orange*) with overlying base material (*yellow*). (**b**) Placement of etch into coronal pulp chamber (*purple*) (37 % phosphoric acid) to allow penetration of bleach in to the dentinal tubules

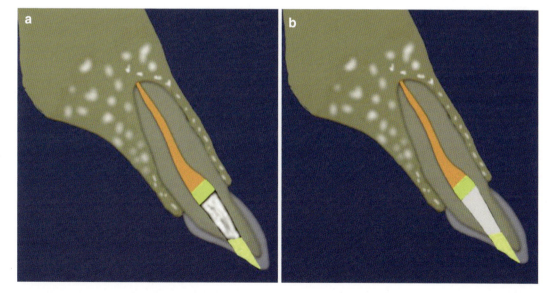

Fig. 18.5 Diagrammatic representation of the non-vital bleach technique showing (**a**) placement of bleach into coronal pulp chamber and overlying temporary restoration. The patient can be reviewed every 3–4 days for replacement of bleach up to 3–4 visits (depending on changes in discoloration). Usually you should aim to over-bleach due to risk of relapse. (**b**) Placement of calcium hydroxide dressing in the coronal pulp chamber when bleaching procedure has been completed. A final definitive tooth colored restoration can then be placed sealing the coronal pulp chamber permanently

18.3 Bleaching Complications

External cervical root resorption has been widely documented as a risk of intra-coronal bleaching. Several hypotheses have been put forward as to the mechanism by which this can occur including cemental defects at the cement-enamel junction, denaturing of dentine provoking an immunological response and the acid environment caused by the bleaching agent resulting in enhanced osteoclastic activity. As a preventive measure against the development of external root resorption, clinical guidelines have been put in place as discussed previously. The key is to coronally seal the root canal with a protective material to prevent cervical leakage of the bleaching agent. The use of sodium perborate mixed with water is a safer alternative to higher-strength bleaching agents and adjunctive use of thermocatalytic methods sometimes employed.

18.4 Clinical Cases

Case 1 Nonvital bleaching of tooth 21 having undergone root canal treatment several years previously (pink-brown discolouration)

A 32-year-old gentleman was seen for consultation regarding nonvital walking bleaching for his front tooth. He was concerned about his discoloured tooth which had been root treated several years ago. His motivation for seeking treatment now was due to his imminent wedding. The patient's chief complaint at time of examination was of the pink-brown discolouration affecting tooth 21. Clinical examination revealed no abnormalities. Tooth 21 was non-tender to percussion and palpation. Probing profile was within normal limits. An intact palatal access restoration was noted. Tooth 21 had obvious pink-brown discolouration associated with the clinical crown. Radiographic examination revealed a homogenous well condensed root filling 0-2 mm from the radiographic apex. No voids were visible. The root filling extended into the coronal pulp chamber. An intact periodontal ligament space was visible at the peri-apex. The patient was advised of the treatment options and informed of alternative treatments including

cast restorations (veneer or ceramic crown). The patient was advised that nonvital bleaching could sometimes reverse requiring further bleaching in the future. Risks were discussed including the possibility of external cervical root resorption with the patient. No previous history of trauma was noted.

The patient was seen for three treatment appointments using sodium perborate and distilled water. A satisfactory result was achieved and the patient referred back to his general dental practitioner to complete the coronal restoration after a 2-week interim period of calcium hydroxide dressing in the coronal pulp chamber (Figs. 18.6, 18.7, 18.8, and 18.9).

Case 2 Nonvital bleaching of tooth 11 following endodontic treatment (grey-brown discolouration)

A fit and healthy 21-year-old Australian defence force member was referred for endodontic management of tooth 11. The patient had been out in the field for some training during which time he sustained trauma to his front tooth. The patient recalled hitting his tooth with a rifle butt resulting in some localized pain and discomfort, which settled over a few days. At the time of consultation, the patient reported the tooth was asymptomatic but had noticed the tooth had discoloured. Clinical examination revealed tooth 11 had obvious grey-brown discolouration (see Fig. 18.12). Percussion tenderness was noted and tooth 11 responded negatively to both electric pulp testing and thermal stimulus (CO_2 snow).

Access preparation confirmed a necrotic pulp chamber. Working length was established and chemomechanical preparation was completed using stainless-steel hand files and 1 % sodium hypochlorite solution. An intra-canal medicament of calcium hydroxide was placed for a 4-week period. At the obturation appointment, tooth 11 remained asymptomatic. Obturation was completed using a warm vertical compaction technique using gutta-percha, AH Plus cement, system B and Obtura. The root filling was cut back 2 mm below the cement-enamel junction (CEJ), and the level was confirmed by measurement of depth by a periodontal probe (see Figs. 18.10, 18.11, and 18.12).

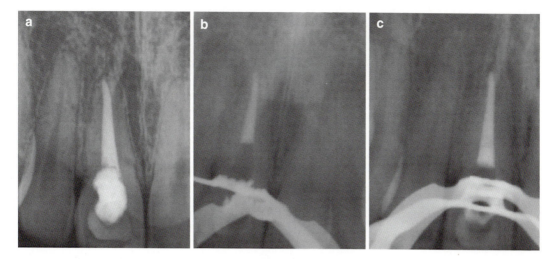

Fig. 18.6 Clinical radiographs showing (**a**) preoperative view, (**b**) gutta-percha root filling cutback below CEJ, and (**c**) IRM base material overlying gutta-percha and sealing to level of CEJ

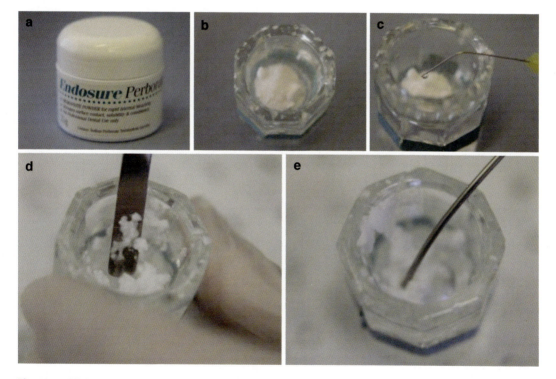

Fig. 18.7 Clinical photographs showing (**a**, **b**) sodium perborate (Bocasan), (**c**) addition of distilled water (ratio 2:1), (**d**) mixture at desired consistency, and (**e**) use of carrier system to deliver bleach to the intra-coronal aspect of the tooth

An IRM restoration was placed above this at the CEJ. The coronal pulp chamber was etched with 37 % phosphoric acid and then washed with saline after 1 min. Sodium perborate bleach was mixed with sterile saline (2:1 ratio) and then packed into the coronal pulp chamber. A temporary glass ionomer restoration was placed over the bleach. The patient was reviewed at 3 days, 7 days and 14 days (see Fig. 18.10). The bleach was replaced at days 3 and 7. At the final

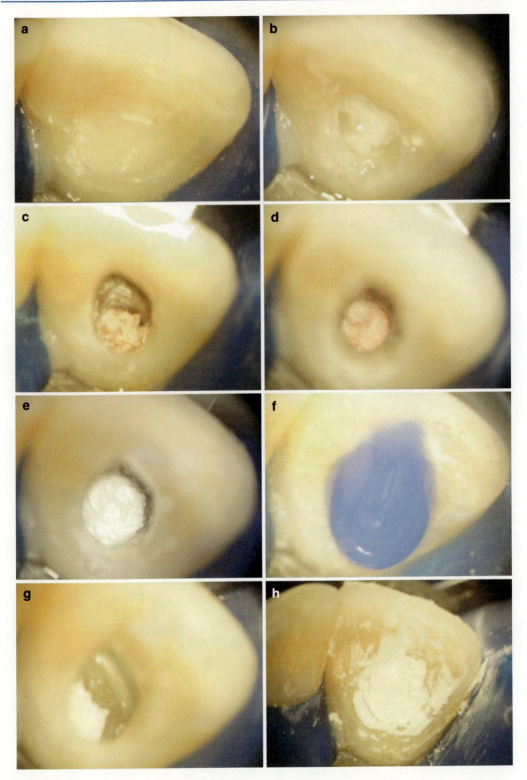

Fig. 18.8 Clinical photographs showing steps for non-vital walking bleach technique. (a) Preoperative view, (b) access cavity preparation and composite removal, (c) gutta-percha exposed, (d) gutta-percha cut back below CEJ, (e) placement of base layer over gutta-percha and to the level of CEJ, (f) acid etch placed in coronal access cavity, (g) placement of bleach, and (h) interim temporary restoration

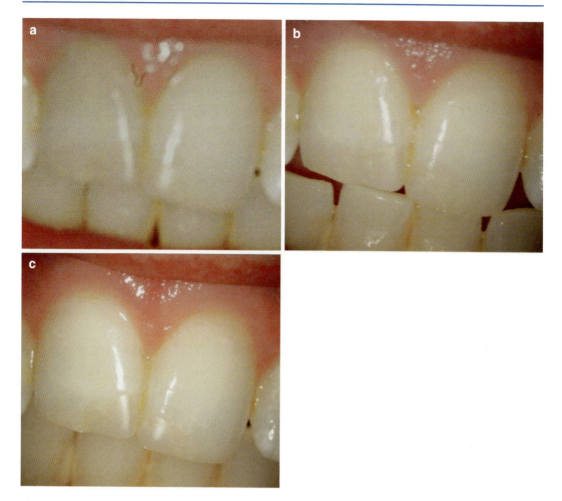

Fig. 18.9 Clinical photograph showing (**a**) preoperative view, (**b**) 7 days following placement of intra-coronal bleaching, and (**c**) 14 days postoperatively

appointment after a satisfactory result was achieved, the coronal pulp chamber was washed with saline prior to temporary double seal IRM/glass ionomer temporary restoration placement. The patient was discharged back to his general dental practitioner for placement of a permanent tooth-coloured coronal restoration.

Case 3 Nonvital bleaching of tooth 22 following endodontic treatment (yellow-brown discolouration)

A fit and healthy 34-year-old female patient was referred for endodontic management of tooth 22. The patient had previously undergone fixed orthodontic appliance therapy in her early teens, but the teeth had relapsed due to retainers not been worn. The patient had been undergoing further orthodontic appliance therapy (Invisalign) with her orthodontist during which time she had noticed some pain and sensitivity with the tooth. Clinical examination at the time of consultation revealed tooth 22 was asymptomatic with no tenderness to percussion. Palpation tenderness was noticed overlying the peri-apex of tooth 22. Tooth 22 responded negatively to both electric pulp testing and thermal stimulus (CO_2 snow). Radiographic examination revealed tooth 22 had obvious root canal narrowing in the apical third (see Fig. 18.13). A decision was made to carry out non-surgical root canal treatment with nonvital bleaching following completion of treatment.

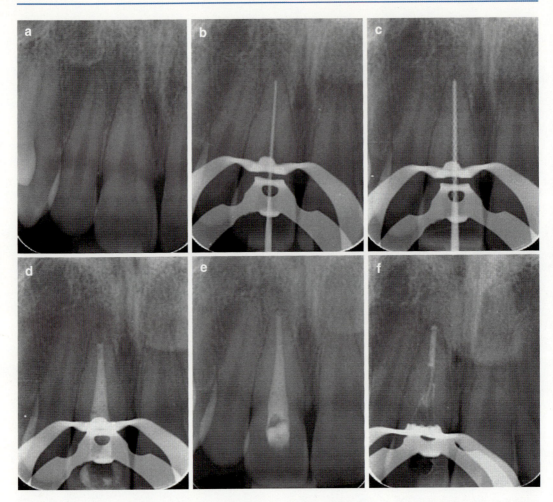

Fig. 18.10 Clinical radiographs showing nonsurgical root canal treatment of tooth 11. Note (**a**) preoperative view of tooth 11. (**b**) Initial apical file placement and confirmation of working length. (**c**) Master apical file radiograph following completion of chemo-mechanical debridement using stainless steel hand files using a 1mm step-back technique. (**d**) and (**e**) Placement of intra-canal calcium hydroxide medicament and double seal temporary restoration. The dressing was left in situ for 4 weeks prior to obturation. (**f**) 1 month later down-pack radiograph demonstrating warm vertical compaction technique using gutta-percha and AH plus cement

The patient was warned of the inherent risks with nonvital bleaching including cervical root resorption, the possibility of no colour changes or reversal of bleaching effects over time.

Access preparation was carried out confirming a necrotic root canal system. Chemomechanical preparation was completed using 1 % sodium hypochlorite solution and rotary files (Pro Taper NEXT). An intra-canal medicament of calcium hydroxide was placed for a 4-week period prior to completion of treatment. Obturation of the canal system was completed using gutta-percha and AH Plus cement using a warm vertical compaction technique. The root filling was cut back to 2 mm below the cement-enamel junction. A sub-seal IRM restoration was placed over the gutta-percha root filling at the level of the cement-enamel junction (see Fig. 18.15).

37 % phosphoric acid was placed in the coronal pulp chamber and rinsed out after 1 min. Intra-coronal bleach (sodium perborate) was placed after mixing to the desired consistency

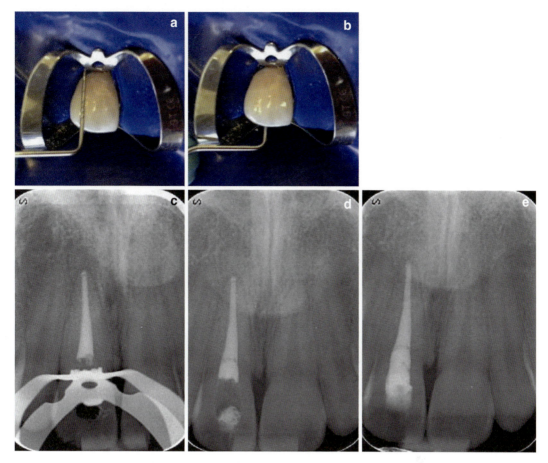

Fig. 18.11 Clinical photographs and radiographs showing (**a**, **b**) confirming level of gutta-percha below the CEJ using a periodontal probe. (**c**) Completed gutta-percha root filling cut back 2 mm below the cement-enamel junction. (**d**) IRM restoration placement at the CEJ, coronal bleach placement, and temporary restoration in place. (**e**) Completed temporary IRM/glass ionomer restoration following 3 sessions of non-vital bleaching using sodium perborate

(2:1 ratio with sterile saline). A temporary glass ionomer restoration was placed as an interim between bleach replacement appointments.

The patient was reviewed at 3 days, 7 days and 14 days. At the 3-day and 7-day appointment, the intra-coronal sodium perborate bleach was replaced and re-temporized using glass ionomer cement. At the 3-day appointment review, significant colour changes had occurred with some yellow discolouration still present at the cervical margin. Further whitening was evident at the 7- and 14-day review appointment (see Fig. 18.14).

At the final review appointment, the coronal pulp chamber was irrigated with sterile saline solution to remove any remnants of bleaching product. A temporary IRM/glass ionomer restoration was replaced (see Fig. 18.15). The patient was advised to see her general dental practitioner for permanent coronal restoration placement. The patient was very happy with the outcome following nonvital bleaching but understood that if any further colour changes were to occur, then she would probably have to consider an aesthetic cast restoration.

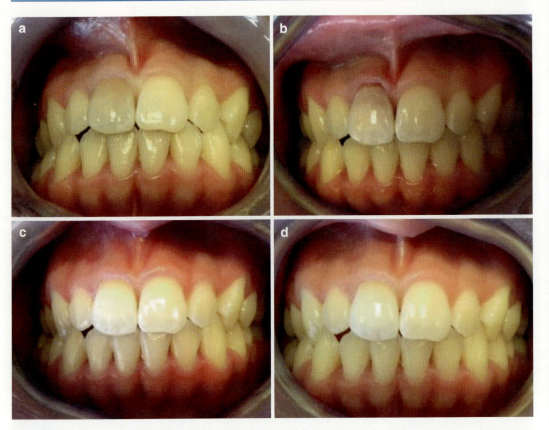

Fig. 18.12 Clinical photographs showing (**a**) preoperative. (**b**) 3-day, (**c**) 7-day, and (**d**) 14-day images of tooth 11 following non-vital bleach technique using sodium perborate

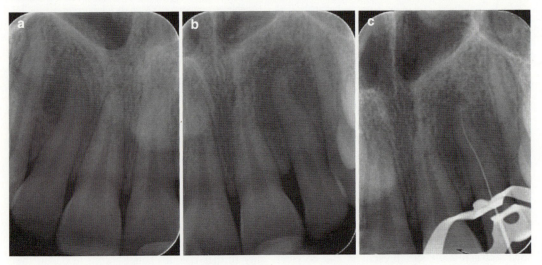

Fig. 18.13 Clinical radiographs showing nonsurgical root canal treatment of tooth 22. Note: (**a**) preoperative view of tooth 12 showing normal canal anatomy. (**b**) Preoperative view of tooth 22 demonstrating apical canal narrowing. (**c**) Initial apical file placement and confirmation of working length. (**d**) Master apical file radiograph following completion of chemo-mechanical debridement using rotary files. (**e, f**) Completed obturation using a warm vertical compaction technique using AH plus cement and gutta-percha using system B and Obtura. Note the gutta-percha has been cut back to 2 mm below the level of the cement-enamel junction

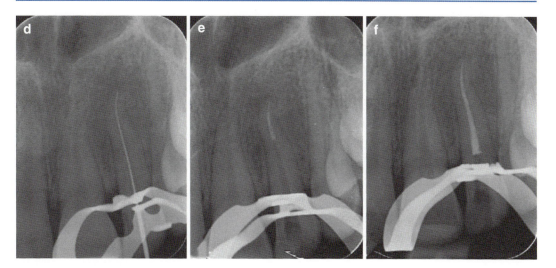

Fig. 18.13   (continued)

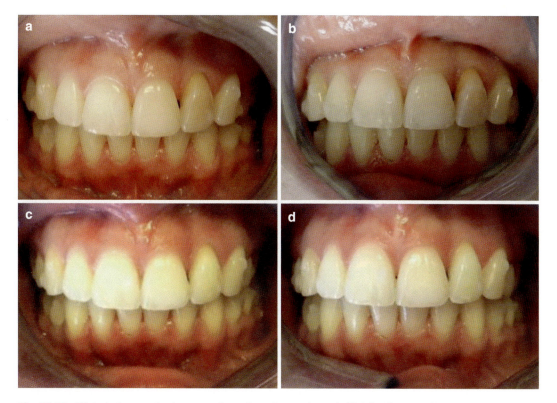

Fig. 18.14   Clinical photographs demonstrating colour changes in tooth 22 following non-vital bleaching procedure using sodium perborate. Note: colour changes at (**a**) pre-operative (**b**) 3 days (**c**) 7 days and (**d**) 14 days

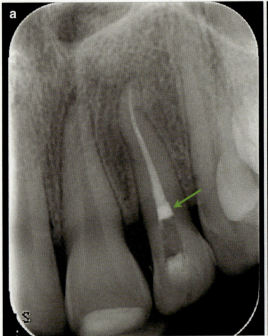 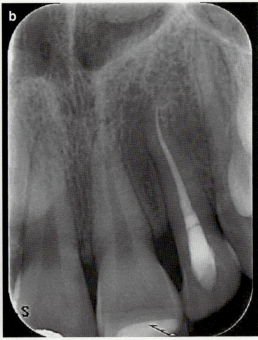

Fig. 18.15 Clinical radiographs demonstrating (**a**) completed obturation with cervical IRM sub-seal overlying gutta-percha (*green arrow*) and intra-coronal bleach. (**b**) IRM/glass ionomer temporary restoration following satisfactory non-vital bleaching of tooth 22

Clinical Hints and Tips for Nonvital Bleaching

- Ensure you have informed the patient that bleaching is not permanent and not guaranteed before starting treatment.
- Always ensure that the endodontic treatment is satisfactory prior to commencing nonvital bleaching.
- Gutta-percha is cut back below the level of the CEJ and all restorative materials are removed from the coronal pulp chamber.
- A seal of at least 2 mm is placed at the cervical region as a barrier.
- Nonvital walking bleach technique requires only 2–4 visits. If at this stage the desired effect is not achieved, then stop and consider alternative options.
- Taking clinical photographs pre-, peri- and postoperatively is useful to demonstrate changes to the patient.
- Use sodium perborate with distilled water as a safer alternative to other bleaching agents and chairside power bleaching techniques.

References

1. Spasser HF. A Simple bleaching technique using sodium perborate. N Y State Dent J. 1961;27: 332–4.
2. Nutting EB, Poe GS. A new combination for bleaching teeth. J South Calif Dent Assoc. 1963;31:289.
3. Nutting EB, Poe GS. Chemical bleaching of discoloured endodontically treated teeth. Dent. Clin. North. Am 1967;11:655–662.
4. Poyser NJ, Kelleher MG, Briggs PF. Managing discoloured non-vital teeth: the inside/outside bleaching technique. Dent Update. 2004;31(204–210): 213–4.
5. Attin T, Paque F, Ajam F, Lennon AM. Review of the current status of tooth whitening with the walking bleach technique. Int Endod J. 2003;36:313–29.
6. Vachon C, Vanek P, Friedman S. Internal bleaching with 10% Carbamide peroxide in vitro. Pract Periodontics Aesthet Dent. 1998;10:1145–54.
7. Ari H, Ungor M. In vitro comparison of different types of sodium perborate used for intra-coronal bleaching of discoloured teeth. Int Endod J. 2002;35:433–6.
8. Rotstein I, Mor C, Friedman S. Prognosis of intra-coronal bleaching with sodium perborate preparations in vitro: 1 year study. J Endod. 1993;19:10–2.

9. Rotstein I, Zalkind M, Mor C, Tarabeah S. In vitro efficacy of sodium perborate preparations used for intracoronal bleaching of discoloured non-vital teeth. Endod Dent Traumatol. 1991;7:177–80.

10. Watts A, Addy M. Tooth discolouration and staining: a review of the literature. Br Dent J. 2001; 190:309–16.

11. Brown G. Factors influencing successful bleaching of the discoloured root-filled tooth. Oral Surg Oral Med Oral Pathol. 1965;20:238–44.

12. Van der Burght TP, Plaesschaert AJM. Bleaching of tooth discolouration caused by endodontic sealers. J Endod. 1986;12:231–4.

13. Harrington GW, Natkin E. External resorption associated with bleaching of pulpless teeth. J Endod. 1979;5:344–8.

14. Lado EA, Stanley HR, Weismann MI. Cervical resorption in bleached teeth. Oral Surg Oral Med Oral Pathol. 1983;55:78–80.

15. Cvek M, Lindwall AM. External root resorption following bleaching of pulpless teeth with oxygen peroxide. Endod Dent Traumatol. 1985;1:56–60.

16. Heithersay GS. Invasive cervical resorption. Endod Topics. 2004;7:73–92.

17. Heithersay GS. Invasive cervical resorption: analysis of potential predisposing factors. Quintessence Int. 1999;30:83–95.

18. Hiethersay GS, Dahlstrom SW, Marin PD. Incidence of invasive cervical resorption in bleached root filled teeth. Aust Dent J. 1994;39:82–7.

19. Feiglin B. A 6-year recall study of clinically chemically bleached teeth. Oral Surg Oral Med Oral Pathol. 1987;63:610–3.

20. Plotino G, Buono L, Grande N, Pameijer C, Francesco S. Non vital tooth bleaching: a review of the literature and clinical procedures. J Endod. 2008;34: 394–407.

Index

© Springer International Publishing Switzerland 2016
B. Patel (ed.), *Endodontic Treatment, Retreatment, and Surgery,*
DOI 10.1007/978-3-319-19476-9

Printed by Printforce, the Netherlands